McGraw-Hill's

PCAT

McGraw-Hill's
PCAT

PHARMACY COLLEGE ADMISSION TEST

George J. Hademenos, Ph.D.

Shaun Murphree, Ph.D.

Jennifer M. Warner, Ph.D.

Kathy A. Zahler, M.S.

Mark A. Whitener, Ph.D.

New York | Chicago | San Francisco | Lisbon | London | Madrid | Mexico City | Milan | New Delhi
San Juan | Seoul | Singapore | Sydney | Toronto

The McGraw·Hill Companies

Library of Congress Cataloging-in-Publication Data

McGraw-Hill's PCAT : pharmacy college admission test / George J. Hademenos . . . [et al.].—1st ed.
    p. ; cm.
  ISBN-13: 978-0-07-160045-3
  ISBN-10: 0-07-160045-0
   1. Pharmacy colleges—United States—Entrance examinations—Study guides.
2. Pharmacy—Examinations, questions, etc.   3. Pharmacy—Vocational guidance.
I. Hademenos, George J.   II. Title: PCAT : pharmacy college admission test.
III. Title: McGraw-Hill's Pharmacy College Admission Test.   IV. Title: Pharmacy College
Admission Test.   [DNLM: 1. College Admission Test—Examination Questions.   2. Pharmacy—
Examination Questions.   3. Schools, Pharmacy—Examination   QV 18.2 M478 2009]
  RS105.M34 2009
  615'.1076—dc22

                              2008018628

1 2 3 4 5 6 7 8 QPD/QPD 0 1 4 3 2 1 0 9 8

ISBN 978-0-07-160045-3
MHID 0-07-160045-0

McGraw-Hill books are available at special quantity discounts to use as premiums and sales promotions, or for use in corporate training programs. For more information, please write to the Director of Special Sales, McGraw-Hill Professional, Two Penn Plaza, New York, NY 10121-2298. Or contact your local bookstore.

Contents

PART IV: REVIEWING PCAT BIOLOGY

PART V: REVIEWING PCAT CHEMISTRY

PART VI: REVIEWING PCAT MATH SKILLS

PART VII: REVIEWING PCAT WRITING

PART VIII: PCAT PRACTICE TEST

How to Use This Book

Welcome to *McGraw-Hill's PCAT*. You've made the decision to pursue a career in pharmacy, you've studied hard, you've taken and passed difficult science courses, and now you must succeed on this very tough exam. We're here to help you.

This book has been created by a dedicated team of scientists, teachers, and test-prep experts. Together, they have helped thousands of students score high on all kinds of exams, from rigorous science tests to difficult essay-writing assignments. They have pooled their knowledge, experience, and test-taking expertise to make this the most effective PCAT preparation program available.

McGraw-Hill's PCAT contains a wealth of features to help you do your best. In the months, weeks, or days before you take the test, you can substantially improve your chances of scoring high by using this book as follows:

➤ In Part I, you'll learn basic facts about the test, be familiarized with the test format, and learn about the kinds of questions that you're going to encounter. You'll also find important tips about pacing and guessing. In addition, you can review some basic test-taking strategies to keep in mind throughout all phases of the exam.

➤ In Part II, you can take a half-length Diagnostic Test. The questions on this test follow the PCAT format and cover the same topics as the actual exam. When you finish the test, use the results to measure how well prepared you currently are to take the PCAT. You can also use the results to decide which topics to focus on during the course of your review.

➤ In Parts III through VII, you can review every subject you must know for the PCAT. Parts III through VII present detailed coverage of all tested topics in verbal skills, biology, chemistry, mathematics, and writing. Concise chapter summaries, "Cram Sessions," at the end of each chapter reiterate key terms and concepts for quick and effective review. Many also offer valuable advice for tackling PCAT questions in the particular topic area. Each science review ends with "On Your Own" practice quizzes that you can use as a fast, efficient way to test your mastery of the subject. Part VII covers the Writing section—the parts of the PCAT most dreaded by many test takers. Here you'll find numerous sample essays illustrating exactly what the graders are looking for. Read the samples carefully—and learn how you can score high on these difficult PCAT sections.

➤ In Part VIII, you'll find a complete sample PCAT for practice. This test presents questions spanning the entire range of subjects and difficulty levels you're likely to find on the PCAT. Take the test under actual testing conditions: set aside the time you'll need to take the entire test at one sitting. Screen out distractions, and concentrate on doing your best. Of course, this practice test can provide only an approximation of how well you will do on the actual PCAT. However, if you approach it as you would the real test, it should give you a very good idea of how well you are prepared. After you take the test, read through the explanations for each question, paying special attention to those you answered incorrectly or had to guess on. If necessary, go back and reread the corresponding sections in the subject reviews in this book.

Different people have different ways of preparing for a test like the PCAT. You must find a preparation method that suits your schedule and your learning style. We have tried to make *McGraw-Hill's PCAT* flexible enough for you to use in a way that works best for you, but to succeed on this rigorous exam, there's no substitute for serious, intensive review and study. The more time and effort you devote to preparing, the better your chances of achieving your PCAT goals.

PART I

ALL ABOUT
THE PCAT

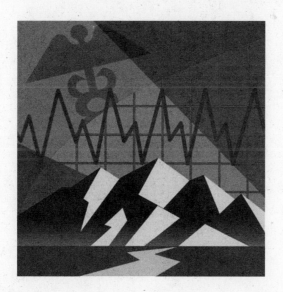

1. **Introducing the PCAT**
2. **Test Format and Structure**
3. **General Test-Taking Strategies**

CHAPTER 1

Introducing the PCAT

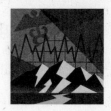

Read This Chapter to Learn About:

➤ PCAT Basics
➤ Where and When to Take the PCAT
➤ How to Register for the PCAT
➤ Your PCAT Scores
➤ How Pharmacy Schools Use PCAT Scores
➤ Reporting Scores to Pharmacy Schools
➤ For Further Information

PCAT BASICS

The Pharmacy College Admission Test (PCAT) is a standardized exam that is used to assess applicants to pharmacy schools. It is required as part of the admissions process by most U.S. pharmacy schools. The test is created and administered by Harcourt Assessment, the oldest commercial test publisher in the nation and a leader in the test development and publishing industry. The American Association of Colleges of Pharmacy (AACP) endorses the PCAT as the official preferred admissions test for entrance into pharmacy school.

The questions on the PCAT are basically designed to measure your problem-solving and critical-thinking skills. Three test sections assess your mastery of basic concepts in biology, chemistry, and quantitative ability. A fourth test section tests general, nonscientific word knowledge and usage. A fifth test section requires you to read passages on general topics and answer questions by applying your reasoning skills to what you have read. Finally, a sixth test section requires you to write two essays that demonstrate an effective use of language conventions and the ability to suggest the solution to a problem.

WHERE AND WHEN TO TAKE THE PCAT

The PCAT is offered at approximately 150 sites in the United States (including the U.S. territory of Puerto Rico) and at 12 sites in Canada. At the time of this writing, the PCAT had international test centers only in Canada and Qatar.

There are four test dates every year, in January, June, August, and October. The test day is always Saturday. Some test centers give the test in the morning only and others, usually larger, also provide an afternoon session.

It is a good idea to take the PCAT in the spring or summer of the year before the fall in which you plan to enroll in pharmacy school. That way, you have enough time to submit your scores to meet the schools' application deadlines.

For up-to-date lists of testing sites and also for upcoming test dates, make sure to check the official PCAT Web site at www.PCATweb.info.

HOW TO REGISTER FOR THE PCAT

You can register for the PCAT online at www.PCATweb.info. Online registration is available until approximately 10 weeks before the test date. If you prefer to register by mail, you must call Harcourt Assessment/PSE Customer Relations to request the form and refer to the official PCAT Web site for test center codes and pharmacy school codes. It is a good idea to register early, because seating at the test centers may be limited and you want to make sure you get a seat at the center of your choice. When you register, you are charged a fee, which you can pay via credit card with online registration or via money order with paper registration.

YOUR PCAT SCORES

When you take the PCAT, your work on each of the six test sections first receives a "raw score." On the five multiple-choice sections (Verbal Ability, Biology, Reading Comprehension, Chemistry, and Quantitative Ability), the raw score is calculated based on the number of questions you answer correctly. No points are deducted for questions answered incorrectly.

Each raw score is then converted into a scaled score. Using scaled scores helps to make test takers' scores comparable from one version of the PCAT to another. For the five multiple-choice sections (also referred to as subtests) and the composite for the whole multiple-choice test, scaled scores range from 200 (lowest) to 600 (highest). One of the writing sections will be experimental, meaning that it is being tested for future use and will not affect your score. The other writing section will have two recorded scores, one for Conventions of Language and one for Problem Solving from 0 (lowest) to 5.0 (highest).

Your score report will be mailed to you within approximately six weeks of your date of testing. PCAT score reports also include percentile rankings for the multiple-choice test and a mean score for the writing section that show how well you did in comparison to others who took the same test.

HOW PHARMACY SCHOOLS USE PCAT SCORES

Pharmacy school admission committees emphasize that PCAT scores are only one of several criteria that they consider when evaluating applicants. When making their decisions, they also consider students' college and university grades, recommendations, personal interviews, and involvement and participation in extracurricular or health-care–related activities. If the committee is unfamiliar with the college you attend, they may pay more attention than usual to your PCAT scores. A high score on the Writing Sample may also compensate for any weaknesses in communication skills noted on the application or at an interview.

There is no hard-and-fast rule about what schools consider to be an acceptable PCAT score. A scaled score of 400 corresponds to the fiftieth percentile of the PCAT. Pharmacy schools have their own judgments about a desirable PCAT score. Contact the programs to which you are applying to gauge what score you will need to be competitive for admission.

Note that PCAT scores are only valid for five years. Consult the pharmacy schools to which you are applying to confirm their individual policies on duration of test score validity.

REPORTING SCORES TO PHARMACY SCHOOLS

Official transcripts of your PCAT scores are sent by Harcourt Assessment to the institutions to which you requested your scores reported. For a fee, additional official transcripts can be requested online or by mail.

FOR FURTHER INFORMATION

For further information about the PCAT, visit the official PCAT Web site at

www.PCATweb.info

For questions about registering for the test, reporting and interpreting scores, and similar issues, you may also contact Harcourt Assessment/PSE Customer Service.

Telephone:
1-800-622-3231
210-339-8710

Fax:
1-888-211-8276
210-339-8711

Mail:
Harcourt Assessment, Inc.
PSE Customer Relations—PCAT
19500 Bulverde Road
San Antonio, TX 78259

CHAPTER 2

Test Format and Structure

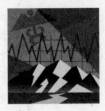

Read This Chapter to Learn About:

➤ The Format of the Test
➤ The Verbal Ability and the Reading Comprehension Sections
➤ The Biology and Chemistry Sections
➤ The Quantitative Ability Section
➤ The Writing Section

THE FORMAT OF THE TEST

The PCAT consists of seven separately timed sections. The test takes approximately four hours, in addition to administrative time for instructions at the beginning and a short rest break about halfway through the test. The morning session begins at 8:30 a.m. and ends at approximately 1:30 p.m. The afternoon session begins at 2:00 p.m.

The seven test sections are always given in the same order. The chart on the following page shows the sections in order, with the number of questions and time allowed for each section. There are a total of 240 questions and 2 essays on the test.

THE WRITING SECTION

According to the testmakers, the purpose of the Writing section is to assess your ability to communicate clearly, logically, and persuasively—a skill that is essential for pharmacists who interact with colleagues and the public. The Writing section of the PCAT is designed to measure effective use of language conventions and the ability to suggest the solution to a problem. The writing topics will address problems related to general health or science, or social, cultural, or political issues.

You are required to write one short essay in each writing section. The time limit for each one is 30 minutes. For each one, you will be given an essay prompt in the form of a statement that presents a problem. Your job is to write an essay in which you accomplish the following tasks:

➤ Suggest a solution to the problem presented
➤ State a clear thesis
➤ Support your thesis with relevant examples from your academic studies, personal experience, etc.
➤ Use correct grammar, punctuation, and word choice
➤ Write legibly
➤ Analyze alternative solutions to the one that you are suggesting
➤ Allow time at the end of this section to proofread your work

Within the 30-minute time limit, you must organize your thoughts, plan your writing (perhaps by jotting down a quick outline on scratch paper), and write your essay. You do not necessarily have to produce a lengthy piece of writing, but you must write enough to accomplish the above tasks in a way that is cogent, logical, and effective.

The PCAT Writing section is given two scores, one for language conventions and one for problem solving. The language conventions score is for grammar, punctuation, sentence structure, diction, and mechanics. The problem solving score is for developing an effectively written argument, sufficiently explaining a solution to a problem, presenting relevant support, analyzing alternate solutions, and refraining from faulty reasoning.

EXAMPLE: The following is an example of a typical PCAT writing prompt.

Discuss a solution to the problem of parental concern about childhood vaccinations.

THE VERBAL ABILITY SECTION

The Verbal Ability section of the PCAT is made up of 48 questions that are designed to measure general, nonscientific word knowledge and usage. This test section contains the following:

➤ Analogies
➤ Sentence completion

See Part III of this book for a complete review of these topics.

Test Section	Description	Time Limit	Number of Questions
Writing	Measures the effective use of language conventions in a written essay. You may write either an argumentative or problem solving essay. <table><tr><td>Conventions of Language</td></tr><tr><td>Problem Solving</td></tr></table>	30 min	1 writing topic
Verbal Ability	Measures general, nonscientific word knowledge using analogies and sentence completion. <table><tr><td>Analogies</td><td>60%</td></tr><tr><td>Sentence Completion</td><td>40%</td></tr></table>	30 min	48 items
Biology	Measures knowledge of the principles and concepts of basic biology with major emphasis on human biology. <table><tr><td>General Biology</td><td>60%</td></tr><tr><td>Microbiology</td><td>20%</td></tr><tr><td>Anatomy & Physiology</td><td>20%</td></tr></table>	30 min	48 items
Chemistry	Measures knowledge of principles and concepts of inorganic and elementary organic chemistry. <table><tr><td>General Chemistry</td><td>60%</td></tr><tr><td>Organic Chemistry</td><td>40%</td></tr></table>	30 min	48 items
Rest Break			
Writing	Measures the effective use of language conventions in a written essay. You may write either an argumentative or problem solving essay. <table><tr><td>Conventions of Language</td></tr><tr><td>Problem Solving</td></tr></table>	30 min	1 writing topic

Test Section	Description	Time Limit	Number of Questions
Reading Comprehension	Measures ability to comprehend, analyze, and interpret reading passages on scientific topics. 	Comprehension	30%
Analysis	40%
Evaluation	30%		50 min	6 passages 48 items
Quantitative Ability	Measures skills in arithmetic processes including fractions, decimals, and percentages, and the ability to reason through and understand quantitative concepts and relationships, including application of algebra. 	Basic Math	15%
Algebra	20%
Probability & Statistics	20%
Precalculus	23%
Calculus	22%		40 min	48 items

EXAMPLES

The following are examples of PCAT analogy and sentence completion questions.

Analogy question:

UMBRELLA : RAIN :: PARASOL :
A. hail
B. sun
C. shade
D. snow

Answer: **B**

Sentence completion question:

Since the mid-1960s, scientists have recognized that every dolphin has a _____ signature whistle, which is used for identification purposes.
A. universal
B. muted
C. superfluous
D. distinctive

Answer: **D**

THE BIOLOGY AND CHEMISTRY SECTIONS

The Biology and Chemistry sections of the PCAT test your mastery of the concepts and principles of biology and chemistry as taught in typical undergraduate college courses with laboratory sessions. In order to correctly answer most PCAT science questions, you need to be able to use that knowledge and your own reasoning skills to analyze scientific information, interpret scientific data, and calculate the solutions to scientific problems. Each of the two sections contains 48 multiple-choice items.

Biology

The testmakers list the following biology concepts as topics for questions in the PCAT Biology section:
➤ General biology
➤ Microbiology
➤ Human anatomy and physiology

See Part IV of this book for a complete review of these topics.

> **EXAMPLE:** The following is an example of a PCAT biology question.
>
> **1.** Which statement is true?
>   **A.** A cell placed in an isotonic solution will swell.
>   **B.** A cell placed in a hypotonic solution will swell.
>   **C.** A cell placed in a hypotonic solution will shrink.
>   **D.** A cell placed in a hypertonic solution will remain the same size.
>
> Answer: **B**

Chemistry

The testmakers list the following chemistry concepts as topics for questions in the PCAT Chemistry section:
➤ General chemistry
➤ Organic chemistry

See Part V of this book for a complete review of these topics.

> **EXAMPLE:** The following is an example of a PCAT chemistry question.
>
> **1.** Compare the Fischer and sawhorse projections below:

Assuming all conformations are available, the two depictions are best described as
- A. enantiomers.
- B. diastereomers.
- C. constitutional isomers.
- D. identical.

Answer: **B**

The Reading Comprehension Section

The Reading Comprehension section of the PCAT is made up of 48 questions that are intended to measure ability to comprehend, analyze, and evaluate reading passages on science-related topics. This test section contains the following:

➤ Six reading passages, each of which is 500 to 600 words long
➤ Between five and eight multiple-choice questions per passage

The passages are taken from texts that you most likely have never seen before and may be on topics with which you are unfamiliar. However, do not be alarmed; you will not be asked questions that require any prior knowledge of the passage topic. Everything you need to know to answer each question will be included in the passage.

The questions in the Reading Comprehension section may ask you to do any of the following:

➤ Identify the main idea of the passage
➤ Analyze an argument presented in the passage and judge its validity
➤ Use information from the passage to solve a given problem
➤ Determine cause-and-effect relationships for events or conditions described in the passage
➤ Evaluate a claim made in the passage based on the strength of the evidence or argument provided to support that claim
➤ Identify the reasons or evidence offered in support of a particular viewpoint
➤ Recognize stated or unstated assumptions that underlie a viewpoint presented in the passage
➤ Identify new facts or results that might undermine a conclusion presented in the passage
➤ Apply information from the passage to a new situation
➤ Determine the meaning of an unfamiliar word based on its context

See Part III of this book for a complete review of these topics.

EXAMPLE

The following is an example of a PCAT reading comprehension passage and related question.

1 For years, anecdotal evidence from around the world has indicated that amphibians were under siege, especially in the Caribbean. Finally, proof of this hypothesis is available, thanks to the concerted, Internet-based effort of scientists involved with the Global Amphibian Assessment.

2 Amphibians have a unique vulnerability to environmental changes thanks to their permeable skin and their need of specific habitats to allow their metamorphosis from larva to adult. Studies indicate that they are at risk due to global climate change, reduction in the ozone layer leading to an increased exposure to ultraviolet rays, interference with migratory pathways, drainage of wetlands, pollution by pesticides, erosion and sedimentation, and exposure to unknown pathogens thanks to the introduction of nonnative species. In other words, human progress is responsible for the losses this population is suffering.

3 Scientists have long considered amphibians a barometer of environmental health. In areas where amphibians are declining precipitously, environmental degradation is thought to be a major cause. Amphibians are not adaptable. They must have clean water in which to lay their eggs. They must have clean air to breathe after they grow to adulthood. Their "double life" as aquatic and land-dwelling animals means that they are at risk of a double dose of pollutants and other hazards.

4 The Global Amphibian Assessment concluded that nearly one-third of the world's amphibian species are under immediate threat of extinction. Nearly half of all species are declining in population. The largest numbers of threatened species are in Colombia, Mexico, and Ecuador, but the highest percentages of threatened species are in the Caribbean. In Haiti, for example, nine out of ten species of amphibians are threatened. In Jamaica, it's eight out of ten, and in Puerto Rico, seven out of ten.

5 Certainly, this is a disaster for amphibians, but scientists rush to point out that it may be equally a disaster for the rest of us on Earth. Even recent pandemics among amphibians may be caused by global changes. True, amphibians are ultrasensitive to such changes, but can reptiles, fish, birds, and mammals be far behind?

1. The main point of the passage is that

    A. the extinction of amphibians is due to global warming.
    B. amphibians really are a barometer of environmental health.
    C. only equatorial amphibians are currently under siege.
    D. amphibians' "double life" on land and in water may end up saving them.

Answer: **B**

THE QUANTITATIVE ABILITY SECTION

The Quantitative Ability section contains 48 questions that test your quantitative skills and understanding of mathematical relationships and concepts. The testmakers list the following mathematical concepts as topics for questions in the PCAT Quantitative Ability section:

➤ Basic math
➤ Algebra
➤ Probability and statistics
➤ Precalculus
➤ Calculus

See Part VI of this book for a complete review of these topics.

EXAMPLES: The following are examples of PCAT quantitative ability questions.

1. Solve for x: $4(2x+20)+3(x-1)=0$

A. 11   **B.** 7   **C.** −7   **D.** −11

Answer: **C**

2. What is the slope of a line that passes through the points (−3, 3) and (3, 3)?

A. positive   **B.** negative   **C.** 0   **D.** undefined

Answer: **C**

CHAPTER 3

General Test-Taking Strategies

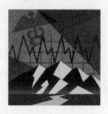

Read This Chapter to Learn About:

➤ General Strategies for Answering PCAT Questions

➤ Coping with Exam Pressure

This chapter presents some general test-taking strategies that apply to all the multiple-choice questions on the PCAT. These strategies can help you gain valuable points when you take the actual test.

GENERAL STRATEGIES FOR ANSWERING PCAT QUESTIONS

Take Advantage of the Multiple-Choice Format

All of the questions on the PCAT (except for the Writing prompts) are in the multiple-choice format, which you have undoubtedly seen many times before. That means that for every question, the correct answer is right in front of you. All you have to do is pick it out from among three incorrect choices, called "distracters." Consequently, you can use the process of elimination to rule out incorrect answer choices. The more answers you rule out, the easier it is to make the right choice.

Answer Every Question

Recall that on the PCAT, there is no penalty for choosing a wrong answer. Therefore, if you do not know the answer to a question, you have nothing to lose by guessing. So make sure that you answer every question. If time is running out and you still have not answered some questions, make sure to enter an answer for the questions that you have not tackled. With luck, you may be able to pick up a few extra points, even if your guesses are totally random.

Make Educated Guesses

What differentiates great test takers from merely good ones is the ability to guess in such a way as to maximize the chance of guessing correctly. The way to do this is to use the process of elimination. Before you guess, try to eliminate one or more of the answer choices. That way, you can make an educated guess, and you have a better chance of picking the correct answer. Odds of one out of two or one out of three are better than one out of four!

Go with Your Gut

In those cases where you are not 100 percent sure of the answer you are choosing, it is often best to go with your gut feeling and stick with your first answer. If you decide to change that answer and pick another one, you may well pick the wrong answer because you have overthought the problem. More often than not, if you know something about the subject, your first answer is likely to be the correct one.

Use the Test Booklet Provided

The PCAT is a paper-and-pencil test, so there is a test booklet for you to write in. Jot down notes, make calculations, and write out an outline for each of your essays. Be aware, however, that you cannot remove the test booklet from the test site. All test items are collected from you before you leave the room. You are not permitted to bring any of your own scratch paper into the test site.

COPING WITH EXAM PRESSURE
Keep Track of the Time

Make sure that you are on track to answer all of the questions within the time allowed. With so many questions to answer in a short time period, you are not going to have a lot of time to spare. Keep an eye on your watch.

Do not spend too much time on any one question. In the Reading Comprehension section, you have only 50 minutes to read 6 passages and answer 48 questions. If you find yourself stuck for more than a minute or two on a question, then you should make your best guess and move on. If you have time left over at the end of the section, you can return to the question and review your answer. However, if time runs out, do not give the question another thought. You need to save your focus for the rest of the test.

Do Not Panic if Time Runs Out

If you pace yourself and keep track of your progress, you should not run out of time. If you do, however, do not panic. Because there is no guessing penalty and you have nothing to lose by doing so, enter answers to all of the remaining questions. If you are able to make educated guesses, you will probably be able to improve your score. However, even random guesses may help you to pick up a few points. In order to know how to handle this situation if it happens to you on the test, make sure you observe the time limits when you take the practice tests. Guessing well is a skill that comes with practice, so incorporate it into your preparation program.

If Time Permits, Review Questions You Were Unsure Of

Within each test section, you are permitted to return to questions you may have skipped or to change your answer. If time permits, you may want to take advantage of this opportunity to review questions you were unsure of, or to check for careless mistakes. However, once you have completed an entire section, you cannot go back to it and make changes.

PART II

PCAT DIAGNOSTIC TEST

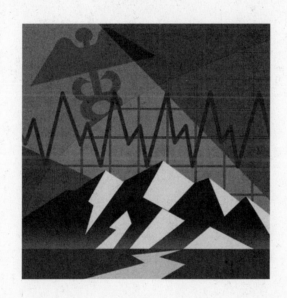

4. Half-Length PCAT Diagnostic Test

CHAPTER 4

Half-Length PCAT Diagnostic Test

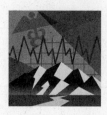

In This Chapter You Will Find
➤ A half-length PCAT Diagnostic Test covering all PCAT subject areas
➤ Sample questions like the ones on the real exam
➤ Answer explanations for every question

The Diagnostic Test in this chapter presents questions in all the subject areas tested on the PCAT. The test is half as long as the actual exam. There are questions on verbal ability, biology, chemistry, reading comprehension, and quantitative ability, all in the multiple-choice format that you will encounter on the PCAT. There is also a writing section with an essay-writing prompt like the ones used on the real test. All of the questions have also been designed to match the actual exam in degree of difficulty. Answer explanations for every question are provided at the end of the test.

This test will give you a very good idea of what you will face on test day. It is called a Diagnostic Test because it will help you to "diagnose" how well prepared you are right now for the real exam, and what subjects you need to review and study.

This test includes an Answer Sheet that you may want to remove from the book. Use this sheet to mark your answers to the multiple-choice questions. For Section 1, the Writing section, you may write your essay on the blank pages provided. When you are finished with the test, carefully read the answer explanations, especially for any questions that you answered incorrectly. Pinpoint your weak areas by determining the topics in which you made the most errors. This knowledge will help you focus your study as you work your way through the subject review chapters in this book.

This test will help you gauge your test readiness if you treat it as an actual examination. Here are some hints on how to take the test under conditions similar to those of the actual exam.

➤ Find a time when you will not be interrupted.

➤ Complete the test in one session, following the suggested time limits.

➤ If you run out of time on any section, take note of where you ended when time ran out. This will help you determine if you need to speed up your pacing.

PCAT Diagnostic Test: Answer Sheet

SECTION 2. VERBAL ABILITY

1 Ⓐ Ⓑ Ⓒ Ⓓ   11 Ⓐ Ⓑ Ⓒ Ⓓ   21 Ⓐ Ⓑ Ⓒ Ⓓ
2 Ⓐ Ⓑ Ⓒ Ⓓ   12 Ⓐ Ⓑ Ⓒ Ⓓ   22 Ⓐ Ⓑ Ⓒ Ⓓ
3 Ⓐ Ⓑ Ⓒ Ⓓ   13 Ⓐ Ⓑ Ⓒ Ⓓ   23 Ⓐ Ⓑ Ⓒ Ⓓ
4 Ⓐ Ⓑ Ⓒ Ⓓ   14 Ⓐ Ⓑ Ⓒ Ⓓ   24 Ⓐ Ⓑ Ⓒ Ⓓ
5 Ⓐ Ⓑ Ⓒ Ⓓ   15 Ⓐ Ⓑ Ⓒ Ⓓ
6 Ⓐ Ⓑ Ⓒ Ⓓ   16 Ⓐ Ⓑ Ⓒ Ⓓ
7 Ⓐ Ⓑ Ⓒ Ⓓ   17 Ⓐ Ⓑ Ⓒ Ⓓ
8 Ⓐ Ⓑ Ⓒ Ⓓ   18 Ⓐ Ⓑ Ⓒ Ⓓ
9 Ⓐ Ⓑ Ⓒ Ⓓ   19 Ⓐ Ⓑ Ⓒ Ⓓ
10 Ⓐ Ⓑ Ⓒ Ⓓ   20 Ⓐ Ⓑ Ⓒ Ⓓ

SECTION 3. BIOLOGY

1 Ⓐ Ⓑ Ⓒ Ⓓ   11 Ⓐ Ⓑ Ⓒ Ⓓ   21 Ⓐ Ⓑ Ⓒ Ⓓ
2 Ⓐ Ⓑ Ⓒ Ⓓ   12 Ⓐ Ⓑ Ⓒ Ⓓ   22 Ⓐ Ⓑ Ⓒ Ⓓ
3 Ⓐ Ⓑ Ⓒ Ⓓ   13 Ⓐ Ⓑ Ⓒ Ⓓ   23 Ⓐ Ⓑ Ⓒ Ⓓ
4 Ⓐ Ⓑ Ⓒ Ⓓ   14 Ⓐ Ⓑ Ⓒ Ⓓ   24 Ⓐ Ⓑ Ⓒ Ⓓ
5 Ⓐ Ⓑ Ⓒ Ⓓ   15 Ⓐ Ⓑ Ⓒ Ⓓ
6 Ⓐ Ⓑ Ⓒ Ⓓ   16 Ⓐ Ⓑ Ⓒ Ⓓ
7 Ⓐ Ⓑ Ⓒ Ⓓ   17 Ⓐ Ⓑ Ⓒ Ⓓ
8 Ⓐ Ⓑ Ⓒ Ⓓ   18 Ⓐ Ⓑ Ⓒ Ⓓ
9 Ⓐ Ⓑ Ⓒ Ⓓ   19 Ⓐ Ⓑ Ⓒ Ⓓ
10 Ⓐ Ⓑ Ⓒ Ⓓ   20 Ⓐ Ⓑ Ⓒ Ⓓ

SECTION 4. CHEMISTRY

1 Ⓐ Ⓑ Ⓒ Ⓓ   11 Ⓐ Ⓑ Ⓒ Ⓓ   21 Ⓐ Ⓑ Ⓒ Ⓓ
2 Ⓐ Ⓑ Ⓒ Ⓓ   12 Ⓐ Ⓑ Ⓒ Ⓓ   22 Ⓐ Ⓑ Ⓒ Ⓓ
3 Ⓐ Ⓑ Ⓒ Ⓓ   13 Ⓐ Ⓑ Ⓒ Ⓓ   23 Ⓐ Ⓑ Ⓒ Ⓓ
4 Ⓐ Ⓑ Ⓒ Ⓓ   14 Ⓐ Ⓑ Ⓒ Ⓓ   24 Ⓐ Ⓑ Ⓒ Ⓓ
5 Ⓐ Ⓑ Ⓒ Ⓓ   15 Ⓐ Ⓑ Ⓒ Ⓓ
6 Ⓐ Ⓑ Ⓒ Ⓓ   16 Ⓐ Ⓑ Ⓒ Ⓓ
7 Ⓐ Ⓑ Ⓒ Ⓓ   17 Ⓐ Ⓑ Ⓒ Ⓓ
8 Ⓐ Ⓑ Ⓒ Ⓓ   18 Ⓐ Ⓑ Ⓒ Ⓓ
9 Ⓐ Ⓑ Ⓒ Ⓓ   19 Ⓐ Ⓑ Ⓒ Ⓓ
10 Ⓐ Ⓑ Ⓒ Ⓓ   20 Ⓐ Ⓑ Ⓒ Ⓓ

SECTION 5. READING COMPREHENSION

1 Ⓐ Ⓑ Ⓒ Ⓓ   11 Ⓐ Ⓑ Ⓒ Ⓓ   21 Ⓐ Ⓑ Ⓒ Ⓓ
2 Ⓐ Ⓑ Ⓒ Ⓓ   12 Ⓐ Ⓑ Ⓒ Ⓓ   22 Ⓐ Ⓑ Ⓒ Ⓓ
3 Ⓐ Ⓑ Ⓒ Ⓓ   13 Ⓐ Ⓑ Ⓒ Ⓓ   23 Ⓐ Ⓑ Ⓒ Ⓓ
4 Ⓐ Ⓑ Ⓒ Ⓓ   14 Ⓐ Ⓑ Ⓒ Ⓓ   24 Ⓐ Ⓑ Ⓒ Ⓓ
5 Ⓐ Ⓑ Ⓒ Ⓓ   15 Ⓐ Ⓑ Ⓒ Ⓓ
6 Ⓐ Ⓑ Ⓒ Ⓓ   16 Ⓐ Ⓑ Ⓒ Ⓓ
7 Ⓐ Ⓑ Ⓒ Ⓓ   17 Ⓐ Ⓑ Ⓒ Ⓓ
8 Ⓐ Ⓑ Ⓒ Ⓓ   18 Ⓐ Ⓑ Ⓒ Ⓓ
9 Ⓐ Ⓑ Ⓒ Ⓓ   19 Ⓐ Ⓑ Ⓒ Ⓓ
10 Ⓐ Ⓑ Ⓒ Ⓓ   20 Ⓐ Ⓑ Ⓒ Ⓓ

SECTION 6. QUANTITATIVE ABILITY

1 Ⓐ Ⓑ Ⓒ Ⓓ   11 Ⓐ Ⓑ Ⓒ Ⓓ   21 Ⓐ Ⓑ Ⓒ Ⓓ
2 Ⓐ Ⓑ Ⓒ Ⓓ   12 Ⓐ Ⓑ Ⓒ Ⓓ   22 Ⓐ Ⓑ Ⓒ Ⓓ
3 Ⓐ Ⓑ Ⓒ Ⓓ   13 Ⓐ Ⓑ Ⓒ Ⓓ   23 Ⓐ Ⓑ Ⓒ Ⓓ
4 Ⓐ Ⓑ Ⓒ Ⓓ   14 Ⓐ Ⓑ Ⓒ Ⓓ   24 Ⓐ Ⓑ Ⓒ Ⓓ
5 Ⓐ Ⓑ Ⓒ Ⓓ   15 Ⓐ Ⓑ Ⓒ Ⓓ
6 Ⓐ Ⓑ Ⓒ Ⓓ   16 Ⓐ Ⓑ Ⓒ Ⓓ
7 Ⓐ Ⓑ Ⓒ Ⓓ   17 Ⓐ Ⓑ Ⓒ Ⓓ
8 Ⓐ Ⓑ Ⓒ Ⓓ   18 Ⓐ Ⓑ Ⓒ Ⓓ
9 Ⓐ Ⓑ Ⓒ Ⓓ   19 Ⓐ Ⓑ Ⓒ Ⓓ
10 Ⓐ Ⓑ Ⓒ Ⓓ   20 Ⓐ Ⓑ Ⓒ Ⓓ

SECTION 1. WRITING

1 Question   Time: 30 minutes

Discuss a solution to the problem of caring for a rapidly increasing number of elderly citizens.

_____
_____
_____
_____
_____
_____
_____
_____
_____
_____
_____
_____
_____
_____
_____
_____
_____
_____
_____
_____
_____
_____
_____
_____
_____
_____
_____
_____
_____

SECTION 2. VERBAL ABILITY

24 Questions   **Time: 15 Minutes**

Directions: Questions 1–10 consist of sentences with one or two blanks where words or phrases have been left out. Choose the word or set of words that **best** completes each sentence from the choices given.

1. The cells that function in body defense are known _____ as leukocytes, or white blood cells.
   A. especially
   B. collectively
   C. permissively
   D. increasingly

2. Graphics such as the Punnett square provide a simple way to _____ complex combinations.
   A. control
   B. integrate
   C. magnify
   D. visualize

3. The _____ that living things can arise from nonliving things under certain conditions is _____ *spontaneous generation*, or *abiogenesis*.
   A. concept . . . conceived
   B. theory . . . documented
   C. potential . . . christened
   D. idea . . . termed

4. Breathing is _____ by altering the size of the chest cavity through movement of the diaphragm.
   A. accomplished
   B. sponsored
   C. indicated
   D. amplified

5. Chemists in laboratories may choose to use a catalyst to make a reaction _____ quickly.
   A. contain
   B. allow
   C. occur
   D. reveal

6. Some _____ of a calcium deficiency might _____ stunted growth, convulsions, or rickets.
   A. indications . . . behold
   B. deficits . . . evince
   C. results . . . include
   D. products . . . contain

7. When the centers of respiration _____ increases in amounts of carbon dioxide, they _____ the muscles involved in breathing to work faster.
   A. allow . . . provide
   B. detect . . . signal
   C. observe . . . apply
   D. achieve . . . alert

8. Dolphins can hear sounds that are two octaves higher than any _____ by humans.
   A. perceived
   B. documented
   C. enabled
   D. conducted

9. All organisms, from the smallest to the largest, have a _____ for reproducing their own kind.
   A. duplicate   C. material
   B. process   D. transfer

10. Pea plants made a _____ experimental resource for Mendel, because they are _____ easy to grow and have a short life cycle.
    A. constructive . . . obstinately   C. troublesome . . . unusually
    B. reliable . . . hardly   D. favorable . . . relatively

Directions: For questions 11–24, choose the word that best completes the analogy so that the third and fourth terms have a relationship parallel to that of the first and second terms.

11. ELECTRICIAN : OHM :: TEST PILOT :
    A. Volt   C. Mach
    B. RPM   D. Anemometer

12. PACIFIC : INDIAN :: SUPERIOR :
    A. Anterior   C. Erie
    B. Atlantic   D. Native American

13. CONNECTION : CORRELATION :: SCHISM :
    A. Granite   C. Bond
    B. Division   D. Vacuum

14. STOMACH : DIGESTION :: STOMATA :
    A. Differentiation   C. Growth
    B. Respiration   D. Circulation

15. PALEOZOIC : REPTILES :: MESOZOIC :
    A. Sponges   C. Birds
    B. Brachiopods   D. Plants

16. SIGHT : VISION :: HEARING :
    A. Tinnitus   C. Otology
    B. Eustachian tube   D. Audition

17. MICRO- : MILLIONTH :: NANO- :
    A. Thousandth   C. Ten-millionth
    B. Ten-thousandth   D. Billionth

18. MUCOUS MEMBRANES : DIPHTHERIA :: NERVE TISSUE :
    A. Botulism   C. Bruxism
    B. Anemia   D. Dengue

19. MUHAMMAD : MECCA :: JESUS :
    A. Jerusalem
    B. Bethlehem
    C. Nazareth
    D. Calvary

20. STAMP : PHILATELIST :: COIN :
    A. Mint
    B. Currency
    C. Financier
    D. Numismatist

21. TAJ MAHAL : AGRA :: GREAT PYRAMID ::
    A. Accra
    B. Aswan
    C. Suez
    D. Giza

22. GLIDER : MOTOR :: INTEGRATED CIRCUIT :
    A. Transistor
    B. Wires
    C. Crystal
    D. Semiconductor

23. DACTYL : FINGER :: CARDIO :
    A. Toe
    B. Heart
    C. Hand
    D. Blood

24. COOL : FEBRILE :: PARCHED :
    A. Heated
    B. Humid
    C. Chilly
    D. Stiff

**STOP. IF YOU HAVE TIME LEFT OVER,
CHECK YOUR WORK ON THIS SECTION ONLY.**

SECTION 3. BIOLOGY

24 Questions   **Time: 15 Minutes**

1. Which statement is true?
   A. A cell placed in an isotonic solution will swell.
   B. A cell placed in a hypotonic solution will swell.
   C. A cell placed in a hypotonic solution will shrink.
   D. A cell placed in a hypertonic solution will remain the same size.

2. A class of drugs known as carbonic anhydrase inhibitors is known to increase the excretion of Na^+, K^+, HCO_3^- ions via urine while allowing for the retention of H^+ ions. This should cause
   A. an increase in urine volume due to osmotic effects
   B. a decrease in urine volume due to increased water reabsorption at the distal convoluted tubule
   C. a decrease in urine pH due to the excretion of HCO_3^- ions
   D. no changes to the normal properties of urine since Na^+, K^+, and HCO_3^- ions are normally secreted in the urine

3. How do mitosis and meiosis differ from each other?
   A. The goal of mitosis is to produce cells which are genetically identical to the original parent cell; the goal of meiosis is to produce cells which contain twice the number of chromosomes as the original parent cell.
   B. The cells formed by mitosis are diploid; the cells formed by meiosis are haploid.
   C. Mitosis results in the production of gametes; meiosis results in the production of cells which are used for the organism's growth and replacement of damaged cells.
   D. Synapsis and crossing over occur in mitosis to assure new combinations of genetic material; there is no synapsis and crossing over in meiosis.

4. Many antibiotics work by blocking the function of bacterial ribosomes, which are structured a little differently from eukaryotic ribosomes. These antibiotics will
   A. block lipid synthesis   C. destroy the cell membrane
   B. block DNA synthesis   D. block protein production

5. The phenotypic ratio obtained in a Punnett square is 1:2:1. Based on this ratio, which genetic "rules" can you conclude were involved?
   A. multiple alleles   C. normal dominance
   B. pleiotropy   D. incomplete dominance

6. When certain synthetic hormones are administered to patients who need them, some are ineffective when given orally. The best explanation for this would be
   A. The hormone is not being absorbed by the stomach.
   B. The hormone is excreted by the large intestine.
   C. The hormone is degraded by enzymes acting in the small intestine.
   D. The hormone is denatured by the stomach acidity.

7. A DNA template reads: T A C G A C. Which of the following is the complementary DNA sequence?
   - **A.** U A C G A C
   - **B.** T A C G A C
   - **C.** A T G C T G
   - **D.** A U G C U G

8. You know that bacterial cells are prokaryotic. In comparison to a typical eukaryotic cell, bacterial cells would
   - **A.** have a greater variety of organelles
   - **B.** have a smaller nucleus
   - **C.** lack a cell membrane
   - **D.** none of the above

9. Pancreatitis is a disorder that causes human pancreas cells to destroy all components in the cell and die. This disorder would involve a problem with which of these cell structures?
   - **A.** lysosomes
   - **B.** ribosomes
   - **C.** cell membrane
   - **D.** mitochondria

10. During pulmonary gas exchange, oxygen and carbon dioxide always move
    - **A.** into the alveoli
    - **B.** into the blood
    - **C.** from high to low concentration
    - **D.** out of the blood

11. In aerobic cellular respiration, what is the "big picture" significance of the first two steps (glycolysis and the Krebs cycle) of the process?
    - **A.** They make lots of ATP for the cell.
    - **B.** They create glucose for the cell.
    - **C.** They allow for electrons and protons to be collected for use in the electron transport chain.
    - **D.** All of the above are significant.

12. The genetic material of mitochondria and chloroplasts resembles that of modern day bacteria as opposed to that of typical eukaryotic genetic material. This would mean that
    - **A.** The DNA in these organelles exists in linear chromosome form.
    - **B.** The DNA in these organelles exists in plasmid form.
    - **C.** The DNA in these organelles exists in a single loop.
    - **D.** The RNA in these organelles is single-stranded.

13. Consider a bacterial cell that performs **anaerobic** respiration. If that bacterial cell had access to 6 molecules of glucose to use, how many ATPs would it be able to produce?
    - **A.** 2 ATP
    - **B.** 12 ATP
    - **C.** 6 ATP
    - **D.** 36 ATP

14. Cystic fibrosis is an autosomal recessive disorder. This means that
   A. It is more common in boys than girls.
   B. A child can only inherit cystic fibrosis if at least one of the parents has the disease.
   C. The allele for cystic fibrosis must be present in two copies in order to show the cystic fibrosis phenotype.
   D. If it runs in a family, it shows up in every generation.

15. It is not uncommon for individuals with leukemia (cancer of the white blood cells) to receive stem cell transplants. Why might this be a productive treatment option?
   A. The stem cells are capable of differentiating into new blood cells, which include the leukocytes, erythrocytes, and platelets.
   B. The stem cells can damage and replace the cancerous leukocytes.
   C. The stem cells can act as immune system modulators, enhancing the function of the entire system.
   D. The stem cells can temporarily replace the function of the cancerous cells and slow down the progression of the disease.

16. Human sperm cells require energy in order to move towards an egg cell. What cell structure would enable the sperm to move?
   A. mitochondria   **C.** flagellum
   B. lysosomes   **D.** smooth endoplasmic reticulum

17. Light hits PSII, which causes electrons to be excited to a high energy level. These electrons are picked up by an electron acceptor and passed through an electron transport chain where _____ is made.
   A. O_2 **C.** NADPH
   B. G3P   **D.** ATP

18. A child is taken to the hospital because she has an extremely high fever. The physician immediately orders an ice bath to lower her body temperature. The most logical explanation for this treatment is that an increased body temperature
   A. could cause denaturation to her enzymes causing critical cellular reactions to be unable to occur
   B. would prevent substances from being transported properly across the cell membrane
   C. would increase the rate of cellular respiration to a dangerous level
   D. could prevent cell division

19. Imbalances in sodium ion concentrations would most likely cause problems with
   A. neuron function   **C.** cell division
   B. aerobic cellular respiration   **D.** muscle contraction

20. You have identified an unusual eukaryotic organism that is multicellular and makes its food. It must belong in the kingdom
   A. Plantae   **C.** Fungi
   B. Animalia   **D.** Protista

21. A diploid human cell that is not dividing will contain _____ chromosomes. These chromosomes will each consist of _____ chromatid(s).
   A. 46 . . . 1   **C.** 46 . . . 2
   B. 23 . . . 1   **D.** 23 . . . 2

22. Which of the following are found in **both** plant and animal cells?
   A. nucleus, Golgi complex, chloroplasts
   B. endoplasmic reticulum, cell wall, nucleus
   C. ribosomes, mitochondria, cell membrane
   D. central vacuole, nucleus, lysosomes

23. Why are we as humans particularly concerned about bacteria that are able to form spores?
   A. because they can survive for long periods of time without food and water
   B. because they are difficult to kill
   C. because they cause human disease
   D. all of the above

24. Erythropoietin is a peptide hormone as opposed to a steroid hormone. This means that EPO's mechanism of action will involve
   A. changes in the gene expression of its target cells
   B. the phosphorylation of ADP
   C. the use of second messenger molecules in its target cells
   D. the entrance of the hormone into the target cells where it will find its receptor

---

**STOP. IF YOU HAVE TIME LEFT OVER,
CHECK YOUR WORK ON THIS SECTION ONLY.**

SECTION 4. CHEMISTRY

24 Questions   **Time: 15 Minutes**

1. What is the correct name of the compound with the formula $(NH_4)_3PO_4$?
   - A. triammonium phosphate
   - B. ammonium(I)phosphate
   - C. ammonium phosphate
   - D. ammonium phosphide

2. How many g of HF can be produced by complete reaction of 33.9 g of BF_3? (atomic masses B = 10.8 ^{g}/$_{mol}$, F = 19 ^{g}/$_{mol}$, and H = 1 ^{g}/$_{mol}$)

   $$BF_3(g) + 3H_2O(l) \longrightarrow 3HF(g) + H_3BO_3(s)$$
   - A. 90 g
   - B. 10 g
   - C. 30 g
   - D. 38 g

3. Which of the following represents a neutralization reaction?
   - A. $2Mg(s) + O_2(g) \longrightarrow 2\,MgO(s)$
   - B. $2H_3PO_4(aq) + 3Ca(OH)_2(s) \longrightarrow Ca_3(PO_4)_2(s) + 6H_2O(l)$
   - C. $Ba(NO_3)_2(aq) + H_2SO_4(aq) \longrightarrow BaSO_4(s) + 2\,HNO_3(aq)$
   - D. $Zn(s) + 2HNO_3(aq) + 2HCl(aq) \longrightarrow ZnCl_2(aq) + 2NO_2(g) + 2H_2O(l)$

4. The following reaction is carried out at 298°C and a pressure of 750 torr. If 17.5 L of O_2 is reacted with excess PbS, how many L of SO_2 are formed at the same temperature and pressure?

   $$2PbS(s) + 3O_2(g) \longrightarrow 2PbO(s) + 2SO_2(g)$$
   - A. 11.7 L
   - B. 17.5 L
   - C. 35 L
   - D. 67 L

5. The enthalpy of combustion for benzene is given by the following equation:

   $$2C_6H_6(l) + 15O_2(g) \longrightarrow 6H_2O(l) + 12CO_2(g) + 6535\ kJ$$

   How much heat is released when 256 g of benzene are completely burned in oxygen?
   (atomic masses C = 12 ^{g}/$_{mol}$, H = 1 ^{g}/$_{mol}$, and O = 16 ^{g}/$_{mol}$)
   - A. 1.07×10^4 kJ
   - B. 2.14×10^4 kJ
   - C. 1.67×10^5 kJ
   - D. 8.37×10^4 kJ

6. Which of the following is a valid set of quantum numbers for an electron in an atom?
   - A. $n = 3, \ell = 3, m_\ell = -2, m_s = +1/2$
   - B. $n = 3, \ell = 2, m_\ell = 4, m_s = -1/2$
   - C. $n = 3, \ell = 2, m_\ell = -2, m_s = -1/2$
   - D. $n = -3, \ell = 2, m_\ell = -2, m_s = -1/2$

7. What is the correct electron configuration of S^{2-}? (Atomic number of sulfur is 16)
   - A. $1s^2 2s^2 2p^6 3s^2 3p^4$
   - B. $1s^2 2s^2 2p^6 3s^2 3p^2$
   - C. $1s^2 2s^2 2p^6 3s^2 3p^5$
   - D. $1s^2 2s^2 2p^6 3s^2 3p^6$

8. How many resonance structures are there for the Lewis structure of SO_4^{2-} with two single bonds between S and O and two double bonds between S and O?

A. 3

B. 1

C. 4

D. 6

9. Which of the following molecules is polar?

A. SO_3

B. PF_3

C. SiF_4

D. CO_2

10. Which transition on the phase diagram will include melting?

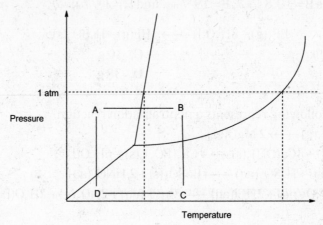

A. $A \rightarrow B$

B. $B \rightarrow C$

C. $A \rightarrow D$

D. $C \rightarrow D$

11. What will the osmotic pressure be in a solution that is 0.5 M $CaCl_2$ at 27°C? $(R = 0.082\ ^{L.atm}/_{mol.K})$

A. 12.3 atm

B. 1.1 atm

C. 3.3 atm

D. 36.9 atm

12. The following reaction is first order in Br_2 and second order in NO. Each of the changes listed will increase the rate of the reaction EXCEPT

$$2NO(g) + Br_2(g) \longrightarrow 2NOBr(g)$$

A. Adding NO to the reaction

B. Increasing the volume

C. Increasing the temperature

D. Adding a catalyst

13. Barium phosphate is a slightly soluble compound that dissolves in water according to the following equilibrium:

$$Ba_3(PO_4)_2(s) \rightleftharpoons 3Ba^{2+}(aq) + 2PO_4^{3-}(aq)$$

What is the correct expression for the K_{sp} of barium phosphate?

A. $K_{sp} = 3 \times [Ba^{2+}]2 \times [PO_4^{3-}]$

B. $K_{sp} = [Ba^{2+}]^3[PO_4^{3-}]^2$

C. $K_{sp} = \dfrac{[Ba^{2+}]^3[PO_4^{3-}]^2}{[Ba_3(PO_4)_2]}$

D. $K_{sp} = \dfrac{3 \times [Ba^{2+}]2 \times [PO_4^{3-}]}{[Ba_3(PO_4)_2]}$

14. Which of the following will have an increased solubility in acidic solution?
    A. $Ni(CN)_2$ C. NH_4Cl
    B. $NaNO_3$ D. $FeCl_2$

15. The standard reduction potentials that make up the two half cells of a Ni/Cd battery are shown below. Cadmium is the anode and nickel oxyhydroxide is the cathode. What is the voltage of this battery?

$$Cd(OH)_2(s) + 2e^- \longrightarrow Cd(s) + 2OH^-(aq) \qquad E° = -0.81 \text{ V}$$
$$NiO(OH)(s) + H_2O(l) + e^- \longrightarrow Ni(OH)_2(s) + OH^-(aq) \qquad E° = 0.49 \text{ V}$$

    A. −0.32 V   C. 1.79 V
    B. 0.17 V   D. 1.30 V

16. In comparing methoxide (MeO^-) and methanethiolate (MeS^-), **methoxide** is
    A. more nucleophilic and more basic   C. less nucleophilic and more basic
    B. more nucleophilic and less basic   D. less nucleophilic and less basic

17. In comparing chloride (Cl^-) and iodide (I^-), **chloride** is
    A. the better leaving group and the better nucleophile
    B. the better leaving group and the poorer nucleophile
    C. the poorer leaving group and the better nucleophile
    D. the poorer leaving group and the poorer nucleophile

18. Consider the substitution reaction of (3R)-3-bromo-1,1-dimethylcyclo-hexane (below), in which the stereochemistry of the product has not been specified.

    The most likely mechanism and stereochemical outcome of this process is
    A. SN1 to give a single enantiomer   C. SN2 to give a single enantiomer
    B. SN1 to give a racemic mixture   D. SN2 to give a racemic mixture

19. For the compound 2,3,4-trimethylpentan-2-ol,

    How many stereocenters are present?
    A. 0   C. 2
    B. 1   D. 3

20. Acetoin (shown below) is used as a flavorant and is obtained in optically pure form from bacterial fermentation of glucose.

The best IUPAC name for acetoin is

A. (3R)-3-hydroxybutan-2-one   **C.** (3S)-3-hydroxybutan-2-one

B. (2R)-3-oxobutan-2-ol   **D.** (2S)-3-oxobutan-2-ol

21. Compare the Fischer and sawhorse projections below:

Assuming all conformations are available, the two depictions are best described as

A. enantiomers   **C.** constitutional isomers

B. diastereomers   **D.** identical

22. Compare the chair and 2-dimensional cyclohexane depictions below:

Assuming all conformations are available, the two depictions are best described as

A. enantiomers   **C.** constitutional isomers

B. diastereomers   **D.** identical

23. Consider the Jones oxidation of heptane-1,6-diol.

The most likely product of this reaction would be

A. a hydroxy ketone   **C.** a dicarbonyl

B. a hydroxy acid   **D.** an oxo acid

24. Consider the PCC oxidation of heptane-1,6-diol.

The most likely product of this reaction would be

A. a hydroxy ketone   **C.** a dicarbonyl

B. a hydroxy acid   **D.** an oxo acid

**STOP. IF YOU HAVE TIME LEFT OVER,
CHECK YOUR WORK ON THIS SECTION ONLY.**

SECTION 5. READING COMPREHENSION

24 Questions   **Time: 25 Minutes**

Directions: Read each passage. Answer the questions that follow by choosing the best answer from the choices given.

PASSAGE 1

1   The use of inhaled anesthetics can be traced back as far as the medieval Moors, who used narcotic-soaked sponges placed over the nostrils of patients. Some 300 years later, in 1275, Majorcan alchemist Raymundus Lullus is supposed to have discovered the chemical compound later called ether. The compound, which would later have a brief but important run as the anesthetic of choice in Western medicine, was synthesized by German physician Valerius Cordus in 1540. Adding sulfuric acid, known at the time as "oil of vitriol," to ethyl alcohol resulted in the compound Cordus called "sweet vitriol."

2   During the next few centuries, ether was used by physicians for a variety of purposes. Its effectiveness as a hypnotic <u>agent</u> was well known, and a favorite pastime of medical students in the early 19th century was the "ether frolic," an early version of the drunken frat party. Nevertheless, no record of ether's being used as an anesthetic in surgery appears until the 1840s.

3   Dr. Crawford Williamson Long of Jefferson, Georgia, removed neck tumors from a patient under ether anesthesia on March 30, 1842. However, he failed to publish the record of his experiment until 1848, by which time Dr. William T. G. Morton, a dentist in Hartford, Connecticut, had conducted a variety of experiments with ether on animals and himself, culminating in the painless extraction of a tooth from a patient under ether on September 30, 1846.

4   After reading about Morton's successful use of ether, doctors at Harvard invited him to demonstrate his technique. At Massachusetts General Hospital on October 16, 1846, Morton administered ether to a patient, and senior surgeon John Collins Warren removed a growth from the patient's neck as a crowd of doctors and dignitaries looked on. The operation is recorded in several paintings of the era, indicating its critical importance. Despite its volatility and side effects, ether continued to be used as an anesthetic until it was overtaken by less harmful potions. Morton, meanwhile, struggled unsuccessfully to be granted a patent for his "discovery" and then, when that failed, for his "technique." After years of litigation, he died penniless at age 49.

1. The statement in the first paragraph that ether would "have a brief but important run as the anesthetic of choice in Western medicine" implies that the author believes that
   A. ether was not a particularly good anesthetic
   B. ether was not used long enough to judge its effectiveness
   C. ether was effective during the period when it was used
   D. ether was a noteworthy import from the East to the West

2. In the context of the second paragraph, the word *agent* is used to mean
   A. manager
   C. instrument
   B. negotiator
   D. arbitrator

3. Which of these would be the **best** title for the passage?
   A. "Inhaled Anesthetics"
   C. "How Anesthetics Have Changed"
   B. "An Important Anesthetic"
   D. "Our Debt to Ancient Physicians"

4. Which of the following statements from the passage provides the **least** support for the author's claim that ether was an important discovery for physicians at the time?
   A. "Dr. Crawford Williamson Long of Jefferson, Georgia, removed neck tumors from a patient under ether anesthesia on March 30, 1842."
   B. "After reading about Morton's successful use of ether, doctors at Harvard invited him to demonstrate his technique."
   C. "The operation is recorded in several paintings of the era, indicating its critical importance."
   D. "Nevertheless, no record of ether's being used as an anesthetic in surgery appears until the 1840s."

5. In the first paragraph, the author probably writes that Lullus "is supposed to have discovered" ether because
   A. There is conflicting evidence about his discovery.
   B. Lullus did not really discover ether at all.
   C. Although Lullus was meant to discover it, someone else did.
   D. No one can really "discover" a chemical compound.

6. How is the information in the fourth paragraph organized?
   A. by reasons and examples
   B. using comparisons and contrasts
   C. in time order
   D. using cause-and-effect relationships

7. What evidence could the author have included that would **best** support the contention that ether was important to the history of medicine?
   A. the chemical makeup of diethyl ether—CH_3-CH_2-O-CH_2-CH_3
   B. names and occupations of the patients on whom Long and Morton worked
   C. a comparison of chloroform to nitrous oxide when used as anesthesia
   D. examples of how ether was used in battlefield medicine during the Civil War

8. The author probably includes information about Dr. Long in the third paragraph to show that
   A. Morton was not the first to use ether in a surgical procedure.
   B. Publishing results can mean the difference between fortune and penury.
   C. Both dentists and doctors used ether to good effect.
   D. Doctors in the Northeast often received more attention than Southern doctors.

PASSAGE 2

1   The Arecibo Observatory, near the north shore of Puerto Rico, is a key component of Cornell University's National Astronomy and Ionosphere Center (NAIC). In a joint venture with the National Science Foundation, the observatory exists to provide observation time and support for scientists worldwide. A panel of judges determines the "most promising" research proposals among the hundreds that are presented to the observatory each year. Those scientists are invited to Puerto Rico for viewing time on Arecibo's giant telescope.

2   Scientists who visit the observatory are typically involved in one of three studies: radio astronomy, which is the study of natural radio energy produced by faraway galaxies and stars; atmospheric science, which is the study of the earth's upper atmosphere, including its temperature, density, and <u>composition</u>; and radar astronomy, which is the study of planets and their moons, asteroids, and comets. The enormous telescope assists with all three studies.

3   The Arecibo telescope does not resemble what most of us think of when we hear the word *telescope*. Its reflective surface covers a remarkable 20 acres. Dangling above it are towers and cables, subreflectors and antennas, all of which can be positioned using 26 motors to transmit radio waves and receive echoes with astonishing precision.

4   Arecibo has been the site of hundreds of fascinating discoveries. Among these are the rate of rotation of the planet Mercury, determined two years after the telescope launched in 1963; two new classes of pulsars; and the first planets ever spotted outside of our solar system. Today, one of the most important goals of the observatory is to document and quantify global climate change by monitoring changes in temperature, hydrogen composition, and wind-fields in the ionosphere.

5   Although at one time, scientists had to travel to Puerto Rico to share viewing time on the giant telescope, today there are new protocols that enable remote viewing. At the University of Texas at Brownsville, students are helping to design a remote-control command center that will control the positioning of the telescope from 2,000 miles away. Students and professors will use the command center to study radio pulsars, rotating neutron stars that release radiation in regular pulses.

9. In the context of the second paragraph, the word *composition* means
   A. structure   **C.** opus
   B. array   **D.** compilation

10. Based on the information in the third paragraph, you can conclude that most telescopes

    A. do not have reflective surfaces

    B. contain radio antennas

    C. are not as large as Arecibo's

    D. cannot be repositioned

11. All of these are typical studies at Arecibo **except**

    A. the nature of the ionosphere

    B. production of remote-controlled devices

    C. radio waves produced by galaxies

    D. investigations of distant asteroids

12. The author's purpose in the fourth paragraph is to

    A. provide the history of the observatory

    B. describe Arecibo in some detail

    C. compare and contrast astronomical studies

    D. list some of Arecibo's successes

13. Which statement expresses a personal **opinion**?

    A. "Those scientists are invited to Puerto Rico for viewing time on Arecibo's giant telescope."

    B. "Scientists who visit the observatory are typically involved in one of three studies."

    C. "Arecibo has been the site of hundreds of fascinating discoveries."

    D. "Students and professors will use the command center to study radio pulsars."

14. The remote-control command center will **most** likely

    A. result in remarkable research findings

    B. save scientists the cost of traveling

    C. fail to achieve its goal of assisting students

    D. be used primarily for atmospheric studies

15. Recently, Arecibo has lost government funding. The part of the passage that could **best** be used to support a call to fund this observatory is found in paragraph

    A. 1

    B. 2

    C. 3

    D. 4

16. The **tone** of the passage suggests that the author finds Arecibo

    A. expensive to maintain

    B. scientifically intriguing

    C. old-fashioned in its approach

    D. too involved in popular science

PASSAGE 3

1 The Red List is published annually by the World Conservation Union to indicate to the world which species are threatened, endangered, and extinct. The most recent list included nearly 16,000 endangered species, including, incredibly, nearly every ape on the planet.

2 The Western Lowland gorilla moved from "endangered" to "critically endangered" in 2007. "Critically endangered" indicates that its population and range are shrinking, and it is in imminent danger of extinction. The Mountain gorilla, once studied by George Schaller and Dian Fossey in the 1960s, has also been endangered for years.

3 The gorilla has the misfortune to be native to an area that has been ravaged by war. Rwanda and the Congo are war-torn nations, and the resulting damage to habitat has affected gorillas as well as humans. Gorilla populations have also been ransacked by the Ebola virus, which has killed an estimated 90 percent of the gorilla population in each area of western and central Africa where it has been found.

4 Like humans, gorillas tend to have a single offspring at one time, with each one gestating for about nine months. Females do not mature until around age six, and nearly half of baby gorillas do not survive till breeding age.

5 The number-one threat to gorillas, however, is human greed. Humans are burning down the forests where the last remaining gorilla families live. They are doing this to harvest charcoal, which is used to fuel cooking fires throughout the region. In addition, they are poaching the last remaining gorillas for meat and for their hands or other parts, which are considered a delicacy in Africa and are used medicinally in parts of Asia.

6 Even the tourist industry, once thought to be a way to preserve the ape population, has proved deadly to the gorillas. Many have died from measles or respiratory infections caught from humans. Despite the best efforts of dedicated conservationists and African rangers, some give these vegetarian cousins of *Homo sapiens* no more than a decade before all wild specimens are eradicated.

17. The author's **tone** indicates that she feels the eradication of apes is
  A. inevitable   **C.** intentional
  B. shocking   **D.** impossible

18. Based on information in the passage, about how many gorillas have survived Ebola in regions where the virus is prevalent?
  A. about 1 percent   **C.** about half
  B. about 1 in 10   **D.** only 9 in 10

19. How are the ideas in the first two sentences of the second paragraph related?
  A. Sentence 2 provides a contrast to sentence 1.
  B. Sentence 2 is the next step after sentence 1.
  C. Sentence 2 defines a term that appears in sentence 1.
  D. Sentence 2 provides support for a theory in sentence 1.

20. The main point of the passage is that
    A. gorillas are not designed for survival
    B. conservation is unrealistic
    C. humans put gorillas at risk
    D. we all must protect our ape cousins

21. The author's purpose in the fifth paragraph is to
    A. introduce a hypothesis and support it with examples
    B. compare some indignities perpetrated on apes
    C. list some possible reasons for the extinction of species
    D. contradict theories suggested in earlier paragraphs

22. By the end of the passage, the author concludes that
    A. Africans care little about gorillas.
    B. The large apes should fight back.
    C. Humans are largely evil.
    D. Gorillas may not survive.

23. Which adds the **most** credibility to the information given in the passage?
    A. the mention of Dian Fossey in the second paragraph
    B. the reference to the 2007 Red List in the second paragraph
    C. the use of words like "war-torn" and "ransacked" in the third paragraph
    D. the reference to the tourist industry in the sixth paragraph

24. Which new information, if true, would **most challenge** the claim that gorillas have only a decade before extinction in the wild?
    A. a new transboundary law outlawing any human incursion into gorilla habitat
    B. the discovery of a vaccine against Ebola in humans
    C. successful breeding of Mountain with Lowland gorillas in a zoo setting
    D. observations of several twin babies in existing gorilla families

---

**STOP. IF YOU HAVE TIME LEFT OVER,
CHECK YOUR WORK ON THIS SECTION ONLY.**

SECTION 6. QUANTITATIVE ABILITY

24 Questions   **Time: 20 Minutes**

Directions: Choose the best answer to each question.

1. $\dfrac{1}{3} \div \dfrac{5}{9} =$

   A. $\dfrac{3}{5}$ **B.** $\dfrac{5}{3}$ **C.** $\dfrac{5}{9}$ **D.** $\dfrac{1}{9}$

2. What is the average of the numbers 24, 53, 70, 89, 34, and 30?

   A. 84   **B.** 39   **C.** 71   **D.** 50

3. Express 239 in scientific notation.

   A. 2.39×10^0 **B.** 2.39×10^1 **C.** 2.39×10^2 **D.** 2.39×10^3

4. $(-5.4 \times 10^7) \div (2.7 \times 10^3) =$

   A. -1.5×10^4 **B.** -2.0×10^4 **C.** -3.5×10^4 **D.** -5.0×10^4

5. What is the solution of the inequality $3x - 9 > 1 - 2x$?

   A. $x > \dfrac{1}{2}$ **B.** $x < \dfrac{1}{2}$ **C.** $x > 2$ **D.** $x < 2$

6. Given the equation $\dfrac{56}{4x+8} = \dfrac{1}{8}$, what is the value of x?

   A. 64   **B.** 110   **C.** 164   **D.** 215

7. Find the roots of the quadratic equation $x^2 - 2x - 1 = 0$.

   A. $x = 1 \pm \sqrt{2}$ **B.** $x = 1 \pm 2$ **C.** $x = \sqrt{2} \pm 1$ **D.** $x = 1 \pm \sqrt{3}$

8. $\left(\dfrac{4}{3}\right)^2 + \left(\dfrac{2}{4}\right)^2 =$

   A. $\dfrac{96}{36}$ **B.** $\dfrac{84}{36}$ **C.** $\dfrac{73}{36}$ **D.** $\dfrac{65}{36}$

9. If $\dfrac{x}{y} = 8$ and $x = 64$, then what is the sum $x + y$?

   A. 56   **B.** 64   **C.** 72   **D.** 81

10. On a single roll of a die, what is the probability of not getting a 2?

    A. $\dfrac{1}{6}$ B. $\dfrac{3}{6}$ C. $\dfrac{4}{6}$ D. $\dfrac{5}{6}$

11. What is the probability of randomly selecting a ten card from a standard deck of cards?

    A. $\dfrac{1}{52}$ B. $\dfrac{1}{13}$ C. $\dfrac{12}{13}$ D. $\dfrac{51}{52}$

12. What is the probability that two cards drawn from a deck of cards are face cards (king, queen, or jack) of any suit if the first card drawn is replaced before the second card is drawn?

    A. $\dfrac{9}{169}$ B. $\dfrac{1}{16}$ C. $\dfrac{3}{13}$ D. $\dfrac{1}{26}$

Questions 13 and 14

A teacher assessed the performance of her class of 15 students on a particular assignment and noted the following distribution of grades:
{94, 71, 68, 83, 80, 86, 76, 86, 91, 97, 88, 77, 85, 70, 78}

13. What is the mean of the data set?

    A. 55   B. 66   C. 78   D. 82

14. What is the median of the data set?

    A. 80   B. 83   C. 85   D. 86

15. Solve for x: $10 + 5x^2 = 135$

    A. ±2   B. ±5   C. ±10   D. ±25

16. Solve for x: $4(2x + 20) + 3(x - 1) = 0$

    A. 11   B. 7   C. −7   D. −11

17. What is the equation of a line that passes through the point $(2, -3)$ and has a slope of $-\dfrac{1}{2}$?

    A. $y = -\dfrac{1}{2}x + 2$ B. $y = -\dfrac{1}{2}x - 2$ C. $y = \dfrac{1}{2}x + 2$ D. $y = \dfrac{1}{2}x - 2$

18. What is the slope of a line that passes through the points $(-3, 3)$ and $(3, 3)$?

    A. −3   B. 3   C. 0   D. undefined

19. What is the slope of a line that passes through the points $(0, 4)$ and $(4, 0)$?

    A. −4   B. −1   C. 0   D. undefined

20. Evaluate the following derivative: $\dfrac{d}{dx}\left(5x^6\right)$

   A. $30x^5$ **B.** $\dfrac{30}{x^5}$ **C.** $\dfrac{15}{x^5}$ **D.** $15x^5$

21. Evaluate the following derivative: $\dfrac{d}{dx}\left(3x^3 - 2x^2\right)$

   A. $3x^2 + 2x$ **B.** $3x^2 - 2x$ **C.** $9x^2 - 4x$ **D.** $9x^2 + 4x$

22. Evaluate the following derivative: $\dfrac{d}{dx}\left(25 - 7x^3\right)$ at $x = -2$

   A. 35 **B.** 84 **C.** -84 **D.** -120

23. Evaluate the following indefinite integral: $\displaystyle\int 10t^4\,dt$

   A. $2t^5 + C$ **B.** $10t^5 + C$ **C.** $\dfrac{2}{5}t^5 + C$ **D.** $\dfrac{10}{3}t^5 + C$

24. Evaluate the following definite integral: $\displaystyle\int_2^4 \left(x^4 - 6x\right)dx$

   A. 123.6 **B.** 162.4 **C.** 183.7 **D.** 250.2

**STOP. IF YOU HAVE TIME LEFT OVER,
CHECK YOUR WORK ON THIS SECTION ONLY.**

Answer Key

Section 2. Verbal Ability

1. B	10. D	19. B
2. D	11. C	20. D
3. D	12. C	21. D
4. A	13. B	22. B
5. C	14. B	23. B
6. C	15. C	24. B
7. B	16. D	
8. A	17. D	
9. B	18. A	

Section 3. Biology

1. B	10. C	19. A
2. A	11. C	20. A
3. B	12. C	21. A
4. D	13. B	22. C
5. D	14. C	23. D
6. D	15. A	24. C
7. C	16. C	
8. D	17. D	
9. A	18. A	

Section 4. Chemistry

1. C	10. A	19. B
2. C	11. D	20. A
3. B	12. B	21. B
4. A	13. B	22. A
5. A	14. A	23. D
6. C	15. D	24. C
7. D	16. C	
8. D	17. D	
9. B	18. B	

Section 5. Reading Comprehension

1. C	10. C	19. C
2. C	11. B	20. C
3. B	12. D	21. A
4. D	13. C	22. D
5. A	14. B	23. B
6. C	15. D	24. A
7. D	16. B	
8. A	17. B	
9. A	18. B	

Section 6. Quantitative Ability

1. A	10. D	19. B
2. D	11. B	20. A
3. C	12. A	21. C
4. B	13. D	22. C
5. C	14. B	23. A
6. B	15. B	24. B
7. A	16. C	
8. C	17. B	
9. C	18. C	

Answer Explanations

SECTION 1. WRITING

Ask a teacher or another student to score your essay, or score it yourself using the following scoring rubrics.

CONVENTIONS OF LANGUAGE SCORING RUBRIC	
0	Paper blank, illegible, or not in English.
1.0	Multiple errors in capitalization, punctuation, grammar, and/or usage, seriously affecting flow and meaning.
2.0	Multiple errors in capitalization, punctuation, grammar, and/or usage, affecting both flow and meaning.
3.0	Several errors in capitalization, punctuation, grammar, and/or usage. Errors may affect flow, but they do not affect meaning.
4.0	Some errors in capitalization, punctuation, grammar, and/or usage, but errors do not affect meaning or flow.
5.0	Few errors in capitalization, punctuation, grammar, and/or usage.

PROBLEM SOLVING SCORING RUBRIC	
0	Paper blank, illegible, on a topic other than that assigned, or not in English.
1.0	Lack of understanding evident. Organization nonexistent or unclear. Ideas undeveloped.
2.0	Organization unclear or scattershot. Ideas underdeveloped and unsupported.
3.0	Organization fairly coherent. Ideas developed and supported with relevant details that lack complexity.
4.0	Organization coherent and focused. Ideas complex, well developed, and clearly supported.
5.0	Organization coherent and focused. Ideas complex, sophisticated, and substantially developed, with logical, convincing support.

SECTION 2. VERBAL ABILITY

1. Answer: B

Choices C and D make little sense in context. The cells might be known especially (choice A) as leukocytes, but it makes more sense for them to be known collectively, or as a group, by that name.

2. Answer: D

Whether or not you recall what a Punnett square is, the word *graphics* should be enough of a clue to help you recognize that it is designed to help make something more visually accessible. A graphic would not control (choice A) combinations, and it is not clear how it would integrate (choice B) or magnify (choice C) them.

3. Answer: D

The first blank might logically be replaced by *concept* (choice A), *theory* (choice B), or *idea* (choice D), but only *christened* (choice C) or *termed* (choice D) make contextual sense in the second blank, meaning that choice D is the best answer.

4. Answer: A

Eliminate choice B, which does not make sense. Then use clues from the sentence to decide which of the remaining words is best. The diaphragm moves, which alters the size of the chest cavity. This does not *amplify*, or enlarge breathing (choice D). It does more than *indicate* breathing (choice C)—it results in, or *accomplishes*, breathing (choice A).

5. Answer: C

If you look only at the end of the sentence, your choice will be clear. A reaction does not *contain* (choice A), *allow* (choice B), or *reveal* (choice D) quickly. It *occurs* quickly, making choice C the best answer.

6. Answer: C

You might have *indications* of a deficiency (choice A), but they would not *behold* the symptoms given. You would not refer to *deficits* of a deficiency (choice B); nor would you call the results of a deficiency its *products* (choice D). In this case, the simplest answer is also the best.

7. Answer: B

It may take a couple of readings to analyze the structure of this sentence. The centers of respiration are doing something to increases in amounts of carbon dioxide, after which they are doing something else to the muscles involved in breathing. The only pair of words that makes sense is choice B.

8. Answer: A

Again, the structure of the sentence is tricky. Dolphins and humans are being compared in regard to their hearing. Humans are not *documenting* (choice B), *enabling* (choice C), or *conducting* (choice D) the sounds; they are *perceiving* them (choice A)—or rather, failing to perceive them.

9. Answer: B

Reduce the sentence to its simplest parts by eliminating the descriptive phrase in the middle. All organisms have a *process* for reproducing. None of the other choices makes sense.

10. Answer: D

Any of the first words would fit the context, as would any of the second words. The trick is to find the pair that makes sense. If the plants were *obstinately*, or stubbornly, easy to grow, they would not be a *constructive* resource (choice A). If the plants were *hardly* easy to grow, they would not be a *reliable* resource (choice B). If the plants were *unusually* easy to grow, they would not be a *troublesome* resource (choice C). If, however, they were *relatively* easy to grow, they would be a *favorable*, or beneficial, resource.

11. Answer: C

The *ohm* is a unit of measure used by electricians to measure resistance. The *mach* is a unit of measure used by test pilots to measure speed.

12. Answer: C

Pacific and *Indian* are the names of two oceans. *Superior* and *Erie* are the names of two of the Great Lakes.

13. Answer: B

Connection and *correlation* are synonyms, as are *division* and *schism*.

14. Answer: B

This is an Object/Action relationship. *Stomata* are pores on the underside of leaves used by the plant in respiration, or gas exchange. The *stomach* is an organ in larger animals used in digestion.

15. Answer: C

The end of the Paleozoic era (453 to 248 million years ago) saw the rise of the first reptiles. The end of the Mesozoic era (248 to 65 million years ago) saw the rise of the first birds.

16. Answer: D

These are simple synonyms. *Vision* is *sight*, and *audition* is *hearing*.

17. Answer: D

The prefix *micro-* means "millionth," as in *microgram*. The prefix *nano-* means "billionth," as in *nanometer*.

18. Answer: A

The disease *diphtheria* attacks the mucous membranes. The toxin *botulism* attacks the nerve tissue.

19. Answer: B

Mecca, in Saudi Arabia, is the birthplace of Muhammad. Bethlehem, on the West Bank in Israel, is the birthplace of Jesus. This is a Characteristic analogy.

20. Answer: D

A collector of stamps is a *philatelist*. A collector of coins is a *numismatist*.

21. Answer: D

The Taj Mahal is a mausoleum in Agra, India. The Great Pyramid is a mausoleum in Giza, Egypt.

22. Answer: B

A glider is marked by its lack of a motor, and an integrated circuit is marked by its lack of wires.

23. Answer: B

The root *dactyl*, as in *pterodactyl*, means "finger." The root *cardio*, as in *cardiovascular*, means "heart."

24. Answer: B

If you are *febrile*, or feverish, you are not *cool*. A place that is *humid* is not *parched*.

SECTION 3. BIOLOGY

1. Answer: B

Cells in hypotonic solutions will gain water and swell. By definition, a hypotonic solution has more water and less solute relative to what it is being compared to. Cells in isotonic solutions will remain the same size since there is no net movement of water. Hypertonic solutions have less water and more solute relative to what they are being compared to. This means a cell in a hypertonic solution would lose water and shrivel.

2. Answer: A

Increasing the levels of Na^+, K^+ and HCO_3^- excreted in the urine should increase the concentration of the urine. As the urine becomes more concentrated, osmotic effects occur and extra water will be excreted with the urine in an attempt to dilute the urine. This will increase the urine volume (choice A). Choice B can be eliminated since it contradicts choice A. Choice C can be eliminated because urine pH would decrease (become more acidic) with an increased concentration of H^+, not HCO_3^-. Na^+, K^+, and HCO_3^- are all excreted normally in the urine but increased concentrations will have an effect on the concentration of urine and the amount of water excreted.

3. Answer: B

This question requires a knowledge of the purposes of mitosis and meiosis. Mitosis is used for growth, repair, and replacement of cells. Mitosis begins with a diploid cell and ends with identical diploid daughter cells. The purpose of meiosis is to produce genetically diverse daughter cells. Meiosis begins with a diploid parent cell and ends with four genetically unique, haploid daughter cells. The only choice that reflects correct statements concerning mitosis and meiosis is choice B.

4. Answer: D

This question is asking about the function of ribosomes. The role of ribosomes is protein synthesis. If an antibiotic blocks ribosome activity, protein synthesis will be affected.

5. Answer: D

The phenotypic ratio contains three numbers, which indicates that three phenotypes are present. Of the choices listed, only one can lead to the presence of three different phenotypes. In the heterozygous condition, incomplete dominance can lead to the expression of an intermediate phenotype.

6. Answer: D

You need to think about the route taken when a substance is taken orally. The medication would have to travel through the digestive system before it would be absorbed into the bloodstream in the small intestine. It would move from the oral cavity to the esophagus to the stomach and then to the small intestine for absorption. Since most substances are absorbed in the small intestine and not the stomach, choice A can be eliminated. In the stomach, the pH is often between 1 and 2. This level of acidity may cause denaturation of the peptide hormones. Further, the stomach is designed with enzymes to digest proteins; these enzymes could also damage the peptide hormone. This makes choice D the most logical explanation. This eliminates choices B and C as options because the damage has been done prior to the hormone entering the small intestine or the large intestine.

7. Answer: C

This question relies on knowing the rules of complementary base pairing. Cytosine always pairs with guanine and adenine always pairs with thymine. The only time uracil is present would be in RNA.

8. Answer: D

None of the other choices works. Choice A suggests bacterial cells would have more organelles than eukaryotic cells. This is false, since bacterial cells do not have organelles. Choice B suggests that the nucleus of bacteria is smaller than that of eukaryotic cells. However, bacterial cells do not have a nucleus. Choice C indicates that bacterial cells lack a cell membrane. This is also false since all cells have a cell membrane.

9. Answer: A

The question asks about a cell structure that would be able to break down (digest) cellular components. Of the structures listed, the lysosomes would be the best option. Ribosomes produce proteins, the cell membrane serves as the outer boundary of the cell, and the mitochondria are used for cellular respiration.

10. Answer: C

Pulmonary gas exchange is always based on simple diffusion. Diffusion allows for the movement of a substance from an area of high concentration of the substance to an area of low concentration of the substance. Depending on the concentrations, oxygen and carbon dioxide will move in variable directions. Choices A, B, and D indicate that the movement of gases always occurs in a fixed direction, which is incorrect.

11. Answer: C

The big ATP payoff in aerobic cellular respiration comes from the electron transport chain. In order for the electron transport chain to work, it requires a source of electrons and hydrogen ions (protons). These items must be collected by molecules such as NAD^+ and FAD. While a little ATP is made in the initial stages of aerobic cellular respiration, the primary purpose of the initial steps such as glycolysis and the Krebs cycle is to allow NAD^+ and FAD to collect electrons and protons for the electron transport chain.

12. Answer: C

This question is asking for a comparison between the organization of DNA in bacteria and eukaryotic cells. Eukaryotic DNA exists in multiple linear pieces termed chromosomes. Bacterial DNA consists of a single loop of DNA. While bacteria can have extra-chromosomal DNA, known as plasmids, this is not the case for all bacteria. While RNA is single-stranded, it is not the primary genetic material of the cells and is only produced during transcription.

13. Answer: B

Anaerobic respiration results in the production of 2 ATP per glucose molecule. These are produced in glycolysis. If the cell had access to 6 molecules of glucose, each one would produce 2 ATP, for a total of 12 ATP.

14. Answer: C

Autosomal traits are carried on the nonsex chromosomes. These are any chromosomes other than the X or Y and consist of human chromosomes 1-22. Recessive traits often skip generations since carriers are unaware that they are carrying a single copy of the disease-causing allele.

15. Answer: A

Stem cells that originate in the bone marrow serve as the precursor to all blood cells. These include the erythrocytes, leukocytes, and platelets. If a person has leukemia and abnormal leukocytes, a stem cell transplant would allow for the differentiation of new and hopefully normal leukocytes. Stem cells do not have the ability to attack other cells, replace the function of abnormal cells, or act as immune system modulators.

16. Answer: C

This question relies on knowledge of cell structures. Mitochondria are used for the process of cellular respiration, which produces ATP. Lysosomes perform cellular digestion.

The smooth endoplasmic reticulum is responsible for lipid synthesis. The only structure that enables a cell to move is the flagellum.

17. Answer: D

During the light-dependent reactions of photosynthesis, electrons will be passed through electron carrier molecules. In PSII, the result will be production of ATP needed for the light-independent reactions.

18. Answer: A

This question presents a situation where a very high fever is increasing temperature in the body. Of the choices listed, some make more sense than others. It does not seem plausible that increased temperature would increase the cellular respiration rates to dangerous levels, that increased temperature would prevent substances from transporting across the membrane, or that increased temperature would alter cell division. However, increased temperature is one factor that can cause denaturation of enzymes if high temperatures are not quickly reduced.

19. Answer: A

Sodium has a variety of roles in the body. Of the choices listed, sodium is highly involved with the function of neurons. Sodium-potassium pumps maintain an unequal balance of ions across the membrane of neurons during resting potential. During action potential, sodium channels open in order to initiate an impulse. If the sodium ion concentration was out of balance, the neuron's function could be compromised.

20. Answer: A

Within the four kingdoms of the domain Eukarya, only one contains individuals that are multicellular and produce their own food. The kingdom Plantae fits these criteria.

21. Answer: A

The diploid number for humans is 46 and the haploid number is 23. When cells are not dividing, each chromosome is present in a single copy. These chromosomes are composed of one chromatid when they are not replicated.

22. Answer: C

Choice A can be eliminated because chloroplasts are unique to plants. Choice B can be eliminated because the cell wall is unique to plants. Choice D can be eliminated because the central vacuole is unique to plants. This leaves us with choice C as the only option.

23. Answer: D

All of these statements are correct. Spores are made by only a few types of bacteria, many of which can cause diseases such as tetanus, botulism, or anthrax. When spores form they can survive for extended periods of time and are difficult to kill by ordinary measures.

24. Answer: C

This question is asking about the general differences in mechanisms of action between steroid and peptide hormones. Steroid hormones are derived from cholesterol, enter their target cells where they bind to a receptor, and act to influence gene expression. Peptide hormones are not lipid-soluble and do not enter their target cells. They act as first messengers to activate second messengers in their target cells.

SECTION 4. CHEMISTRY

1. Answer: C
In ionic compounds in which the cation and anion have only one possible charge, the name of the compound is the cation name followed by the name of the anion. The indications of the number of ions or the ions' charge are not necessary. The cation in this case is the ammonium ion, NH_4^+, and the anion is phosphate, PO_4^{3-}.

2. Answer: C
The steps in solving this problem are:
$$g\ BF_3 \longrightarrow mol\ BF_3 \longrightarrow mol\ HF \longrightarrow g\ HF$$

The molar masses needed are $BF_3 = 67.8$ g/mol and $HF = 20$ g/mol.

$$33.9g\ of\ BF_3 \times \frac{1\ mol\ BF_3}{67.8g\ BF_3} = 0.50\ mol\ BF_3$$

$$0.50\ mol\ BF_3 \times \frac{3\ mol\ HF}{1\ mol\ BF_3} = 1.5\ mol\ HF$$

$$1.5\ mol\ HF \times \frac{20g\ HF}{1\ mol\ HF} = 30g\ HF$$

Common mistakes are omitting the stoichiometry step (the middle one above) or multiplying by three times the molar mass of HF in the last step.

3. Answer: B
A neutralization reaction is the reaction of an acid (H_3PO_4) and a base ($Ca(OH)_2$) to produce a salt ($Ca_3(PO_4)_2$) and water. Reaction A is a combination reaction that is also an oxidation reduction reaction. Reaction C is a precipitation reaction. Reaction D is an oxidation reduction reaction.

4. Answer: A
The only gas on the reactants side is oxygen. The only gas on the products side is the sulfur dioxide. For every mole of oxygen that reacts, there will be ⅔ (the molar ratio from the balanced equation) moles of sulfur dioxide. The temperature and pressure are fixed, so the volume of the gas will be proportional to the number of moles of gas; therefore the ratio of the volumes of the gases will also be ⅔.

$$17.5L\ O_2 \times \frac{2L\ SO_2}{3L\ O_2} = 11.7L\ SO_2$$

5. Answer: A
For this thermochemical equation the number representing the heat is for the number of moles listed in the balanced equation. The molar mass of C_6H_6 is 78 g/mol.

The steps are:

$$g\ C_6H_6 \rightarrow mol\ C_6H_6 \rightarrow heat$$

$$256\,g\ of\ C_6H_6 \times \frac{1\,mol\ C_6H_6}{78\,g\ C_6H_6} = 3.28\ mol\ C_6H_6$$

$$3.28\,mol\ C_6H_6 \times \frac{6535\,kJ}{2\,mol\ C_6H_6} = 1.07 \times 10^4\ kJ$$

A common error is to forget the factor of 2 in the last step from the balanced equation.

6. Answer: C

To check the validity of quantum numbers, check in the order from n to ℓ to m_ℓ to m_s. Valid values are n = a positive integer (1,2,3,4, . . .), ℓ = an integer from 0 to a maximum of n−1 (0, 1, 2, . . . , n−1), m_ℓ = integers between −ℓ and +ℓ (−ℓ, . . . 0 . . . , +ℓ), and m_s must be either + ½ or − ½.

   A. n = 3, ℓ = 3, m_ℓ − 2, m_s = + ½ (incorrect, For n = 3, the maximum value of ℓ is 2.)
   B. n = 3, ℓ = 2, m_ℓ = −4, m_s − ½ (incorrect, for ℓ = 2, the m_ℓ value must be between −ℓ and +ℓ or between −2 and +2
   C. n = 3, ℓ = 2, m_ℓ = −2, m_s = − ½ (all numbers are correct)
   D. n = − 3, ℓ = 2, m_ℓ = −2, m_s = − ½ (incorrect, n cannot be a negative number).

7. Answer: D

To form anions, electrons are added to atoms. To form cations, electrons are removed from an atom. The anion S^{2-} is a sulfur atom (16 electrons) plus two electrons (a total of 18 electrons). Choice D has the correct number of electrons. Choice A is the electron configuration of a neutral sulfur atom (16 electrons). Choice B is 14 electrons (removal of two electrons), and choice C has 17 electrons.

8. Answer: D

The resonance structures possible for sulfate must have two double bonds and two single bonds. The number of possible resonance structures is the number of unique pairs of O atoms that can have the double bond. If you label the O atoms A, B, C, and D as shown below, the possible pairs are A-B, A-C, A-D, B-C, B-D, and C-D.

9. **Answer: B**

For a molecule to be polar, the molecule must have polar bonds and the bond vectors must not cancel out. All the molecules have polar bonds, but the vectors cancel, except in PF_3, which is trigonal pyramidal. The VSEPR structures of the molecules (lone pairs except those on the central atom have been omitted) and the orientations of the bond vectors are shown below each structure.

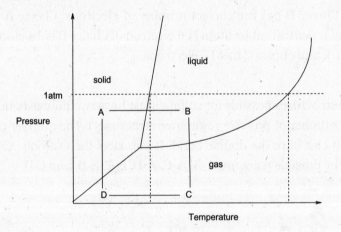

10. **Answer: A**

Melting is the phase transition from solid to liquid. The phase diagram with the regions labeled is shown below. Only the transition from $A - B$ would include melting when the substance crosses the solid-liquid line.

11. **Answer: D**

The osmotic pressure (Π) for a solution is $\Pi = MRT$ where M is the molarity of particles, R is the gas constant, and T is the Kelvin temperature. $CaCl_2$ is an ionic solid that separates into ions: $CaCl_2(aq) \rightarrow Ca^{2+}(aq) + 2Cl^-(aq)$. For each mole of $CaCl_2$ that dissolves, three moles of particles are formed. A 0.50 M solution of $CaCl_2$ will have a molarity of 1.5 M in particles. The temperature must be converted to K ($27 + 273 = 300$ K). The osmotic pressure will be:

$$\Pi = 1.5 \, \frac{mol}{L} \times 0.082 \, \frac{L \cdot atm}{mol \cdot K} \times 300 \, K = 36.9 \, atm$$

Choice A uses a molarity of 0.5 M. Choice C uses the temperature in Celsius. Choice B combines the errors in A and C.

12. Answer: B

The rate of a reaction can be increased by increasing the concentration of the reactants (which allows more collisions), by increasing the temperature (which increases the fraction of molecules with sufficient energy to react successfully), or by adding a catalyst (which lowers the activation energy of the reaction). Increasing the volume of the reaction will decrease the concentration of the reactants, which will slow the reaction rate.

13. Answer: B

The equilibrium constant is the product of the concentrations of the products raised to the power equal to the coefficients in the balanced equation divided by the product of the concentrations of the reactants raised to the power equal to the coefficients in the balanced equation. Pure solids and liquids are left out of the expression. This is why choices C and D are incorrect.

14. Answer: A

A substance will be more soluble in acidic solution if the anion reacts with the acid. This will happen if the anion is a base that reacts with acids. Hydroxide is a strong base, so sparingly soluble metal hydroxides are more soluble in acidic solutions. The anions Cl^- and NO_3^- are the conjugate bases of the strong acids HCl and HNO_3, respectively. Conjugate base strength is inversely related to the acid from which the base is derived, so Cl^- and NO_3^- are very weak bases. The weak acid CN has a relatively strong conjugate base CN^- which will react with acids according to the reaction below.

$$H^+(aq) + CN^-(aq) \rightarrow HCN(aq)$$

By removing the CN^- ion from solution, the solubility equilibrium shifts to the right allowing more $Ni(CN)_2$ to dissolve.

15. Answer: D

The reactions given in the problem are reductions, so one must be reversed to be the oxidation of the reaction. Reduction occurs at the cathode and oxidation occurs at the anode. The problem states that Cd is the anode, so this reaction must be reversed. If the reaction is reversed, the sign of E° must also be reversed. The cathode half reaction must be multiplied by 2 to balance the number of electrons transferred, but the E° is not multiplied by this number. Remember the $V = J/c$, so multiplying charge also multiplies energy, but the ratio J/c is still the same value. The incorrect answers arise from not reversing the Cd half reaction, multiplying the Ni reaction E° by 2, or a combination of these two errors.

$$Cd(s) + 2OH^-(aq) \longrightarrow Cd(OH)_2(s) + 2e^- \qquad E° = +0.81\,V$$

$$2NiO(OH)(s) + 2H_2O(l) + 2e^- \longrightarrow 2Ni(OH)_2(s) + 2OH^-(aq) \qquad E° = +0.49\,V$$

$$Cd(s) + 2NiO(OH)(s) + 2H_2O(l) \longrightarrow Cd(OH)_2(s) + 2Ni(OH)_2(s) \quad E°cell = +1.30\,V$$

16. **Answer: C**

Sulfur is lower on the periodic table, therefore methanethiolate is both more polarizable (thus, more nucleophilic) and larger (less basic).

17. **Answer: D**

Iodine is lower on the periodic table than chlorine; therefore, iodide is more polarizable and more nucleophilic than chloride. The same top-to-bottom trend makes iodide less basic than chloride. Neither are terribly basic—nevertheless, inasmuch as chloride is the stronger base (i.e., weaker conjugate acid), it is the poorer leaving group.

18. **Answer: B**

The substrate has an excellent leaving group (bromide) attached to a secondary center. Therefore, from the substrate's standpoint both S_N1 and S_N2 would be viable options. However, the conditions are very mild—methanol is a poor nucleophile, and therefore would not engage in S_N2 chemistry. Failing that, the leaving group will leave (ionization) to give a planar carbocation, which can be captured from the front or back in equal probability; therefore, a racemic mixture will be formed.

19. **Answer: B**

While all three interior carbons (C2, C3, and C4) look suspicious, closer inspection reveals that only the middle carbon (C3) is connected to four different groups—both C2 and C4 are connected to two methyl groups; therefore, they are not asymmetric centers.

20. **Answer: A**

There are two functional groups on the molecule—only one can define the main chain. The ketone is of higher priority, therefore the compound is a hydroxybutanone, not an oxobutanol. The stereochemistry at C3 can be quickly determined by assigning CIP priorities to the substituents: -OH takes a; -C=O, takes b; -CH$_3$ takes c; and H (not shown) takes d. The progression of a → b → c is counterclockwise, but d is coming out at us (it should be pointing away from us); thus, the center must be R.

21. **Answer: B**

To establish the elements of commonality, notice that in the comparison sawhorse structure, the carboxylic acid is to the right and pointing up, and the conformation is staggered (zigzag). By definition, a Fischer projection is eclipsed, so this will have to be reconformed to make an intuitive evaluation (shown following). One center is the same configuration (C2) and one is different (C3); therefore, the two are diastereomers.

22. Answer: A

To establish the elements of commonality, notice that in the comparison two-dimensional representation, the hydroxyl group is at 10 o'clock and the chloro substituent is at 6 o'clock. After two simple manipulations (shown below), we see that both centers are of opposite configuration, thus enantiomers.

23. Answer: D

Jones conditions will oxidize the secondary alcohol to the ketone and the primary alcohol to the carboxylic acid.

24. Answer: C

PCC will oxidize the secondary alcohol to the ketone and the primary alcohol to the aldehyde.

SECTION 5. READING COMPREHENSION

1. Answer: C

Ether's run is described as "brief but important," implying that despite its short reign as the anesthetic of choice, it was an effective choice. There is no support in the passage for any of the other answer choices.

2. Answer: C

The word *agent* has multiple meanings, but only one works in context here. The author speaks of ether's use as "a hypnotic agent," meaning an instrument that causes hypnosis. Only choice C is a synonym that works in the context given.

3. Answer: B

Choice A is far too broad for the four-paragraph passage given here, which really focuses on a single anesthetic (choice B). Choice C is not relevant to the passage, which focuses more on how anesthetics have been similar from century to century than on how they have changed. Although the passage opens with reference to ancient physicians (choice D), this is not the main idea of the passage.

4. Answer: D

Your answer will be the statement that **least** indicates that ether was important. To find it, you must read each statement with that key idea in mind. Choice A supports the idea by showing how one doctor used ether. Choice B supports the idea by showing that doctors were eager to learn about ether. Choice C supports the idea by showing that artists of the day captured the important event. Only choice D does not fit; it states only that the usefulness of ether had not been discovered for many years.

5. Answer: A

"Supposed to have discovered" means that Lullus is "said to have discovered." It implies that there is not a lot of corroborating evidence; if there were, the author would have simply said "discovered." Choice B may be true, but for the time being, the author is implying that Lullus may or may not have made the discovery.

6. Answer: C

The fourth paragraph is a narrative that tells about Morton's demonstration, followed by his attempts to win a patent. It is told in story form, in the order in which events occurred.

7. Answer: D

If ether was truly important to the history of medicine, it would be nice to see some examples of its use that support that claim. Of the suggestions given, only choice D provides such examples. Ether's chemical makeup (choice A) has nothing to do with its importance. The names and occupations of patients (choice B) are unlikely to offer evidence of this kind—unless they proved to be famous historical figures. Since there is no evidence that they were, choice B is not the best answer. A comparison of two other anesthetic agents (choice C) would not add or subtract useful evidence about ether's importance. The best answer is choice D.

8. Answer: A

Use what is given to you in the passage to answer this question. The inclusion of information about Long may in part be a cautionary tale about the importance of publishing results (choice B), but since Morton himself died in penury, it is not a very good cautionary tale. Choice C is true, but it is not the primary reason the author included this information. There is no evidence to support choice D; in fact, the author makes clear that Long's being overlooked was largely his own fault. The best answer is choice A; Long performed an operation using ether before Morton did.

9. Answer: A

Scientists are studying the composition of the upper atmosphere—its makeup or structure. None of the other synonyms fits the context in which the word is found.

10. **Answer: C**

It is not the reflective surface (choice A) that the author finds remarkable; rather, it is the size of that surface (choice C). Neither choice B nor choice D is supported by the paragraph.

11. **Answer: B**

The three typical courses of study at Arecibo are described in the second paragraph. They include radio astronomy (choice C), atmospheric science (choice A), and radar astronomy (choice D). Since you are asked to find the exception, the correct answer is choice B.

12. **Answer: D**

To answer this kind of question, simply return to the paragraph in question and think about its main idea. The main idea of the fourth paragraph is established in the initial topic sentence: "Arecibo has been the site of hundreds of fascinating discoveries." The author then proceeds to list a few of these. The correct answer is choice D.

13. **Answer: C**

You can often locate an opinion by searching for adjectives or adverbs that are subjective. Although *giant* (choice A) or *typically* (choice B) might fall into this category, they are not as clearly subjective as *fascinating* (choice C) is. Not everyone would agree that the discoveries were fascinating. It is a statement of opinion that cannot be proved.

14. **Answer: B**

There is no way to predict whether the command center will succeed (choice A) or fail (choice C). The passage states that it will be used to study pulsars, not for atmospheric studies (choice D). The best answer is choice B—the remote-control command center will mean that scientists in Texas need not travel to Puerto Rico to use the telescope.

15. **Answer: D**

Here you are asked a hypothetical question: If you were to choose part of this passage to support the notion that Arecibo deserved funding, which part would you choose? The answer will be the paragraph that most clearly states the positive value of Arecibo. The fourth paragraph (choice D) lists important discoveries that have been made using the telescope. This is the best answer.

16. **Answer: B**

The author never indicates that Arecibo is anything other than a useful tool for scientists. All of the passage seems dedicated to that theme. There is no support for choices A, C, or D in the passage.

17. **Answer: B**

The author uses the word *incredibly* to describe the fact that nearly every ape on the planet appears on the Red List. Her tone is that of someone who is shocked at this information. She surely does not feel that this is inevitable (choice A), or she would not blame it so straightforwardly on human behavior. Nor does she think it is impossible (choice D); it is clearly happening. There is nothing to indicate that she thinks it is intentional (choice C); it is more a side effect of human behavior and not entirely deliberate, except in the case of poaching.

18. **Answer: B**
According to the third paragraph, in areas with Ebola, it wipes out 90 percent of the gorillas. That leaves 1 in 10.

19. **Answer: C**
The only way to answer this question is to refer back to the sentences indicated. Here they are: 1) "The Western Lowland gorilla moved from 'endangered' to 'critically endangered' in 2007." 2) " 'Critically endangered' indicates that its population and range are shrinking, and it is in imminent danger of extinction." Sentence 2 defines the term *critically endangered* that is used in sentence 1. The correct answer is choice C.

20. **Answer: C**
The main point of the passage will be the point around which every paragraph in the passage is centered. The author never states that gorillas are not designed for survival (choice A). Although conservation does not seem to be working at present, the author never suggests that it is an unrealistic goal (choice B). Choice D may be a tacit conclusion one may draw from the passage, but it is not overtly suggested and is not the main point. Every part of the passage indicates that human behavior is harming the great apes in general and gorillas in particular. The best answer is choice C.

21. **Answer: A**
Return to the fifth paragraph and compare it to the answer choices. The author begins with the statement: "The number-one threat to gorillas, however, is human greed." The other sentences in the paragraph give examples of this, including the burning of forests for fuel and the killing of gorillas for meat and medicine. Although indignities are mentioned (choice B), the author does not "compare" them. Nor does the author list reasons for extinction of species (choice C); the list gives examples of harm done to gorillas but does not imply that they have caused extinction. The fifth paragraph does not contradict what has come before (choice D); it confirms it and adds examples.

22. **Answer: D**
The best answer will be clearly supported by the information in the passage. Choice A is contradicted by the fact that African rangers are trying to protect gorillas. Choice B is not suggested anywhere in the passage. Choice C is again contradicted by the fact that conservationists and rangers are doing their best. The only conclusion that is supported is choice D. The author ends with the grim assessment: "Some give these vegetarian cousins of *Homo sapiens* no more than a decade before all wild specimens are eradicated."

23. **Answer: B**
Credibility is support that comes from a convincing source. Dian Fossey, as an expert on gorillas, might be a credible source (choice A), but she is not ever quoted; she is only mentioned in passing. The use of specific words (choice C) does not lend credibility to the passage; nor does the mention of the tourist industry (choice D). The best answer is choice B; the Red List is an important source of information about endangered species.

24. Answer: A

If an answer is to challenge the assertion that gorillas will die out in a decade, the answer must give gorillas hope for a longer existence. Of the answer choices given, choice B would potentially end Ebola in humans, but it is not clear that this would assist gorillas. Choice C, the breeding of different subspecies, might help gorillas, but it would not help those "in the wild," as the question demands. Twin babies (choice D) might indicate better odds for survival, but it is not as clear a benefit as choice A, which would keep all humans from getting near the gorillas to harm them by hunting, clearing land, or passing on diseases.

SECTION 6. QUANTITATIVE ABILITY

1. Answer: A

The quotient of the two fractions can be found by writing the fractions as:

$$\frac{1}{3} \div \frac{5}{9} = \frac{\frac{1}{3}}{\frac{5}{9}} = \left(\frac{1}{3}\right) \cdot \left(\frac{9}{5}\right) = \frac{3}{5}.$$

2. Answer: D

The average of a set of numbers is calculated by:

$$Avg = \frac{24 + 53 + 70 + 89 + 34 + 30}{6} = \frac{300}{6} = 50.$$

3. Answer: C

The number 239 is expressed in scientific notation by first expressing the value in terms of a real number such that $1 \le a < 10$. In this case, the number becomes 2.39. In order to retain the original number, the number must be multiplied by 100 which, in terms of exponents, is 10^2. Thus, in scientific notation,

$$239 = 2.39 \times 100 = 2.39 \times 10^2.$$

4. Answer: B

To divide the two numbers in scientific notation, you have:

$$-5.4 \times 10^7 \div 2.7 \times 10^3 = \frac{-5.4 \times 10^7}{2.7 \times 10^3} = -\frac{5.4}{2.7} \times \frac{10^7}{10^3} = -2.0 \times 10^4.$$

5. Answer: C

To solve the inequality $3x - 9 > 1 - 2x$, you need to collect like terms of x on one side of the inequality and all other values to the other side. You first add 9 to both sides of the inequality:

$$3x - 9 + 9 > 1 - 2x + 9$$

$$3x > 10 - 2x.$$

You then add $2x$ to both sides of the inequality:

$$3x + 2x > 10 - 2x + 2x$$

$$5x > 10.$$

Dividing both sides by 5 yields $x > 2$.

6. Answer: B

To solve for the unknown in the equation $\dfrac{56}{4x+8} = \dfrac{1}{8}$, the goal is to isolate the unknown variable x on one side of the equation with all other terms on the other side. You begin by multiplying both sides of the equation by $4x + 8$:

$$\left(4x+8\right) \cdot \frac{56}{4x+8} = \frac{1}{8} \cdot \left(4x+8\right)$$

$$56 = \frac{1}{8} \cdot \left(4x+8\right)$$

You then divide both sides by $\dfrac{1}{8}$ which, in essence, means you multiply both sides of the equation by its reciprocal $\dfrac{8}{1}$:

$$\frac{8}{1} \cdot 56 = \frac{1}{8} \cdot \left(4x+8\right) \cdot \frac{8}{1}$$

$$448 = \left(4x+8\right).$$

You then subtract 8 from both sides with the final step of dividing both sides by 4, giving you the desired result.

$$448 - 8 = 4x$$

$$\frac{440}{4} = x$$

$$x = 110.$$

7. Answer: A

The equation is in the form of a quadratic equation $ax^2 + bx + c = 0$, where a = 1, b = −2, and c = −1. To solve this problem, you use the quadratic formula or

$$x = \frac{-b \pm \sqrt{b^2 - 4ac}}{2a} = \frac{-(-2) \pm \sqrt{(-2)^2 - 4(1)(-1)}}{2(1)} = \frac{2 \pm 2\sqrt{2}}{2} = 1 \pm \sqrt{2}.$$

8. Answer: C

The sum of $\left(\dfrac{4}{3}\right)^2 + \left(\dfrac{2}{4}\right)^2$ can be found by first computing the value of each term.

$$\left(\frac{4}{3}\right)^2 = \left(\frac{4^2}{3^2}\right) = \frac{16}{9}$$

$$\left(\frac{2}{4}\right)^2 = \left(\frac{2^2}{4^2}\right) = \frac{4}{16} = \frac{1}{4}$$

$$\left(\frac{4}{3}\right)^2 + \left(\frac{2}{4}\right)^2 = \frac{16}{9} + \frac{1}{4} = \frac{64+9}{36} = \frac{73}{36}.$$

9. **Answer: C**

From the first equation, multiply both sides by y resulting in

$$x = 8y.$$

Because $x = 64$, you can write

$$64 = 8y$$

$$\text{or } y = \frac{64}{8} = 8.$$

Substituting the given information regarding x and y into its sum yields:

$$x + y = 64 + 8 = 72.$$

10. **Answer: D**

The probability of not getting a 2 on the roll of the dice can be found using the equation

$q = \dfrac{f}{n} = \dfrac{n-s}{n}$, where n is the total number of possible outcomes ($n = 6$) and s is the

number of outcomes considered a success ($s = 1$). So

$$q = \frac{n-s}{n} = \frac{6-1}{6} = \frac{5}{6}.$$

Another way of looking at this problem would be that the probability of not rolling a 2 is equal to the probability of rolling a 1, 3, 4, 5, and 6, which is five out of a possible six outcomes.

11. **Answer: B**

To determine the probability that a selected card is a ten, you should first note that a card can be selected from a deck in $n = 52$ different ways. Since there are four ten cards, one ten for each of the four suits, a ten can be drawn from the deck in $s = 4$ different ways.

Thus, the probability that the selected card is a ten is: $p = \dfrac{s}{n} = \dfrac{4}{52} = \dfrac{1}{13}$.

12. **Answer: A**

Because the two drawings are made from a complete deck of cards, the two events are independent of one another. We first need to determine the probability of drawing a face card of any suit from a deck of cards. Out of a total of 52 cards, there are 3 face cards of any suit and a total of 12 face cards. The probability of drawing a face card of any suit, P(A), is $\dfrac{12}{52}$. Because the first card is replaced before the second drawing, the probability of drawing a face card of any suit, P(B), is also $\dfrac{12}{52}$. Thus, the probability of drawing two face cards of the same suit is:

$$P(A \text{ and } B) = P(A) \cdot P(B) = \frac{12}{52} \cdot \frac{12}{52} = \frac{144}{2704} = \frac{9}{169}.$$

13. Answer: D

The mean of a data set is the arithmetic average of the values of the data set when arranged in ascending numerical order or

$$\frac{94+71+68+83+80+86+76+86+91+97+88+77+85+70+78}{15} = \frac{1230}{15} = 82.$$

14. Answer: B

The median is the middle or center value of the data set when arranged in ascending numerical order, or 83.

15. Answer: B

In order to solve the equation $10 + 5x^2 = 135$ for x, you need to isolate x:

$$5x^2 = 135 - 10 = 125$$

$$x^2 = \frac{125}{5} = 25.$$

Taking the square root of each side of the equation yields $x = \pm 5$.

16. Answer: C

This equation can be solved by simplifying each side of the equation, combining like terms, isolating x on one side of the equation and then solving for x:

$$4(2x + 20) + 3(x - 1) = 0$$
$$8x + 80 + 3x - 3 = 0$$
$$11x + 77 = 0$$
$$x = -\frac{77}{11} = -7.$$

17. Answer: B

You can use the information provided by the specific point and the value of the slope to derive the equation for the line:

$$m = \frac{y_2 - y_1}{x_2 - x_1}$$

$$-\frac{1}{2} = \frac{y_2 - (-3)}{x_2 - 2} = \frac{y_2 + 3}{x_2 - 2}$$

$$y_2 + 3 = -\frac{1}{2} \cdot (x_2 - 2)$$

$$y_2 + 3 = -\frac{1}{2}x_2 + 1$$

$$y_2 = -\frac{1}{2}x_2 + 1 - 3$$

$$y_2 = -\frac{1}{2}x_2 - 2$$

or

$$y = -\frac{1}{2}x - 2.$$

18. Answer: C

The slope of a line that passes through the points $(-3, 3)$ and $(3, 3)$ can be found by:

$$m = \frac{y_2 - y_1}{x_2 - x_1} = \frac{3 - 3}{3 - (-3)} = \frac{0}{6} = 0.$$

19. Answer: B

The slope of a line that passes through the points $(0, 4)$ and $(4, 0)$ can be found by:

$$m = \frac{y_2 - y_1}{x_2 - x_1} = \frac{0 - 4}{4 - 0} = -\frac{4}{4} = -1.$$

20. Answer: A

The derivative of this function can be evaluated by:

$$\frac{d}{dx}\left(5x^6\right) = 30x^5.$$

21. Answer: C

The derivative of a polynomial is the sum of the derivatives of the terms of the polynomial, or:

$$\frac{d}{dx}\left(3x^3 - 2x^2\right) = \frac{d}{dx}\left(3x^3\right) + \frac{d}{dx}\left(-2x^2\right)$$

$$= \frac{d}{dx}\left(3x^3\right) - \frac{d}{dx}\left(2x^2\right)$$

$$= 9x^2 - 4x.$$

22. Answer: C

You first must calculate the derivative before you can evaluate the derivative at a given point.

$$\frac{d}{dx}\left(25 - 7x^3\right) = -21x^2.$$

The derivative can now be evaluated at $x = -2$ by plugging in the value of -2 for x in the derivative or

$$\frac{d}{dx}\left(25 - 7x^3\right)\bigg|_{x=-2} = -21 \cdot (-2)^2 = -21 \cdot 4 = -84.$$

23. **Answer: A**

Evaluating this integral yields:

$$\int 10t^4 \, dt = \frac{10}{5}t^5 = 2t^5 + C.$$

24. **Answer: B**

You begin by solving the integral and then evaluating the result between the limits of 2 and 4.

$$\int_2^4 \left(x^4 - 6x\right) dx = \left(\frac{x^5}{5} - \frac{6x^2}{2}\right) = \left(\frac{x^5}{5} - 3x^2\right)\bigg|_2^4 = \left(\frac{(4)^5}{5} - 3(4)^2\right) - \left(\frac{(2)^5}{5} - 3(2)^2\right)$$

$$= \left(\frac{1024}{5} - 48\right) - \left(\frac{32}{5} - 12\right) = \frac{812}{5} = 162.4$$

PART III

REVIEWING PCAT VERBAL SKILLS

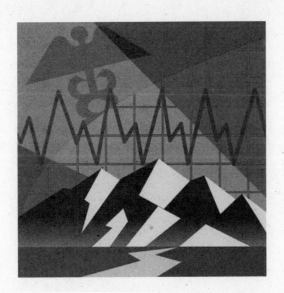

CHAPTER 5

Verbal Ability

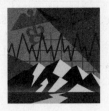

Read This Chapter to Learn About:

➤ What the Verbal Ability Section Tests

➤ Sentence Completions and How to Solve Them

➤ Analogical Thinking

➤ Types of Analogies

➤ Affixes and Roots

WHAT THE VERBAL ABILITY SECTION TESTS

It may seem odd to find Sentence Completions and Analogies in a test for would-be pharmacists. Surely knowledge of biology and chemistry is far more important than the ability to choose the correct word in a word puzzle.

However, your comfort level in English is essential to your achievement in any graduate program, where the amount of reading and writing you will do may be greater than at any other time in your professional life. Analogies have proved a useful indicator of success in college to the extent that some colleges even accept the Miller Analogies Test as a substitute for the SAT.

Sentence Completions test your vocabulary knowledge, your understanding of basic English grammar and sentence structure, and your reading comprehension. Analogies test your general knowledge as well as your skill in logical thinking. Put together, the Verbal Ability part of the PCAT tests your facility with the English language. You will have 30 minutes to complete 48 items.

HOW VERBAL ABILITY IS SCORED

As with all the multiple-choice sections of the PCAT, your score is scaled on a scale ranging from 200 to 600, where 400 is the mean.

SENTENCE COMPLETIONS

PCAT Sentence Completions are cloze sentences in which one or two meaningful words or phrases are omitted. Your job is to choose among four possible choices to complete the sentence in a way that makes sense. You do this by using both the structure of the sentence and the context of the sentence to make the best choice.

Here is an example:

Since the mid-1960s, scientists have recognized that every dolphin has a _____ signature whistle, which is used for identification purposes.
   A. universal
   B. muted
   C. superfluous
   D. distinctive

To answer this question, you go through a rapid series of steps. Let us dissect the process you would use if those steps were slowed way down.

Dissecting the Process

➤ **Think about structure.** The structure of the sentence is (1) the order in which words appear and (2) the grammar used to form the sentence. You first need to figure out what part of speech is missing. In the example above, since the blank precedes an adjective that precedes a noun, it might be either an adverb modifying that adjective (*signature*) or an adjective modifying that noun (*whistle*). Since all of the word choices are adjectives, that is not a huge help. So next, you should look at the clauses and phrases that form the sentence. The blank is in the main clause. An adverbial phrase begins the sentence:*Since the mid-1960s*. An adjectival clause ends the sentence:*which is used for identification purposes*. Many of these clues will help you solve the word puzzle.

➤ **Think about context.** Context has to do with meaning. First, consider the main idea of the sentence, which might be restated as "Dolphins' Whistles." Next, think about what you are told about the whistles: (1) Every dolphin has one. (2) The whistles are used for identification purposes. At this point, you might be able to think of a word of your own that fills the blank and makes sense in context. An example might be: *Since the mid-1960s, scientists have recognized that every dolphin has a* **unique** *signature whistle, which is used for identification purposes.*

➤ **Compare the answer choices.** Last, you must take what you have learned and apply each answer choice to the structure and context of the sentence. If the whistle were *universal* (A), it would be the same for every dolphin. In that case, it would not be very useful for identification purposes. If the whistle were *muted* (B), it would be quiet. Again, this might not be useful. If the whistle were *superfluous* (C), it would be extra, or unnecessary. However, the sentence tells you that the whistles are necessary—for identification purposes. You are left with (D): the whistles are *distinctive,* meaning that each one is different, which makes them indeed useful for identification purposes. Notice that *distinctive* is similar in meaning to the word *unique* mentioned above.

Test-Taking Tips for Sentence Completions

1. **Use sentence structure** to determine the part of speech missing.
2. **Use context clues** to brainstorm a word that makes sense in place of the blank.
3. **Compare** your word to the answer choices and pick the choice that fits best.

TWO-STEP SENTENCE COMPLETIONS

Most sentence completions will have a single blank. A few will have two blanks. You use the same process to solve a two-step sentence completion that you use to solve a one-step sentence completion. The difference is that in a two-step sentence completion, some of the answer choices may work for one blank but not for the other, so you need to make sure that you choose the answer that works for both. Here is an example:

> Tornadoes are most _____ to occur during the latter half of the day in the spring and fall, when the air is _____ stable.
> A. often . . . not
> B. unlikely . . . thinly
> C. apt . . . least
> D. never . . . completely

The first word in each choice is to fill in the first blank in the sentence; the second word is to fill in the second blank.

In this case, using structural clues tells you that both words will be adverbs, and indeed all of the choices are adverbs. Using structural clues also tells you that the first word is something that can be modified by the word *most.* That eliminates (D); you would never say "most never." Although you would say "most often" in some contexts, you would not say "most often to occur," which is ungrammatical in English. You can eliminate (A) as a choice. That leaves (B) and (C). In both cases, the first word makes sense in context. Tornadoes might be "most unlikely" to occur (B), or they might be "most apt" to occur (C). It is the second half of the sentence that will tell you which word pair works better. The air would not be "thinly stable," but it might be "least stable." The best choice is (C).

ANALOGIES

An **analogy** is a relationship between or among words or concepts. When you take a test of analogies, you are looking for parallel relationships among four words or phrases, often called *terms.*

Analogies may be set up like mathematical ratios:

OSTRICH : BIRD :: BLUE WHALE : MAMMAL

You read the analogy above this way: "Ostrich is to bird as blue whale is to mammal." An ostrich is a bird, and a blue whale is a mammal. The relationships are parallel.

On the PCAT, you will not be given all four pieces of the analogy. You will be given three and asked to choose the fourth from a set of four options. PCAT Analogies look like this:

UMBRELLA : RAIN :: PARASOL :
A. hail
B. sun
C. shade
D. snow

To solve the analogy, you select the letter of the choice that fits. Here, you might think: "An umbrella blocks the rain." Now look for a parallel relationship between the third term and the answer choices. A parasol blocks the sun, so the correct answer is (B).

Analogical Thinking

When you first see an analogy, sometimes you may immediately infer how the two pairs correspond. When the connection is not immediately obvious, you need to fill in the blanks between the words in each pair. Filling in the blanks accurately will help you solve the analogy. Take this analogy:

FRANCE : PARIS :: SWITZERLAND : GENEVA

You might think: "Paris is a city in France. Geneva is a city in Switzerland." Since the second term names a city in the first term, and the fourth term names a city in the second term, the analogy works.

Now suppose the analogy looks like this:

FRANCE : PARIS :: SWITZERLAND :
A. Geneva
B. Bern
C. Zurich
D. Gstaad

Suddenly, your "Blank is a city in blank" correspondence does not work. All four of the answer choices name cities in Switzerland. You need to dig deeper to fill in the blanks. What special relationship does Paris have to France? Think: "Paris is the capital city of France. Bern is the capital city of Switzerland." Now you can choose (B) and have a valid analogy.

Try filling in the blanks between each pair of words below. In each case, you may find that there are several ways to do it, but one is the most likely and therefore the most logical.

1. CAR : AUDI   (Example: An Audi is one kind of car.)
2. BANANA : PEEL
3. MERLIN : WIZARD
4. CANADA : NORTH AMERICA
5. REVEAL : CONCEAL
6. WHISKER : CAT
7. POTATO : EYE
8. MEASLES : RASH
9. FORTUNATE : LUCKY
10. KANSAS : TOPEKA
11. ARCH : FOOT
12. SALAMANDER : AMPHIBIAN
13. CZAR : RULER
14. BUCK : DOE
15. CITRUS : LEMON
16. PLUMBER : SNAKE
17. SALT : WHITE
18. EDISON : PHONOGRAPH
19. KILO- : THOUSAND
20. FOUGHT : FIGHT

STAY PARALLEL

The logic of an analogy has to do with its parallelism. You may see answer choices on the PCAT that are stuck in expressly to fool you. They might have a connection with one part of the analogy but not with the others. For the analogy to be valid, all four parts must connect.

Try this analogy:

ATTORNEY : CLIENT :: GUIDANCE COUNSELOR :
A. school
B. privilege
C. student
D. customer

Here, the distractors, or incorrect answer choices, are all designed to throw you off. A *guidance counselor* does work in a *school* (A). *Attorney-client privilege* is a matter of law (B). A *client* is synonymous with a *customer* (D).

To get the right answer, you need to recall the original connection. Fill in the blanks. Think: "An attorney gives advice to a client. A guidance counselor gives advice to a student." The only answer that maintains the logic of the analogy is (C).

MATCH PARTS OF SPEECH

The parallelism on the PCAT is even more rigid than that. The first term will always be the same part of speech as the third term. The second term will always be the same part of speech as the fourth term. Take this analogy:

LIAR : DECEITFUL :: SAGE : WISE

A liar is deceitful, and a sage is wise. Terms one and three are nouns. Terms two and four are adjectives.

What you would never see is this:

FLEW : SOARED :: CRASHED : COLLISION

Here, the first three terms are clearly verbs in the past tense, but the fourth is a noun.

MAINTAIN ORDER

Remember that there is only one kind of relationship in analogies on the PCAT: Term one is to term two as term three is to term four.

LARK : SING :: FROG : CROAK

The PCAT will never reverse a relationship. In other words, you will never see term one is to term two as term four is to term three. That does not mean that the testmaker won't throw in some distractors to fool you, as in this example:

TROUT : FISH :: DUCK :
A. mallard
B. swan
C. swim
D. bird

If you were not thinking, you might fill in the blanks this way: "A *trout* is a kind of *fish*. A *mallard* is a kind of *duck*. The answer is (A)." Wrong! Term one is to term two as term three is to term four, not as term four is to term three. The right way to fill in the blanks is this: "A *trout* is a kind of *fish*. A *duck* is a kind of *bird*. The answer is (D)."

Types of Analogies

There are as many possible relationships between words and concepts as there are words and concepts. However, the PCAT tests only a select few.

SYNONYMS

The first and second terms are synonyms, as are the third and fourth terms. For example:

RHYTHM : BEAT :: RHYME : VERSE

Rhythm means about the same as *beat*. *Rhyme* means about the same as *verse*.

ANTONYMS

The first and second terms are antonyms, as are the third and fourth terms. For example:

HUNGRY : REPLETE :: SLEEPY : ALERT

Hungry means the opposite of *replete*. *Sleepy* means the opposite of *alert*.

DEGREE

Degree analogies are much like synonym analogies. However, in a degree analogy, one word in each pair is greater in some way than the other:

HUNGRY : RAVENOUS :: HAPPY : ECSTATIC

To be *ravenous* is to be very, very *hungry*. To be *ecstatic* is to be very, very *happy*.

CATEGORY

In this kind of analogy, one word in each pair is the category into which the other word falls, as here:

DOCTOR : SURGEON :: FISH : STURGEON

A *surgeon* is one kind of *doctor*. A *sturgeon* is one kind of *fish*.

PART/WHOLE

In a part/whole analogy, one word in each pair may be part of the other:

GENESIS : OLD TESTAMENT :: MATTHEW : NEW TESTAMENT

The Book of *Genesis* is part of the *Old Testament*. The Book of *Matthew* is part of the *New Testament*.

CHARACTERISTIC

There are various sorts of characteristic analogies. One word in each pair may be a description of the other, as here:

MOURNER : SORROWFUL :: SCOUNDREL : WICKED

A *mourner* may be described as *sorrowful*. A *scoundrel* may be described as *wicked*.

One word in each pair may be either a feature of the other or a feature that the other lacks:

MOURNER : JOY :: SCOUNDREL : CONSCIENCE

A *mourner* lacks *joy*. A *scoundrel* lacks a *conscience*.

One word in each pair may name the location of the other:

MOURNER : CEMETERY :: SCOUNDREL : REFORMATORY

A *mourner* might be found in a *cemetery*. A *scoundrel* might be found in a *reformatory*.

Finally, one word in each pair might name the material from which the other is made. This kind of analogy is similar to a part/whole analogy:

BEET : BORSCHT :: TOMATO : SALSA

Borscht is a Russian soup made of *beets*. *Salsa* is a Spanish sauce usually made of *tomatoes*.

OBJECT/ACTION

This final type of relationship involves an object or agent that causes or uses another. This relationship may involve invention or creation, as here:

PASCAL : ADDING MACHINE :: NEWTON : TELESCOPE

Blaise *Pascal* invented an *adding machine*. Isaac *Newton* invented a *telescope*.

The relationship may involve cause and effect:

VICTOR : DEFEAT :: INVADER : INCURSION

A *victor* causes the loser's *defeat*. An *invader* causes an *incursion*.

Sometimes, one word in the pair is a tool used by the other:

FENCER : FOIL :: SKIER : POLE

A *fencer* uses a *foil* to fence. A *skier* uses a *pole* to ski.

Often, one word has to do with the function of the other. This may be posed in the form of a measurement unit and whatever it measures:

CENTIMETER : LENGTH :: CENTILITER : CAPACITY

A *centimeter* measures *length*. A *centiliter* measures *capacity*.

VOCABULARY AND VERBAL ABILITY

An extensive vocabulary clearly gives you an advantage in answering Sentence Completion and Analogy questions. There is no easy way to expand your vocabulary except by reading widely and internalizing new words. However, studying this chart of common English-language roots and affixes will help you gain an understanding of the underpinnings of English vocabulary. Knowing roots and affixes can help you deduce the probable meanings of unfamiliar words.

Prefix	Meaning	Examples
a-, ac-, ad-, af-, ag-, al-, an-, ap-, as-, at-	to, toward, in addition to, according to	ahead, accompany, adhere, affix, aggravate, alarm, announce, appall, assent, attempt
a-, an-	without	amoral, analgesic
ab-, abs-	away from	abdicate, absence
ante-	before	antebellum, anterior
anti-	against	antiwar, antipathy
auto-	self	automobile, autobiography
bi-	two	biannual, bicycle
circum-	around	circumnavigate, circumvent
co-, cog-, col-, com-, con-, cor-	with, together, mutually	coherent, cognizant, collapse, companion, concur, correspond
contra-	against, opposite	contradict, contravene
de-	to do the opposite of	decriminalize, degenerate
dis-	not, opposite of	disagree, disfavor
e-, ex-	out of, away from	egress, extension
em-, en-	to put into, to cause to be	embody, endear
epi-	upon, over	epidermis, epitaph
extra-	outside, beyond	extracurricular, extraordinary
il-, im-, in-, ir-	not	illicit, impossible, incorrect, irresponsible
inter-	between, among	intercom, international

Prefix	Meaning	Examples
intro-	into	introduce, introvert
mal-	bad	maladjusted, malformed
mis-	wrong	misnomer, misunderstood
mono-	one	monotone, monogamy
multi-	many	multifaceted, multimillions
non-	no, not	nonentity, nonsensical
ob-, oc-, of-, op-	toward, against	object, occlude, offend, opposite
over-	above, more than	overachieve, overcharge
para-	beside	paradigm, paragraph
per-	through, throughout	perambulate
peri-	around, about	peripatetic, periodic
post-	after	postdate, posthumous
pre-	before	prediction, preexist
pro-	for, supporting	procreate, promotion
re-	back, again	recall, recapture
retro-	backward	retrofit, retrospective
semi-	half	semicircle, semiconscious
sub-, suc-, suf-, sup-, sus-	below, under	subarctic, succumb, suffer, suppress, suspend
super-	over, above	superfluous, superscript
sur-	over, above	surpass, surrealism
sym-, syn-	together	sympathetic, synthesize
trans-	across	transatlantic, transmission
tri-	three	tricycle, trilogy
un-	not, opposite of	unlikely, unravel
uni-	one	uniform, unisex
Suffix	**Function and Meaning**	**Examples**
-able, -ible	adjective-forming; capable of, worthy of	laudable, flexible
-acy, -cy	noun-forming; state, quality	literacy, bankruptcy

Suffix	Function and Meaning	Examples
-age	noun-forming; action	breakage, blockage
-al	adjective-forming; state, quality	communal, supplemental
-an, -ian	noun-forming; one who	artisan, librarian
-ance, -ence	noun-forming; action, state, quality	performance, adherence
-ancy, -ency	noun-forming; state, quality	buoyancy, fluency
-ant, -ent	noun-forming; one who	deodorant, antecedent
-ant, -ent, -ient	adjective forming; indicating	compliant, dependent, lenient
-ar, -ary	adjective-forming; related to	solar, imaginary
-ate	verb-forming; cause to be	percolate, graduate
-ation	noun-forming; action	hibernation, strangulation
-dom	noun-forming; place, condition	kingdom, freedom
-en	adjective-forming; made of	flaxen, wooden
-en	verb-forming; cause to be	cheapen, dampen
-er, -or	noun-forming; one who	painter, sailor
-fold	adverb-forming; divided or multiplied by	threefold, hundredfold
-ful	adjective-forming; full of	joyful, playful
-ful	noun-forming; amount	cupful, bucketful
-fy, -ify	verb-forming; cause to be	liquefy, justify
-ia	noun-forming; disease	anemia, anorexia
-iatry	noun-forming; medical treatment	psychiatry, podiatry
-ic	adjective-forming; having the qualities of	futuristic, academic
-ician	noun-forming; one who	physician, mortician
-ics	noun-forming; science of	genetics, physics
-ion	noun-forming; action	completion, dilution
-ish	adjective-forming; having the quality of	foolish, boyish

Suffix	Function and Meaning	Examples
-ism	noun-forming; doctrine	pacifism, jingoism
-ist	noun-forming; person who	jurist, polemicist
-ity, -ty	noun-forming; state, quality	reality, cruelty
-ive, -ative, -itive	adjective-forming; having the quality of	supportive, talkative, definitive
-ize	verb-forming; cause to be	demonize, dramatize
-less	without	careless, hopeless
-ly	adverb-forming; in the manner of	loudly, suddenly
-ment	noun-forming; action	argument, statement
-ness	noun-forming; state, quality	kindness, abruptness
-ous, -eous, -ose, -ious	adjective-forming; having the quality of	porous, gaseous, jocose, bilious
-ship	noun-forming; condition	scholarship, friendship
-ure	noun-forming; action, condition	erasure, portraiture
-ward	adverb-forming; in the direction of	forward, windward
-wise	adverb-forming; in the manner of	otherwise, clockwise
-y	adjective-forming; having the quality of	chilly, crazy
-y	noun-forming; state, condition	jealousy, custody

Root	Meaning	Examples
ami, amo	to love	amiable, amorous
aud, audit, aur	to hear	audible, auditory, aural
bene, ben	good	benevolent, benign
bio	life	biography, biology
biblio	book	bibliography, bibliophile
brev	short	abbreviate, brevity
chron	time	chronology, synchronize
cogn, gnos	to know	cognitive, agnostic

Root	Meaning	Examples
corp	body	corpulent, corporation
cred	to believe	credible, incredulous
dict	to say	indictment, dictation
doc, doct	to teach	docile, indoctrinate
duc, duct	to lead	conducive, induction
fac, fact	to make, to do	efface, factory
fid	belief	confide, fidelity
fluct, flux	to flow	fluctuation, influx
form	shape	format, cuneiform
fract, frag	to break	infraction, fragment
gen	to produce	generation, congenital
geo	earth	geographer, geology
grad, gress	to step, to move	graduate, ingress
graph	to write	photograph, graphics
ject	to throw	project, rejection
junct	to join	conjunction, adjunct
lect	to choose, to gather	select, collection
loc	place	locale, locomotion
log	to say	logical, analog
luc, lum, lust	light	lucid, luminous, illustrate
man	to make, to do	manager, manufacture
mem	to recall	remember, memorable
mit, miss	to send	remit, admission
mob, mov, mot	to move	mobile, remove, motion
nasc, nat	to be born	nascent, prenatal
nom, nym	name	nominal, homonym
nov	new	renovate, novice
oper	to work	operate, inoperable
path	feeling	empathy, sympathetic
ped, pod	foot	pedal, podiatrist
pel, puls	to push	repel, impulse

Root	Meaning	Examples
pend	to hang	pendant, impending
phil	love	philosophy, necrophilia
phon	sound	phonograph, telephone
pict	to paint	picture, depict
port	to carry	export, portage
psych	mind	psychology, psychic
quer, quest	to ask	query, request
rupt	to break	interrupt, rupture
scrib, scrip	to write	inscribe, script
sent, sens	to feel	sentient, sensation
sequ	to follow	sequence, consequential
soci	companion	society, associate
sol	alone	solo, solitude
solv, solu, solut	to loosen, to release	solve, soluble, solution
spec, spect	to look	special, inspection
spir	to breathe	spirit, respiration
stab, stat	to stand	stability, statue
tact	to touch	tactile, contact
tele	far	telescope, teleport
tend, tens	to stretch	extend, tensile
tain, tent	to hold	maintain, contents
term	end	terminal, exterminate
terr	earth	territory, subterranean
therm	heat	thermal, thermometer
tors, tort	to twist	torsion, contort
tract	to pull	contract, tractable
uni	one	universe, unicycle
vac	empty	vacuous, evacuate
ven, vent	to come	convene, venture
ver	true	verify, verisimilitude
verb	word	verbal, adverbial

Root	Meaning	Examples
vers, vert	to turn	reverse, convert
vid, vis	to see	video, invisible
vit, viv	to live	vital, convivial
voc, voke	to call	vocal, invoke
volv, volt, vol	to roll	volvox, revolt, convoluted

ON YOUR OWN

Try your hand at these Sentence Completions and Analogies.

1. Bone tumors once had a _____ prognosis because, unlike many other tumors, they tend to shed cancerous cells into the blood.
   - A. synthetic
   - B. survivable
   - C. surgical
   - D. dismal

2. Because a squid's tentacle has no joints, it has the _____ to bend at any point and in any _____.
   - A. capacity . . . direction
   - B. ability . . . area
   - C. tendency . . . form
   - D. will . . . trajectory

3. INVASION : MOAT :: INFECTION :
   - A. bacillus
   - B. injury
   - C. bandage
   - D. seepage

4. TRY : STRUGGLE :: SUCCEED :
   - A. fight
   - B. fail
   - C. thrive
   - D. manage

5. ORANGE : YELLOW :: PURPLE :
   - A. green
   - B. blue
   - C. lavender
   - D. royal

Answers and Explanations

1. **Answer (D)**
Contextually, the answers that make the most sense are (B) and (D). A closer look at the structure and context of the sentence shows that bone tumors shed cancerous cells into the blood, which would tend toward a *dismal* prognosis, not a *survivable* one.

2. Answer (A)

In this two-step sentence completion, the first word in answer choices (A), (B), and (C) fits contextually, but only *direction* makes sense in the second part of the sentence.

3. Answer (C)

A *moat* can prevent an *invasion*, and a *bandage* can prevent an *infection*. This is an example of an Object/Action analogy.

4. Answer (C)

This is a Degree analogy. To *struggle* is to *try* very hard. To *thrive* is to *succeed* very well.

5. Answer (B)

In this Part/Whole analogy, *yellow* is a component of the color *orange*, and *blue* is a component of the color *purple*.

Verbal Ability

You will have 30 minutes to complete 48 questions in the Verbal Ability section of the test. These questions test general knowledge, vocabulary, and your facility with the English language.

Sentence Completions (40%)   Solve Sentence Completions by analyzing the structure and context of the sentence and choosing the word or words from the four answer choices that make the most sense structurally and contextually.

Analogies (60%)   In Analogies, you are given three parts of the analogy and asked to find the fourth. The relationship of the fourth term to the third is equivalent to the relationship between the second term and the first:

   STONE : WALL :: TILE : ROOF

A *stone* (first term) is part of a *wall* (second term) as a *tile* (third term) is part of a *roof* (fourth term).

Types of analogies include the following: Synonyms, Antonyms, Degree, Category, Part/Whole, Characteristic, and Object/Action.

A strong mastery of English vocabulary helps you answer Sentence Completion and Analogy questions correctly. You can apply your knowledge of common roots and affixes to help identify the meanings of unfamiliar words.

Reading Comprehension

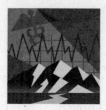

WHAT READING COMPREHENSION TESTS

In contrast to the sections on Chemistry or Biology, the Reading Comprehension section of the PCAT does not test specific knowledge. Instead, it assesses your ability to comprehend, analyze, and evaluate information from an unfamiliar written text. Its format will be familiar to anyone who has attended school in the United States. Most reading comprehension tests look just like it.

The PCAT Reading Comprehension section consists of six passages of about 300 to 400 words, each of which is followed by a set of multiple-choice questions. The passages are nonfiction and are usually on areas of the natural or physical sciences that are not routinely tested elsewhere in the exam. The expectation is that you will not be familiar with the content of a given passage, or that if you are familiar with it, you will not be an expert.

For this reason, it is not possible to *study* for the Reading Comprehension section of the PCAT. That being said, however, there are some things you may do to *prepare* for it.

HOW READING COMPREHENSION IS SCORED

As with all the multiple-choice sections of the PCAT, your score is scaled on a scale ranging from 200 to 600, where 400 is the mean.

PREPARING FOR READING COMPREHENSION

By this stage in your educational career, you should have a pretty good sense of your test-taking skills. If you have achieved solid scores on reading comprehension tests in the past, the PCAT Reading Comprehension section should be no problem at all. If your comprehension skills are subpar, if you freeze when faced with difficult reading passages, if you read very slowly, or if English is not your first language, you should take the time to work through this section of the book.

Read

The best way to learn to read better is to read more. If you read only materials in your chosen discipline, you are limiting yourself in a way that may show up on your PCAT score. Reading broadly in subject areas that do not, at first glance, hold much appeal for you will train you to focus your attention on what you are reading. Pick up a journal in a field you do not know. Read an article. Summarize the key ideas. Consider the author's purpose. Decide whether the author's argument makes sense to you. Think about where the author might go next with his or her argument. Think about the author's tone.

All of this sounds like a chore, but it is the key to making yourself read actively. An active reader interacts with a text rather than bouncing off it. Success on the PCAT's Reading Comprehension section requires active reading.

You can use any of the strategies below to focus your attention on your reading. You may use many of them already, quite automatically. Others may be just what you need to shift your reading comprehension into high gear.

ACTIVE READING STRATEGIES

➤ **Monitor your understanding.** When faced with a difficult text, it is all too easy to zone out and skip through challenging passages. You will not have that luxury when the text you are reading is only 350 words long, and it is followed by eight questions that require your understanding. Pay attention to how you are feeling about a text. Are you getting the author's main points? Is there something that makes little or no sense? Are there words that you do not know? Figuring out what makes a passage hard for you is the first step toward correcting the problem. Once you figure it out, you can use one of the following strategies to improve your connection to the text.

➤ **Predict.** Your ability to make predictions is surprisingly important to your ability to read well. If a passage is well organized, you should be able to read the introductory paragraph and have a pretty good sense of where the author is going with the text. Practice this one starting with newspaper articles, where the main ideas are supposed to appear in the first paragraph. Move on to more difficult reading. See whether your expectation of a text holds up through the reading of the text. Making predictions about what you are about to read is an immediate way to engage with the text and to keep you engaged throughout your reading.

➤ **Ask questions.** Keep a running dialogue with yourself as you read. You do not have to stop reading; just pause to consider, "What does this mean? Why did the author use this word? Where is he or she going with this argument? Why is this important?" This will become second nature after a while. When you become acclimated to asking yourself questions as you read a test passage, you may discover that some of the questions you asked appear in different forms on the test itself.

➤ **Summarize.** You do this when you take notes in class or when you prepare an outline as you study for an exam. Try doing it as you read unfamiliar materials, but do it in your head. At the end of a particularly dense paragraph, try to reduce the author's verbiage to a single, cogent sentence that states the main idea. At the end of a longer passage, see whether you can restate the theme or message in a phrase or two.

➤ **Connect.** Every piece of writing is a communication between the author and the reader. You connect to a text first by bringing your prior knowledge to that text and last by applying what you learn from the text to some area of your life. Even if you know nothing at all about architecture or archaeology, your lifetime of experience in the world carries a lot of weight as you read an article about those topics. Connecting to a text can lead to "Aha!" moments as you say to yourself, "I knew that!" or even "I never knew that!" If you are barreling through a text passively, you will not give yourself time to connect. You might as well tape the passage and play it under your pillow as you sleep.

Pace Yourself

The Reading Comprehension section is timed. If you are a slow reader, you are at a decided disadvantage. You will have 50 minutes to read six passages and answer 48 questions. That gives you about eight minutes for each question set. It would be a shame to lose points because you failed to complete a passage or two.

You do not need to speed-read to perform well on the Reading Comprehension section, but you might benefit from some pointers that speed readers use.

SPEED-READING STRATEGIES

➤ **Avoid subvocalizing.** It is unlikely that you move your lips while you read, but you may find yourself "saying" the text in your head. This slows you down significantly, because you are slowing down to speech speed instead of revving up to reading speed. You do not need to "say" the words; the connection between your eyes and your brain is perfectly able to bypass that step.

➤ **Do not regress.** If you do not understand something, you may run your eyes back and forth and back and forth over it. Speed readers know this as "regression," and it is a big drag on reading speed. It is better to read once all the way through and then reread a section that caused you confusion.

➤ **Bundle ideas.** Read phrases rather than words. Remember, you are being tested on overall meaning, which is not derived from single words but rather from phrases, sentences, and paragraphs. If you read word by word, your eye stops constantly, and that slows you down. Read bundles of meaning, and your eyes will flow over the page, improving both reading speed and comprehension.

Preview

When it comes to taking tests, knowing what to expect is half the battle. The PCAT's Reading Comprehension section assesses a variety of reading skills, from the most basic comprehension skills to the higher-level analysis and evaluation skills. Here is a breakdown of skills you should expect to see tested.

THREE KINDS OF QUESTIONS

➤ **Comprehension.** These questions look at the author's main idea and support for his or her hypothesis. Expect questions on Finding the Main Idea, Locating Supporting Details or Evidence, and Interpreting Vocabulary. Comprehension questions make up approximately 30 percent of the Reading Comprehension section of the PCAT.

SAMPLE QUESTION STEMS

The main point of the passage is . . .
The central thesis of the passage is . . .
*Which would be the **best** title for . . .*
According to the passage . . .
In the context of the second paragraph, X means . . .

Interpreting Vocabulary

On the PCAT, words that will be assessed in Interpreting Vocabulary questions are underlined in the passage. You will need to use the context of the sentence and paragraph to determine which of the four answer choices is the best definition of the underlined word. Often, all four choices will be multiple meanings of the word; but always, only one of those multiple meanings will fit the context used in the passage. You should try to replace the underlined word with each answer choice to find the one that works best in context.

➤ **Analysis.** These questions deal with the purpose and structure of the passage. Expect questions on Making Predictions, Drawing Conclusions, Recognizing or Analyzing Organization, and Identifying Author's Purpose. Analysis questions make up approximately 40 percent of the Reading Comprehension section of the PCAT.

SAMPLE QUESTION STEMS

Based on the passage, you can tell that . . .
The passage implies that . . .
The passage suggests that . . .
The ideas in the first and second paragraphs relate by . . .
The passage is organized in . . .
The author's purpose in the third paragraph is . . .
The author includes X to show . . .

Analyzing Organization

A paragraph or passage may be organized in a number of different ways. Some modes of organization support an author's purpose better than others. In the PCAT, paragraphs are numbered, and those numbers are often referred to in questions to make it easier for you to scan or skim the passage and find out what you need to know. Some organizational modes frequently used in nonfiction passages include time order or sequence; spatial order; order of importance; and organization by causes and effects, opinion and reasons, thesis statement and examples, or comparisons and contrasts.

➤ **Evaluation.** These questions deal with your understanding of the author's assumptions and viewpoints. Expect questions on Analyzing an Argument, Judging Credibility, Assessing Evidence, Distinguishing Between Fact and Opinion, and Evaluating Tone. Evaluation questions make up approximately 30 percent of the Reading Comprehension section of the PCAT.

SAMPLE QUESTION STEMS

*Which of the following statements provides the **least** support . . .*
Which of the following assertions does the author support . . .
The author's claim that X is supported by . . .
*Which adds the **most** credibility to the information . . .*
Which statement expresses a personal opinion about . . .
*The **tone** of the passage suggests that . . .*
What evidence could the author have added to show . . .

Since the format of the test is a familiar one, you may not need to preview the format itself. However, you may benefit from these tips on taking reading comprehension tests.

Evaluating Tone

The tone of a passage is the expression of the author's feelings about the topic. You can discern tone by looking broadly at an author's purpose and specifically at the author's word choice. For example, suppose the shared purpose of two different articles is to reveal the effects of global warming on the Arctic. Through the use of very technical terms, one article may end up with a didactic tone. Through the use of loaded words such as *tragic* or *appalling*, the other article may end up with a pessimistic tone. Most words that describe people's emotional states may be used to describe a passage's tone; some examples are *humorous, flippant, solemn, critical, angry,* and *cynical.*

Test-Taking Tips for Reading Comprehension

1. **Preview** the passage. Read the first paragraph. Skim the passage.
2. **Skim** the question stems (the part of each question that does not include the answer choices.) This will give you a quick idea of what to look for as you read.
3. **Read** the passage, using your active reading strategies.
4. **Answer** the questions. If a question stumps you, skip ahead and come back to it at the end of the question set.

ON YOUR OWN

It is certainly true that the more you practice reading comprehension, the better you are likely to perform on the PCAT. Here is a practice passage followed by a question set and explanatory answers. Follow along and see how well your comprehension jibes with the answers given. Try to use your active reading strategies as you read the passage. Can you make it through the question set in about eight minutes?

Sample Passage

1   For years, anecdotal evidence from around the world indicated that amphibians were under siege, especially in the Caribbean. Finally, proof of this hypothesis is available, thanks to the concerted, Internet-based effort of scientists involved with the Global Amphibian Assessment.

2   Amphibians have a unique vulnerability to environmental changes thanks to their permeable skin and their need of specific habitats to allow their metamorphosis from larva to adult. Studies indicate that they are at risk due to global climate change, reduction in the ozone layer leading to an increased exposure to

ultraviolet rays, interference with migratory pathways, drainage of wetlands, pollution by pesticides, erosion and sedimentation, and exposure to unknown pathogens thanks to the introduction of nonnative species. In other words, human progress is responsible for the losses this population is suffering.

3 Scientists have long considered amphibians a barometer of environmental health. In areas where amphibians are declining precipitously, environmental degradation is thought to be a major cause. Amphibians are not adaptable. They must have clean water in which to lay their eggs. They must have clean air to breathe after they grow to adulthood. Their "double life" as aquatic and land-dwelling animals means that they are at risk of a double dose of pollutants and other hazards.

4 The Global Amphibian Assessment concluded that nearly one-third of the world's amphibian species are under immediate threat of extinction. Nearly half of all species are declining in population. The largest numbers of threatened species are in Colombia, Mexico, and Ecuador, but the highest percentages of threatened species are in the Caribbean. In Haiti, for example, nine out of ten species of amphibians are threatened. In Jamaica, it is eight out of ten, and in Puerto Rico, seven out of ten.

5 Certainly, this is a disaster for amphibians, but scientists rush to point out that it may be equally a disaster for the rest of us on Earth. Even recent pandemics among amphibians may be caused by global changes. True, amphibians are ultrasensitive to such changes, but can reptiles, fish, birds, and mammals be far behind?

1. The main point of the passage is that
   A. The extinction of amphibians is due to global warming.
   B. Amphibians really are a barometer of environmental health.
   C. Only equatorial amphibians are currently under siege.
   D. Amphibians' "double life" on land and in water may end up saving them.

2. The passage implies that the Global Amphibian Assessment has done science a favor by
   A. setting forth a hypothesis that connects the environment to species decline
   B. eliminating the need to study the connection between extinction and environment
   C. refuting a contention that had existed purely through anecdotal evidence
   D. collecting data to prove something that was previously just a hypothesis

3. The author's point in the first paragraph that amphibians are especially at risk in the Caribbean is **best** supported by evidence presented in which paragraph?
   A. 2   C. 4
   B. 3   D. 5

4. The author's purpose in the third paragraph is to
   A. provide background on the Assessment study
   B. explain why amphibians are especially vulnerable
   C. list types of amphibians that are most at risk
   D. present examples of dangers from around the world

5. What evidence could the author have included that would **best** support the main idea?
   A. statistics involving numbers of frog species in Haiti
   B. personal observations about the hazards of pollution
   C. names of people involved in the Assessment study
   D. comparisons between amphibians and reptiles

Answers and Explanations

1. Answer: B

This **Comprehension** question asks you to **Find the Main Idea**. You will find questions of this sort frequently on the PCAT Reading Comprehension Test, and they often appear first in a question set. To find the main idea, you need to read actively and summarize as you go. There are no titles on PCAT passages to give away the central thesis; it is up to you as a reader to derive it from the text.

Review the answer choices. The author does indicate that (A) is a possibility. Just because this detail is included does not make it the central thesis. Although the major threat is to equatorial amphibians (C), it is not true that "only" those species are in danger, nor is that the main idea. There is no support for (D). The main idea, instead, revolves around (B). The new study indicates that previous anecdotal evidence was correct: Amphibians really *are* a barometer of environmental health.

2. Answer: D

This **Analysis** question requires you to **Draw Conclusions** about an assertion that is not directly stated. The answer may be inferred from the opening paragraph, which thanks the scientists involved for offering "proof of this hypothesis" through their "concerted, Internet-based efforts." The Assessment did not set forth the hypothesis (A); that had already been done via anecdotal evidence. They certainly did not eliminate the need for more study (B); nor did they refute the contention (C). They proved it (D).

3. Answer: C

This is an **Evaluation** question that asks you to **Assess Evidence**. To answer it correctly, you must skim the paragraphs mentioned to see which one best supports the contention that amphibians are especially at risk in the Caribbean. Paragraphs 2, 3, and 5 do not mention the Caribbean at all. Paragraph 4 includes the information "the highest percentages of threatened species are in the Caribbean," followed by three examples: "In Haiti, for example, nine out of ten species of amphibians are threatened. In Jamaica, it is eight out of ten, and in Puerto Rico, seven out of ten." Because the evidence appears in paragraph 4, the best answer is (C).

4. Answer: B

This **Analysis** question has you **Identify Author's Purpose**—not in the passage as a whole, but in a single paragraph of the passage. Return to the third paragraph and think about why the author included it. Compare your thoughts to the four answer choices. The author is not providing background on the Assessment study (A). This particular paragraph does not contain a list of amphibians that are most at risk (C). Nor does it give examples of dangers (D); instead, it explains why certain environmental factors (clean water, clean air) are especially important for amphibians. The point of the paragraph is to indicate what qualities amphibians have that put them at risk, so (B) is the best answer.

5. Answer: A

This **Evaluation** question asks you to **Assess Evidence** in a different way. You are given hypothetical additions to the passage and asked to determine which one would best support the central thesis. The passage has to do with amphibians and how susceptible they are to environmental degradation. Although (B) has to do with pollution, personal anecdotes would not tell a reader much about the effect on amphibians. The names of participants in the study (C) might interest some readers, but again, it would not support the main idea. Bringing reptiles into the mix (D) would just confuse the issue. The best answer is (A); statistics on numbers of species in Haiti, where amphibians are apparently under siege, might provide strong evidence for the author's contentions.

Reading Comprehension

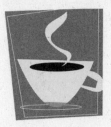

Passages in the Reading Comprehension section consist of 300 to 400 words. They are nonfiction passages on a scientific theme. There are six passages with 48 multiple-choice questions to be read and completed in 50 minutes.

You cannot **study** for Reading Comprehension, but you can **prepare**. Here are some suggestions you can use to prepare:

➤ **Read,** using Active Reading Strategies.
➤ **Pace yourself**, using Speed-Reading Strategies.
➤ **Preview** the test.

Questions in the Reading Comprehension section test the following skills:

➤ **Comprehension** (30%), including Finding the Main Idea, Locating Supporting Details or Evidence, and Interpreting Vocabulary
➤ **Analysis** (40%), including Making Predictions, Drawing Conclusions, Recognizing or Analyzing Organization, and Identifying Author's Purpose
➤ **Evaluation** (30%), including Analyzing an Argument, Judging Credibility, Assessing Evidence, Distinguishing Between Fact and Opinion, and Evaluating Tone

PART IV

REVIEWING PCAT BIOLOGY

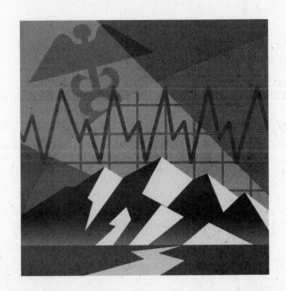

General Biology

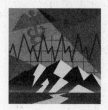

PART I. CLASSIFICATION AND CELL STRUCTURE

With so much diversity among living organisms, it can be difficult to classify them into groups based on appearance alone. Characteristics of the cells that compose the organism are relied heavily upon when classifying organisms. There are three domains to which all living organisms can be classified: **Bacteria**, **Archaea**, and **Eukarya**.

CLASSIFICATION OF LIVING ORGANISMS

Classification is based on many factors but three major criteria exist: 1) the number of cells that compose the organism, 2) the structure of the cells, and 3) how the organism obtains nutrients. A summary of the typical characteristics of each domain can be seen in Table 7.1:

Table 7.1: Characteristics of Each Domain			
	Bacteria	**Archaea**	**Eukarya**
Number of cells	unicellular	unicellular	variable
Complexity of cells	prokaryotic	prokaryotic	eukaryotic
Method of obtaining nutrients	absorbed	absorbed	variable

Within the domain Eukarya, there is a tremendous amount of diversity. This domain is subdivided into four kingdoms: Animalia, Plantae, Fungi, and Protista. The characteristics of each kingdom can be seen in Table 7.2. While there is a great deal of diversity within this group, there are also many similarities, particularly in cell structure, amongst members of this group.

Table 7.2: Characteristics of the Kingdoms of Eukarya				
	Plantae	**Animalia**	**Protista**	**Fungi**
Number of cells	multicellular	multicellular	usually unicellular	variable
Method of obtaining food	made through photosynthesis	ingested	usually absorbed	absorbed
Example organisms	grass, trees, flowering plants	humans, starfish, birds, and fish	algae, protozoa, slime molds	yeasts, mushrooms, and molds

PROKARYOTIC AND EUKARYOTIC CELLS

The cell is the basic unit of life. As a general rule, all cells are small in size in order to maintain a large **surface area to volume ratio**. Having a large surface area relative to a small volume allows cells to perform vital functions at a reasonably fast rate, which is necessary for survival. Cells that are too large have small surface area to volume ratios and have difficulties getting the nutrients that they need and expelling wastes in a timely manner.

The two major categories of cells are **prokaryotic** and **eukaryotic**. All organisms in the domains Bacteria and Archaea are composed of prokaryotic cells while all members of the domain Eukarya are composed of eukaryotic cells. There are some similarities between the two cell types, but there are also some significant differences. Table 7.3 depicts the major structural differences between prokaryotic and eukaryotic cells.

Table 7.3: Major Differences between Eukaryotic and Prokaryotic Cells

Characteristic	Eukaryotic cells	Prokaryotic cells
Cell size	relatively larger	relatively smaller
Presence of organelles	present	absent
Organization of genetic material	linear pieces of DNA organized as chromosomes housed within the nucleus	a single loop of DNA floating in the cytoplasm
Oxygen requirements	generally need oxygen to produce energy during cellular respiration	may not require oxygen to produce energy during cellular respiration

One primary factor that differentiates eukaryotic cells from prokaryotic cells is the presence of **organelles**. Organelles are membrane-bound compartments within the cell that have specialized functions. They help with cellular organization and efficiency by ensuring that specific reactions have specific organelles in which to occur. The structure of a typical eukaryotic cell can be seen in Figure 7.1.

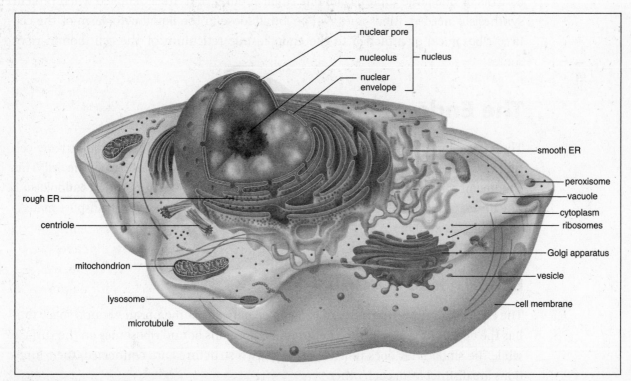

FIGURE 7.1: Animal cell structure. A typical animal cell contains a variety of structures and membrane-bound organelles.

The Cytoplasm

The liquid portion of the cell is the cytoplasm. The organelles and other structures of the cell are suspended within the cytoplasm. The cytoplasm consists of water, nutrients, ions, and wastes, and can be the site of a variety of chemical reactions within the cell.

The Nucleus

All eukaryotic cells contain a membrane-bound **nucleus**. The nucleus houses the genetic material of the cell in the form of chromosomes. The outer boundary of the nucleus is referred to as the nuclear membrane (also termed the nuclear envelope) and it keeps the contents of the nucleus separate from the rest of the cell. The nuclear membrane has pores that allow certain substances to enter and exit the nucleus. Within the nucleus, there is a **nucleolus**. The job of the nucleolus is to make the ribosomal ribonucleic acid (rRNA) needed to produce ribosomes.

Ribosomes

Ribosomes are made from rRNA (produced in the nucleolus) and protein. A ribosome consists of one large subunit and one small subunit that are assembled when protein synthesis is needed. Ribosomes can be found loose in the liquid cytoplasm of the cell (free ribosomes) or attached to the endoplasmic reticulum of the cell (bound ribosomes).

The Endomembrane System

The endomembrane system consists of several organelles within the eukaryotic cell that work together as a unit to synthesize and transport molecules within the cell. This endomembrane system consists of: smooth endoplasmic reticulum, rough endoplasmic reticulum, Golgi complex, lysosomes, peroxisomes, and vesicles that transport materials within the system.

ENDOPLASMIC RETICULUM

The **endoplasmic reticulum** (ER) is a folded network of membrane-bound space that has the appearance of a maze. The rough ER contains bound ribosomes on the surface while the smooth ER does not. While these two structures are connected, their functions are distinct from each other.

In the smooth ER, the primary function is the production of lipids needed by the cell. In certain types of eukaryotic cells (such as the liver), the smooth ER plays a critical role in the production of detoxifying enzymes.

Since the rough ER has bound ribosomes, its function is related to protein synthesis. The ribosomes produce proteins which enter the rough ER. Once inside the rough ER, these proteins are chemically modified and moved to the smooth ER. The combined contents of the smooth ER and the rough ER will now be shipped by vesicles to the Golgi complex for sorting. Vesicles are tiny pieces of membrane that will break off and carry the contents of the ER throughout the endomembrane system.

GOLGI COMPLEX

Vesicles from the ER arrive at the **Golgi complex** (also called the Golgi apparatus) and deliver their contents, which include proteins and lipids. These molecules will be further modified, repackaged, and tagged for their eventual destination. The contents of the Golgi complex leave via vesicles and many of them will be moved to the cell membrane for secretion out of the cell.

LYSOSOMES

Lysosomes are membrane-bound **vacuoles** (large sacs) that contain digestive enzymes used to break down any substances that enter the lysosomes. Cellular structures that are old, damaged, or unnecessary can be degraded in the lysosomes. Further, substances taken into the cell by endocytosis (the process of cells taking in molecules by enclosing them in a vesicle pinched off of the cell membrane) can be transported to the lysosomes for destruction. In order to function properly, the pH of the lysosomes must be acidic. In some cases, cells purposefully rupture their lysosomes in an attempt to commit cellular suicide in a process known as apoptosis.

PEROXISOMES

Peroxisomes are another type of vacuole found within the endomembrane system. They are capable of digesting fatty acids and amino acids. They also degrade toxic hydrogen peroxide, a metabolic waste product, to water and oxygen gas.

Mitochondria

Mitochondria are the organelles responsible for energy production in the cell. They perform aerobic cellular respiration that ultimately creates **adenosine triphosphate** (ATP), which is the preferred source of energy for cells. Since all cells require energy to survive, the process of cellular respiration is a vital one for the cell. Mitochondria have some interesting and unusual features: they are bound by an inner and outer membrane, they contain their own DNA distinct from the nuclear DNA, and they can self-replicate. These unique features have led to the development of **endosymbiotic theory,** which suggests that mitchondria are the evolutionary remnants of bacteria that were engulfed by other cells long ago in evolutionary time.

The Cytoskeleton

The **cytoskeleton** is composed of three types of fibers that exist within the cytoplasm of the cell. These fibers have a variety of functions including structural support, maintenance of cell shape, and cell division. **Microtubules** are one type of hollow fiber, made of the protein tubulin, that are responsible for structural support and the maintenance of cell shape. They also provide tracks that allow for the movement of organelles within the cell. During cell division, microtubules are used to help direct chromosomes through the cell. **Microfilaments** are made of the protein actin; they assist with cellular movement. The final type of fiber found in the cytoskeleton is **intermediate filaments**, the composition of which varies greatly from one cell type to the next. The primary purpose of the intermediate filaments is structural support for the cell.

Structures that Allow for Movement

Certain types of animal cells contain additional structures such as cilia and flagella. **Cilia** are hairlike structures on the surface of some cells that move in synchronized motion. For example, cilia on the surface of cells lining the respiratory tract constantly move in an attempt to catch and remove bacteria and particles that may enter the respiratory tract. Some animal cells such as sperm contain **flagella,** which essentially act as tails to allow for movement.

Cell Structures in Plant Cells

Plant cells are a particular type of eukaryotic cell that generally have all of the structures and organelles described to this point. However, there are a few additional structures that are unique to plant cells. These include a cell wall, chloroplasts, and a central vacuole. The **cell wall** is composed of cellulose (fiber) and serves to protect the cell from its environment and from desiccation. The **chloroplasts** within a plant cell contain the green pigment chlorophyll, which is used in the process of photosynthesis. Chloroplasts are similar to mitochondria in that they have their own DNA and replicate independently. Endosymbiotic theory is also used to explain their existence in plants. Finally, plant cells contain a large **central vacuole** which serves as reserve storage for water, nutrients, and waste products. The central vacuole typically takes up the majority of space within a plant cell.

The cell membrane

The outer boundary of the cell is the **cell membrane** (plasma membrane); its purpose is to form a selectively permeable barrier between the cell and its external environment. The membrane itself is composed of a bilayer of phospholipids containing proteins scattered within the bilayer. **Phospholipids** are unique molecules because they have polar and nonpolar regions. The head of a phospholipid is composed of a glycerol and phosphate group (PO_4) that carries a charge and is **hydrophilic**. The tails of the phospholipid are fatty acids that are not charged and are **hydrophobic**. Phospholipids spontaneously arrange themselves in a bilayer where the heads align themselves towards the inside and outside of the cell where water is located, and the fatty acid tails are sandwiched between the layers. Nonpolar molecules have an easier time crossing the bilayer than other types of molecules.

In addition to the phospholipid bilayer, there are some other substances present in the cell membrane. The **fluid mosaic model** seen in Figure 7.2 shows the basic membrane structure. **Cholesterol** is found embedded within the interior of the membrane; its primary purpose is to regulate the fluidity of the membrane. Proteins are scattered within the bilayer; they may serve multiple purposes such as membrane transport, enzymatic activity, cell adhesion, and communication; they may also serve as receptors for specific substances that may need to cross the membrane. Some proteins and lipids within the cell membrane contain carbohydrates on the exterior surface. These carbohydrates, or glycoproteins and glycolipids, often serve as identifying markers, or antigens, for the cell.

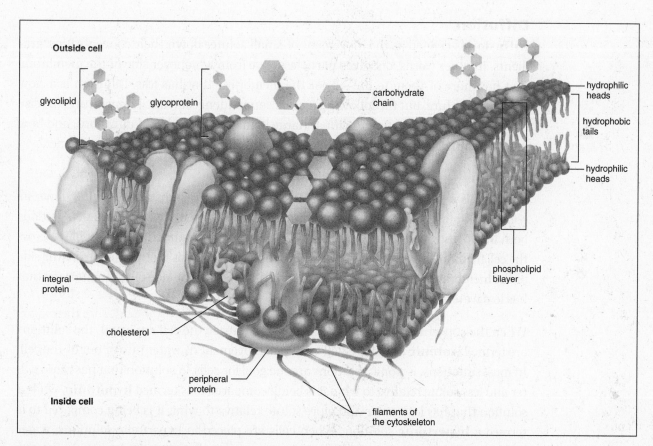

FIGURE 7.2: The fluid-mosaic model. The cell membrane is composed of a phospholipid bilayer in which proteins are embedded. The membrane is anchored to the cell via cytoskeleton fibers.

Movement of Substances across the Cell Membrane

There are a variety of ways that substances can cross the cell membrane. The three main membrane transports are passive transport, active transport, and bulk transport. **Passive transport** occurs spontaneously without energy while **active transport** requires energy in the form of adenosine triophosphate (ATP).

Concentration gradients are a key consideration with movement across the cell membrane. The **concentration gradient** refers to a relative comparison of solutes and overall concentrations of fluids inside and outside the cell. Without the influence of outside forces, substances tend to move down their concentration gradient towards equilibrium. Only with an energy input can items move against their concentration gradient.

PASSIVE TRANSPORT

Passive transport mechanisms consist of diffusion and osmosis, both of which move a substance from an area of high concentration to an area of low concentration. Diffusion and osmosis are spontaneous processes and do not require ATP.

Diffusion

Diffusion is defined as the movement of small solutes down their concentration gradients. In other words, dissolved particles move from whichever side of the membrane that has more of them to the side of the membrane that has less. Diffusion is a slow process by nature, but the following factors can influence its rate: temperature, the size of the molecule attempting to diffuse (large items are incapable of diffusion), and how large the concentration gradient is. Diffusion continues until **equilibrium** is met.

Osmosis

Osmosis is a very specific type of diffusion in which the substance moving down its concentration gradient is water. In an attempt to have equally concentrated solutions both inside and outside the cell, osmosis will occur if the solute itself is unable to cross the cell membrane because it is too large. Simply put, osmosis moves water from the side of the membrane that has more water (and less solute) to the side of the membrane that has less water (and more solute).

When the concentrations of solutes inside and outside the cell are equal, the solutions are termed **isotonic** and there will be no net movement of water into or out of the cell. In most situations, isotonic solutions are the goal for cells. A solution that has more water and less solute relative to what it is being compared to is termed **hypotonic,** while a solution that has less water and more solute relative to what it is being compared to is termed a **hypertonic** solution. When cells are placed in hypertonic solutions, water will leave the cell via osmosis, which can cause cells to shrivel. Cells placed in hypotonic solutions will gain water via osmosis and may swell and burst. The osmotic effects of each type of solution can be seen in Figure 7.3.

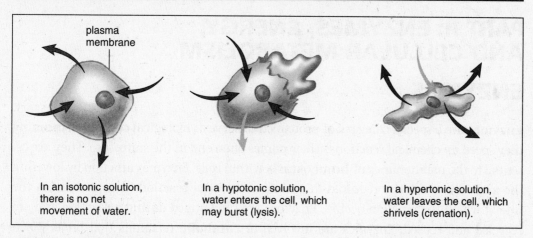

In an isotonic solution, there is no net movement of water.

In a hypotonic solution, water enters the cell, which may burst (lysis).

In a hypertonic solution, water leaves the cell, which shrivels (crenation).

FIGURE 7.3: Osmotic effects on animal cells. The arrows indicate the movement of water. In an isotonic solution, a cell neither gains nor loses water; in a hypertonic solution, the cell loses water; in a hypotonic solution, the cell gains water.

ACTIVE TRANSPORT

Active transport is in direct contrast to passive transport and is used to move solutes against their concentration gradient from the side of the membrane that has less solute to the side that has more. The solutes move via transport proteins in the membrane that act as pumps. Because this is in contrast to the spontaneous nature of passive transport, energy in the form of ATP must be invested to pump solutes against their concentration gradients.

BULK TRANSPORT

The methods for membrane transport described thus far are limited by the size of molecules and do not affect the movement of large items (or large quantities of an item) across the membrane. Endocytosis and exocytosis are used to move large items across the cell membrane.

Endocytosis is used to bring items into the cell. The membrane surrounds the item to form a vesicle which pinches off and moves into the cell. When liquids are moved into the cell this way, the process is termed **pinocytosis**. When large items, such as other cells, are brought into the cell, the process is termed **phagocytosis**.

Exocytosis is used to transport molecules out of the cell. In this case, vesicles containing the substance to be transported move towards the cell membrane and fuse with the membrane. This releases the substance to the outside of the cell.

PART II: ENZYMES, ENERGY, AND CELLULAR METABOLISM

ENZYMES

Enzymes are a special category of proteins that serve as biological **catalysts,** meaning they speed up chemical reactions. Their names often end in the suffix -ase. They are essential to the maintenance of **homeostasis** within cells. Enzymes function by lowering the **activation energy** required to initiate a chemical reaction, thus increasing the rate at which the reaction occurs. Enzymes are unchanged during a reaction and are recycled and reused. Enzymes are involved in **catabolic** reactions that break down molecules, as well as **anabolic** reactions that are involved in biosynthesis. Most enzymatic reactions are reversible.

Enzyme Structure

As is true of all forms of proteins, the shape of an enzyme is critical to its ability to catalyze a reaction. The area on the enzyme where the **substrates** interact is termed the **active site**. Any changes to the shape of the active site will render the enzyme unable to function. Enzyme specificity is based on shape; a single enzyme typically only interacts with a single substrate or single class of substrates.

Enzyme Function

The induced fit model is used to explain the mechanism of action for enzyme function seen in Figure 7.4. Once a substrate binds loosely to the active site of an enzyme, a conformational change in shape occurs to cause tight binding between the enzyme and the substrate. This tight binding allows the enzyme to facilitate the reaction.

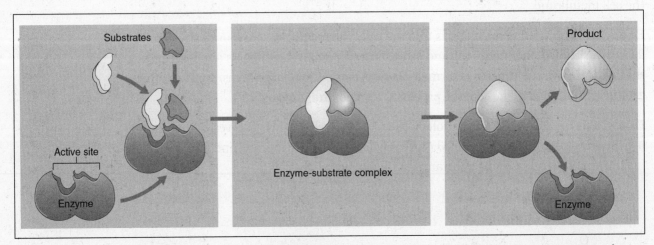

FIGURE 7.4:   The induced fit model. Enzymes interact with their substrates to form an enzyme-substrate complex. This complex allows the chemical reaction to occur.

Some enzymes require assistance from other substances to work properly. If assistance is needed, the enzyme will have binding sites for cofactors or coenzymes. **Cofactors** are various types of ions such as Fe^{++} and Zn^{++}. **Coenzymes** are organic molecules usually derived from vitamins obtained in the diet. For this reason, mineral and vitamin deficiencies can have serious consequences on enzymatic functions.

Factors that Affect Enzyme Function

There are several factors that can influence the activity of a particular enzyme. The first is the concentration of the substrate and the concentration of the enzyme. Reaction rates stay low when the concentration of the substrate is low, while the rates increase when the concentration of the substrate increases. Temperature is also a factor that can alter enzyme activity. Each enzyme has an optimal temperature for functioning. In humans this is typically body temperature ($37°C$). At lower temperatures, the enzyme is less efficient. Increasing the temperature above the optimal point can lead to enzyme **denaturation,** which renders the enzyme useless. Extreme changes in pH can also lead to enzyme denaturation. The denaturation of an enzyme is not always reversible.

Control of Enzyme Activity

It is critical to be able to regulate the activity of enzymes in cells to maintain efficiency. This regulation can be carried out in several ways. Feedback or **allosteric inhibition** acts somewhat like a thermostat to regulate enzyme activity. Many enzymes contain allosteric binding sites and require signal molecules to function. As the product of a reaction builds up, repressor molecules can bind to the **allosteric site** of the enzyme, causing a change to the shape of the active site. The consequence of this binding is that the substrate can no longer interact with the active site of the enzyme and the activity of the enzyme is temporarily slowed or halted. When the product of the reaction declines, the repressor molecule dissociates from the allosteric site, which allows the active site of the enzyme to resume its normal shape. The enzyme is now capable of resuming its normal activity.

Another mechanism of enzyme regulation is the use of inhibitor molecules. A **competitive inhibitor** is a molecule that resembles the substrate in shape so much that it binds to the active site of the enzyme, thus preventing the substrate from binding. **Noncompetitive inhibitors** bind to allosteric sites, changing the shape of the active site and decreasing the functioning of the enzyme.

ENERGY

The preferred source of energy for cells is **adenosine triphosphate** (ATP). The structure of ATP can be seen in Figure 7.5. ATP is a hybrid molecule consisting of the nitrogenous base adenine (found in nucleotides), the sugar ribose, and three phosphate groups (PO_4). The breaking of the bond that attaches the last PO_4 to the molecule results in the release of energy that is used in a variety of cellular processes. The resulting

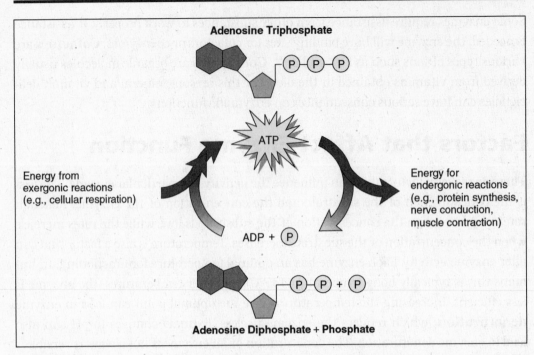

FIGURE 7.5: The ATP cycle. When a PO$_4$ is removed from ATP, energy is released and ADP is the resulting product. Cellular respiration is a primary means of adding a PO$_4$ to ADP to generate ATP.

molecule is **adenosine diphosphate** (ADP). Unfortunately, the process of adding a PO$_4$ to ADP is not a simple one. The chemical reactions of cellular respiration are used to achieve this goal.

Photosynthesis

Since cellular respiration involves the breakdown of glucose to produce ATP, it is critical first to understand the synthesis of glucose that occurs during photosynthesis. Photosynthesis can be performed by traditional plants, algae, and certain types of bacteria. During this two-step process, solar energy is converted to chemical energy via a series of electron transfers that produce oxygen gas as a byproduct. This chemical energy is then used to fix carbon (from CO$_2$), ultimately to produce glucose for the plant. The overall equation for photosynthesis is:

$$6H_2O + 6CO_2 + sunlight + energy \rightarrow C_6H_{12}O_6 + 6O_2 + 6H_2O$$

CHLOROPLASTS, CHLOROPHYLL, AND LIGHT

The reactions of photosynthesis occur in the chloroplasts of the typical plant cell. This structure can be seen in Figure 7.6. The green pigment chlorophyll exists in the thylakoids; its job is to absorb solar energy. However, many wavelengths of visible light are reflected (and thus useless to the plant). The most valuable wavelengths of light for photosynthesis are those that correspond to blue and red light. The less useful green and yellow wavelengths are reflected, making plants appear green to our eyes.

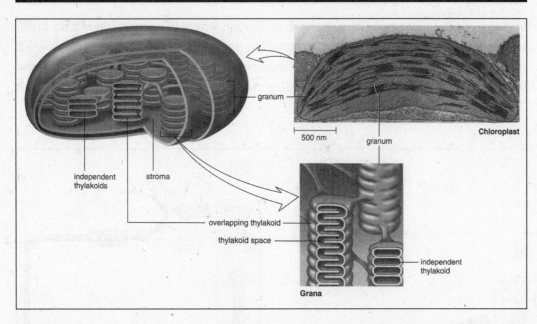

FIGURE 7.6: The chloroplasts each contain thylakoids, which contain chlorophyll for the light-dependent reactions to occur, and stroma for the light-independent reactions to occur.

Chlorophyll molecules and other pigments in the thylakoids arrange themselves as part of photosystems (abbreviated PS). The photosystems attract and absorb solar energy and facilitate the passage of electrons through carrier molecules. There are two types of photosystems: PSII (also called P680) and PSI (also called P700).

THE LIGHT-DEPENDENT REACTIONS

During the light-dependent reactions, solar energy will be converted to chemical energy. This process happens in the thylakoids of the chloroplasts. Solar energy will be used to split water molecules, which will provide a source of electrons for a series of redox reactions. A byproduct of the splitting of the water molecules is that oxygen gas is released. The electrons from water will be moved to PSII, where they will be boosted to high energy levels and passed through electron carrier molecules, ultimately resulting in the production of ATP that will be used in the light-independent reactions. The electrons then move to PSI, where they will again be boosted to a high energy level and passed through another set of electron carrier molecules. This time, NADP$^+$ will be reduced to NADPH, which will carry the energy of the electrons to the light-independent reactions. Figure 7.7 shows the steps involved in the light-dependent reactions.

The Light-Independent Reactions

The light-independent reactions are also known as the Calvin cycle. These reactions occur in the stroma of the chloroplast, as seen in Figure 7.8. Carbon dioxide is let into the plant by stomata on the surface of leaves, which are like pores that can open and close to regulate the entrance of CO_2 into (and the exit of water from) the plant. The first step of the Calvin cycle involves carbon fixation where CO_2 is combined with RuBP with assistance from the enzyme rubisco. The remainder of the cycle involves ATP (produced in the light-dependent reactions) energizing molecules and NADPH (also from the light-dependent reactions) donating electrons to molecules. The eventual result

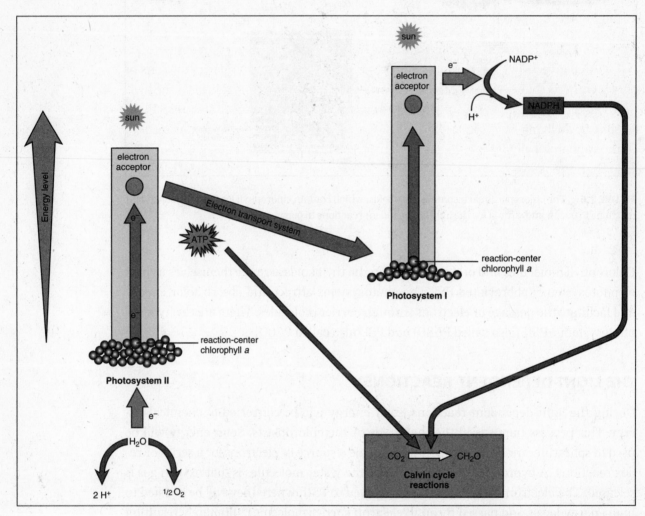

FIGURE 7.7: The light-dependent reactions. As energized electrons leave Photosystem II, they are replaced by electrons as water molecules are split. The electrons that leave Photosystem II proceed through an electron transport system, where ATP is ultimately produced. Energized electrons then leave Photosystem I, where they are eventually passed to NADPH. The ATP and NADPH produced in this step will be used in the light-independent reactions.

is that a molecule of G3P is released from the cycle and the remaining molecules are used to regenerate RuBP (the starting point of the cycle). The significance of G3P is that two of these molecules can be joined to form glucose (food) for the plant. This glucose can be used to build molecules such as starch and cellulose in the plant, or it can be broken down to produce large amounts of ATP in the process of cellular respiration.

CELLULAR RESPIRATION AND METABOLISM

Cellular metabolism encompasses the sum total of all anabolic and catabolic reactions that occur within the cell. These critical reactions rely on a variety of enzymes to increase their rate to an appropriate level. Anabolic reactions require energy, while catabolic reactions release energy. These reactions are coupled so that the energy released from a catabolic reaction can be used to fuel an anabolic reaction.

A critical catabolic reaction in cells is the breakdown of glucose to release energy which is used to convert ADP back to ATP. This glucose is made in the anabolic reactions of photosynthesis that occurs in plants. In animals, the glucose is obtained from the diet. The breakdown of glucose occurs in the process of **cellular respiration,** which must be done by all living organisms. Cellular respiration can be done aerobically (using oxygen) or anaerobically (without oxygen). The aerobic pathway has a much higher ATP yield than the anaerobic pathway. The production of ATP in either pathway relies on the addition of a PO_4 to ADP. This can be achieved through **substrate-level phosphorylation,** in which ATP synthesis is directly coupled to the breakdown of glucose, or via **oxidative phosphorylation,** in which ATP synthesis involves an intermediate molecule.

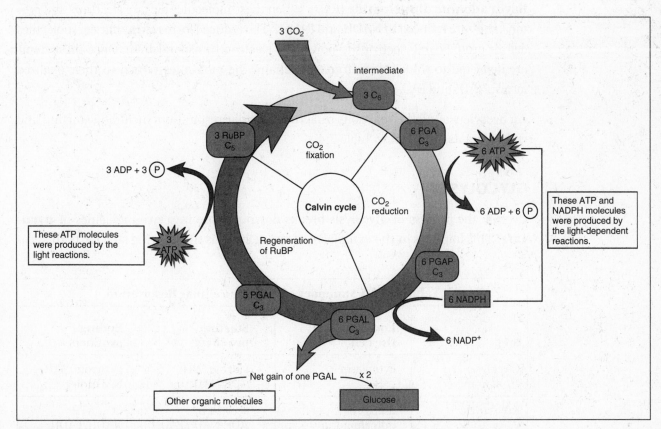

FIGURE 7.8:   The Calvin cycle. The Calvin cycle is divided into carbon fixation, reduction of carbon dioxide, and regeneration of RuBP. The cycle releases one PGAL per turn. Two PGALs are used to produce a glucose molecule.

Aerobic Respiration

The aerobic pathway can be demonstrated by the following reaction in which glucose and oxygen interact to produce carbon dioxide, water, and ATP:

$$C_6H_{12}O_6 + 6O_2 \rightarrow 6CO_2 + 6H_2O + ATP$$

Aerobic cellular respiration begins with the process of **glycolysis,** followed by the **Krebs Cycle** (also called the citric acid cycle), and concludes with the **electron transport chain**. The electron transport chain is fueled by protons (H^+) and electrons and is the step that produces the majority of ATP.

During glycolysis and the Krebs cycle, glucose will be systematically broken down and small amounts of ATP will be generated by substrate-level phosphorylation. Carbon dioxide will be released as a waste product. However, the most important part of these steps is that the breakdown of glucose allows for electron carrier molecules to collect protons and electrons needed to run the electron transport chain in which ATP is produced in mass quantities.

Electron carrier molecules are a critical part of aerobic cellular respiration. These electron carrier molecules include **nicotinamide adenine dinucleotide** (NAD^+) and **flavin adenine dinucleotide** (FAD). When these molecules pick up electrons and protons, they are reduced to NADH and $FADH_2$. The reduced forms of the carrier molecules deliver protons and electrons to power the electron transport chain. Once these items are delivered to the electron transport chain, the molecules return to their oxidized forms, NAD^+ and FAD.

An overview of all the reactions of aerobic cellular respiration, including starting and ending points, is shown in Table 7.4.

GLYCOLYSIS

Overall, the process of glycolysis breaks down glucose into two molecules of **pyruvate**. This happens in the cytoplasm of the cell and is the starting step for both aero-

Table 7.4: A Summary of Aerobic Cellular Respiration			
Step	**Location in the cell**	**Starting products**	**Ending products**
Glycolysis	cytoplasm	glucose, ATP, ADP, NAD^+	pyruvate, ATP, NADH
Krebs cycle	matrix of mitochondria	acetyl-CoA, ADP, NAD^+, FAD	CO_2, ATP, NADH, $FADH_2$
Electron transport chain	cristae membrane of mitochondria	NADH, $FADH_2$, O_2, ADP	NAD^+, FAD, H_2O, ATP

bic and anaerobic cellular respiration. During the process, two ATP molecules are invested while four ATP molecules are gained via substrate level phosphorylation. This leaves a net gain of two ATP for the process. In addition, NAD^+ is reduced to NADH that will be used in a later step (the electron transport chain) for oxidative phosphorylation. Figure 7.9 shows the major chemical reactions of glycolysis. At the end of glycolysis, the pyruvate molecules can be further broken down either aerobically or anaerobically. In the aerobic pathway, the subsequent reactions will occur in the mitochondria. The pyruvate from glycolysis must be moved to the mitochondria via active transport.

MITOCHONDRIAL STRUCTURE

A key feature of the mitochondrion is its double membrane. The folded inner membrane is called the **cristae membrane;** it is the site of the electron transport chain. The space between the inner and outer membrane is termed the **intermembrane space**. The space bounded by the inner membrane is a liquid called the **matrix**; it is the location where the Krebs cycle occurs.

KREBS CYCLE

In aerobic respiration, the two pyruvate molecules remaining at the end of glycolysis will be actively transported to the matrix of the mitochondria. They will be modified in order to enter into the reactions of the Krebs cycle. This modification, termed **pyruvate decarboxylation**, involves the oxidation of pyruvate and the release of CO_2. The remnants of pyruvate are a two-carbon acetyl group. Coenzyme A (CoA) will be added to the acetyl group, creating **acetyl-CoA,** which is capable of entering the Krebs cycle. These modifications to pyruvate also allow for the reduction of NAD^+ to NADH that will be used later in the electron transport chain. Because there are two pyruvate molecules, this step produces two CO_2, two acetyl-CoA, and two NADH.

Now that acetyl-CoA has been formed, this molecule will enter the Krebs cycle by combining with a four-carbon molecule (oxaloacetate) to form the six-carbon molecule, citric acid. The remaining reactions of the Krebs cycle are seen in Figure 7.10. The Krebs cycle involves the removal of the two carbons that entered as acetyl-CoA, which are released as CO_2, the production of one ATP molecule via substrate level phosphorylation, and the rearrangement of the intermediate products to form the starting molecule of oxaloacetate. In this way, the cycle is able to continue. In addition, the rearrangement of intermediates in the process allows for the reduction of NAD^+ to NADH and FAD to $FADH_2$. Because there are two acetyl-CoA molecules, this cycle must turn twice. The end result is the production of four CO_2, two ATP, six NADH, and two $FADH_2$. At this point, glucose that has been fully broken down into CO_2 will be exhaled by animals and released through the stomata in plants or further used in photosynthesis. At this point, the process continues with the electron transport chain.

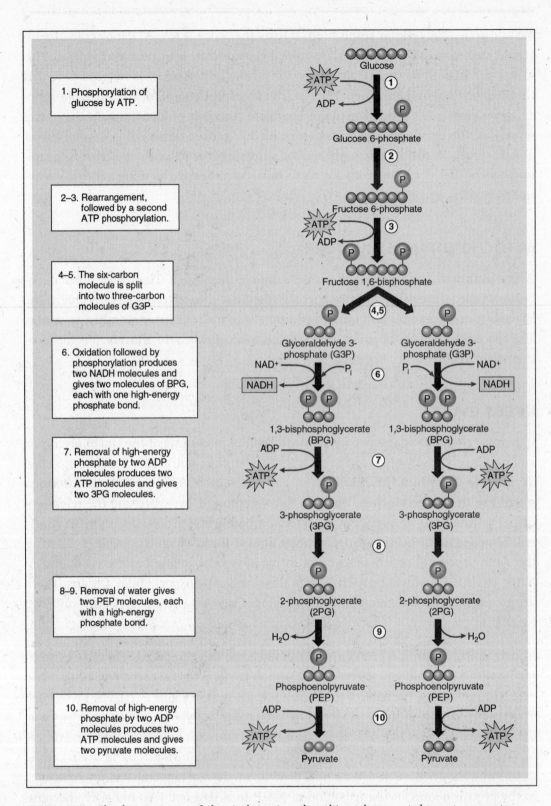

FIGURE 7.9: Glycolosis is a series of chemical reactions that ultimately convert glucose to pyruvate.

THE ELECTRON TRANSPORT CHAIN

During glycolysis and the Krebs cycle, NAD^+ and FAD have been reduced to NADH and $FADH_2$. Once they are reduced, they will move towards the electron transport chains located in the cristae membrane of the mitochondria. Here, they will be oxidized by releasing the electrons and protons that they are carrying to the chain. At this point, the oxidized forms of NAD^+ and FAD will return to the glycolysis and the Krebs cycle to be used again and again.

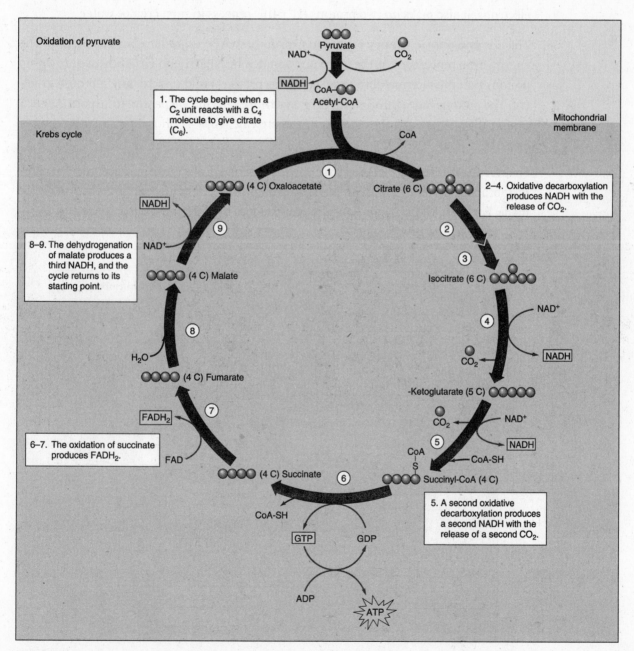

FIGURE 7.10: The Krebs cycle consists of a series of oxidative and decarboxylation reactions that occur in the matrix of the mitochondria.

The electron transport chain (Figure 7.11) is structurally a series of three carrier molecules including **cytochromes** that are associated with an ATP synthase enzyme. The ATP that is generated in this process will be made by oxidative phosphorylation. There are multiple electron transport chains located throughout the cristae membrane. The electrons from NADH and $FADH_2$ will enter the chain and be passed through the three carrier molecules. NADH delivers its electrons to the first complex in the chain; those electrons are passed to the second and third complexes. $FADH_2$ delivers its electrons to the second complex and then passes the electrons to the third complex. Eventually the electrons are accepted by the terminal electron acceptor, which is the oxygen inhaled through the respiratory system (hence the aerobic label). As the oxygen picks up the electrons, it also picks up two protons (H^+); this process in turn creates water.

The **chemiosmotic theory** is used to explain how ATP is produced in this process. The energy from movement of the electrons donated by NADH and $FADH_2$ is used to pump protons into the intermembrane space. These protons build up, creating a proton gradient. The protons move through the **ATP synthase** enzyme via passive transport. As each proton moves through the ATP synthase enzyme, ADP is phosphorylated producing one ATP.

For every NADH that donates electrons to the chain, 3 protons are pumped into the intermembrane space and 3 protons reenter through the ATP synthase; thus three ATP are made. For every $FADH_2$, 2 protons are pumped into the intermembrane space and 2 pro-

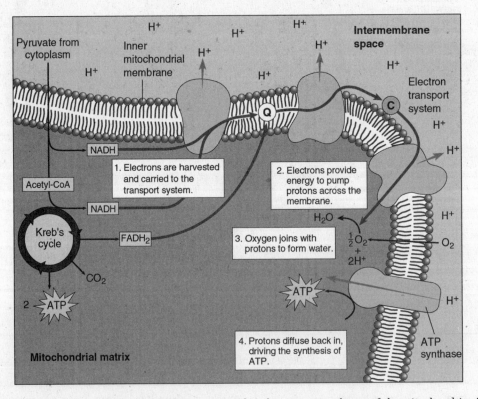

FIGURE 7.11: The electron transport chains exist within the cristae membrane of the mitochondria. ATP is produced via chemiosmosis.

Table 7.5:   A Summary of ATP Production in Aerobic Cellular Respiration

	Products of previous steps	**ATP made during chemiosmotic phosphorylation in the electron transport chain**
Glycolysis	2 NADH 2 ATP	2 NADH = 6 ATP (however, the net gain will be 4 ATP due to the use of ATP to actively transport pyruvate to the mitochondria)
Krebs cycle (including pyruvate decarboxylation)	8 NADH 2 FADH2 2 ATP	8 NADH = 24 ATP 2 FADH2 = 4 ATP
Total	4 ATP (substrate level phosphorylation from glycolysis and Krebs cycle)	32 ATP (oxidative phosphorylation from the electron transport chain)

tons reenter through the ATP synthase, so that 2 ATP are made. A total of 32 ATP are produced in the electron transport chain. Combining this number of ATP with the 4 ATP produced by substrate level phosphorylation in glycolysis and the Krebs cycle leads to a grand total of 36 ATP per glucose molecule made in aerobic cellular respiration. A summary of ATP made throughout the process of aerobic respiration can be seen in Table 7.5.

If oxygen is not available to accept electrons, the electrons in the electron transport chain will build up, essentially shutting down the electron transport chain. Not only will ATP production drastically decline, but now that NADH cannot be oxidized to NAD^+ by the electron transport chain, there will not be enough NAD^+ to continue glycolysis. In this case, the use of fermentation will be necessary to complete the oxidation of NADH to NAD^+ in order to continue glycolysis.

Anaerobic Pathways

There are times that oxygen is either not available or not utilized by cells to perform aerobic respiration. For animals, this may occur for brief episodes when the oxygen demands of the cells cannot be met. Unfortunately, the use of anaerobic respiration produces very little ATP as compared to aerobic cellular respiration, and thus cannot meet the ATP demands of larger organisms for extended periods of time. In other organisms, such as certain bacteria and yeasts that are single celled, anaerobic respiration is used permanently or for lengthy periods of time.

The first step in the anaerobic pathway is glycolysis. Once glycolysis occurs and pyruvate is generated, the anaerobic pathway continues with a second step, **fermentation**. Depending on the organism, fermentation can occur in one of two ways: lactic acid fermentation or alcoholic fermentation. The primary benefit of either type of fermentation is that it allows for the oxidation of NADH to NAD^+, which is necessary for glycolysis to continue in the absence of a functional electron transport chain. It is important to note that fermentation itself produces no ATP. The only ATP created during anaerobic respiration (glycolysis and fermentation) is from the glycolysis step. Therefore it is absolutely critical to regenerate the NAD^+ needed to continue with glycolysis. The total net gain of ATP from anaerobic respiration is 2 ATP as compared to 36 from complete aerobic respiration.

LACTIC ACID FERMENTATION

Lactic acid fermentation occurs in some types of bacteria and fungi, as well as in the muscle cells of animals when oxygen levels are not sufficient to meet the demands of aerobic respiration. In this step, pyruvate is reduced to lactic acid, thus regenerating the NAD^+ needed to continue glycolysis. In humans, large amounts of lactic acid are responsible for muscle fatigue after major exertion.

ALCOHOLIC FERMENTATION

Some organisms, such as certain bacteria and yeast, use **alcoholic fermentation**. In this step, pyruvate is decarboxylated, which produces CO_2 gas, and then reduced to form ethanol. As with lactic acid fermentation, NAD^+ is recycled so that glycolysis may continue.

PART III: DNA STRUCTURE AND REPLICATION

THE GENETIC MATERIAL

Deoxyribonucleic acid (DNA) is the genetic material of the cell. The information encoded in DNA ultimately directs the synthesis of particular proteins within cells. These proteins determine all of our biological characteristics. When a cell divides, DNA will self-replicate to ensure that progeny cells receive the same DNA instructions as the parent cell.

DNA Structure

DNA is a nucleic acid polymer consisting of the **nucleotide** monomers. A nucleotide is a hybrid molecule consisting of deoxyribose (a sugar), a phosphate group (PO_4), and a nitrogenous base. There are four nitrogenous bases used to make nucleotides: adenine (A), thymine (T) cytosine (C), and guanine (G). Each nucleotide differs only by the nitrogenous base used. In total, there are four possible nucleotides used in DNA.

The nitrogenous bases of each nucleotide can be classified as a purine or pyrimidine based on their chemical structure. A **purine** is a double-ringed structure while **pyrimidines** are single-ring structures. The nitrogenous bases A and G are purines while C and T are pyrimidines.

James Watson and Francis Crick proposed their famous model for DNA structure in 1953. By using information from other studies, they knew that DNA existed in a double-stranded conformation and that the amount of A and T in a DNA molecule was always the same, as was the amount of C and G. Using this information, they developed the model of DNA structure seen in Figure 7.12. A single stand of DNA has a sugar-phosphate backbone. Two strands of DNA are hydrogen-bonded together via their nitrogenous bases. The idea of complementary base pairing is essential to this model. This means that a purine must pair with a pyrimidine. An A on one strand of DNA will always bond to a T on another strand of DNA, using two hydrogen bonds. A C on one strand will always bond to a G on another strand, using three hydrogen bonds. This base pairing holds together the two strands of DNA, which then twist around themselves to take on the double helix conformation.

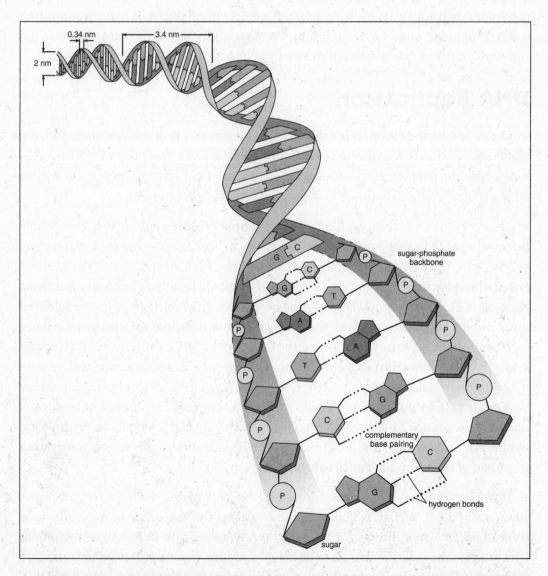

FIGURE 7.12: DNA double helix. The Watson and Crick model of DNA structure shows two strands of DNA that run antiparallel to each other.

Each strand of DNA has a specific polarity or direction in which it runs. This polarity is referred to as 5' and 3', referring to particular carbon atoms in the ribose molecule. The complementary strand of DNA always runs antiparallel, in the opposite direction of the original strand. So if one DNA strand runs 5' to 3', the other strand of the double helix runs 3' to 5'.

Chromosome Structure

In eukaryotic cells, DNA is organized in linear **chromosomes**. Humans have 23 pairs or a total of 46 chromosomes per **somatic** (nonreproductive) cell. A single chromosome consists of one DNA double helix wrapped around specialized **histone** proteins that form **chromatin**. Each of these chromosomes consists of an enormous amount of DNA, all of which must fit into the nucleus of the cell. Organizing the DNA around histones and other specialized proteins helps compact the DNA. During cell division, the chromatin then coils even more to form a compact chromosome. When chromosomes replicate in preparation for cell division, the new copies stay attached to the original copies at a location called the **centromere**.

DNA Replication

During normal cell division, it is essential for all components of the cell, including the chromosomes, to replicate so that each progeny cell receives a copy of the chromosomes from the parent cell. The process of replicating DNA must happen accurately to ensure that no changes to the DNA are passed on to the progeny cells.

The process of DNA replication is termed **semiconservative replication**. One double helix will need to be replicated so that two double helices result—one for each progeny cell. Because the DNA double helix has two strands, each strand can serve as a template to produce a new strand. The process of semiconservative replication has three basic steps. First, the original DNA double helix must unwind. This process is achieved using the enzyme **helicase**. Next, the hydrogen bonds that hold the nitrogenous bases together must be broken. This "unzips" the double helix in a localized area of the chromosome called the **origin of replication.** Finally, each template strand will be used to produce a complementary strand of DNA using the normal rules of complementary base pairing. **DNA polymerase** binds to the DNA template and chemically reads the nucleotide sequence while assembling the complementary nucleotides to produce the new strand. The synthesis of DNA occurs in both directions, moving outwards from the origin of replication in **replication forks**.

As DNA is synthesized during replication, the DNA polymerase reads the template DNA strand from the 3' to 5' direction, which means that the new DNA being synthesized will run in the 5' to 3' direction. Since one DNA template runs in the 3' to 5' direction, DNA polymerase will be able to read it and produce a continuous complementary strand called the **leading strand**. However, the other DNA template runs in the 5' to 3' direction, so the complementary strand (the **lagging strand**) will be synthesized in a discontinuous manner since the replication fork is moving against the direction of DNA synthesis. In order to synthesize the discontinuous strand of DNA, a primer (a short sequence of nucleotides) must bind to the DNA; DNA polymerase will begin to synthesize the new DNA strand until it runs into the next primer. This results in small pieces of DNA termed **Okazaki fragments** that must eventually be linked together. The primers will eventually be degraded and the Okazaki fragments will be linked using the enzyme **DNA ligase**.

DNA Repair

During the process of DNA replication, it is possible for DNA polymerase to make mistakes by adding a nucleotide that is not complementary to the DNA template or by adding or deleting nucleotides on the new DNA strand. Luckily, DNA polymerase has a proofreading ability which usually detects these errors and repairs them. However, if these errors are not corrected, there will be a permanent change to the DNA. This change is termed a **mutation**. In some cases, the mutation that cannot be successfully repaired will trigger the process of cellular suicide (apoptosis) to destroy the damaged cell. When this mechanism does not initiate, the mutation remains and can be passed on to progeny cells.

PART IV. PROTEIN SYNTHESIS
THE CENTRAL DOGMA

A gene is a segment of DNA located on a chromosome that has information to encode for a single protein. Proteins are made in the cytoplasm of the cell with assistance from ribosomes. The DNA and genes of a cell are located in the nucleus. Unfortunately, the DNA cannot leave the nucleus, nor can the ribosomes enter the nucleus. To get around this problem, the DNA message in the nucleus is converted to an intermediate **ribonucleic acid** (RNA) message that can travel to the cytoplasm and be read by the ribosomes to produce a protein. Protein synthesis is a two-step process: the conversion of DNA to RNA is **transcription**, and the conversion of RNA to a protein is **translation**. The **central dogma** of molecular biology describes the flow of genetic information in the cell:

$$DNA \rightarrow RNA \rightarrow protein$$

RNA

RNA is another form of nucleic acid and is a critical player in the process of protein synthesis. RNA molecules are another form of nucleic acid; they are very similar to DNA, with the few exceptions seen in Table 7.6.

Within the cell, there are three types of RNA: **ribosomal RNA** (rRNA), **transfer RNA** (tRNA), and **messenger RNA** (mRNA). Each type has a specific role in the process of protein synthesis. The functions of each type of RNA can be seen in Table 7.7.

Table 7.6: Differences between DNA and RNA (Nucleic Acids)		
	DNA	**RNA**
Number of strands	2, double helix	Single
Sugar used in the nucleotide	Deoxyribose	Ribose
Nitrogenous bases used	adenine, thymine, guanine, cytosine	adenine, uracil, guanine, cytosine

Table 7.7: Types of RNA	
Type of RNA	**Function**
Ribosomal (rRNA)	rRNA is made in the nucleolus of the nucleus. It is a structural component of ribosomes.
Transfer (tRNA)	tRNA is located in the cytoplasm of the cells. It is used to shuttle amino acids to the ribosome during the process of translation.
Messenger (mRNA)	mRNA is copied from DNA in the nucleus and serves as the messenger molecule to carry the DNA message to the ribosomes in the cytoplasm.

Transcription

The first step of protein synthesis is to produce mRNA from the DNA. The process of transcription initially resembles the process of semiconservative DNA replication. At the point where transcription is to begin, the DNA double helix must unwind. In this local area, the hydrogen bonds holding together the base pairs must break. Since only one strand of mRNA needs to be produced, only one strand of the DNA will serve as a template. The enzyme **RNA polymerase** will recognize sequences of DNA called **promoters** and bind to them. The RNA polymerase will chemically read the sequence of DNA and assemble the complementary RNA nucleotides in the 5' to 3' direction. The rules of complementary base pairing during transcription are similar to those of DNA replication, with one major change; RNA uses the base uracil (U) instead of thymine (T). If the DNA molecule contains the base A, then the complementary RNA molecule will contain the base U, while C and G will pair. RNA polymerase will continue to synthesize the complementary RNA strand until it reaches a termination sequence on the DNA. At this point, the RNA molecule will be released and the DNA double helix will reform. The process of transcription can be seen in Figure 7.13.

RNA Modification

Once RNA has been produced from the DNA template, it must be modified before it can be translated into a protein. First, a **5' cap** will be added to the 5' end of the RNA. This

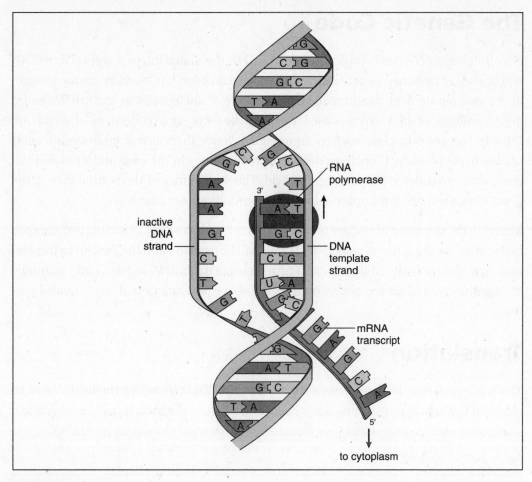

FIGURE 7.13: During transcription, complementary RNA is made from a DNA template using the enzyme RNA polymerase.

cap is a chemically modified nucleotide that will help regulate translation. Next, a **poly-A tail** will be added to the 3' end of the RNA. This tail consists of many A nucleotides placed on the end of the RNA. The purpose of the tail is to prevent degradation of the RNA molecule.

While some of the chromosomal DNA has information that is needed to code for proteins, the majority of the DNA does not. The coding DNA molecules are termed **exons,** and the noncoding DNA molecules are termed **introns** or "junk DNA." Unfortunately, the introns are located within the exons, disrupting their sequence.

During transcription, the RNA that is copied from the DNA contains the sequences of both the introns and the exons. Prior to translation, the introns must be removed, and the exons must be spliced together to form functional mRNA. Several unique RNAs can be produced by splicing the same exons in different sequences. This **RNA splicing** occurs in the nucleus. Once the splicing is complete, the mRNA molecule moves through the nuclear pores to the cytoplasm, where translation will occur.

The Genetic Code

Now that the mRNA has been produced, it must be translated into a protein. The mRNA will be read as **codons**, 3 nucleotides at a time. Each codon has the information to specify for one amino acid. Mathematically, there are 4 nucleotides in the mRNA and if every combination of 3 letters is used, there will be 64 possible codons, all of which are listed in the **genetic code** seen in Figure 7.14. Since there are only 20 amino acids used to make proteins, there is an overlap or redundancy in the code in that more than one codon can code for the same amino acid. The significance of the redundancy of the genetic code will become apparent later when mutations are discussed.

Knowing the sequence of codons on the mRNA makes it possible to use the genetic code to decipher the sequence of amino acids that will be used to build the protein in translation. Any change to the DNA, which in turn changes the mRNA codons, can potentially change the order of amino acids and thus the shape and function of the intended protein.

Translation

The process of translation occurs in the cytoplasm. The codons on the mRNA will be read and the appropriate amino acids needed to produce the protein will be assembled. This process will require assistance from various enzymes, ribosomes, and tRNA.

		Second letter			
	U	**C**	**A**	**G**	
U	UUU ⎫ Phe UUC ⎭ UUA ⎫ Leu UUG ⎭	UCU ⎫ UCC ⎪ Ser UCA ⎪ UCG ⎭	UAU ⎫ Tyr UAC ⎭ UAA Stop UAG Stop	UGU ⎫ Cys UGC ⎭ UGA Stop UGG Try	U C A G
C	CUU ⎫ CUC ⎪ Leu CUA ⎪ CUG ⎭	CCU ⎫ CCC ⎪ Pro CCA ⎪ CCG ⎭	CAU ⎫ His CAC ⎭ CAA ⎫ Gln CAG ⎭	CGU ⎫ CGC ⎪ Arg CGA ⎪ CGG ⎭	U C A G
A	AUU ⎫ AUC ⎬ Ile AUA ⎭ AUG Met or start	ACU ⎫ ACC ⎪ Thr ACA ⎪ ACG ⎭	AAU ⎫ Asn AAC ⎭ AAA ⎫ Lys AAG ⎭	AGU ⎫ Ser AGC ⎭ AGA ⎫ Arg AGG ⎭	U C A G
G	GUU ⎫ GUC ⎪ Val GUA ⎪ GUG ⎭	GCU ⎫ GCC ⎪ Ala GCA ⎪ GCG ⎭	GAU ⎫ Asp GAC ⎭ GAA ⎫ Glu GAG ⎭	GGU ⎫ GGC ⎪ Gly GGA ⎪ GGG ⎭	U C A G

First letter (left side) — *Third letter* (right side)

FIGURE 7.14: The genetic code. The codons on mRNA can be read on the genetic code to predict the sequence of amino acids produced by a particular mRNA.

RIBOSOMES

Eukaryotic ribosomes are composed of two subunits, one large and one small, of rRNA and various proteins. Once the ribosome assembles on the mRNA, there will be two RNA binding sites inside the ribosome: the peptidyl (P) site and the aminoacyl (A) site.

tRNA

The purpose of the tRNA molecules is to shuttle the appropriate amino acids to the ribosomes, as dictated by the codons on the mRNA. The tRNA itself is a piece of RNA folded into a specific configuration. On one end, the tRNA contains an **anticodon**. This sequence is complementary to the codon on the mRNA. On the other end of the tRNA, a specific amino acid will be attached.

THE STEPS OF TRANSLATION

Translation occurs as a three-step process. First, the ribosome must assemble on the mRNA. Next, the amino acids dictated by the codons must be brought to the ribosome and bonded together. Finally, the resulting protein must be released from the ribosome. The entire process of translation can be seen in Figure 7.15.

INITIATION

The process of translation begins when the ribosome assembles on the mRNA. The location for ribosomal assembly is signaled by the **start codon** (AUG) found on the mRNA. The small ribosomal subunit then binds to the mRNA. The first tRNA will enter the P site of the ribosome. This tRNA must have the appropriate anticodon (UAC) to hydrogen bond with the start codon (AUG). As seen in the genetic code, the amino acid specified by the start codon is methionine. Thus the first amino acid of every protein will be methionine. Now, the large subunit of the ribosome can assemble on the mRNA.

ELONGATION

At this point, the P site of the ribosome is occupied but the A site is not. A tRNA bearing the appropriate anticodon to bind with the next codon of the mRNA will enter the ribosome and hydrogen bond to the codon. A key enzyme, **peptidyl transferase,** will be used at this point to form a peptide bond between the two amino acids in the P and A sites. The two amino acids will now be attached to the tRNA in the A site. The tRNA in the P site will break off (leaving behind its amino acid) and leave the ribosome. The ribosome will now move over one codon to the right, putting the remaining tRNA in the P site and leaving an empty A site. This process—a new tRNA entering, a peptide bond forming between amino acids, the tRNA in the P site leaving, and the ribosome shifting over by one codon—will occur over and over again.

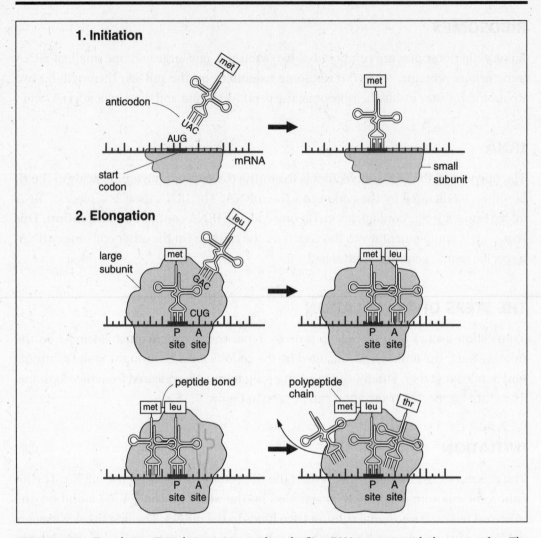

FIGURE 7.15: Translation. Translation initiates when the first tRNA interacts with the start codon. The tRNAs continue to deliver their amino acids to the ribosome during elongation.

TERMINATION

There are three mRNA codons (UAA, UAG, and UGA) that act as **stop codons** and do not code for amino acids. When one of these codons reaches the A site of the ribosome, no more tRNAs enter and the protein will be released from the ribosome. The ribosomal subunits will dissociate. This signals the end of translation. In some cases, it is necessary for the released protein to be modified before it can be functional. This often occurs in the endoplasmic reticulum or the Golgi complex.

MUTATIONS

Mutations change the coding sequence of DNA from that which was originally intended. When the DNA changes, the mRNA codons change, and the amino acid sequence of the protein made may change. This may produce a protein that functions better than the one coded for by the original sequence of DNA (thus providing an advantage), one that functions equivalent to the intended protein, or, in the worst case, a protein that functions worse than the intended protein or does not function at all. Recall that mutations happen spontaneously and that the rate of mutation is increased by exposure to mutagens.

Point Mutations

When a single nucleotide is swapped for another, this is termed a **point** (substitution) **mutation**. This will ultimately change a single codon on the mRNA. In some cases, this mutation will be silent; that is, if the codon is changed and still codes for the intended amino acids, there will be no detectable consequence. However, sometimes even a single point mutation can have major consequences. If the new codon codes for a different amino acid than what was intended (a **missense mutation**), the new protein may not function properly. This can lead to a genetic disease such as sickle-cell anemia. It is also possible for a change in a single nucleotide to produce a stop codon in a new location, causing a **nonsense mutation**. In this case, the protein produced would be too short and most likely nonfunctional.

Frameshift Mutations

A **frameshift mutation** is the result of the addition or deletion of nucleotides. Unlike the point mutation, in which the overall number of nucleotides does not change, adding or deleting changes the number of nucleotides. Since mRNA is read in codons, an addition or deletion will alter all of the codons from the point of the mutation onwards. This disrupts the reading frame of the mRNA. Since many codons are changed, the frameshift mutation generally produces a damaged or nonfunctional protein.

REGULATION OF GENE EXPRESSION

Gene expression refers to the process that controls which genes are transcribed and translated. Each cell has many genes, and it is not necessary for every cell to express every gene it has. In order to be efficient, cells are selective about which genes they express, making only the proteins that are necessary at a given time.

Gene expression can be regulated on a permanent level due to a process called **differentiation**. Because nearly all of the cells within the body are specialized, it makes sense that these cells really only need to express the genes related to that cell's particular function. Even though all cells have the same genes, each specialized cell is only capable of expressing a small subset of those genes. So while brain cells have the gene to produce the protein insulin, they are unable to express this gene; it is not needed for the functioning of a brain cell, and it would be inefficient to make an unnecessary protein. The process of differentiation happens early in development and is thought to be irreversible. Cells that have yet to differentiate are referred to as **stem cells**.

Once a cell has differentiated and committed to a set of genes that it needs to express, genes within this set can be regulated on a minute-to-minute basis. There are a number of ways to regulate the process of transcription and translation. These methods can completely prevent gene expression. If gene expression does occur, there are methods to control the rate of the process, in turn influencing the amount of protein that is produced. Table 7.8 summarizes the major mechanisms for the control of gene expression.

Table 7.8: Mechanisms for Regulating Gene Expression	
Stage at which regulation occurs	**Mechanisms used**
Transcriptional regulation	➤ Coiling of chromosomes to physically prevent or allow the access of transcription factors and RNA polymerase to the promoter regions of DNA
Posttranscriptional regulation	➤ mRNA splicing
	➤ Control over the rate at which mRNA leaves the nucleus via nuclear pores
Translational regulation	➤ Lifespan of mRNA, which is influenced by the length of the poly-A tail added during RNA modification in the nucleus
Posttranslational regulation	➤ Degradation of protein immediately following synthesis
	➤ Failure to properly modify the protein, rendering it useless

PART V. GENETICS
BASIC MENDELIAN CONCEPTS

The basic principles of genetics were proposed by Gregor Mendel in the 1860s. His work with traits in pea plants led him to propose several theories of inheritance. Mendel did all his work and postulated his theories at a time when the genetic material had not even been discovered, so the fact that his theories hold true today could be considered quite a stroke of luck.

Several pieces of terminology are essential in order to discuss genetics. The exact genetic makeup of an individual for a specific trait is referred to as the **genotype,** while the physical manifestation of the genetic makeup is referred to as a **phenotype** for a specific trait. A **gene** has information to produce a single protein or enzyme: however, genes can exist in different forms termed **alleles**. In some cases, mutations can cause the production of alleles that produce faulty versions of the enzymes needed for metabolism, leading to a class of genetic disorders known as **inborn errors of metabolism.**

Mendel's law of segregation

There are several important ideas found in Mendel's **law of segregation**. These ideas can be summarized in the following way:

➤ For every given trait, an individual inherits two alleles for the trait.
➤ As an individual produces egg and sperm cells (gametes), the two alleles segregate so that each gamete contains only a single allele per trait. During fertilization, each gamete contributes one allele per trait, providing the offspring with two alleles per trait.

There are exceptions to the law of segregation. These include the alleles carried on sex chromosomes in males. Because males contain one X chromosome and one Y chromosome, the male will not have two alleles per trait for genes on the sex chromosomes.

Complete Dominance

Individuals can inherit two of the same allele (**homozygous individuals**) or two different alleles (**heterozygous individuals**) for any given trait. In the heterozygous individual, only one allele is normally expressed, while the other allele is hidden. The **dominant** allele will be the one expressed; the **recessive** allele will be hidden in the presence of a dominant allele. When an individual is heterozygous for a particular trait, his or her phenotype will appear dominant, yet they still carry and can pass on the recessive allele via their gametes. A recessive phenotype is only observed when the individual is homozygous for the recessive allele. Keep in mind that dominant traits are not necessarily more common or more advantageous than recessive traits. Those labels only refer to the pattern of inheritance that the allele follows. The most common allele in the population is usually referred to as **wild type**. By convention, a single letter is selected to represent a particular trait. The dominant allele is always notated with a capital letter while the recessive allele is notated with a lowercase letter.

A **monohybrid cross** is a breeding between two parents (the P generation) where a single trait is analyzed. The offspring of this cross are called the F_1 **generation**. A breeding between two F_1 offspring will produce the next generation, F_2, and so on. When the genotypes of parents are known for a specific trait, a Punnett square can be used to predict the genotypes of the offspring.

In order to use a Punnett square, the genotypes of both parents must be known. The potential gametes of each parent are determined and every possible combination of gametes is matched up in a matrix in order to determine every genotype of the potential offspring. A ratio of the phenotypes of the offspring is expressed as dominant:recessive.

Mendel worked with many traits in the pea plant. He found that when he crossed a true-breeding (homozygous) plant of a dominant phenotype to a true-breeding plant of a recessive phenotype, 100% of the F_1 offspring had the dominant phenotype. However, when he bred two of the F_1 offspring, he found that 75% of the F_2 offspring had the

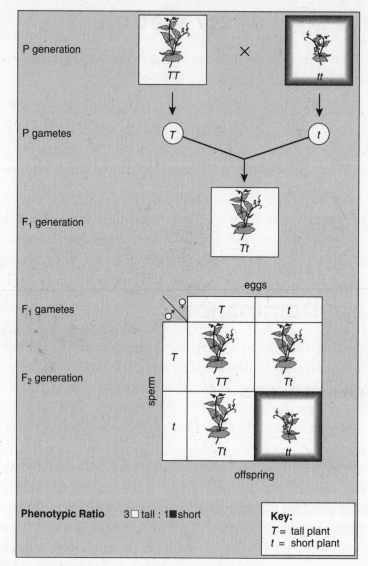

FIGURE 7.16: Monohybrid cross. The crossing of two heterozygous individuals leads to the typical 3:1 phenotypic ration observed by Mendel.

dominant phenotype, while 25% had the recessive phenotype. While the recessive phenotype had disappeared in the F_1 generation, it had reappeared in the F_2 generation. The F_1 offspring were all heterozygous. When two heterozygotes are bred to produce the F_2 generation, the offspring will always show Mendel's observed 3:1 **phenotypic ratio**. A cross between two heterozygotes that results in a 3:1 phenotypic ratio can be seen in Figure 7.16.

TEST CROSSING

Using a **testcross** (also called a backcross) is a method to determine the genotype of a parent with a dominant phenotype. An organism with the dominant phenotype may be either homozygous or heterozygous. In the testcross, the parent with the dominant phenotype is always crossed to a homozygous recessive mate. The outcome of the phenotypic ratio of the offspring will reveal the genotype of the unknown parent. If 100% of the offspring have the dominant phenotype, then the unknown parent was homozygous dominant. If the offspring display a 1:1 ratio, the genotype of the unknown parent was heterozygous.

Mendel's Law of Independent Assortment

A dihybrid cross considers the inheritance of two different traits at the same time. The rules of the monohybrid cross apply as long as the traits involved meet certain criteria. Mendel's **law of independent assortment** states the following:

➤ The alleles must assort independently during gamete formation, meaning that the distribution of alleles for one trait has no influence on the distribution of alleles for the other trait.

➤ If two genes are linked—that is, they occur on the same chromosome—they will not assort independently and thus will be inherited together, changing the expected outcomes in the offspring.

Dihybrid crosses

Two unlinked traits can be considered together in a Punnett square. When two traits are involved in a **dihybrid cross**, each trait is assigned a different letter. In order to predict the possible offspring, all possible gamete combinations of each trait for the parents must be considered. A Punnett square is used as a matrix to match up all possible gamete combinations for the offspring. Suppose two parents have the genotypes AABB and aabb. All F_1 offspring will be AaBb. If two F_1 offspring are bred, a 9:3:3:1 phenotypic ratio will be seen in the F_2 generation. See Figure 7.17 for an example of a dihybrid cross.

EXCEPTIONS TO MENDEL'S LAWS

While Mendel's laws tend to be good predictors of inheritance for some genetic situations, sometimes these laws do not apply. Not every trait operates according to a simple dominant/recessive pattern or in a completely predictable manner.

Linked Genes

The location of a gene on a chromosome is referred to as the **locus** of the gene. Genes that are linked occur on the same chromosome, which means that if one allele is found in a gamete, the other will be too. In the case of linkage, the combination of gametes produced will not be as diverse as would be the case with nonlinked alleles. In some cases, the loci of the alleles are so close together that they will always be inherited together. However, if the loci of the alleles are far away from each other on the chromosome, then there is a possibility for crossing over or genetic recombination to occur.

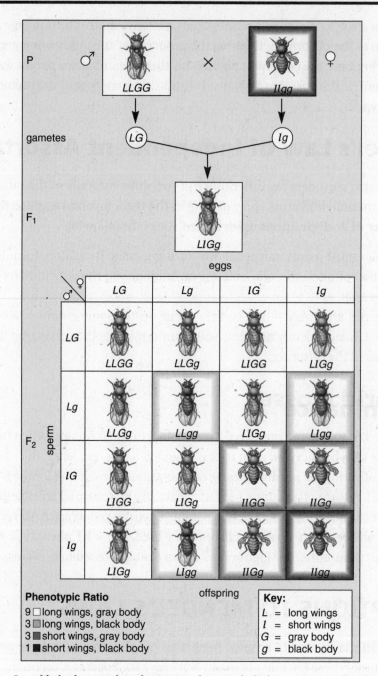

FIGURE 7.17: In a dihybrid cross, the inheritance of two unlinked traits is considered simultaneously. In this cross, Mendel's 9:3:3:1 phenotypic ratio is observed.

Multiple Alleles

For the traits Mendel observed with pea plants, there were always two alleles. One was dominant and one was recessive. However, while an individual can only inherit two alleles (one from each parent) for any given trait, there may be more than two alleles to select from in the **gene pool** that consists of all genotypes in the population. These new alleles arise due to mutation and increase diversity in the population.

Human blood type is an example of **multiple alleles**. The ABO system has three alleles: I^A, I^B, and i. The alleles I^A and I^B are dominant, while the allele i is recessive. Each allele codes for either the presence or absence of particular **antigens** on the surface of red blood cells. Any time multiple alleles are involved with a trait, more than two potential phenotypes will be expected. This is the case in blood type, where four phenotypes can be observed: Type A, Type B, Type AB, and Type O.

Incomplete Dominance

According to Mendelian rules, a heterozygous individual always expresses the dominant phenotype. If alleles behave by **incomplete dominance**, this will not be the case. Using flower color in snapdragons is a classic example. If the allele R codes for red flowers and the allele r codes for white flowers, Mendelian rules would suggest that the heterozygote (Rr) would have red flowers. However, because this trait behaves according to incomplete dominance, both alleles will be expressed to some degree, leading to a pink (intermediate) phenotype in the heterozygous offspring. In the case of incomplete dominance, only two alleles are involved, yet there are three potential phenotypes that can arise.

Codominance

Codominance is similar to incomplete dominance. For this to occur, the trait involved must have multiple alleles and more than one of them must be dominant. If a heterozygous individual inherits two different dominant alleles both alleles will be expressed, leading to an individual that has both phenotypes (as opposed to the blended phenotype seen with incomplete dominance).

Human blood type is an example of codominance as well as multiple alleles. Should an individual inherit the genotype of $I^A I^B$ it will express the A phenotype as well as the B phenotype. In this case, the result is Type AB blood. See Table 7.9 for more details on human blood type.

Table 7.9: The Genetic Basis of Human Blood Types		
Blood Type	**Potential Genotypes**	**Antigens found on the red blood cell surface**
Type A	$I^A I^A$ or I^Ai	A
Type B	$I^B I^B$ or I^Bi	B
Type AB	$I^A I^B$	A and B
Type O	Ii	None

Polygenic traits

Generally, a single gene influences one trait. **Polygenic traits** involve gene interaction. This means that more than one gene acts to influence a single trait. Skin color and hair color are both examples of polygenic traits. Because more than one gene is involved, the number of potential phenotypes is increased as a result of continuous variation.

Epistasis

Epistasis is a unique genetic situation in which one gene interferes with the expression of another gene. In many cases, epistasis can lead to the masking of an expected trait. An example is coat color in Labrador retrievers. These dogs have black, chocolate, or yellow fur. In addition to the gene that controls fur color, the B gene, there is another allele that controls how pigment is distributed in the fur, the E gene. The B gene produces an enzyme that processes brown pigment to black pigment. Dogs that have the genotype BB or Bb will produce black pigment while those with the genotype bb will produce brown pigment. The E gene allows the pigment to be deposited into the hair follicle. If the Labrador is EE or Ee, it will be able to deposit the pigment. However, dogs with the genotype ee will not. Therefore, the gene B determines if a dog will produce black or brown pigment, but these phenotypes can only be expressed if the dog is homozygous dominant or heterozygous for the E gene. Any dog that is homozygous recessive for the E gene, ee, will be yellow.

Pleiotropy

Pleiotropy occurs when a single gene influences two or more other traits. Most frequently, the effects of pleiotropy are seen in genetic diseases. In sickle-cell disease, the mutation in the hemoglobin gene results in the production of hemoglobin protein with a reduced oxygen-carrying ability. In turn, this affects multiple organ systems in the body, explaining the multiple symptoms of the disease.

Sex Linkage

When alleles are found on the X and Y sex chromosomes, the normal rules of genetics may not apply. While the sex chromosomes do contain genes to influence gender, there are other traits found on these chromosomes that have nothing to do with gender. Women inherit an XX genotype, while men inherit an XY genotype. In men, traits that occur on the sex chromosomes are the exception to the normal rule of always having two alleles per trait. Because the sex chromosomes in men are not a true pair, they do not have two alleles per trait on their sex chromosomes. The Y chromosome in men is always inherited from the father and contains relatively few genes compared to the X chromosome.

When a recessive trait is located on the X chromosome, women must receive two copies of the recessive allele (one from each parent) to express the recessive trait. However, men who inherit a recessive allele on their only X chromosome will express the recessive phenotype. Color blindness and hemophilia are examples of traits that are sex linked. While women can express these traits, they must receive the recessive alleles on both X chromosomes (meaning they must receive these alleles from both of their parents). Therefore, these traits are more commonly observed in men, who need only receive the recessive trait on their single X chromosome.

Women who are heterozygous for a trait on the X chromosome do not express the trait, yet they are carriers for the trait and can pass it to their sons. Since women are genotypically XX, every egg cell they make contains the X chromosome. Men are XY, and thus half their sperm contain the X chromosome and half contain the Y. In males, the Y chromosome must come from the father; the X comes from the mother.

Environmental Influences on Genes

While some genes behave according to very predictable rules, there are many cases where some external or internal environmental factor can interfere with the expression of a particular genotype. **Penetrance** of a genotype is a measure of the frequency with which a trait is actually expressed in the population. If a trait has 80 percent penetrance, 80 percent of the people with the genotype for the particular trait have the phenotype associated with the genotype. While some traits always show 100 percent penetrance, others do not. Within an individual, **expressivity** is a measure of the extent of expression of a phenotype. This means that in some cases expression of a phenotype is more extreme than others.

There are many examples of how the environment affects the expression of a particular phenotype. Hydrangea plants may have the genotype to produce blue flowers, but depending on the acidity of the soil they are grown in (an environmental factor), they may express a different phenotype than expected (for example, they may produce pink flowers). Women who have the BRCA 1 and 2 alleles are at a high but not guaranteed risk for developing breast cancer, meaning that something other than the allele determines the expression of the allele.

There are many traits that cannot be predicted by genotype alone, such as intelligence, emotional behavior, and susceptibility to cancer. In many cases, the interaction of genes and the environment is a complicated relationship that is impossible to predict. Factors in humans such as age, gender, diet, and so forth are all known to influence the expression of certain genotypes.

PART VI. CELL DIVISION

CELL DIVISION AND CHROMOSOMES

Cell division in eukaryotes happens by one of two processes. **Mitosis** is normal cell division that takes place in growth and the replacement of cells. In mitosis, a parent cell is copied in order to produce two identical offspring (daughter) cells. However, there are times that producing genetically identical offspring cells is not appropriate, such as sexual reproduction. During the process of sexual reproduction, genetically diverse gametes must be created. These gametes will be produced by the process of **meiosis**. Mitosis and meiosis have many features in common.

During either form of cell division, it is critical that the chromosomes be replicated and properly allocated to each of the daughter cells. Chromosomes occur in **homologous pairs**. For each pair of chromosomes found in an individual, one member of the pair came from the maternal parent and the other member of the pair came from the paternal parent.

The total number of chromosomes found in an individual is called the **diploid** (2N) number. When individuals reproduce, this number must be cut in half to produce **haploid** (N) egg and sperm cells. The human diploid number is 46 and the human haploid number is 23. The process of mitosis begins with a diploid cell and ends with two identical diploid cells. In the process of meiosis, a diploid cell will begin the process and will produce four haploid gametes.

When a cell is not dividing, each chromosome exists in single copy called a **chromatid**. However, when the cell is preparing to divide, each chromosome must be replicated so that it contains two chromatids, sometimes called **sister chromatids**. Each chromosome has a compressed region called the **centromere.** When the chromosomes replicate the sister chromatids stay attached to each other at the centromere.

Mitosis

Mitosis is the process of normal cell division in eukaryotic cells. It occurs in most cells except for gametes and mature nerve and muscle cells in animals. It begins with a single parent cell that replicates all components within the cell, divides the components into two piles, and then splits to form two genetically identical daughter cells. The most critical components for replication and division are the chromosomes, so particular care must be taken to ensure an equal distribution of chromosomes to each daughter cell.

The Cell Cycle

Mitosis is necessary for the growth of organisms, because it takes an increased number of cells for an organism to get bigger. When an individual has stopped growing, mitosis is only needed to replace cells that have died or been injured. For this reason, mitosis needs to be a regulated process that only occurs when new cells are needed. The **cell cycle** regulates the process of cell division in each individual cell. A normal cell cycle has the following stages, seen in Figure 7.18:

➤ G_1: This is the first gap phase of the cell cycle. In this stage, the parent cell is growing larger and is adding cytoplasm and replicating organelles.
➤ S: During this phase of DNA synthesis, the chromosomes are all being replicated. Once this stage is complete, each chromosome will consist of two sister chromatids connected at the centromere.

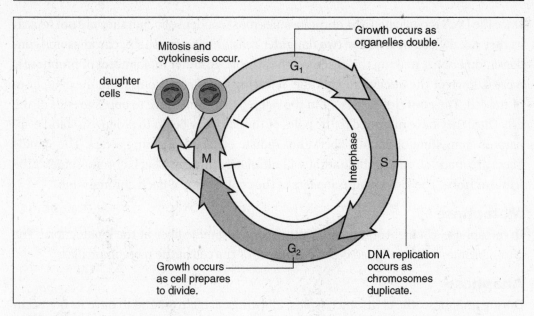

FIGURE 7.18:   The cell cycle. Cells go through a cycle that regulates their division. Interphase is prepara-tion for cell division and consists of the G_1, S, and G_2 phases of the cycle. The M phase is where the cells ac-tually divide.

➤ G_2: This is the second gap phase. The cell will continue to grow in size and make fi-nal preparations for cell division.

➤ M: During the M phase, mitosis actually occurs. The replicated chromosomes and other cellular components will be divided up to ensure that each daughter cell re-ceives equal distributions. The division of the cytoplasm at the end of the M phase is referred to as **cytokinesis**.

The first three phases of the cell cycle, G1, S, and G2, are collectively called **interphase**. Interphase simply means preparation for cell division. The actual cell division occurs during the M phase of the cycle.

Some cells lose the ability to progress through the cell cycle and are thus unable to divide. Mature human nerve and muscle cells are an example. Cells without the ability to divide are considered to be in the G_0 phase of the cell cycle where division will never resume.

M PHASE

The M phase of the cell cycle is subdivided into four stages: **prophase**, **metaphase**, **anaphase**, and **telophase**. The primary concern in these stages will be alignment and splitting of sister chromatids to ensure that each daughter cell receives an equal contri-bution of chromosomes from the parent cell. A visual summary of the events of the M phase can be seen in Figure 7.19.

Prophase

Chromosomes are located in the nucleus. Prior to division, the chromosomes are not condensed and thus are not visible. Leaving the chromosomes in an uncondensed state makes it easier to copy the DNA but makes the chromosomes very stringy and fragile.

Once the DNA is replicated, the chromosomes must condense so that they are not broken as they are divided up into the two daughter cells. During prophase, chromosome condensation occurs, making the chromosomes visible. Another major event of prophase is a breakdown of the nuclear membrane, releasing the chromosomes into the cytoplasm of the cell. The **centrioles** present in the cell replicate and move to opposite ends of the cell. Once they have migrated to the poles of the cell, they begin to produce a spindle apparatus, consisting of spindle fibers that radiate outwards forming asters. The spindle fibers are made of microtubules that will ultimately attach to each chromosome at the **kinetochore**. The kinetochore appears at the centromere of each chromosome.

Metaphase

In metaphase, each chromosome is attached to a spindle fiber at the kinetochore. The chromosomes will be aligned down the center of the cell at the metaphase plate.

Anaphase

During anaphase, the centromere splits, allowing each chromatid to have its own centromere. At this point, the chromatids can be separated from each other and are pulled

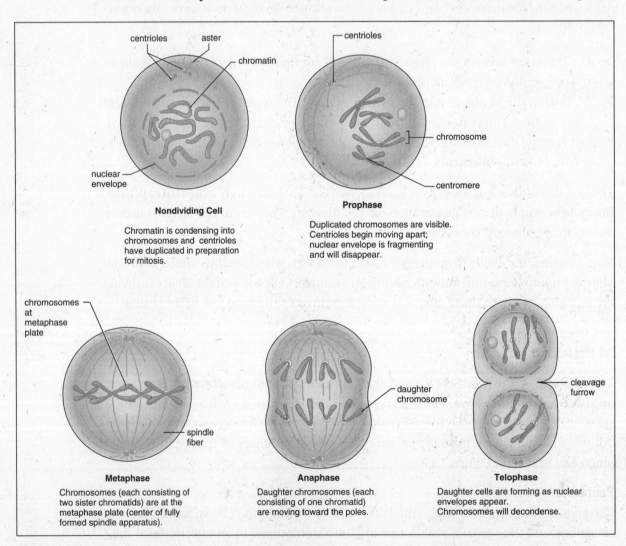

FIGURE 7.19: Mitosis consists of four phases: prophase, metaphase, anaphase, and telophase.

towards opposite poles of the cell, separating the chromosomes into two distinct piles—one for each daughter cell.

Telophase

Now that the chromosomes have been divided into two groups, the spindle apparatus is no longer needed and disappears. A new nuclear membrane forms around each set of chromosomes, and the chromosomes uncoil back to their original state. Finally, **cytokinesis,** where the cytoplasm is divided between the cells, occurs. In animal cells, a cleavage furrow forms that pinches the cells apart from each other. A cell plate (made of cellulose) divides the two daughter cells in plants. The end result is two daughter cells ready to begin interphase of their cell cycles.

MEIOSIS

Because mitosis produces genetically identical diploid daughter cells, it is not appropriate for sexual reproduction. The process of meiosis begins with a diploid parent cell in the reproductive system that has completed interphase and then follows stages similar to mitosis, twice. The result is four haploid gametes that are genetically diverse. A summary of the events of meiosis can be seen in Figure 7.20.

Meiosis I

Meiosis I encompasses stages similar to mitosis with two major changes. The first involves genetic recombination between homologous pairs; the second involves the alignment of chromosome pairs during metaphase.

Prophase I

During Prophase I of meiosis, there are many similarities to prophase of mitosis. The chromosomes condense, the centrioles divide and move towards the poles of the cell, spindle fibers begin to form, and the nuclear membrane dissolves. The unique event seen in Prophase I is crossing over. Homologous pairs of chromosomes associate and twist together in **synapsis**. This configuration consists of two replicated chromosomes, or a total of four chromatids, and is often called a **tetrad**. At this point, **crossing over** can occur, where pieces of one chromatid break off and exchange with another. Crossing over can occur in more than one location and can unlink genes that were previously linked on the same chromosome. It is also an important source of genetic diversity, creating combinations of alleles that were not seen previously.

Metaphase I

In metaphase of mitosis, chromosomes align single file down the center of the cell. In metaphase I of meiosis, the chromosomes align as pairs down the center of the cell.

This alignment of pairs is the critical factor in creating haploid daughter cells. Recall from genetics the law of independent assortment. The alignment of each member of the homologous pair during metaphase I is random, so each daughter cell will have a unique combination of maternal and paternal alleles.

Anaphase I

The homologous pairs will separate from each other during anaphase I and be pulled to the poles of the cells. This separation is referred to as **disjunction**.

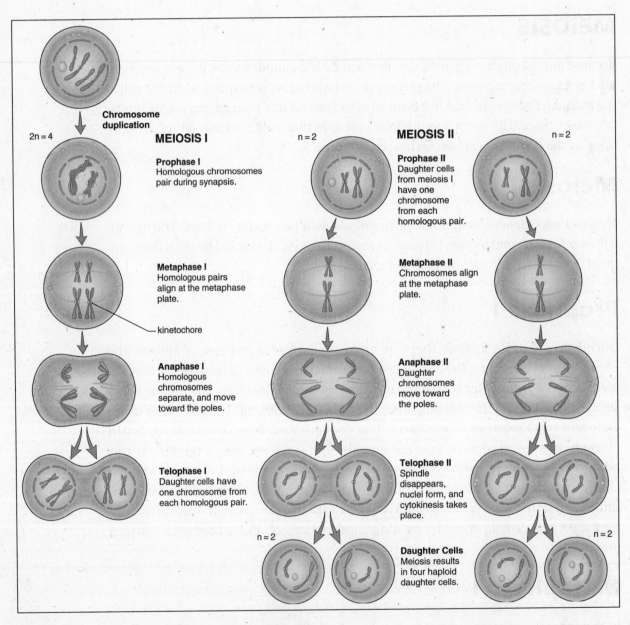

FIGURE 7.20: Meiosis consists of two rounds of cell division.

Telophase I

The events of telophase I are similar to mitosis. The spindle apparatus dissolves, nuclear membranes form around each set of chromosomes, and cytokinesis occurs to form the two daughter cells. At this point, each daughter cell is genetically unique and contains half the number of chromosomes of the parent cell. However, these chromosomes are still in their replicated form, consisting of two chromatids.

Meiosis II

Meiosis II is only necessary to split the chromatids present in the daughter cells produced during meiosis I. There will not be an interphase between meiosis I and II, because the chromosomes are already replicated. The events of meiosis II are as follows:

➤ Prophase II: Centrioles replicate and move towards the poles of the cell, chromosomes condense, and the nuclear membrane dissolves.

➤ Metaphase II: Chromosomes align down the center of the cell.

➤ Anaphase II: Sister chromatids are separated and move towards the poles of the cell.

➤ Telophase II: Nuclear membranes re-form and cytokinesis occurs to produce daughter cells.

At the end of meiosis II, there are four daughter cells. Each is haploid with a single copy of each chromosome. Each cell is genetically diverse as a result of crossing over and independent assortment.

Gametogenesis

Meiosis results in four gametes. In men, all four of these gametes will become sperm. In women, only one of these gametes will become a functional egg cell; functional eggs are released once every 28 days, during ovulation. If all four gametes became functional eggs and were released each cycle, there would be the potential for four embryos. The three gametes that do not become functional eggs in women are termed **polar bodies**. This will be discussed in more detail in Chapter 9.

Mistakes in Meiosis

Mistakes that happen during meiosis can have drastic consequences. Because the gametes are used for reproduction, any chromosomal damage to the gametes will be passed on to the next generation. If chromosomes fail to separate properly during meiosis, a **nondisjunction** has occurred. This will lead to gametes that have the wrong number of chromosomes. If those gametes are fertilized, the resulting embryo will have the wrong diploid number. An example of this is Down syndrome, which often is the result of a nondisjunction in the female gamete which received an extra chromosome.

This condition is referred to as a **trisomy**. When a gamete is missing a chromosome as the result of a nondisjunction and is fertilized by a normal gamete, the result is an embryo with 45 chromosomes. This is termed a **monosomy**. With the exception of Down syndrome, which is a trisomy of human chromosome 21 (which is very small) and certain trisomies and monosomies of the sex chromosomes (X and Y), most embryos with trisomies and monosomies do not survive development.

There are other forms of chromosomal damage that can occur in meiosis. They typically have serious, if not fatal, consequences. They are as follows:

➤ **Deletion**: This occurs when a portion of a chromosome is broken off and lost during meiosis. While the total chromosome number is normal, some alleles have been lost.

➤ **Duplication**: This occurs when a chromosome contains all of the expected alleles and then receives a duplication of some alleles.

➤ **Inversion**: When a portion of a chromosome breaks off and reattaches to the same chromosome in the opposite direction, this is termed inversion.

➤ **Translocation**: This occurs when a piece of a chromosome breaks off and reattaches to another chromosome.

PART VII. EVOLUTION

EVOLUTION

Evolution simply means change. The changes referred to are genetic ones; thus the concept of mutation is at the center of the process of evolution. Evolution is something that occurs over generations of time; thus a single individual does not evolve but populations of individuals do evolve. **Microevolution** deals with genetic changes to a specific population of individuals in a given area, while **macroevolution** is concerned with changes that occur to a species on a larger scale over a longer period of time.

Mechanisms for Evolution

There are a variety of factors that are responsible for the microevolution of a particular population. Natural selection, based on mutation, tends to be the major driving force for evolution, while genetic drift and gene flow can also influence the process.

Mutation

New alleles are created by mutation. Some of these new alleles code for proteins that are beneficial, neutral, or detrimental as compared to the original protein intended by the allele. New alleles that code for beneficial proteins can provide advantages that are ultimately selected for by natural selection and are passed to the next generation, while detrimental alleles will be selected against.

Natural Selection

A central concept to the explanation of how evolution occurs is that of Darwin's natural selection. **Natural selection** explains the increase in frequency of favorable adaptations from one generation to the next. This results from differential reproductive success, in which some individuals reproduce more often than others, thus selecting for particular traits and increasing the frequency of their alleles in the next generations. Those that reproduce less decrease the frequency of their alleles in the next generation.

FITNESS CONCEPT

The concept of evolutionary **fitness** is key to natural selection. In this context, fit refers to the reproductive success of an individual and its contribution to the next generation. Those individuals that are more fit, are more evolutionarily successful, in that their genetic traits will be passed to the next generation; this increases the frequency of specific alleles in the gene pool.

Over generations, selective pressures that are exerted on a population can lead to **adaptations**. When selective pressures change, some organisms that may have been considered marginally fit before may now be extremely fit under the new conditions. Further, those individuals that may have been very fit previously may no longer be fit. Their genetic adaptations will be selected against. While an individual cannot change their genetics, over time, the population has changed genetically which is termed adaptation.

DIFFERENTIAL REPRODUCTIVE SUCCESS AND COMPETITION

Competitive interactions within a population are another critical factor for natural selection. The ability to outcompete other individuals for resources, including mates, is a key feature of fitness. In any given population, some individuals are better able to compete for resources and are considered more fit than others, leading to differential reproductive success. This concept assumes that mating in the population is random. In some cases, such as with humans, mating is nonrandom, which leads to another form of selection to be discussed shortly.

Competition between species can also influence the evolutionary progression of all species involved. In some cases, **symbiotic** relationships exist in which two species exist together for extended periods of time. In **mutualistic** relationships, both species benefit from the association. In **parasitic** relationships, one species benefits at the expense of the other species. In **commensalism**, one species benefits while the other species is relatively unharmed. When two species are competing for the same ecological requirements or **niche**, the reproductive success and fitness, as well as the growth, of one or both populations may be inhibited based on its ability to compete for resources. This will change the microevolutionary course of the population.

Gene Flow

When individuals leave a population, they take their alleles with them, resulting in **gene flow**. This can decrease genetic variation within the gene pool, ultimately affecting the evolution of the population. **Outbreeding** occurs with the individuals that left the population. The new populations that these individuals enter can increase diversity in their gene pool by adding new alleles to it.

Genetic Drift

Genetic drift involves changes to the allelic frequencies within a population due to chance. While this is generally negligible in large populations, it can have major consequences in smaller populations. The **bottleneck effect** and the **founder effect** are examples of genetic drift to be discussed shortly.

GENETIC BASIS FOR EVOLUTION AND THE HARDY-WEINBERG EQUATION

The **Hardy-Weinberg equation** can be used to calculate allelic frequencies within a population given that the population is large and microevolution is not occurring, which is not necessarily a realistic situation. In the equation, p represents the frequency of a dominant allele and q represents the frequency of a recessive allele, such that $p + q = 1$. Further, the equation $p^2 + 2pq + q^2 = 1$ can be used to show the frequency of homozygous dominant individuals (p^2), heterozygotes ($2pq$), and homozygous recessive individuals (q^2). Given information on the frequency of a single allele, all other pieces within the equation can be determined. While these frequencies are accurate at a given time, any evolution occurring within the population would shift these predicted values.

Violations of Hardy-Weinberg

In order for Hardy-Weinberg allelic frequencies to hold true, it is necessary for certain criteria to be met. If any of these criteria are violated, the allelic frequencies will change over time. Any of the following will negate Hardy-Weinberg equilibrium: 1) nonrandom mating, 2) gene flow, 3) populations with a small number of individuals, 4) mutations, 5) bottleneck effect, and 6) founder effect. The **bottleneck effect** is a form of genetic drift in which catastrophic events wipe out a large percentage of a population. When the population is small, the few remaining alleles in the gene pool may not be characteristic of the larger population. Generally, genetic diversity is lost due to inbreeding by the remaining members of the population. The **founder effect** is a form of genetic drift that occurs when a small number of individuals leave a larger population and form their own small population where inbreeding is necessary. The new population only has the diversity brought to it by the founding members.

TYPES OF NATURAL SELECTION

For any given trait, there can be several different phenotypes. If two phenotypes are present for a particular trait, **dimorphism** is the case. If three or more phenotypes are seen for a particular trait, **polymorphism** is at work. For example, flower color in snapdragons exhibits polymorphism with red, white, and pink phenotypes. Some phenotypes can be considered intermediates (like pink flowers); others are extremes from either end of the intermediate phenotype (like red and white flowers). When natural selection occurs, it may select for intermediate phenotypes, either extreme phenotype, or both extreme phenotypes, as seen in Figure 7.21.

Directional Selection

In **directional selection**, an allele that is considered advantageous is selected for. The allelic frequency continues to shift in the same direction generation after generation. In this case, one allele that produces an extreme phenotype is selected for. The selection of antibiotic resistance alleles in bacteria is an example of directional selection. Over time, selective pressures can result in an entire population possessing the same alleles for a particular trait.

Stabilizing Selection

Stabilizing selection leads to favoring of the alleles that produce an intermediate phenotype. Human birth weight would be an example of stabilizing selection. Babies of an intermediate weight are favored over those that are too small to survive or too large to be easily delivered.

Disruptive Selection

In some cases, the environment favors two extreme phenotypes at the same time. In this case, **disruptive selection** occurs. Individuals with either extreme phenotype are

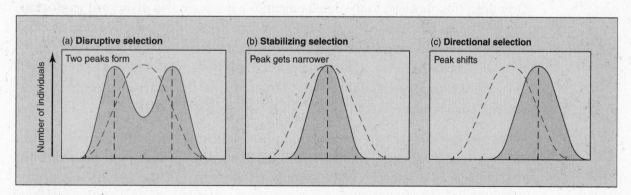

FIGURE 7.21: Types of natural selection. (*a*) In disruptive selection, the extreme phenotypes are selected for, whereas the intermediate phenotype is selected against. (*b*) In stabilizing selection, the intermediate phenotype is favored. (c) In directional selection, one extreme phenotype is favored.

favored, while those with the intermediate forms of the alleles are selected against. Over time, the continued selection of both extremes may lead to the evolution of two distinct species.

Artificial Selection

When particular alleles are purposely selected for through nonrandom mating, **artificial selection** occurs. The breeding of domesticated dogs is an excellent example of the results of artificial selection. All breeds of dogs are members of the same species, having been selectively bred from wolves for specific traits that are appealing to the breeder. Both toy poodles and Great Danes are examples of the extreme phenotypes that can be selected for when artificial selection is used. Traits that are artificially selected for are not necessarily the result of the most fit alleles. Many breeds of dog have medical conditions or predispositions as a result of artificial selection.

TYPES OF EVOLUTION

The evolutionary process can proceed in a variety of directions or patterns: convergent, divergent, and parallel evolution. When two populations exist in the same type of environment that provides the same selective pressures, the two populations will evolve in a similar manner via **convergent evolution**. While the populations may not be closely related, they may develop similar, analogous structures to allow them to function in similar environments. Fish in Antarctica have evolved the ability to produce specialized glycoproteins which serve as a sort of antifreeze to prevent their tissues from freezing in the low-temperature water. Fish on the opposite side of the world, in the Arctic, have evolved the same kind of antifreeze protection mechanism. Genetic studies show that the two species of fish produce antifreeze proteins that are very different from each other, which strongly suggests that two independent events led to the evolution of these mechanisms.

In an individual population, individuals within the population may evolve differently. Over time, this may lead to the development of new species via **divergent evolution**. In many cases, changes to the population or geographic isolation may cause different adaptations within the population. This sort of evolution can lead to homologous structures. Vertebrate limbs are an excellent example of divergent evolution. The forearms of different vertebrate species have different structures and functions; however, they all diverged from a common origin.

When two species share the same environment, the evolution of one species can affect the evolution of the other species. This is called **parallel evolution** or **coevolution**. Any changes to one species will require adaptations to the other species in order for them to continue to exist in the same environment. An example might be how the predation patterns of birds influence the evolution of butterfly species sharing the same space. Some butterflies have evolved the ability to store poisonous chemicals that deter birds from eating them, while other butterflies simply mimic the poisonous ones to avoid being preyed upon.

EVIDENCE FOR EVOLUTION

There is a large body of evidence to support evolutionary theory. Most evidence comes from studies of paleontology, biogeography, molecular biology, comparative anatomy, and comparative embryology.

➤ **Paleontology**: The field of paleontology provides evidence for evolution in the form of the fossil record. **Fossilization** occurs when a whole organism or parts of an organism become embedded in sediments and petrified over thousands of years. These fossils serve as physical evidence of organisms that lived in the past.

➤ **Biogeography**: The study of the natural distribution of organisms, **biogeography**, can also lend credence to evolutionary theory. Looking at similarities and differences between different organisms living in different locations can help decipher evolutionary relationships between organisms as well as common ancestors.

➤ **Molecular Biology**: The ability to compare DNA and other molecules, such as proteins, made by various organisms also helps support evolutionary theory. Organisms that are more closely related share more DNA similarities than organisms that are distantly related. Evolutionary time can be measured by genetic changes over time. Comparisons of mutation rates in conserved gene sequences can be used to construct **molecular clocks**, which can be used to estimate when specific lineages emerged.

➤ **Comparative anatomy**: An analysis of anatomical features in organisms can be used to make comparisons between different species. **Homologous structures**, such as the forelimbs of mammals, are similar in structure between various organisms and they share a similar function, indicating that these structures came from a common ancestral species. **Analogous structures** have similar functions between various organisms, but these structures have different lines of descent. **Vestigial structures** seen in organisms have no functional value, yet are evolutionary remnants from ancestral species. Examples of vestigial structures are the human appendix, bone structure for hindlimbs in whales, and the coccyx (tailbone) in humans. Since these structures remain, even without apparent functions, they are evidence of prior evolutionary forces at work.

➤ **Comparative embryology**: While many organisms look distinctly different in their adult forms, they may share striking similarities during their developmental periods. Comparative embryology is used to study these similarities during the developmental process. A modification of Haeckel's theory that ontogeny recapitulates phylogeny (or **recapitulation**) suggests that species that have an evolutionary relationship generally share characteristics during embryonic development.

THE ORIGIN OF LIFE

The origin of life encompasses an enormous number of detailed events. The major events will be briefly summarized in this section. Life began approximately four billion years ago when the solar system formed and the Earth cooled. The **big bang theory** is used to explain how the universe, including our solar system, might have come about. This theory supposes that a large, hot mass of material in the galaxy broke apart to distribute matter and energy throughout the universe. This distribution of material caused a major cooling of temperature. Nuclear fusion created many of the major elements which, over time, collided and condensed into stars that provided light and heat. As stars died, heavier elements were released, eventually producing suns (including our sun).

The primitive atmosphere of Earth consisted of a variety of organic and inorganic substances such as ammonia, methane, water, carbon monoxide, carbon dioxide, nitrogen gas, and hydrogen gas. What was lacking was oxygen gas. Water vapor formed rain, which collected into pools containing mineral runoff from rocks. A source of energy within these bodies of water, perhaps derived from lightning or sunlight, fueled the reactions needed to create organic molecules such as sugars, amino acids, nucleotides, and fatty acids. As these monomers collected in clay, they may have polymerized to form molecules such as proteins, carbohydrates, and nucleic acids.

Some proteins produced within clay had enzymatic properties, allowing them to interact with other molecules. The formation of a membrane around these primitive enzymes produced the first **protocell** that had the ability to self-replicate. An association of the protocell with RNA may have produced the first actual cell that resembled modern prokaryotes. These cells lacked organelles and lived in an anaerobic environment. Mutations that occurred in some populations of the first cells provided **photoautotrophic** abilities. The development of photosynthesis had an important impact in that it produced oxygen gas, making an aerobic environment in which aerobic cellular respiration evolved as the dominant energy producing process.

Eukaryotic cells evolved from the prokaryotic-like cells. The theory of **endosymbiosis** explains the presence of organelles within eukaryotic cells. The engulfment of bacterial cells led to mitochondria and the engulfment of photosynthesizing prokaryotes led to the development of chloroplasts, as seen in modern day plants. **Membrane infolding** explains the presence of organelles such as the nucleus and endoplasmic reticulum in eukaryotic cells. Internalizing some of the cell membrane provided greater surface area for reactions to occur, and thus this adaptation was selected for. These first eukaryotic cells resembled **protists** in structure.

Over time, symbiotic relationships occurred between eukaryotic cells that led to specialization and the division of labor needed to eventually produce multicellular organisms. All modern plants, animals, and fungi evolved from these primitive eukaryotic cells.

General Biology

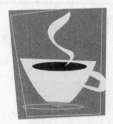

- ➤ The two major cell types are prokaryotic and eukaryotic. The organelles found in eukaryotic cells are the nucleus, smooth ER, rough ER, Golgi complex, lysosomes, peroxisomes, and mitochondria. Cell walls, chloroplasts, and the central vacuole are unique to plant cells.
- ➤ The cell membrane is a phospholipid bilayer which is selectively permeable. Substances can move across the membrane via passive, active, or bulk transport.
- ➤ Enzymes speed chemical reactions by lowering activation energy.
- ➤ Adenosine triphosphate (ATP) is the preferred energy source for all organisms.
- ➤ Photosynthesis provides glucose and oxygen gas for other organisms. The light-dependent reactions convert solar energy to chemical energy, producing oxygen as a byproduct, while the light-independent reactions convert carbon dioxide to glucose.
- ➤ Cellular respiration is used to generate ATP as glucose is broken down. Aerobic cellular respiration breaks down glucose to CO_2. It involves glycolysis, the Krebs cycle, and the electron transport chain. Oxygen serves as the terminal electron acceptor and ultimately binds to protons to produce water. The net yield of ATP from aerobic cellular respiration far exceeds that from anaerobic respiration.
- ➤ DNA is structured as a double helix. Semiconservative replication is used to synthesize complementary strands of DNA.
  - ➤ The central dogma of molecular biology dictates the flow of genetic material in the cell: DNA → RNA → protein. Protein synthesis is a two-step process. Transcription converts DNA to mRNA. Translation converts mRNA to a protein.
- ➤ Mendelian laws assume that one allele is dominant, asserting itself over a recessive allele.
  - ➤ Punnett squares predict offspring given the genotypes of parents. Monohybrid crosses consider one trait, while dihybrid crosses consider two traits together.
  - ➤ Mendel's theories do not consider certain genetic situations, such as incomplete dominance, codominance, polygenic inheritance, pleiotropy, epistasis, or environmental influences.
- ➤ Cell division occurs in two forms: mitosis and meiosis.
  - ➤ Mitosis is used for growth, repair, and replacement of cells.
  - ➤ Meiosis is used for sexual reproduction to produce gametes.
- ➤ Evolution means change. Individuals do not evolve, populations do. Natural selection is the primary mechanism for evolution.
  - ➤ The Hardy-Weinberg equation is used to calculate allelic frequencies population. The two equations are: $p+q=1$ and $p^2+2pq+q^2=1$.
  - ➤ Evidence for evolution occurs in the form of the fossil record, biogeography, comparative anatomy, and comparative embryology.
  - ➤ The origin of life is explained by several key theories including the big bang theory, endosymbiotic theory, and membrane infolding theory.

Microbiology

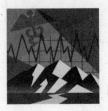

PART I. BACTERIA

PROKARYOTES

There are three domains in which living organisms are classified: **Eukarya**, **Bacteria**, and **Archaea**. All eukaryotic organisms are classified in the domain Eukarya, leaving all prokaryotic cells to be classified as either Bacteria or Archaea. While both domains share the characteristics of being single celled, absorbing their nutrients, having a single loop of DNA, and lacking organelles, there are some differences between the two groups. While Archaea used to be mistakenly classified as bacteria, their molecular and cellular structures were found to be quite different. They have a unique cell wall, ribosomes, and membrane lipids. Archaea live in very diverse environments and some species are termed extremophiles due to their habitats such as polar ice caps, thermal vents, extreme salt concentrations, jet fuel, and others. Most Archaea species are **anaerobes** and none are known to be **pathogens**.

Because of their medical and environmental significance, the focus of this chapter will be on bacteria.

CLASSIFICATION OF BACTERIA

Bacteria are extremely diverse. The classification of bacteria is generally based on the mechanisms used by the particular species to obtain nutrients from the environment. The following are the basic bacterial classifications:

➤ **Photoautotrophs**: There are some bacterial species that produce their own nutrients through the process of photosynthesis, using carbon dioxide from the environment.

➤ **Photoheterotrophs**: Bacteria that perform photosynthesis but cannot use carbon dioxide from the environment are considered photoheterotrophs. In order to get the carbon needed for photosynthesis (which normally comes from carbon dioxide), they extract carbon from a variety of other sources.

➤ **Chemoautotrophs**: These species get their energy from inorganic compounds, and their carbon needs are obtained from carbon dioxide.

➤ **Chemoheterotrophs**: Energy is obtained for these species from inorganic substances while carbon is obtained from a variety of sources other than carbon dioxide. These species are further subdivided based on the source of carbon they use. Some species can extract carbon through parasitic or symbiotic interactions with a host or through the decomposition of other organisms.

Bacteria can also be classified based on their oxygen requirements, or lack thereof, for cellular respiration. Some bacteria are **obligate aerobes**, always requiring oxygen for aerobic cellular respiration. Other bacteria are **obligate anaerobes**, never needing oxygen, generally not dividing, and in some cases being killed by exposure to oxygen. Finally, some bacteria are considered **facultative anaerobes**, requiring oxygen at times and not at other times.

BACTERIAL STRUCTURE

As compared to eukaryotic cells, the structure of bacteria is less complex due to a lack of membrane-bound organelles. Some structures, such as the cytoplasm and ribosomes, have the same structure and function as they do in eukaryotic cells. Table 8.1 shows the major structures present in bacterial cells as well as their functions. These structures can also be seen in Figure 8.1.

BACTERIAL SHAPES

Most bacteria have shapes that correspond to one of three typical conformations. These shapes and organization amongst cells can be used as diagnostic features. The shapes exhibited by most bacteria are as follows:

➤ **Cocci**: are circular in shape; they may exist singly, in pairs (diplococci), in clusters (staphylococci) or in chains (streptococci).

➤ **Bacilli**: are rod or oblong shaped; they may occur in chains.

➤ **Spirilli**: have a spiral shape.

Table 8.1:   Major Bacterial Structures

Structure	Function
Cytoplasm	Liquid portion of the cell where chemical reactions occur
Ribosomes	Protein synthesis
Chromosome	Contains the genes needed to produce proteins required for the cell. The bacterial chromosome consists of a single loop of DNA located in the nucleoid region of the cell.
Plasmids	Some bacterial cells contain small additional loops of DNA called plasmids. The plasmids often contain genes to code for resistance.
Cell wall	Most bacteria have a cell wall that contains peptidoglycan. The cell wall is found on the outer surface of the cell membrane. The cell wall typically can occur in one of two conformations, which can be identified using the Gram staining method. Some bacteria are Gram positive, with their cell wall consisting of a single layer of peptidoglycan, while other bacteria are Gram negative, having two layers in their cell wall: one layer of peptidoglycan and another layer of lipids.
Capsule and slime layers	The capsule is a layer of sugars and proteins on the outer surface of some bacterial cells. It forms a sticky layer that can help the cell attach to surfaces.
Flagella	Bacteria may have a single flagellum, multiple flagella or no flagella. Those with one or more flagella are motile as the flagella rotate to propel the cell. The bacterial flagella are different from eukaryotic flagella in structure. Bacterial flagella consist of the protein flagellin in a hollow, helical conformation which anchors into the cell membrane. A proton pump in the membrane provides power to rotate each flagellum.
Pili	Pili are tiny proteins that generally cover the surface of some types of bacterial cells. They assist the cell in attaching to surfaces.
Spores	A few species of bacteria are capable of creating spores when environmental conditions are not favorable. When bacteria exist in spore form, they are capable of surviving adverse conditions for years. When conditions become favorable again, the spores germinate into the vegetative cell form again.

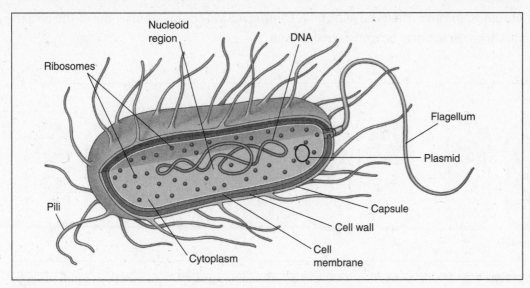

FIGURE 8.1: Bacterial structure. Bacterial cells lack membrane-bound organelles but have a variety of cell structures.

MECHANISMS FOR BACTERIAL REPRODUCTION

Bacteria lack the structures needed to perform mitosis, and because they only have a single chromosome they really do not have a need for cell division as complex as mitosis. Instead, bacteria divide by the process of **binary fission**. It involves the replication of the single loop of DNA, a copy of which is then provided to each of two daughter cells. This process can occur fairly quickly, in some cases as often as once every 20 minutes. Because bacteria are unicellular, creating a new cell means creating a new organism. This process qualifies as asexual reproduction, as each division produces genetically identical offspring. The only way to introduce variation into the population is by mutation, conjugation, or transformation.

Bacterial Conjugation

Some bacteria have another means of passing genetic material to other bacteria. During the process of **conjugation** seen in Figure 8.2, one bacterial cell may copy its **plasmid** to be passed to another cell. The most commonly studied type of plasmid to be passed is called the F plasmid or F factor (the F standing for fertility). In order to pass the plasmid to another cell, a physical connection must be established. This connection is referred to as the **sex pilus** and it is made by the cell that contains the plasmid (termed the male or F+). The sex pilus connects to a cell lacking the plasmid (the female or F−) and serves as a bridge to pass a copy of the plasmid to the female. Once complete, both cells are male and contain the plasmid. Using conjugation provides a rapid mechanism to pass plasmids within a population. Occasionally, plasmids become integrated into the chromosome and when the plasmid is transferred via conjugation, some of the bacterial chromosome may be transferred as well.

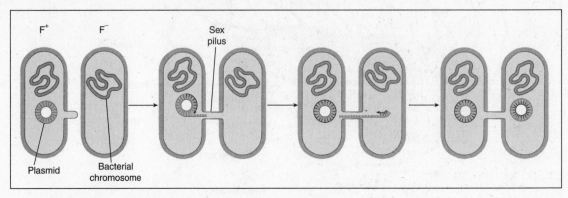

FIGURE 8.2: During conjugation, a bacterial cell containing a plasmid forms a sex pilus, which allows for the transfer of a copy of the plasmid to another bacterial cell that is lacking the plasmid.

Because many plasmids encode for resistance to things such as antibiotics, rapid conjugation can quickly render an entire bacterial population resistant to a particular antibiotic under the right selective pressures. This phenomenon has important medical significance, in that an antibiotic is used to kill bacteria causing infections, and if the bacteria are resistant to that antibiotic it is useless in stopping the infection. Some bacteria are resistant to multiple antibiotics as a result of picking up several plasmids via conjugation.

Bacterial Transformation

Another way that bacteria can pick up genetic variations is through **transformation**. Some bacteria are able to pick up DNA from their environment and incorporate it into their own chromosomal DNA. Bacteria that are able to pick up foreign DNA are termed competent. While some bacteria are naturally competent, others can be coerced to develop competence by artificial means within the lab.

BACTERIAL GENE EXPRESSION AND REGULATION

Just like other organisms, bacteria go through the processes of transcription and translation. The regulation of bacterial gene expression is primarily by **operons,** seen in Figure 8.3, which control the access of RNA polymerase to the genes to be transcribed primarily via repressor proteins. There are many different operons that have been described, but they all have certain basic features:

➤ A **promoter** sequence on the DNA where RNA polymerase must bind. If the promoter is inaccessible, the gene will not be transcribed.

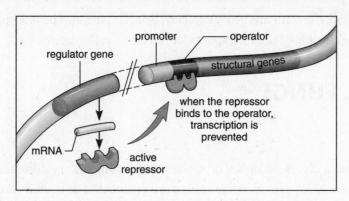

FIGURE 8.3: The operon system is used to regulate gene expression in prokaryotic cells.

➤ An **operator** sequence on the DNA where a repressor protein can bind, if present. When a repressor is bound to the operator, the promoter sequence will be blocked such that RNA polymerase cannot access the site.
➤ A **regulator** gene that produces a repressor protein when expressed.
➤ **Structural** genes, which are the actual genes being regulated by the operon.

Operons come in two basic categories: inducible and repressible. **Inducible operons** are normally "off" while **repressible operons** are normally "on." In an inducible operon, the repressor always binds to the operator so that transcription is always prevented unless an inducer molecule is present. When the inducer is present, it binds to the repressor, preventing the repressor from binding to the operator. This allows transcription to occur. In repressible operon systems, the repressor is always inactive such that transcription always occurs. Only when a corepressor is present to interact with the repressor can transcription be inhibited. When the repressor and corepressor are bound, they can then interact with the operator site and prevent access by RNA polymerase, thus turning off transcription.

THE BACTERIAL GROWTH CYCLE

Bacteria have a typical growth cycle that is limited by environmental factors as well as the amount of nutrients available. The growth cycle consists of the following stages:
➤ **Lag:** There is an initial lag in growth that occurs when a new population of bacteria begins to reproduce. This lag time is normally brief.
➤ **Logarithmic growth:** As bacteria begin to perform binary fission at a very rapid rate, logarithmic growth occurs. This can only last for a limited amount of time.
➤ **Stationary phase:** As the number of bacteria increase, resources decrease and while some bacteria are still dividing, some are dying, which evens out the population count.
➤ **Decline:** As the population hits its maximum, the lack of nutrients, along with the presence of a variety of toxins, means that the population will begin to decline—

more cells will die than are being replaced by cell division. The few species of bacteria that are capable of making spores would do so at this point.

PART II. FUNGI

FUNGI

Fungi constitute a diverse number of species within the Eukarya domain. Some fungi are unicellular, such as yeasts, while others are multicellular, such as mushrooms and molds. Many are harmless, while some are pathogenic. All are heterotrophs, gaining their nutrients from other organisms. They secrete enzymes that break down organic molecules to a small enough size that they can be absorbed through the cell membrane. They may do this by feeding on dead and decaying organisms or by parasitic relationships with living organisms.

Basic Fungal Structure

While some fungi such as yeasts are unicellular, most are multicellular and fairly complex, as seen in Figure 8.4. Within a multicellular fungus, the **mycelium** is the structure that grows near food sources in order to obtain nutrients for the fungus. Within the mycelium, there are **hyphae,** filaments where the nucleus of each cell is located. Other structures such as those needed for reproduction are present, yet their structure will be different depending on the species of fungus. In fact, fungi are classified according to their reproductive structures and mechanisms of reproduction.

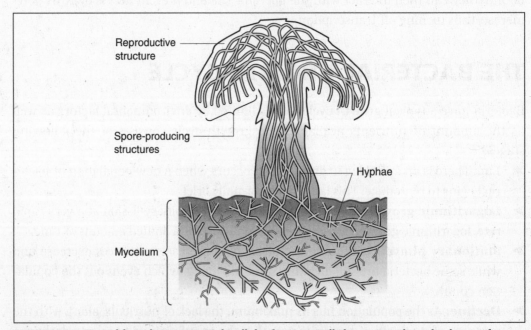

FIGURE 8.4: Typical fungal structure. Multicellular fungi typically have a mycelium, hyphae, and reproductive structures.

Life Cycles and Reproduction of Fungi

Depending on the species, fungi are able to reproduce sexually, asexually, or sometimes by both methods. During asexual reproduction, **spores** are formed in specialized structures in the fungus and perform mitosis to generate offspring. The structure of spores used for fungal reproduction is very different from that of the spores used as survival structures in certain species of bacteria. In some cases, fungal spores are not used at all and the cells fragment to form new cells in the process of budding.

Sexual reproduction is a less common means of reproduction in fungi and often occurs only when environmental conditions are poor. During sexual reproduction, gametes are made by specialized structures in the fungus. The two gametes fuse, leaving a diploid cell which performs meiosis and produces haploid spores.

Fungal Classification

Fungi are classified according to their method of reproduction. The following are the major groups of fungi:

➤ **Yeasts**: single celled, reproduce by budding.
➤ **Ascomycetes**: the "sac fungi" that contain asci, which are sacs that contain haploid spores; most yeasts and some molds fall in this group.
➤ **Basidomycetes**: the "club fungi" which form basidia (club-shaped structures) that contain haploid spores; all reproduction is sexual via conjugation and nuclear fusion; mushrooms are an example.
➤ **Zygomycetes**: perform sexual reproduction by gamete fusion, meiosis, and the production of haploid spores; most bread molds fall into this group.
➤ **Chytrids**: produce flagellated spores; most species are parasites or decomposers that live in water.
➤ **Deuteromycetes**: the "imperfect fungi"; always reproduce asexually (or at least a sexual reproductive phase cannot be identified).
➤ **Lichens**: formed from an interaction between a fungus and a photosynthesizer such as algae.

PART III. VIRUSES

VIRUSES

Viruses are a unique biological entity in that they do not resemble typical cells nor are they classified into any of the domains previously discussed. There is debate whether viruses are living organisms at all, because they are unable to reproduce without a host cell; nor can they perform many of the functions associated with living organisms without the help of a host. Because viruses lack typical cell structures such as organelles, they are much smaller than any form of prokaryotic or eukaryotic cells.

While some viruses contain more sophisticated structures, the only items required for a virus are a piece of genetic material, either DNA or RNA, and a protective protein coating for the genetic material. The viral **genome** (a collection of all the genes present) can consist of only a few genes or can range up to a few hundred genes. Viruses are categorized as animal viruses, plant viruses, or bacteriophages.

Viral Life Cycles

Viruses are specific to the type of host cell that they infect. In order for a virus to infect a cell, that cell must have a receptor for the virus. If the receptor is absent, the cell cannot be infected by the virus. While it seems odd that cells would evolve receptors for viruses, it is usually a case of mistaken identity. The viruses can actually mimic another substance for which the cell has a legitimate need and thus has a receptor for. The process of viral infection is seen in Figure 8.5.

Once a virus binds to a receptor on the membrane of the host cell, the viral genetic material enters the host either by injecting itself across the cell membrane or by being taken in via endocytosis. At some point, the viral genes will be transcribed and translated by the host cell. The nucleic acid of the virus will also be replicated. Eventually new viruses will be produced and released from the host cell. Because each virus contains a copy of the original genetic material, they should all be genetically identical. Mutations are the primary way to induce variation into the viral population.

Animal Viruses

As the name implies, animal viruses are designed to infect the host cells of various animals. Their genetic material may be DNA or RNA depending on the virus. Animal viruses are usually categorized according to the type of nucleic acid they possess, as well as whether the nucleic acid is single-stranded or double-stranded. Once the DNA or RNA of the virus is taken in by the host cell, the virus may immediately become active, using the host cell machinery to transcribe and translate the viral genes. New viruses are assembled and released from the host cell. The release of new viruses can be via **lysis** of the cell membrane, which immediately kills the host cell, or by **budding,** where the new viruses are shipped out of the host cell via exocytosis. Budding does not immediately kill the host cell but may eventually prove fatal to the host. Once the new viruses are released from the original host cell, they seek out new host cells to infect.

Alternatively, the virus may become **latent**, integrating itself into the chromosomes of the host cell, where it may stay for varying amounts of time. Eventually, the latent virus will excise from the host chromosome, and it will become active to produce and release new viruses. Some viruses are capable of alternating between active and latent forms multiple times. Infections caused by specific herpes viruses, such as cold sores and genital herpes, are notorious for alternating between active and latent forms.

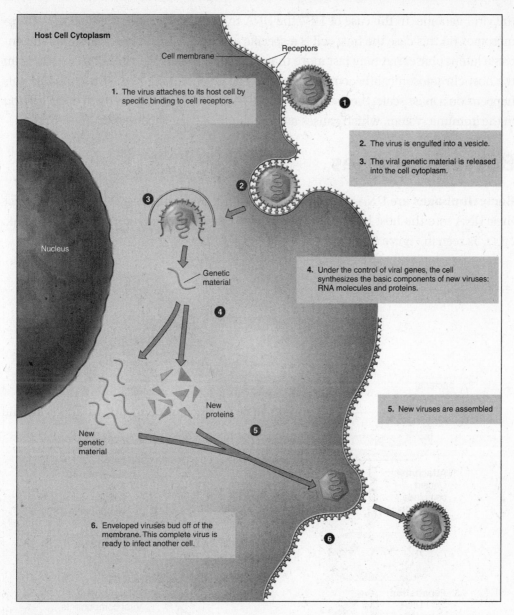

FIGURE 8.5: Viral infection.

Retroviruses

Retroviruses are a unique category of RNA viruses. The Human Immunodeficiency Virus (HIV) was the first retrovirus to be discovered. The key characteristic of retroviruses is that they enter the cell in RNA form that must be converted to DNA form. This is the opposite of the normal flow of information in the cell, which dictates that DNA produces RNA during transcription. The process of converting viral RNA backwards into DNA is called reverse transcription and is achieved by an enzyme called **reverse transcriptase**. This enzyme is encoded for on the viral genome. When the retrovirus enters the host cell, its RNA is immediately transcribed and one result of this is the production of reverse transcriptase. The reverse transcriptase then produces a DNA copy of the viral genome. In the case of HIV, the DNA then integrates into the host cell's chromosomes (in this case the host cell is a specific cell type in the immune system) and enters a latent phase that may last more than ten years. When the viral DNA excises from the host chromosome, it becomes active and begins producing new viruses. When this happens on a mass scale, the death of host cells will signal the beginning of deterioration in the immune system, which causes acquired immunodeficiency syndrome (AIDS).

Bacteriophages

Bacteriophages are DNA viruses that exclusively infect bacteria. They always inject their DNA into the host bacterial cell and then enter either a lytic cycle or a lysogenic cycle, as seen in Figure 8.6.

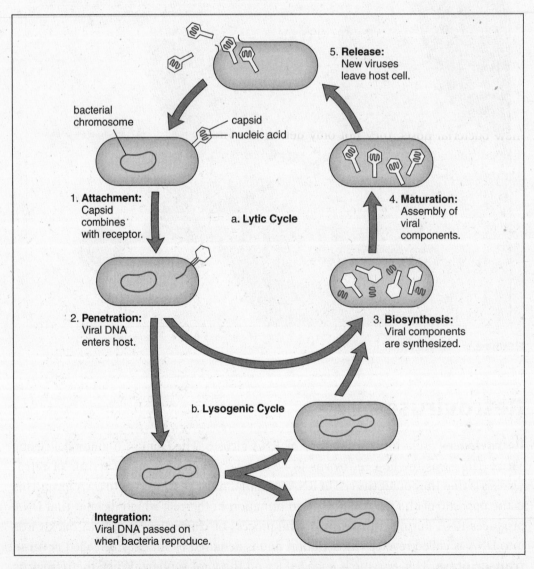

FIGURE 8.6: Bacteriophage life cycles. (*a*) In the lytic cycle, viral particles are released when the cell is lysed. (*b*) In the lysogenic cycle, viral DNA integrates into the host cell chromosome. The lysogenic cycle can be followed by the lytic cycle.

THE LYTIC CYCLE

A bacteriophage that uses the **lytic cycle** immediately activates once in its host to produce viral proteins and replicate viral nucleic acid. New viruses are synthesized and leave the host cell via lysis, always killing their bacterial host. The new viruses then go out and infect new host cells.

THE LYSOGENIC CYCLE

The **lysogenic cycle** is a variation that some viruses use. Viral DNA injected into the host integrates into the bacterial chromosome. The viral DNA may stay integrated for varying lengths of time. Each time the bacterial cell divides by binary fission, the progeny receive a copy of the viral genome. Eventually, the viral DNA that has integrated into the chromosome will excise and enter the lytic cycle, releasing new viruses and killing the host.

TRANSDUCTION

When new viruses are being packaged in a bacterial host, sometimes portions of the bacterial chromosome get packaged with the new viruses. When these viruses infect new bacterial hosts, they not only deliver the viral genome but also some bacterial genes that can recombine with the new host's chromosome. This is the process of **transduction**.

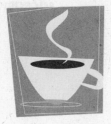

CRAM SESSION

Microbiology

➤ Organisms in the domains Bacteria and Archaea consist of prokaryotic cells. Archaea have unique habitats and unusual cell structures that differentiate them from bacteria.

➤ Bacteria are classified based on how they obtain nutrients and energy. Phototrophs perform photosynthesis while chemotrophs do not. Autotrophs use carbon dioxide as a carbon source while heterotrophs receive carbon from a source other than carbon dioxide.

➤ Bacteria contain a variety of structures that assist in their ability to attach to surfaces and survive adverse conditions. The bacterial structures can be reviewed in Table 8.1.

➤ Bacteria come in the following shapes: cocci, bacilli, and spirilli.

➤ Reproduction in bacteria is by binary fission. Mutation, conjugation, and transformation serve as mechanisms to introduce variation into bacterial populations.

➤ Bacterial gene expression is controlled by the operon system. The genes of repressible operons are always expressed unless a repressor and corepressor block the operator sequence. The genes of inducible operons are never expressed unless an inducer removes the repressor from the operator sequence.

➤ Bacterial population growth is limited by environmental factors.

➤ Fungi can be unicellular or multicellular, and always consist of eukaryotic cells. Their classification is based on their methods of reproduction and reproductive structures, such as spores.

➤ Fungal reproduction can involve asexual and sexual reproductive cycles. Certain fungi have haploid and diploid phases of the life cycle.

➤ Viruses can exhibit complex structures, but many are simplistic in nature.
   ➤ The two required materials for a virus are a piece of genetic material (either DNA or RNA) and a protective protein coat.

➤ Viruses are specific in that they can only infect host cells that have a receptor for that virus.

➤ Animal viruses may take over the host cell immediately following infection or become latent, integrating into the chromosomes of the host.

➤ Retroviruses are a unique class of animal viruses. They are latent viruses that use RNA as their genetic material.
   ➤ The viral genome codes for the production of reverse transcriptase, which allows the virus to convert itself to DNA form, enabling it to insert into the host-cell chromosomes.

➤ Bacteriophages are viruses that infect bacteria. They can enter the lytic or lysogenic cycles.
   ➤ Viruses in the lytic cycle immediately take over their host, produce new viruses, and kill the host as the cell is lysed to release new viruses.

- ➤ Viruses that enter the lysogenic cycle insert into the bacterial chromosome and are transmitted to all progeny during binary fission. The bacteriophage eventually excises and enters the lytic cycle.
- ➤ Transduction occurs when a virus in the lysogenic cycle excises from the bacterial chromosome, taking a portion with it. The new viruses that are packaged contain viral DNA and bacterial DNA that can be transferred to new host cells.

Human Anatomy and Physiology

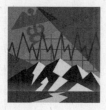

PART I. THE NERVOUS SYSTEM AND SENSES

THE NERVOUS SYSTEM

The nervous system has the daunting task of coordinating all of the body's activities. The **central nervous system** (CNS) is composed of the brain and spinal cord. The **peripheral nervous system** (PNS) is composed of any nervous tissue located outside of the brain and spinal cord. **Nerves** are the primary structures within the PNS. In order to understand the functioning of the CNS and PNS, it is necessary to look at the detailed function of neurons.

Neurons

The basic structure of neurons can be seen in Figure 9.1. **Sensory** (afferent) **neurons** exist in the PNS and direct their messages towards the CNS, while **motor** (efferent) **neurons** exist in the PNS and direct their messages away from the CNS. **Interneurons** are found only in the CNS. While neurons perform the critical function of transmitting messages throughout the body, there are also a large number of **glial cells** present in the nervous system. Glial cells provide support to neurons and are capable of mitosis, unlike mature neurons. The major structures within the neuron are as follows:

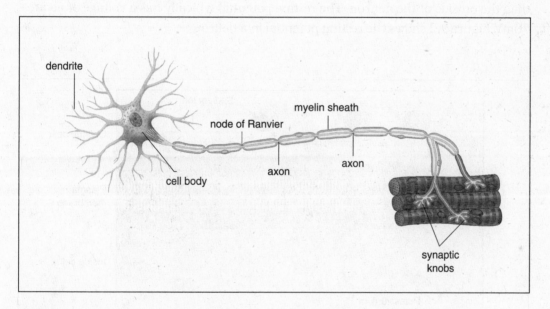

FIGURE 9.1: Neuron structure. A typical neuron consists of dendrites, a cell body, and an axon.

➤ **Dendrites**: projections that pick up incoming messages
➤ **Cell body**: processes messages and contains the nucleus and other typical cell organelles
➤ **Axon**: carries electrical messages down its length
➤ **Synaptic knobs**: occur at the ends of an axon; where electrical impulses are converted to chemical messages in the form of neurotransmitters
➤ **Myelin** sheath: produced by **Schwann cells** (specialized glial cells) that surround the axon of some neurons; there are gaps between the myelin called **nodes of Ranvier**
➤ **Synapse**: the space between the synaptic knobs of one neuron and the dendrites of another neuron

RESTING POTENTIAL

The **resting potential** is the state of the neurons when they are not generating messages. It requires the maintenance of an unequal balance of ions on either side of the membrane to keep the membrane polarized. The resting potential requires a great deal of ATP to maintain.

During resting potential, **sodium-potassium (Na$^+$/K$^+$) pumps** within the membrane of the axon are used to actively transport ions into and out of the axon. The Na$^+$/K$^+$ pumps bring two K$^+$ ions into the axon while sending out three Na$^+$ ions. This results in a high concentration of Na$^+$ outside the membrane and a high concentration of K$^+$ inside the membrane. There are also many negatively charged molecules, such as proteins, within the neuron, so that ultimately the inside of the neuron is more negative than the outside of the neuron. The resting potential typically has a voltage of about −70mV. Figure 9.2 shows the resting potential in a neuron.

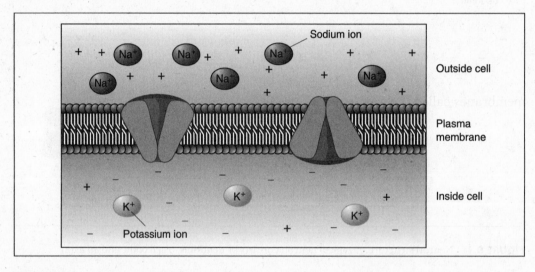

FIGURE 9.2: During resting potential, the Na$^+$/K$^+$ pump is used to maintain an unequal balance of ions inside and outside the cell.

ACTION POTENTIAL

In order to transmit a message, the resting potential of the neuron must be disrupted and depolarized so that the inside of the cell becomes slightly less negative. In order for this **action potential** to occur, a threshold voltage of about −50mV must be achieved. Once the action potential has initiated, **voltage-gated channels** in the membrane of the axon will open. Specifically, Na$^+$ channels open, allowing Na$^+$ to flow passively across the membrane into the axon in a local area. This local flow of Na$^+$ causes the next Na$^+$ channel to open. This continues down the length of the axon towards the synaptic knobs like a wave. While the speed of the axon potential can vary depending on the axon diameter and whether the axon is myelinated or not, its strength cannot. Action potentials are an all-or-nothing event.

As soon as the Na$^+$ channels open and depolarize a small area of the axon, K$^+$ channels open allowing K$^+$ to leak passively out of the axon. This restores the more negative charge within the axon, temporarily preventing the initiation of another action potential during a refractory period. The Na$^+$/K$^+$ pump can then be used to completely restore the resting potential by repolarization.

Communication between Neurons

Each neuron specializes in specific types of **neurotransmitters** and contains vesicles full of them within its synaptic knobs. When an action potential reaches the synaptic knobs and calcium is present, the vesicles containing neurotransmitters fuse with the membrane by exocytosis and release their contents to the synapse. The neurotransmitter will bind to the receptors on the postsynaptic neurons.

The Central Nervous System

The CNS is composed of the **brain** and **spinal cord**. The brain and spinal cord both consist of many neurons and supporting glial cells. **White matter** within the brain and spinal cord consists of myelinated axons. **Gray matter** consists of clusters of cell bodies of neurons. Cranial bones and vertebrae protect the CNS, as do protective membranes called the **meninges**. Between the meninges, and within cavities of the brain, there is **cerebrospinal fluid**. This fluid has some critical functions, such as providing nutrients, removing wastes, and providing cushioning and support for the brain.

STRUCTURE AND FUNCTION OF THE BRAIN

The brain processes conscious thought and sensory information, it coordinates motor activities of skeletal muscle and other organ systems within the body, and it maintains vital functions such as heart rate and ventilation. The brain can be divided into the structures seen in Figure 9.3: **cerebrum**, **cerebellum**, **brain stem**, and **diencephalon**.

The cerebrum in particular has extremely diverse functions. The right and left hemispheres process information in different ways. The right side of the brain tends to specialize in spatial and pattern perception, while the left side of the brain tends to specialize in analytical processing and language. The connection of the two hemispheres via the **corpus callosum** is essential to integrating the functions of both sides of the brain.

The functions of each of the parts of the brain including the cerebrum can be seen in Table 9.1.

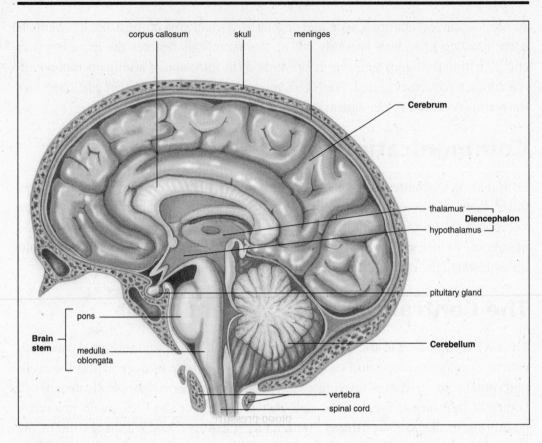

FIGURE 9.3: Brain structure. The cerebrum of the brain is divided into right and left hemispheres connected by the corpus callosum.

The Spinal Cord and Reflex Actions

The spinal cord serves as a shuttle for messages going towards and away from the brain. It also acts as a reflex center that can process certain incoming messages and provide an autonomic response without processing by the brain.

A **reflex arc** is a set of neurons that consists of a receptor, a sensory neuron, an interneuron, a motor neuron, and an effector. The receptor transmits a message to a sensory neuron, which routes the message to an interneuron located in the spinal cord. The interneuron processes the message in the spinal cord and sends a response out through the motor neuron. The motor neuron passes the message to an effector, which can carry out the appropriate response.

The Peripheral Nervous System

The PNS is composed of pairs of nerves that are bundles of axons. There are 12 pairs of **cranial nerves** branching off the brain stem and 31 pairs of **spinal nerves** branching off the spinal cord. The nerves that exist in the PNS are categorized into one of two divisions: the **somatic nervous system** or the **autonomic nervous system**.

Table 9.1:   Major Structures of the Brain and Their Functions

Structure	Function
Cerebrum	The cerebrum is the largest portion of the brain; it is divided into a right and left hemisphere as well as into four lobes (frontal, parietal, occipital, and temporal). Within the cerebrum there are specific areas for each of the senses, motor coordination, and association areas. All thought processes, memory, learning, and intelligence are regulated via the cerebrum. The cerebral cortex is the outer tissue of the cerebrum.
Cerebellum	The cerebellum is located at the base of the brain. It is responsible for sensory-motor coordination for complex muscle movement patterns and balance.
Brain stem	The brain stem is composed of several structures; it ultimately connects the brain to the spinal cord.
	➤ The pons connects the spinal cord and cerebellum to the cerebrum and diencephalon. ➤ The medulla oblongata (or medulla) has reflex centers for vital functions such as the regulation of breathing, heart rate, and blood pressure. Messages entering the brain from the spinal cord must pass through the medulla. ➤ The reticular activating system (RAS) is a tract of neurons that runs through the medulla into the cerebrum. It acts as a filter to prevent the processing of repetitive stimuli. The RAS is also an activating center for the cerebrum. When the RAS is not activated, sleep occurs.
Diencephelon	The diencephalon is composed of two different structures.
	➤ The hypothalamus is used to regulate the activity of the pituitary gland in the endocrine system. In addition, the hypothalamus regulates conditions such as thirst, hunger, sex drive, and temperature. ➤ The thalamus is located near the hypothalamus and serves as a relay center for sensory information entering the cerebrum. It routes incoming information to the appropriate parts of the cerebrum.

The somatic nervous system controls conscious functions within the body such as sensory perception and voluntary movement due to innervation of skeletal muscle. The autonomic nervous system controls the activity of involuntary functions within the body in order to maintain homeostasis. The autonomic nervous system is further subdivided into the **sympathetic** and **parasympathetic** branches. Most internal organs are innervated by both branches. The sympathetic branch is regulated by acetylcholine, epinephrine, and norepinephrine. When activated, the sympathetic branch produces the fight or flight response, in which heart rate increases, ventilation increases, blood pressure increases, and digestion decreases.

The parasympathetic branch is antagonistic to the sympathetic branch and is the default system used for relaxation. Generally, it decreases heart rate, decreases ventilation rate, decreases blood pressure, and increases digestion. The neurotransmitter acetylcholine is the primary regulator of this system.

PART II: MUSCULAR AND SKELETAL SYSTEMS

MUSCULAR TISSUE

Muscles provide structural support, help maintain body posture, regulate openings into the body, assist in thermoregulation via contractions (shivering) that generate heat, and contract to help move blood in veins towards the heart, assisting in peripheral circulation. Skeletal and cardiac muscle is striated, while smooth muscle is not. Cardiac and smooth muscles are involuntary, while skeletal muscle is under voluntary control.

Skeletal Muscle

The cells in **skeletal muscle** have multiple nuclei as the result of the fusing of multiple cells. The muscle cells also contain high levels of mitochondria to provide ATP needed for contraction and the protein **myoglobin** that acts as an oxygen reserve for muscles.

STRUCTURAL ORGANIZATION OF SKELETAL MUSCLE

Muscles are a bundle of muscle cells held together by connective tissue, as seen in Figure 9.4. The muscle cells have **sarcoplasm** (cytoplasm), a modified endoplasmic reticulum called the **sarcoplasmic reticulum**, and a cell membrane called the **sarcolemma** that interacts with the nervous system via the **transverse tubule system** (T tubule). This system provides channels for ion flow through the muscle and has anchor points for sarcomeres. Within the muscle cells are bundles of muscle fibers called myofibrils made of the proteins actin, troponin, tropomyosin, and myosin. **Actin** fibers

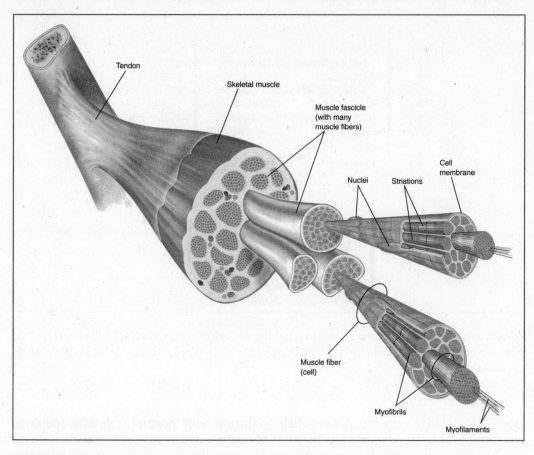

FIGURE 9.4: Skeletal muscle structure. Skeletal muscles are composed of bundles of muscle cells or fibers. Each fiber is composed of myofibrils, which are in turn composed of myofilaments.

have a thin diameter and associate with the proteins **troponin** and **tropomyosin** to produce thin filaments. **Myosin** fibers have a thick diameter with protruding heads and are called thick filaments. In skeletal muscles, the actin and myosin fibers overlap each other in highly organized, repeating units called **sarcomeres**. The overlapping of the fibers is what leads to striation of the muscle. The shortening of sarcomeres is what causes muscle contraction. The structure of a sarcomere can be seen in Figure 9.5.

The Sliding Filament Model

Muscle tissues have regions where the sarcolemma is in contact (via a synapse) with the synaptic knobs of a motor neuron from the somatic branch of the peripheral nervous system. This area is the neuromuscular junction. A neurotransmitter called **acetylcholine** is released from the motor neuron and binds to receptors on the sarcolemma, causing the initiation of an action potential that will result in shortening of the sarcomeres.

The action potential that occurs based on stimulation from the motor neuron will cause the release of calcium from the sarcoplasmic reticulum into the sarcoplasm. The

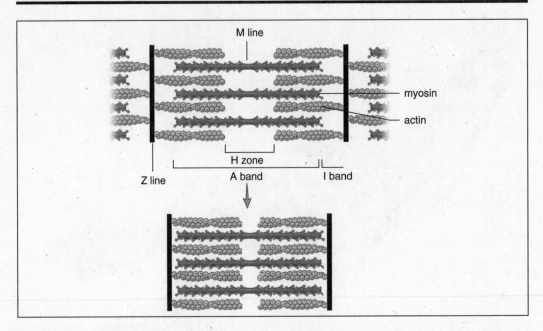

FIGURE 9.5: Sarcomere structure. Shortening of the sarcomere occurs when actin filaments cove toward the center of the sarcomere. The shortening of the sarcomere is responsible for skeletal muscle contraction.

calcium binds to the troponin in the thin filaments, which causes a conformational shift in the tropomyosin protein in the thin filament. This change in shape allows for the exposure of myosin binding sites on the actin. The myosin heads can now bind to the myosin binding sites on the actin forming crossbridges. Hydrolysis of ATP allows for the powerstroke to occur, which pulls the thin filaments towards the center of the sarcomere. The release of the myosin heads from the actin will occur when another ATP binds to the myosin heads. Calcium again exposes the myosin binding sites on actin so that the myosin heads can bind and the powerstroke can occur. The process repeats, each time pulling the thin filaments closer in towards the center of the sarcomere.

Smooth Muscle

Smooth muscle can be found in many parts of the body, including the bladder, digestive tract, and reproductive tract, as well as surrounding blood vessels. The cells that compose smooth muscle contain a single nucleus, as opposed to the multiple nuclei found in skeletal muscle. Smooth muscle contains actin and myosin but it is not organized as sarcomeres, which is why smooth muscle lacks striations. The actin and myosin slide over each other; this process is regulated by calcium and also requires energy provided by ATP. The autonomic branch of the peripheral nervous system innervates smooth muscle via sympathetic and parasympathetic stimulation, producing involuntary contractions. Smooth muscle can perform **myogenic activity,** meaning it can contract without stimulation from the nervous system.

Cardiac Muscle

Cardiac muscle is only found in the myocardium of the heart. It is striated due to the presence of sarcomeres, but is not multinucleated like skeletal muscle. Cardiac muscle is innervated by the autonomic branch of the peripheral nervous system. Like smooth muscle, it can also perform myogenic activity, contracting without stimulation from the nervous system.

THE SKELETAL SYSTEM

The human skeleton, shown in Figure 9.6, is an **endoskeleton** divided into two major parts: the **axial skeleton** and the **appendicular skeleton**. The skull, vertebrae, and rib cage compose the axial skeleton, while the pelvic and shoulder girdles and limbs in the body are part of the appendicular skeleton. The skeleton is used for protection of internal organs, support, storage of calcium and phosphates, production of blood cells, and movement. The skeleton itself is made of bones and associated cartilage.

Cartilage structure

Cartilage is a connective tissue. The matrix is termed **chondrin** and the primary cell type is the **chondrocyte**. During embryonic development, the skeleton begins as cartilage. During the developmental period, much of the cartilage is subject to **ossification,** whereby it is turned into bone by calcification. The primary areas where cartilage is found in the adult skeleton are the nose, ears, discs between vertebrae, rib cage, joints, and trachea. Cartilage is unique in that it contains no blood vessels, nor is it innervated.

Bone Structure

Bone tissue occurs as compact bone and spongy bone. **Compact bone** is very dense, while **spongy bone** is less dense and contains marrow cavities. Within marrow cavities, there is yellow and red bone marrow. **Red bone marrow** contains the stem cells that differentiate into red blood cells, white blood cells, and platelets. **Yellow bone marrow** is primarily a reserve for adipose (fat) tissue.

Long bones within the body have a characteristic structure. The ends of the bone are typically covered in cartilage and are termed the **epiphyses**. The ends are made primarily of spongy bone covered in a thin layer of compact bone. The shaft of the bone (the **diaphysis**) is made of compact bone surrounding a marrow cavity. The **epiphyseal plate** is a disc of cartilage that separates the diaphysis from each epiphysis; this is where bone lengthening and growth occurs. The **periosteum** surrounds the bone in a fibrous sheath and acts as a site for the attachment of muscles via **tendons**.

The microscopic structure of bone consists of the matrix that is found within **osteons,** illustrated in Figure 9.7. There is a **Haversian canal** within each osteon that contains

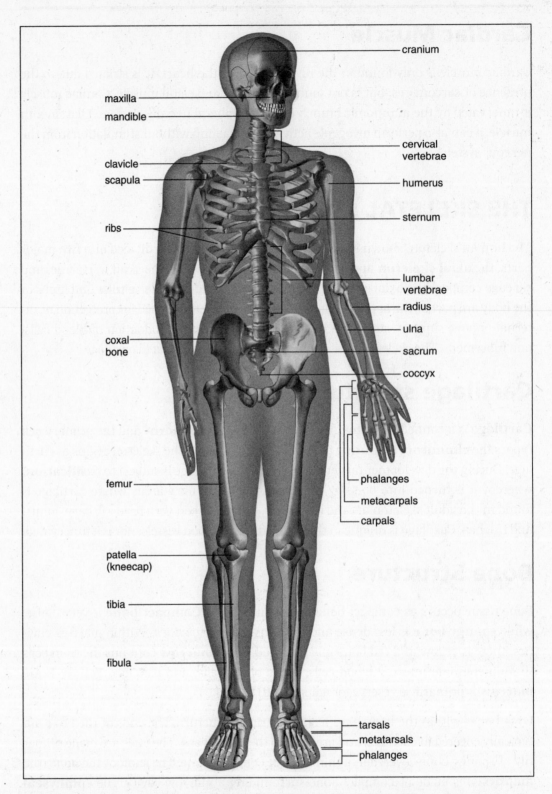

FIGURE 9.6: The human skeleton. The axial skeleton is composed of the skull, vertebral column, sternum, and ribs. The remaining bones in the body are part of the appendicular skeleton.

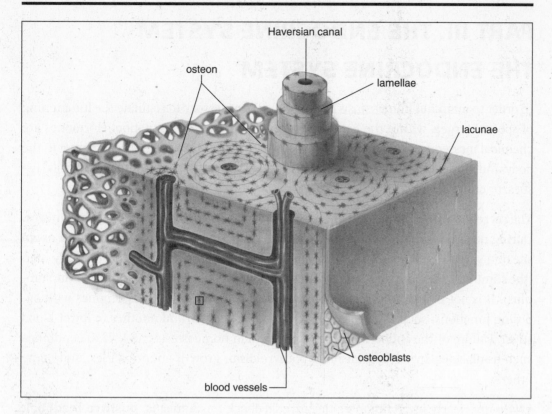

FIGURE 9.7: Bone tissue structure.

blood vessels, nerves, and lymphatic vessels. The canal is surrounded by **lamellae**, which are concentric circles of hard matrix. Within the matrix of the lamellae, there are small spaces called **lacunae** where mature bone cells reside.

Bone Cells

Within the bone, there are three major cell types: osteocytes, osteoblasts, and osteoclasts. The **osteocytes** are found within the lacunae of osteons. They are mature bone cells involved in the maintenance of bone tissue. **Osteoblasts** and **ostoeclasts** are found within bone tissue as well, and are immature cells involved in **bone remodeling**. Osteoblasts build bone by producing components of the matrix, while osteoclasts break down bone in the process of bone reabsorption. Eventually, osteoblasts and osteoclasts will become trapped within matrix of bone tissue and become osteocytes. Osteoblasts are also responsible for bone growth and ossification during development.

The hormones calcitonin from the thyroid gland and parathyroid hormone from the parathyroid glands are responsible for the process of bone remodeling. The levels of blood calcium must be carefully regulated, as calcium is needed for muscle contraction, nervous system communication, and other functions.

PART III. THE ENDOCRINE SYSTEM
THE ENDOCRINE SYSTEM

In order to maintain homeostasis in the body, it is necessary to regulate the functioning of specific targets within the body. **Hormones** achieve this regulation. Hormones are chemical messengers secreted into the bloodstream that travel to a specific target in the body and change the functioning of that target. The target can be individual cells, tissues, or entire organs.

The secretion of hormones is usually regulated via **negative feedback** mechanisms. During negative feedback, the response of the endocrine system or a target is the opposite of a stimulus. For example, if the level of a specific hormone gets particularly high (the stimulus), then the secretion of that hormone will be reduced (opposite of the stimulus). It is not uncommon to see **antagonistic hormones**—two hormones with opposing functions, such as a hormone to raise blood sugar and another to lower blood sugar. Failure of the endocrine system to maintain homeostasis can lead to conditions such as diabetes, hyperthyroidism, hypothyroidism, growth abnormalities, and many others.

While not nearly as common as negative feedback mechanisms, **positive feedback** mechanisms do exist. In this case, the stimulus causes actions in the body, regulated by hormones, that further amplify that stimulus moving the body away from homeostasis. Positive feedback mechanisms are short-lived and eventually homeostasis is regained via lack of stimulus.

The **hypothalamus** in the brain is the main link between the endocrine and nervous systems. The hypothalamus monitors body conditions and makes changes as needed. It produces regulatory hormones that influence glands such as the pituitary, which in turn regulates other glands in the endocrine system.

Endocrine Glands

Hormones are generally secreted from an **endocrine gland** into the bloodstream. The endocrine system is composed of endocrine glands located throughout the body. The major endocrine glands can be seen in Figure 9.8.

Hormone Specificity

The specificity of hormones is based on their interaction with a receptor on the target cells. Only cells that have a receptor for a specific hormone will be affected by that hormone. Once a hormone binds to the receptor, the cell's functioning will be changed in some way. These changes can involve gene expression, chemical reactions, membrane changes, metabolism, and so forth. Because the hormones must travel through the blood, making these changes is a relatively slow process.

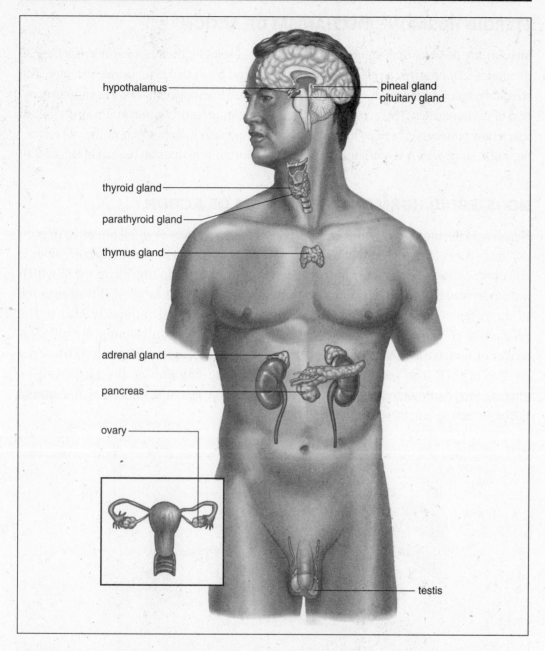

hypothalamus

pineal gland
pituitary gland

thyroid gland

parathyroid gland

thymus gland

adrenal gland

pancreas

ovary

testis

FIGURE 9.8: The endocrine system. Anatomic location of major endocrine structures of the body.

There are two major categories of hormones: **steroids** (which are lipid-soluble) and **non-steroids** (which are water-soluble and classified as **peptides**). Steroid hormones are derivatives of **cholesterol,** while nonsteroid hormones are made of modified amino acids or small proteins. The target cell receptors for steroid hormones exist in the cytoplasm of the cell, while the receptors for nonsteroid hormones exist on the cell membrane of the cell.

A third category of chemical messengers is the **prostaglandins**. These are lipid-based molecules released from cell membranes. Prostaglandins function as a sort of local hormone involved in functions as diverse as regulation of body temperature, blood clotting, the inflammatory response, and menstrual cramping caused by uterine contractions.

STEROID HORMONE MECHANISM OF ACTION

Steroids are derivatives of cholesterol that are lipid soluble; they can easily cross the cell membrane. Once inside a cell, the steroid locates and binds to a cytoplasmic receptor. The steroid-receptor complex moves into the nucleus and interacts with DNA to cause activation of certain genes. This serves as the signal to initiate transcription and translation, so that a new protein is expressed by the cell. This new protein will change how the cell is functioning in some way. A visual summary of steroid hormone action can be seen in Figure 9.9.

NONSTEROID HORMONE MECHANISM OF ACTION

Nonsteroid hormones are composed of amino acid derivatives or small proteins; they do not cross the cell membrane. The hormone itself is termed a **first messenger**, since it will never enter the cell; it only triggers a series of events within the cell, many of which are moderated by **G proteins** found in the cell membrane. The binding of the hormone to the receptor initiates a series of reactions in the cell that ultimately lead to the production of a **second messenger** molecule within the cell. A common second messenger of nonsteroid hormones is **cyclic adenosine monophosphate** (cAMP), a derivative of ATP. The second messenger changes the function of the target cell by altering enzymatic activities and cellular reactions. A visual summary of nonsteroid hormone action can be seen in Figure 9.10.

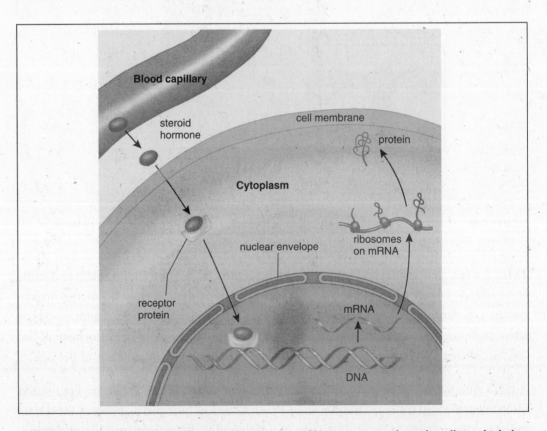

FIGURE 9.9: Steroid hormone mechanism of action. Steroid hormones act only on the cells in which they find their receptors in the cytoplasm of the cell.

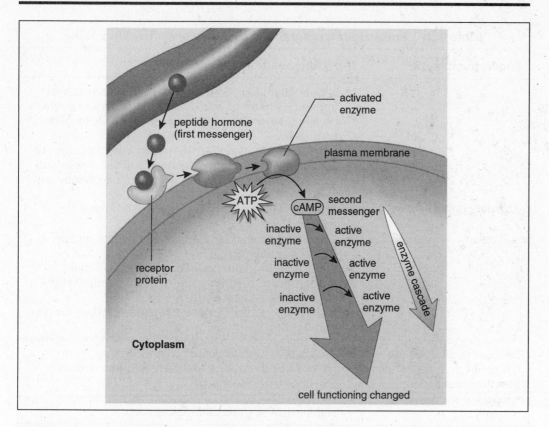

FIGURE 9.10: Nonsteroid hormone mechanism of action. Nonsteroid (peptide) hormones serve as first messengers and find their receptors on the cell membrane of the cell.

Major Endocrine Glands and Their Products

The major endocrine glands of the body include the hypothalamus, pituitary gland (separated into the anterior lobe and posterior lobe), pineal gland, thyroid gland, parathyroid glands, and adrenal glands. Some organs within the body also have endocrine functions and these include the thymus gland, ovaries, testes, pancreas, heart, placenta, kidneys, stomach, and small intestine.

The hypothalamus and pituitary gland have a unique relationship based on their proximity to each other in the brain. The pituitary gland secretes many hormones, some of which influence the secretion of hormones from other endocrine glands. The regulatory hormones made by the hypothalamus control the secretion of hormones from the anterior pituitary. The hypothalamus produces releasing hormones that stimulate the release of anterior pituitary hormones, as well as inhibiting hormones which inhibit the release of hormones from the anterior pituitary. The hypothalamus also makes antidiuretic hormone and oxytocin, but both are stored and released from the posterior pituitary.

Table 9.2 lists the major hormones and the glands that produce them. Unless marked otherwise, each of these hormones is a nonsteroid.

Table 9.2: Endocrine Structures and the Hormones that They Make	
Endocrine structure	**Hormones made and function**
Anterior pituitary	➤ Follicle stimulating hormone (FSH): in women, stimulates the secretion of estrogen in the ovaries and assists in egg production via meiosis; in men, has a role in sperm production ➤ Luteinizing hormone (LH): in women, stimulates the production of estrogen and progesterone by the ovaries and causes ovulation; in men, is involved in testosterone secretion from the testes ➤ Thyroid stimulating hormone (TSH): stimulates the thyroid gland ➤ Growth hormone (GH): stimulates growth of muscle, bone, and cartilage ➤ Prolactin (PRL): stimulates the production of milk ➤ Adrenocorticotropic hormone (ACTH): stimulates the cortex of the adrenal glands ➤ Endorphins: act on the nervous system to reduce the perception of pain
Posterior pituitary (these hormones are made by the hypothalamus but are released by the posterior pituitary)	➤ Antidiuretic hormone (ADH): allows for water retention by the kidneys and decreases urine volume; also known as vasopressin ➤ Oxytocin (OT): causes uterine contractions during childbirth; also stimulates milk ejection
Pineal gland	➤ Melatonin: influences patterned behaviors such as sleep, fertility, and aging
Thyroid gland	➤ Thyroid hormones (TH): regulate metabolism throughout the body; also act on the reproductive, nervous, muscular, and skeletal systems to promote normal functioning; T3 and T4 require iodine to function properly ➤ Calcitonin (CT): influences osteoblasts, which build bone in response to high blood calcium levels; ultimately lowers blood calcium levels
Parathyroid glands	➤ Parathyroid hormone (PTH): influences osteoclasts, which break down bone in response to low blood calcium levels, ultimately increasing blood calcium levels; antagonistic to CT
Adrenal medulla (inner portion of the adrenals)	➤ Epinephrine: released in response to stress; causes fight or flight response; also known as adrenaline ➤ Norepinephrine: released in response to stress; causes fight or flight response; also known as noradrenaline
Adrenal cortex (outer portion of the adrenals)	➤ Glucocorticoids*: help cells convert fats and proteins into molecules that can be used in cellular respiration to make ATP; high levels inhibit the inflammatory response of the immune system; examples are cortisol and cortisone ➤ Mineralocorticoids*: increase sodium retention and potassium excretion by the kidneys; an example is aldosterone ➤ Gonadocorticoids*: secreted in small amounts; examples are androgens and estrogens

Thymus	➤ Thymopoietin: stimulates the maturation of certain white blood cells involved with the immune system (T cells); decreases with age as the thymus gland atrophies ➤ Thymosin: stimulates the maturation of certain white blood cells involved with the immune system; decreases with age as the thymus gland shrivels
Ovaries	➤ Estrogen*: involved in the development of female secondary sex characteristics as well as follicle development and pregnancy ➤ Progesterone*: involved in uterine preparation and pregnancy
Testes	➤ Testosterone*: a type of androgen needed for the production of sperm as well as for the development and maintenance of male secondary sex characteristics
Pancreas	➤ Insulin: decreases blood sugar after meals by allowing glucose to enter cells to be used for cellular respiration; a lack of insulin or lack of response by cell receptors to insulin is the cause of diabetes mellitus; made by the beta islet cells ➤ Glucagon: increases blood sugar levels between meals by allowing for the breakdown of glycogen; antagonistic to insulin; made by the alpha islet cells
Heart	➤ Atrial natriuretic peptide (ANP): made by the heart to lower blood pressure
Kidneys	➤ Renin / angiotensin: Used to regulate blood pressure by altering the amount of water retained by the kidneys ➤ Erythropoietin (EPO): stimulates the production of red blood cells from stem cells in the red bone marrow
Stomach	➤ Gastrin: released when food enters the stomach; causes the secretion of gastric juice needed to begin the digestion of proteins
Small intestine	➤ Cholecystokinin (CCK): stimulates the release of pancreatic digestive enzymes to the small intestine; also stimulates the release of bile from the gallbladder to the small intestine ➤ Secretin: stimulates the release of fluids from the pancreas and bile that are high in bicarbonate to neutralize the acids from the stomach
Placenta (temporary organ during pregnancy)	➤ Human chorionic gonadotropin (HCG): signals the retention of the lining of the uterus (endometrium) during pregnancy ➤ Relaxin: releases ligaments attaching the pubic bones to allow for more space during childbirth ➤ Estrogen: needed to maintain pregnancy ➤ Progesterone: needed to maintain pregnancy

*steroid hormones

PART IV. THE CARDIOVASCULAR SYSTEM
THE CARDIOVASCULAR SYSTEM

The cardiovascular system in humans consists of a four-chambered **heart** to pump blood and a series of vessels needed to transport blood in the body. **Blood** is a connective tissue used to deliver oxygen, nutrients, water, hormones, and ions to all the cells of the body. It is also used to pick up the carbon dioxide and wastes produced by cells and to move these to the appropriate areas for elimination. Further, it assists in thermoregulation in the body as well as fighting infectious agents. The cardiovascular system is closely linked to the following organ systems in the body:

➤ the respiratory system, for the elimination of carbon dioxide, the pickup of oxygen, and assistance regulating blood pH

➤ the urinary system, for the filtration of blood, removal of nitrogenous wastes, regulation of blood volume and pressure, and regulation of blood pH

➤ the digestive system, for the pick up of nutrients to be distributed to the body

The critical functions of the cardiovascular system are achieved by blood transported through the system. For this reason, the composition of blood needs to be examined more closely.

Blood

Blood consists of a liquid matrix, plasma, and formed elements or cells. Humans contain between 4 and 6 liters of blood; this entire volume can be circulated through the body in less than one minute. The pH of blood is 7.4 (slightly basic), and the temperature is slightly warmer than body temperature. Because blood is warmer than the body, changing patterns of circulation can help distribute heat to where it is needed in the body.

Vasoconstriction decreases the diameter of vessels keeping blood closer to the core to warm the body, while **vasodilation** increases the diameter of the vessels, allowing them to release heat towards the surface of the skin to cool the body.

PLASMA

Plasma is the liquid portion of the blood; it makes up approximately 55 percent of the total volume of blood. The primary component of plasma is water. In order to adjust the volume of blood in the body, the water levels of plasma can be altered. This is one role for the kidneys. They can retain or release water via urine to adjust the blood volume. An increase in blood volume will increase blood pressure, while a decrease in blood volume will decrease blood pressure.

In addition to water, plasma also contains nutrients, cellular waste products, respiratory gases, ions, hormones, and proteins. There are three classes of plasma proteins produced by the liver. **Immunoglobulins** are primarily used in the immune response, **albumins** are used to transport certain molecules within the blood, and **fibrinogen** is an inactive form of one protein that is needed to clot blood.

FORMED ELEMENTS

The **formed elements** or cells of the blood are all derived from stem cells in the bone marrow. The three types of cells that are found within the blood are **erythrocytes** (red blood cells), **leukocytes** (white blood cells), and **thrombocytes** (platelets). The **hematocrit** value of blood is a relative comparison of cell volume to plasma volume. The percentage of blood occupied by cells is called the hematocrit value. It is generally about 45. Because red blood cells are by far the most abundant blood cell, hematocrit values are primarily influenced by red blood cells.

Erythrocytes

Erythrocytes are the most abundant type of blood cell. As they mature from stem cells in the bone marrow, they do something odd; they lose their organelles. Without organelles, these cells are unable to perform aerobic cellular respiration and they cannot perform mitosis to replace themselves. Further, they only live about 120 days, at which point they are destroyed by the liver and spleen. The end product of red blood cells' hemoglobin breakdown is **bilirubin,** which is ultimately excreted into the small intestine via bile from the liver. In order to make new red blood cells, more stem cells in the bone marrow must be coerced to differentiate into red blood cells by the hormone **erythropoietin** (EPO). Red blood cells also have an unusual biconcave disc shape that provides them with increased surface area and the ability to be flexible as they move through small vessels.

Transport of Gases

The critical component of red blood cells is the protein **hemoglobin**. Each cell contains about 250 million hemoglobin molecules. Functional hemoglobin consists of four protein chains each wrapped around an iron (heme-) core. This molecule is capable of carrying four molecules of oxygen (O_2). In total, a single red blood cell can carry about a billion O_2 molecules.

As hemoglobin binds to one oxygen molecule, a conformational change in the shape of hemoglobin occurs to allow for the loading of the next three O_2. The same process occurs during the unloading of O_2. Once O_2 is unloaded in the capillary beds of the body, some of the CO_2 produced by the cells will be carried by hemoglobin. Carbon dioxide combines with water to produce carbonic acid, which dissociates into **hydrogen ions** and **bicarbonate ions.** The hemoglobin carries the hydrogen ions while the bicarbonate ions are carried by plasma. The **Bohr effect** states that increasing concentrations of hydrogen ions (which decrease blood pH) and increasing concentrations of carbon dioxide will decrease hemoglobin's affinity for O_2. This allows O_2 to unload from hemoglobin into tissues of the body such as muscle when CO_2 levels are high in tissues. In the lungs, a high level of O_2 will encourage the dissociation of hydrogen ions from hemoglobin, which will join with bicarbonate ions in the plasma to form CO_2 and water. The CO_2 will be exhaled. The enzyme **carbonic anhydrase** catalyzes the formation and disassociation of carbonic acid.

Leukocytes

Leukocytes are a diverse collection of cells, all of which are derived from stem cells in the red bone marrow; all of them function within the immune system. They are found in much lower levels than red blood cells; however, the white blood cell level can fluctuate greatly, particularly when a person is fighting infection. White blood cells can be categorized in the following manner, based on their microscopic appearance:

➤ **Granulocytes** have cytoplasm with a granular appearance. These cells include **neutrophils**, **basophils**, and **eosinophils**. Neutrophils are used to perform phagocytosis. Basophils and eosinophils are involved in inflammation and allergies.

➤ **Agranulocytes** have cytoplasm that does not have a grainy appearance. They include **monocytes**, which mature into **macrophages**, and **lymphocytes**, which are further subdivided into T cells and B cells. Monocytes and macrophages perform phagocytosis, while lymphocytes function as the specific defenses of the immune system.

Thrombocytes

Thrombocytes or platelets are fragments of bone marrow cells called **megakaryocytes**. Platelets only live 10–12 days once mature, so they are replaced often. During injury to blood vessels, a complex series of reactions is initiated. The platelets release **thromboplastin** which converts an inactive plasma protein, **prothrombin**, to the active form, **thrombin**. Thrombin then converts **fibrinogen** to **fibrin**. Fibrin forms a meshwork around the injury that serves to trap other cells, forming a clot. The process of blood clotting requires multiple plasma proteins as well as calcium and vitamin K.

Blood Vessels

Blood flow progresses in unidirectional loops, as illustrated in Figure 9.11. One loop is the **systemic circuit,** which moves blood from the heart, throughout the body, and back to the heart. The other loop is the **pulmonary circuit,** which moves blood from the heart, to the lungs, and back to the heart.

Arteries are large blood vessels leaving the heart. The arteries have thick walls and are very elastic to accommodate blood pressure. As arteries leave the heart, they branch into smaller vessels called **arterioles**. The arterioles become more and more narrow, eventually forming the **capillaries,** which are the smallest vessels. **Capillary beds** are the site of gas exchange within tissues; they are so small that red blood cells have to line up single file to pass through them. Once gas has been exchanged, the capillaries widen and become **venules** that head back towards the heart. The venules become larger **veins,** which ultimately merge into the heart. Veins are not as thick-walled as arteries, since they do not have to deal with the forces exerted by blood pressure. While blood pressure pushes blood through arteries and arterioles, the

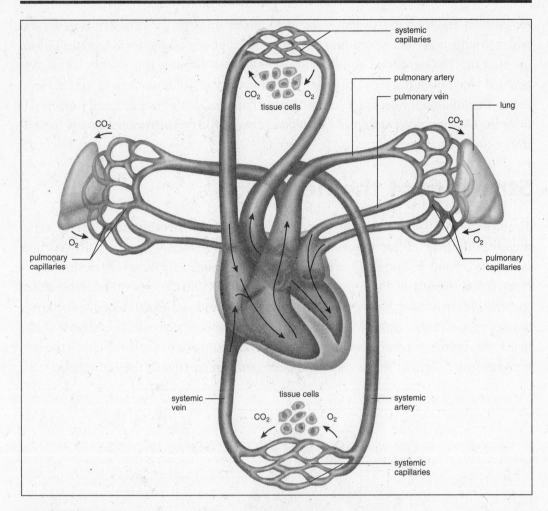

FIGURE 9.11: Blood flows through the body. The right side of the heart pumps blood to the lungs, where external respiration occurs, whereas the left side of the heart pumps blood to the body, where internal respiration occurs.

movement of blood in venules and veins is facilitated by muscles that contract to push the blood along and valves that close to prevent backflow of blood. **Vasoconstriction** and **vasodilation** of arteries serves as a means to regulate blood flow, pressure, and temperature.

The arteries of the systemic circuit branch off the left side of the heart and carry oxygenated blood to the capillaries of the body where gas exchange occurs. Deoxygenated blood returns to the right side of the heart via systemic veins. The pulmonary circuit involves pulmonary arteries that branch off the right side of the heart and carry deoxygenated blood towards the lungs. The pulmonary capillaries allow for gas exchange with the alveoli (air sacs) of the lungs. The newly oxygenated blood now moves back towards the left side of the heart via pulmonary veins.

CAPILLARY BEDS

A capillary bed is a collection of capillaries, all branching off a single arteriole, which serves a specific location in the body. The blood entering the systemic capillary bed is oxygenated and high in nutrients. As blood moves through the capillary bed, oxygen and nutrients must diffuse out into tissues and carbon dioxide and wastes must diffuse in. After this has happened, the capillaries merge into a venule that carries the deoxygenated blood back towards the heart. In pulmonary circulation, deoxygenated blood enters the pulmonary capillary bed where carbon dioxide diffuses out and oxygen diffuses in, causing oxygenation of the blood. **Precapillary sphincters** guard the entrance to the capillary beds.

Structure of the Heart

The structure of the heart can be seen in Figure 9.12. The **myometrium** is the cardiac muscle of the heart. Other tissues are present to compose supporting structures such as valves and chamber linings. The right and left side of the heart have very distinct functions. Blood essentially flows in two loops or circuits within the body. The right side of the heart receives deoxygenated blood from the body and pumps this blood to the lungs to be oxygenated. The right side is considered the pulmonary circuit. The left side of the heart receives oxygenated blood from the lungs and pumps it to the body. This is the systemic circuit. A fluid-filled sac called the **pericardium** surrounds the entire heart.

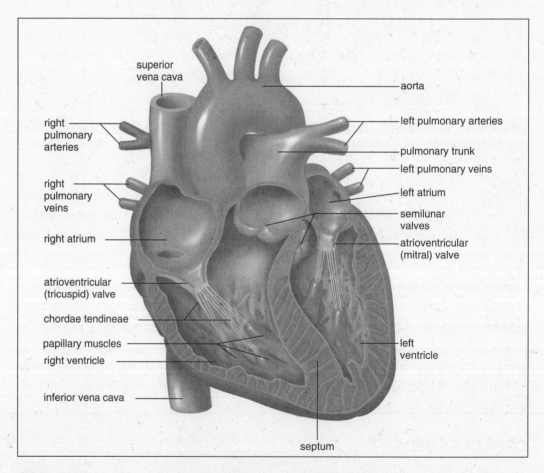

FIGURE 9.12: Heart structure. The vena cava carries deoxygenated blood into the right side of the heart. The aorta carries oxygenated blood out of the left side of the heart.

The right and left sides of the heart must be kept separate from each other. This is achieved by the septum, which is a thick barricade between the two sides of the heart. Each side of the heart has two chambers. The upper chamber is the **atrium** and the lower chamber is the **ventricle**. The atrium and ventricle are separated by **atrioventricular** (AV) **valves**. **Semilunar valves** regulate the flow of blood out of the ventricles.

The pulmonary circuit begins when veins within the body merge into the **venae cavae,** which lie on the dorsal wall of the thoracic and abdominal cavities. The superior vena cava comes from the head and neck, while the inferior vena cava comes from the lower extremities. These vessels carry deoxygenated blood and merge into the right atrium of the heart. As the atrium contracts, blood will pass through an AV valve (the **tricuspid valve**) into the right ventricle. As the ventricle contracts, blood passes through a semilunar valve (the **pulmonary semilunar valve**) into the **pulmonary arteries**. These arteries carry blood to the lungs and are the only arteries in the body that do not carry oxygenated blood. The pulmonary arteries branch into capillaries that surround the **alveoli** (air sacs) in the lungs. Gas exchange occurs to oxygenate the blood.

Once gas exchange has occurred, **pulmonary veins** carry the oxygenated blood towards the left side of the heart into the systemic circuit. The pulmonary veins in the body are the only veins to carry oxygenated blood. Blood reenters the heart through the left atrium. As the atrium contracts (in synch with contraction of the right atrium), blood is pushed through another AV valve (the **bicuspid valve**) to the left ventricle. When the ventricle contracts (similarly in synch with the right ventricle) the blood is pushed into the aorta via a semilunar valve (the **aortic semilunar valve**). The **aorta** is the largest artery in the body, running along the dorsal wall of the body next to the inferior vena cava. The aorta splits into arteries, arterioles, and eventually capillaries, where the blood is once again deoxygenated and must be pushed back to the right side of the heart to begin the process all over again.

The first branches off the aorta are the **coronary arteries,** which serve to provide circulation to the surface of the heart. Blockage of the coronary arteries can stop blood flow to the cardiac muscle, causing death of that muscle. This is characteristic of a heart attack. After blood flows through the coronary arteries, deoxygenated blood is returned to the right side of the heart by **coronary veins**.

REGULATION OF HEART RATE

Cardiac muscle is involuntary and has the ability to contract on its own without stimulation from the nervous system. The impulses that generate heart contraction have to be spread through the conducting system of the heart. The **sinoatrial** (SA) **node**, also known as the pacemaker, is a bundle of conducting cells in the top of the right atrium that initiates contractions. The SA node sends electrical impulses through the two atria, causing them to contract. The impulse arrives at the **atrioventricular** (AV) **node**. The impulse is spread through the **bundle of His** and through **Purkinje fibers** in the walls of the ventricles, causing ventricular contraction.

BLOOD PRESSURE

Blood pressure is a measurement of the force that blood exerts on the walls of a blood vessel. Typically it is measured within arteries, which have enough pressure to overcome the **peripheral resistance** of the arterioles and capillaries. It is expressed with two values: a systolic pressure and a diastolic pressure. The **systolic pressure** is the higher value and is the pressure exerted on arteries as the ventricles contract. The **diastolic pressure** is the lower number and is a measurement of pressure on the arteries during ventricular relaxation. The primary means of regulation of blood pressure is by regulation of blood volume through the kidneys. The higher the blood volume, the higher the blood pressure is.

PART V. THE RESPIRATORY SYSTEM

OVERVIEW OF THE RESPIRATORY SYSTEM

The respiratory system has the primary jobs of providing the body with oxygen and eliminating carbon dioxide. Pulmonary arteries, coming off the right side of the heart, carry deoxygenated blood, which is low in oxygen and high in carbon dioxide, to the lungs. Oxygen that enters the lungs will be distributed to hemoglobin in the erythrocytes within the capillaries that branch off the pulmonary arteries that surround the alveoli. Carbon dioxide will diffuse into the alveoli from the pulmonary arteries to be exhaled. Now blood is oxygenated and will travel back to the left side of the heart via pulmonary veins. In addition to oxygenating blood, the respiratory structures are responsible for pH regulation, vocal communication, the sense of smell, and protection from infectious agents and particles.

Structures of the Respiratory System

The respiratory system is essentially a series of tubes that conduct air into the alveoli located in the lung tissues. The major structures of the system can be seen in Figure 9.13. Air is inhaled through the nose or mouth. Because the respiratory system is an open system, it is particularly vulnerable to infection. In the nose and **pharynx** (back of the throat), air is warmed to body temperature, moisturized so that gas exchange can occur, and filtered. Both areas are covered with a mucous membrane that helps prevent desiccation of the tissues and collects particles and microbes that may enter the system. The nose is particularly well suited to filtration because it has cilia and hair to help trap substances that enter the respiratory system. While filtration in the nose and pharynx will not catch all particles, it will catch many of them. The nose has the additional function of olfaction.

Air flows into the nose or mouth and through the pharynx where there are two passageways: the **esophagus** and the **larynx.** During breathing, air will flow through the **glottis,** which is the opening of the larynx. The larynx is the voice box; it is made of

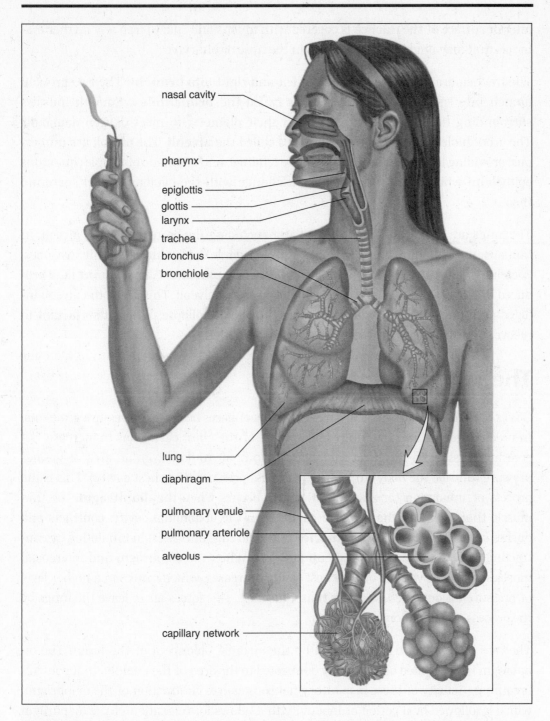

nasal cavity

pharynx

epiglottis
glottis
larynx
trachea
bronchus
bronchiole

lung

diaphragm

pulmonary venule

pulmonary arteriole

alveolus

capillary network

FIGURE 9.13: The respiratory system. Gas exchange occurs between the alveoli of the lungs and the surrounding capillaries.

cartilage and vocal cords that produce sound as they vibrate. Unless a person is swallowing, the esophagus will be closed off and the glottis will be open. But if a person is swallowing, a small piece of cartilage called the **epiglottis** will cover the glottis and stop food from entering the larynx.

As air flows through the larynx, it eventually makes its way into the trachea and the lower respiratory tract. The trachea is supported by C-shaped rings of cartilage. The interior surface of the trachea is covered with mucus and cilia to trap any further materials that may not have been caught in the nose or pharynx.

The trachea branches off towards the left and right into **bronchi**. The two bronchi branch into smaller and smaller tubes called the **bronchioles**. Smooth muscles surrounding the bronchioles can adjust their diameter to meet oxygen demands. The bronchioles terminate in tiny air sacs called the **alveoli**. The alveoli are numerous, providing lots of surface area for gas exchange, and are made of simple squamous epithelium which allows for easy gas exchange with the capillaries that surround them.

The lungs are a collection of resilient tissue including the bronchioles and alveoli. In humans, the right lung has three lobes of tissue, while the left lung has only two lobes. Each lung is surrounded by a fluid-filled **pleural membrane**. A **surfactant** fluid produced by the tissues decreases surface tension in the alveoli. This keeps the alveoli inflated and functioning, which helps prevent alveolar collapse. Without surfactant to relieve surface tension, the lungs are unable to function.

The Act of Ventilation

Gas exchange in the lungs results from the flow of gases because of pressure gradients. In order to get air into the lungs, the volume of the chest cavity has to increase, decreasing pressure in the chest cavity. This allows air to flow from an area of greater pressure (outside the body) to an area with less pressure (the chest cavity). This is the process of inhalation (or inspiration) and it occurs when the **diaphragm**, the thin muscle that separates the thoracic cavity from the abdominal cavity, contracts and pushes down. The **intercostal muscles** of the rib cage also assist in inhalation by contracting to help move the ribcage up and out. When the diaphragm and intercostal muscles relax, the volume of the chest cavity decreases, which results in a higher level of pressure inside the chest cavity than outside it. This forces air to leave the lungs by the process of exhalation (expiration).

The rate of ventilation is controlled by the medulla oblongata of the brain. The diaphragm is innervated and neurally connected to the area of the medulla that controls breathing. Activity of these inspiratory neurons causes contraction of the diaphragm, which is followed by a period of inactivity that allows for relaxation of the diaphragm and exhalation. In a relaxed situation, the diaphragm is stimulated between 12 and 15 times per minute. During times of increased oxygen demand and excessive carbon dioxide production, this rate can increase significantly. While it might be expected that oxygen levels are the primary influence on breathing rate, it turns out that the primary trigger is carbon dioxide levels, monitored by chemoreceptors located in the brain and certain large blood vessels. As carbon dioxide levels increase, the pH decreases (remember carbonic acid levels increase as carbon dioxide levels rise) and thus the breathing rate must increase to eliminate the excess carbon dioxide, which in turn increases the oxygen levels.

GAS EXCHANGE

The concentration of gases can be measured as **partial pressures**. After an inhalation, the amount of oxygen or partial pressure of oxygen in the alveoli is greater than the amount of oxygen or partial pressure in the capillaries surrounding the alveoli, which are branches of the pulmonary arteries. Gases will flow from an area of high concentration (partial pressure) to an area of low concentration (partial pressure), so oxygen will move from the alveoli into the capillaries and bind to hemoglobin. Further, immediately following inhalation, carbon dioxide levels will be low in the alveoli and high in the capillaries. Diffusion will move the carbon dioxide into the alveoli. At this point, the blood in the pulmonary capillaries is oxygenated and ready to move back to the left side of the heart via the pulmonary veins. The gases that diffused into the alveoli will be exhaled.

Carbon dioxide exchange has an important role in the maintenance of acid-base balance within the body. When carbon dioxide interacts with water, it forms carbonic acid. The carbonic acid is converted to the bicarbonate ion and hydrogen ions. The bicarbonate ions help buffer pH in the body. When the pH of the body becomes too alkaline, the reaction can be reversed. The bicarbonate and hydrogen ions join together to produce carbonic acid, which is then converted to water and carbon dioxide. The carbon dioxide is exhaled in order to adjust pH.

PART VI. THE DIGESTIVE SYSTEM
THE DIGESTIVE SYSTEM

The digestive system is designed to extract nutrients from food and eliminate wastes. The system is set up as a series of modified tubes to keep food and digestive enzymes sequestered from the body. It is also known as the **gastrointestinal** (GI) **tract.** In addition to the GI tract, there are several accessory structures (the liver, gallbladder, and pancreas) which perform functions vital to the digestive system. The GI tract and accessory structures can be seen in Figure 9.14.

The three primary components of the diet that require digestion are carbohydrates, proteins, and fats. The digestive system has the following functions: mechanical digestion of food achieved by chewing, chemical digestion of food achieved by assorted digestive enzymes, absorption of nutrients into the bloodstream, and elimination of waste products.

GENERAL STRUCTURE
OF THE DIGESTIVE SYSTEM

Any contact of the digestive enzymes with the rest of the body could actually result in the self -digestion of tissues. Further, the digestive system is an open system into which

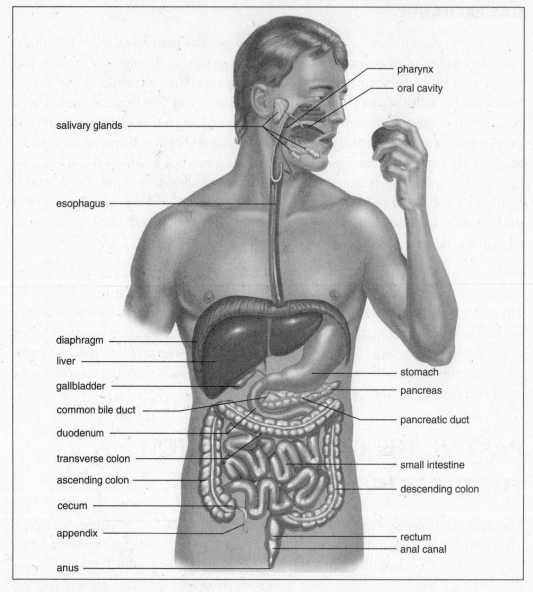

pharynx
oral cavity
salivary glands
esophagus
diaphragm
liver
gallbladder
common bile duct
duodenum
transverse colon
ascending colon
cecum
appendix
anus
stomach
pancreas
pancreatic duct
small intestine
descending colon
rectum
anal canal

FIGURE 9.14: The digestive system. The digestive system includes the gastrointestinal tract as well as the accessory structures of the liver and pancreas.

infectious organisms can enter. The contents of the system need to be kept away from the rest of the body. In order to ensure this, the digestive tubes are composed of four tissue layers, as follows:

➤ The **mucosa** layer is a mucous membrane that actually comes in contact with food. It serves as a lubricant and protects against desiccation, abrasion, and digestive enzymes. The mucosa lack blood vessels and nerve endings.

➤ The **submucosa** layer is below the mucosa. It contains blood vessels, lymphatic vessels, and nerve endings. Its primary function is to support the muscosa and to transport materials to the bloodstream.

➤ The **muscularis** layer is composed of two layers of smooth muscle that run in opposing directions. The nerve endings in the submucosa serve to stimulate the muscularis layer to produce contractions that propel food through the system. These muscular contractions are termed peristalsis.

➤ The **serosa** is a thin connective tissue layer that is found on the surface of the digestive tubing. Its purpose is to reduce friction with other surfaces in contact with the GI tract.

The Pathway of Food through the Digestive Tract

Food enters the digestive tract at the oral cavity. From there, it moves to the esophagus and then the stomach. Small bits of the stomach contents are released to the small intestine, which completes digestion with some help from secretions from the liver and pancreas. In the small intestine, nutrients are absorbed into the bloodstream. Finally, the waste products of digestion are solidified in the large intestine and are released.

THE ORAL CAVITY

As food is ingested and enters the mouth, three sets of salivary glands begin to secrete **saliva**. The teeth are responsible for mechanical digestion of food, breaking it into smaller pieces by chewing. As saliva mixes with the chewed food, chemical or enzymatic digestion begins. In addition to its lubricating function, saliva contains the digestive enzyme **amylase,** which begins the chemical breakdown of carbohydrates such as starch. Since food does not stay in the mouth for long, amylase rarely gets to complete its job in the oral cavity.

THE ESOPHAGUS

As food is ready to be swallowed, it must pass by the **pharynx**. Recall that the pharynx has two openings—one to the larynx and one to the esophagus. Normally, the esophagus is closed during breathing so that air passes through the larynx. When food touches the pharynx, a reflex action occurs that pushes the epiglottis over to cover the **glottis** of the **larynx**. This allows food to proceed down the esophagus. Once in the esophagus, muscular contractions will force the food towards the stomach by **peristalsis**.

THE STOMACH

The **stomach** is a relatively small, curved organ when empty but is capable of great expansion when full of food, due to the presence of many folds in its interior lining. The top and bottom of the stomach are each guarded by a muscular **sphincter**. The stomach is unique in that it has a very acidic environment; it must retain its own secretions. Tightly closing sphincters make sure this happens. The top sphincter opens to allow the bolus of food to enter. Once food is inside the stomach, it will be mixed with **gastric juice** for the purpose of liquefying it as well as initiating the chemical digestion of proteins. The hormone **gastrin** signals the gastric glands of the stomach to begin producing gastric juice as well as for the stomach to start churning. Gastric juice is composed of a mixture of mucus to protect the stomach lining from being digested itself, **pepsinogen,** which is an inactive form of the enzyme that digests protein, and hydrochloric acid, which is needed to activate the pepsinogen. The active form of pepsinogen is called **pepsin**. The hydrochloric acid secreted in the stomach provides an overall pH of 1–2, which is highly acidic. Normally a pH this low would denature enzymes, but pepsin is unusual in that it is inactive except at a low pH. The low pH of the stomach also kills most infectious agents that entered the digestive tract with the food.

As the food mixes with gastric juice, the resulting liquid is called **chyme**. Depending on the size and nutritional content of the meal, it takes on average about four hours for the stomach to empty its contents into the small intestine. The chyme leaves the stomach in small bursts as the bottom sphincter opens.

THE SMALL INTESTINE

The **small intestine** is a tube approximately six meters in length. Its primary job is to complete the chemical digestion of food and to absorb the nutrients into the bloodstream. The small intestine relies on secretions from the liver and pancreas to complete chemical digestion. As the bottom sphincter of the stomach opens, small amounts of chyme enter the top region of the small intestine, the **duodenum**. It is important to neutralize the acidity from gastric juice by the secretion of sodium bicarbonate from the pancreas into the small intestine. In addition to receiving secretions made from the pancreas, the duodenum also receives secretions from the liver. These secretions help with chemical digestion, which occurs in the middle region of the small intestine (the **jejunum**) and its the lower end (the **ileum**).

THE LIVER AND GALLBLADDER

The **liver** is composed of several lobes of tissue and is one of the larger organs in the body. The liver has countless functions. In the case of the digestive system, the liver produces **bile,** which is a fat emulsifier. While bile is not an enzyme, it helps break fats into smaller pieces so that they are more susceptible to digestion by enzymes secreted from the pancreas. Bile contains water, cholesterol, bile pigments, bile salts, and some ions. Bile from the liver is stored in the **gallbladder** (a small structure on the underside of the liver) and is released to the small intestine, based on signals from the hormones **secretin** and cholecystokinin (**CCK**), via the common bile duct as food enters the small intestine.

The liver has some other functions within the digestive system. After the absorption of nutrients, blood from the capillaries in the small intestine will travel directly to the liver via the hepatic portal vein. Once in the liver, the glucose levels of the blood will be regulated. When blood glucose levels get high, the liver will store the excess as glycogen under the influence of insulin. When blood sugar levels are low, the liver will break down glycogen to release glucose under the influence of glucagon. The liver will also package lipids in lipoproteins to allow them to travel throughout the body. The smooth endoplasmic reticulum within the liver can produce enzymes to detoxify certain harmful substances. The liver also stores vitamins A, E, D, and K (the fat-soluble vitamins). After these functions occur in the liver, blood reenters general circulation.

THE PANCREAS

The **pancreas** secretes pancreatic juice into the small intestine via the pancreatic duct. While the pancreas has cells involved in endocrine functions, producing insulin and glucagon, it also has exocrine cells that produce **pancreatic juice**. The pancreas secretes pancreatic juice when food enters the small intestine as signaled by the hormones secretin and CCK. Pancreatic juice contains the following elements:

➤ **Bicarbonate ions**: act as a neutralizer of stomach acid
➤ **Amylase**: completes carbohydrate (starch) digestion that began in the oral cavity to release glucose
➤ **Proteinases**: complete protein digestion that was started in the stomach to release amino acids; three specific proteinases—trypsin, chymotrypsin, and carboxypeptidase—found in pancreatic juice.
➤ **Lipase**: breaks down fats to fatty acids and glycerol
➤ **Nucleases**: break down DNA and RNA to nucleotides

ABSORPTION OF NUTRIENTS

Once the food has been exposed to the secretions of the pancreas, liver, and small intestine it is necessary to absorb the nutrients and eliminate the wastes. It can take anywhere from 3 to 10 hours for nutrients to be absorbed from the small intestine. The small intestine has an internal anatomy that makes it well suited for absorption, because of its tremendous surface area. The mucosa in the small intestine are folded into **villi,** which form the brush border. The villi are then further folded into microscopic **microvilli**. Within each villus, there are capillaries and a **lacteal** (a lymphatic capillary). Nutrients such as glucose and other simple sugars, amino acids, vitamins, and minerals diffuse into the capillaries within each villus, where they are carried into the bloodstream. The end products of fat digestion take another route. The fat products are assembled into a triglyceride and packaged in a special coating including cholesterol, which creates a **chylomicron**. These structures cannot diffuse into capillaries, so they enter the lacteals. The lymphatic fluids will carry the chylomicrons to the blood stream at the thoracic duct (a merger between the two systems).

THE LARGE INTESTINE

Now that the nutrients have been absorbed into the bloodstream, the remnants of digestion have made their way to the **large intestine**. Now water must be reclaimed by the body, which will in turn solidify the waste products. These waste products will be stored by the large intestine and released at the appropriate time. In addition, the large intestine contains a large population of **normal flora** or harmless resident bacteria. These bacteria are responsible for the synthesis of certain vitamins that the body needs.

The large intestine has a much larger girth than the small intestine, but it is shorter. The large intestine is about 1.5 meters long. There are four regions within the large intestine:

➤ The **cecum** is a small area where the large intestine connects with the small intestine on the right side of the body. There is an outgrowth of this area that constitutes the **appendix**. The appendix is a vestigial structure thought to play a noncrucial role in the lymphatic system.

➤ The **colon** constitutes the majority of the large intestine. The primary role of the colon is water absorption in order to solidify the feces. Vitamin absorption can also occur in the colon.

➤ The **rectum** is the ultimate destination for feces in the large intestine. Stretching of this area stimulates nerves and initiates the defecation reflex.

➤ The **anal canal** receives the contents of the rectum for elimination. There are two sphincters regulating exit from the anal canal. The first internal sphincter operates involuntarily and the second external sphincter is under voluntary control.

PART VII. THE URINARY SYSTEM

THE URINARY SYSTEM

The urinary system consists of the kidneys, which produce urine, and supporting tubing to store and eliminate urine from the body. The kidneys are the main excretory organ of the body; however, the skin can also act as an excretory organ. In addition to producing urine as a means of eliminating nitrogenous cellular waste products, the urinary system also regulates blood pressure by means of blood volume, adjusts blood pH, and regulates the osmotic concentrations of the blood.

Structures of the Urinary System

The two **kidneys** of the urinary system filter blood to produce urine. The urine then moves toward the bladder via two **ureter**s, tubes that connect each kidney to the **bladder**. Once urine moves to the bladder, it will be stored. Eventually, urine will leave the body through the **urethra**. The anatomy of the urethra is different in males and females. In males, the urethra is relatively long and must be shared with the reproductive system so that sperm can move through it when appropriate. In females, the urethra is shorter, and it is only used for urine passage. The structures of the urinary system can be seen in Figure 9.15.

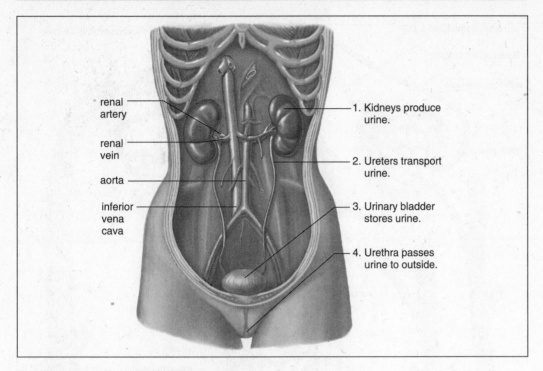

FIGURE 9.15: The urinary system. The kidneys produce urine, which is carried to the bladder by the ureters, where it is eliminated from the system.

Kidney structure

Since the kidneys are the workhorse of the urinary system, their structure and function need to be examined in more detail. The kidneys are placed along the dorsal surface of the abdominal wall, above the waist, and are secured by several layers of connective tissue including a layer of fat. Each kidney has an **adrenal gland** that is located on top of it.

The outer region of the kidney is the **renal cortex**, the middle portion is the **renal medulla**, and the inner portion is the **renal pelvis**. The kidneys are responsible for filtering blood, so they have an excellent blood supply. The **renal arteries** are branches off the aorta and carry blood into the kidneys while the **renal veins** carry blood away from the kidneys towards the inferior vena cava. The indentation where the ureter, renal artery, and renal vein attach to each kidney is the **renal hilus**.

NEPHRON STRUCTURE AND FUNCTION

Within the renal medulla of each kidney, there are triangular chunks of tissue called **renal pyramids**. Within these renal pyramids and extending into the renal cortex, there are about one million **nephrons** per kidney. The nephrons, shown in Figure 9.16, are microscopic tubules that actually produce urine. In reality a nephron is twisted along itself, but for ease of viewing the nephron drawing presented here has

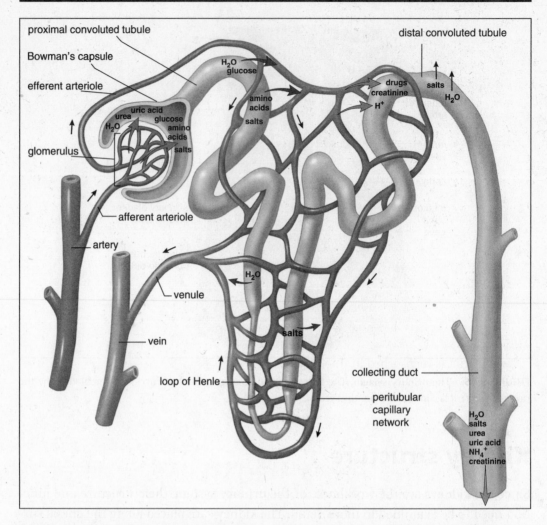

FIGURE 9.16: Nephron structure. Urine is produced as filtrate moves through the nephron. In reality, a nephron is twisted along itself, but for ease of viewing the nephron shown here has been untwisted.

been untwisted. Each nephron is surrounded by a network of capillaries. Any items leaving the nephron will be picked up by the capillaries and returned to the bloodstream. The important parts of the nephron are as follows:

➤ The **renal corpuscle** has two parts. The first is the **glomerulus** which is a network of capillaries. The glomerulus is surrounded by the **Bowman's capsule**. There is no direct connection between the glomerulus and the Bowman's capsule, but instead there is a space between the two. Afferent arterioles carry blood into the glomerulus where blood pressure pushes certain components of the blood into the Bowman's capsule. Efferent arterioles carry blood out of the glomerulus. Only components of the blood that are small (plasma components such as water, ions, small nutrients, nitrogenous wastes, gases, and others) should enter the Bowman's capsule; blood cells and plasma proteins should not. The materials that enter the Bowman's capsule are referred to as **filtrate,** and have approximately the same osmotic concentration as the plasma. A large percentage (approximately 99%) of filtrate that enters the nephron should be reabsorbed back into the bloodstream. Any components remaining in the nephron once filtration and reabsorption is complete will be lost as urine and will be much more concentrated than the plasma.

➤ The **proximal convoluted tubule** allows for the reabsorption of nutrients such as glucose and amino acids, water, salt, and ions. The majority of reabsorption occurs here.

➤ The **loop of Henle** also allows for reabsorption, primarily of salt (NaCl) and water by osmosis. A fairly complex **countercurrent multiplier system** is in effect in the loop of Henle. This area is a loop with a descending side and an ascending side located in close proximity to each other. Each limb of the loop has a different osmotic concentration. As salt is actively pumped out of the ascending limb, it creates a high osmotic pressure that draws water out of the descending limb via osmosis. Fresh filtrate then enters the loop of Henle, pushing the existing filtrate from the descending limb into the ascending limb. The process of pumping salt out of the ascending limb and the osmotic movement of water out of the descending limb is repeated several times.

➤ The **distal convoluted tubule** is where the fine tuning of filtrate concentration begins. Its activities are regulated by specific hormones described below. The more water that is reabsorbed in this section of the nephron, the more concentrated the urine, the lower the urine volume, and the higher the blood volume.

➤ The **collecting duct** can be shared by several nephrons. The remaining urine empties into the collecting duct where it will move towards the renal pelvis and ultimately into the ureters to be carried to the bladder. Hormones can also be used in the collecting duct to allow for the reabsorption of more water, concentrating the urine even more.

REGULATION OF BLOOD VOLUME AND PRESSURE

If **antidiuretic hormone** (ADH) is present, more water will be reabsorbed in the distal convoluted tubule and the collecting duct. This increases the concentration of urine and decreases urine volume. If **aldosterone** is present, more salt will be reabsorbed from the distal convoluted tubule and collecting ducts. Water will follow the movement of salt by osmosis. This results in an increased concentration of filtrate and a decrease in urine volume. Both ADH and aldosterone have the same effects on filtrate concentration. By increasing water reabsorption, blood volume is increased. The increase in blood volume is one way to increase blood pressure.

The secretion of ADH and aldosterone is regulated by renin produced by the kidneys. Renin secretion is triggered by low blood pressure in the afferent arterioles. Renin converts a protein made by the liver called **angiotensin I** into **angiotensin II**. Angiotensin II then triggers release of ADH by the posterior pituitary gland and aldosterone by the adrenal cortex.

One last hormone that alters nephron function is ANP (**atrial natiuretic peptide**), which is secreted by the heart. When the heart stretches due to elevated blood pressure,

ANP is released. ANP decreases water and salt reabsorption by the nephrons. This results in less concentrated urine, a higher urine volume, and a lower blood volume. The reduced blood volume means a decrease in blood pressure.

MAINTENANCE OF ACID-BASE BALANCE

As the kidneys filter blood, they also balance the pH of blood, which is one of their most important functions. Even a relatively minor change to blood pH can have drastic consequences, which is one of the reasons that kidney failure can be deadly. Luckily, **dialysis** methods are available to mimic normal kidney functions for patients whose kidneys do not work properly. Recall that carbon dioxide interacts with water to produce carbonic acid. Carbonic acid can then dissociate into hydrogen ions and bicarbonate ions, both of which influence pH. The pH of blood can be adjusted by changing the amount of bicarbonate ions reabsorbed and altering the amount of hydrogen ions retained in the nephron. When the blood pH drops and becomes acidic, more bicarbonate ions will return to circulation and hydrogen ions will be released in urine, which gives urine an acidic pH.

PROPERTIES OF URINE

The substances remaining at the end of the distal convoluted tubule or collecting duct constitute urine. Urine will always contain water, ions (such as Ca^{++}, Cl^-, Na^+, and K^+), and nitrogenous wastes. Depending on the diet and the functioning of other organs in the body, other components might be present in the urine. Because it was filtered directly from blood, the urine should be sterile. The presence of proteins, blood cells, or nutrients within the urine would be considered abnormal. The three primary nitrogenous wastes, all produced by cells, are as follows:

➤ **Urea**: As cells deaminate amino acids during protein metabolism, the resulting product is **ammonia,** which is highly toxic. The liver will convert ammonia to a less toxic waste called urea. The kidneys will concentrate urea and release it in the urine. Urea is the most abundant of nitrogenous waste products.

➤ **Uric acid**: During nucleic acid metabolism in the cell, uric acid is produced as the waste product.

➤ **Creatinine**: As muscle cells utilize creatine phosphate to produce ATP needed to fuel muscular contraction, creatinine is produced as a waste product.

Other Functions of the Kidneys

In addition to their role in blood filtration and urine production, the kidneys have two additional jobs. First, the kidneys act to convert vitamin D from the diet into an active form that can be used by the cells. The kidneys are able to convert vitamin D to **calcitriol,** which helps the body absorb calcium and phosphorous. Secondly, the kidneys secrete the hormone erythropoietin (EPO) which is used to stimulate red blood cell production in the red bone marrow.

PART VIII. THE LYMPHATIC AND IMMUNE SYSTEMS

THE LYMPHATIC SYSTEM

The **lymphatic system** consists of a series of vessels running throughout the body, lymph, and lymphoid tissue, as seen in Figure 9.17. The system serves to return fluids that were unclaimed at the capillary beds to the circulatory system, picks up chylomicrons from the digestive tract and returns them to circulation, and fights infection via leukocytes.

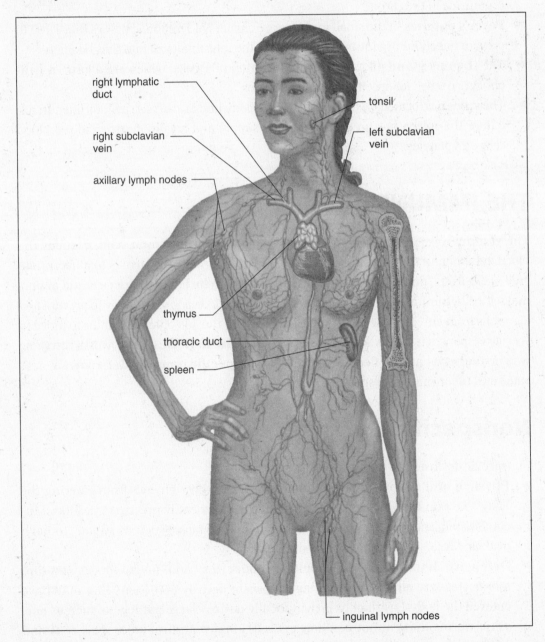

right lymphatic duct

tonsil

right subclavian vein

left subclavian vein

axillary lymph nodes

thymus

thoracic duct

spleen

inguinal lymph nodes

FIGURE 9.17: The lymphatic system is composed of vessels, lymph nodes, the tonsils, spleen, and thymus gland.

The vessels of the lymphatic system carry the fluid **lymph,** which has the same composition as plasma and interstitial fluid. Lymph moves through the vessels primarily due to the influence of muscular contractions that push it and valves that prevent its backflow. The lymphoid tissues within the system are as follows:

➤ **Lymph nodes** are swellings along lymphatic vessels that contain macrophages for phagocytosis of pathogens and cancer cells, and lymphocytes for immune defenses. The lymph is filtered through the nodes before moving on in the system. Clusters of lymph nodes exist in the neck, under the arms, and in the groin. Swelling of the lymph nodes is a sign of infection.

➤ **Tonsils** resemble a lymph node in their ability to prevent infection by pathogenic organisms in the throat.

➤ **Peyer's patches** in the small intestine are clusters of lymphatic tissues that serve to prevent infectious organisms from crossing the intestinal wall into the abdomen.

➤ The **thymus gland** allows for the maturation of T cells, which are a form of lymphocyte needed for specific immune defenses.

➤ The **spleen** is located on the left side of the body and also acts as a blood filter. In addition, the spleen has an excellent blood supply and acts to destroy old red blood cells and platelets.

THE IMMUNE SYSTEM

The immune system exists anywhere white blood cells are found. This includes the blood, lymph, and tissues of the body. The job of the immune system is to differentiate "self" cells from "nonself" (foreign cells) and to eliminate both foreign cells and abnormal self cells. Immune defenses begin with nonspecific responses that try to prevent foreign cells from entering the body and attack them if they do enter, and later to move to specific responses if needed. A **nonspecific immune defense** always works the same way, no matter what the offending invader, while **specific immune defenses** are activated and tailor-made to a specific invader.

Nonspecific Defenses

Nonspecific defenses come in several varieties:

➤ **Physical and chemical barricades** that prevent foreign cells from entering the body. The skin is an example of a barricade that generally prevents infection. Mucous membranes are another good barricade. Chemicals such as sweat, stomach acid, and lysozyme generally prevent infection.

➤ **Defensive leukocytes**: Neutrophils, monocytes, and macrophages (mature monocytes) are all capable of phagocytosis to destroy pathogens that may have entered the body. Eosinophils enzymatically destroy large pathogens such as parasitic worms that cannot be phagocytized. Finally, natural killer (NK) cells find self cells that seem to have odd membrane properties and destroy them. Cancerous cells are notorious for having altered cell membranes and are usually destroyed by NK cells.

➤ **Defensive proteins**: In the case of viral invaders, infected cells can secrete proteins called **interferons**. A virally infected cell releases these proteins as messengers to other cells that are yet to be infected. This limits the spread of the virus within the body by signaling uninfected cells to increase their defenses. Interferons are not specific to certain types of viruses—they work against all types of viruses. The **complement system** is a series of plasma proteins that are effective at killing bacteria by causing lysis of their cell membrane. The complement system also enhances phagocytosis within the area of invasion.

➤ **Inflammation**: When there is damage to tissues, the inflammatory response will initiate. It is characterized by redness and heat due to increased blood flow, swelling, and pain. Increased blood flow to the area is caused by the chemical **histamine,** which is secreted by basophils. This increased blood flow brings in other white blood cells, proteins, and other components needed to fight infection. Histamine makes capillaries more permeable than normal, which results in increased fluid in the area, causing swelling. This swelling can put pressure on pain receptors, creating the sensation of pain.

➤ **Fever**: When the body temperature is reset to a higher level by chemicals called **pyrogens**, fever is the result. Controlled fevers are beneficial, as they increase metabolism and stimulate other immune defenses. When fevers get too high, they are dangerous and can cause the denaturing of critical enzymes needed to sustain life.

Specific Defenses

When nonspecific defenses fail to control infection, specific defenses must be used. Since these are customized to the specific invader, they take at least a week to be created in order to respond strongly to a new antigen (a substance, including microbes, that elicits an immune response). There are two types of specific defenses, both of which use **lymphocytes**. Lymphocytes are derived from stem cells in the red bone marrow. B cells complete their maturation in the bone marrow, while T cells mature in the thymus gland. Both types of cells are designed to recognize foreign antigens and destroy invading microbes. **Humoral immunity** involves B cells, which ultimately secrete antibodies to destroy foreign antigens. **Cellular** (or cell-mediated) **immunity** involves the use of T cells to destroy infected or cancerous cells. A specific variety of T cell known as the helper T cell is the key coordinator of both humoral and cellular responses, which happen simultaneously.

HUMORAL IMMUNITY

Humoral immunity involves the production of specific **antibody** proteins from B cells that have been activated. Each B cell displays an antibody on its cell membrane and each of the million or more B cells in the body has a different antibody on its membrane.

The activation of a particular B cell by a specific antigen is based on shape recognition between the antibody on the B cell membrane and the antigen. The activation process is also dependent on chemicals from a helper T cell, which will be discussed in the next section. This activation causes proliferation of that B cell which leads to a population of **plasma cells** (B cells that actively secrete antibodies) and **memory B cells** that produce the same type of antibody as the original cell from which they were derived. This is referred to as **clonal selection;** it is the key event of the **primary immune response,** which leads to **active immunity**. It takes at least a week for this response to reach peak levels. Once antibodies are produced in large quantities by plasma cells, they circulate through blood, lymph, and tissues, where they seek out their antigen and bind to it, forming a complex. Once an antibody binds to an antigen, the complex will either be phagocytized or will agglutinate and later be removed by other phagocytic cells.

The primary immune response and active immunity can be achieved by natural exposure to an antigen or by vaccination. On secondary and subsequent exposures to the same antigen, the memory B cells that were created during the primary exposure can proliferate into plasma cells that produce antibodies, which provide a much faster response to the antigen. While antibodies do not circulate for long once an antigen has been destroyed, memory B cells can last for years if not forever.

Sometimes antibodies are passed from one person to another, which leads to **passive immunity**. This occurs during pregnancy when maternal antibodies cross the placenta, and during breast feeding. Breast milk contains antibodies that are transmitted to the newborn. Passive immunity can be induced by the injection of antibodies from one individual to another. Passive immunity is short-lived and declines within a few months.

CELLULAR IMMUNITY

Cellular immunity is based on the actions of T cells, which come in several varieties. T cells have a cell membrane receptor that, like antibodies on the surface of B cells, recognizes the shape of one particular antigen. However, T cells cannot be directly activated by contact with the antigen. The antigen must be presented to a **helper T cell** by a self cell that is infected with the antigen or by a macrophage that has engulfed the antigen. The cell presenting the antigen secretes the chemical **interleukin-1** as it binds to the helper T cell. The helper T cell then secretes **interleukin-2**. This step is crucial for both humoral and cellular responses. The activation of the helper T and secretion of interleukin-2 allows for activation of B cells as well as the activation of a **cytotoxic** (killer) **T cell** that can now bind to the antigen. The cytotoxic T cell proliferates and produces effector cells by clonal selection that all have the ability to seek and destroy the foreign antigen. As with plasma cell activation, this primary response takes at least a week to occur. **Memory T cells** are also produced. Once the antigen has been completely destroyed, **suppressor T cells** are used to stop the response of killer T cells. Only memory T cells remain; they can be quickly activated to cytotoxic T cells on secondary and subsequent exposures to the same antigen.

PART IX. REPRODUCTION AND DEVELOPMENT

THE REPRODUCTIVE SYSTEMS

The female and male reproductive systems have the common function of producing gametes for sexual reproduction. Egg cells in females and sperm cells in males are produced by the **gonads**. In addition, the female reproductive system has to be structured to accept sperm from the male system and to allow for embryonic and fetal development.

The Female Reproductive System

The female reproductive system is enclosed within the abdominal cavity and is open to the external environment. While having an opening to the outside environment is necessary for reproduction and childbirth, it presents some unique problems in terms of the ability of pathogens to enter the system.

The structures of the internal female reproductive system consist of the **ovaries,** where egg production occurs, as well as supporting structures, as seen in Figure 9.18. After an egg is released from an ovary, it is swept into the fallopian tube (oviduct) that is associated with that ovary. If sperm are present, they should meet with the egg in the fallopian tube where fertilization will occur. The fallopian tubes merge into the uterus, which is composed of the muscular **myometrium** and the vascularized lining called the **endometrium**. If the egg has been fertilized, the embryo will implant into the endometrium, where development will continue. If fertilization has not occurred, the egg will be lost with the shedding of the endometrium, which occurs about every 28 days during menstruation. The **vagina** serves as an entry point for sperm to enter the system, an exit point for menstrual fluids, and the birth canal during childbirth. The pH of the vagina is acidic, which can discourage the growth of certain pathogens. The **cervix** regulates the opening of the uterus into the vagina and is normally very narrow.

THE MENSTRUAL CYCLE

The female reproductive cycle lasts about 28 days on average. There are characteristic changes within the uterus that occur during this time. These changes are referred to as the menstrual (or uterine) cycle, which goes through three phases (seen in Figure 9.21) as follows:

➤ **Menses**: During the first five or so days of the cycle, the existing endometrium is lost via menstrual fluid as arteries serving the endometrium constrict; this causes tissue death as the cells are cut off from oxygen and nutrients.

➤ The **proliferative** phase: During the second week of the cycle, the primary event in the uterus is the proliferation of cells to replace the endometrium that was lost during menstruation.

➤ The **secretory** phase: During the last two weeks of the cycle, hormones are secreted to prepare the endometrium for implantation, if an embryo is present. As the twenty-eighth day of the cycle approaches, the endometrium deteriorates and menses will soon begin as the cycle restarts.

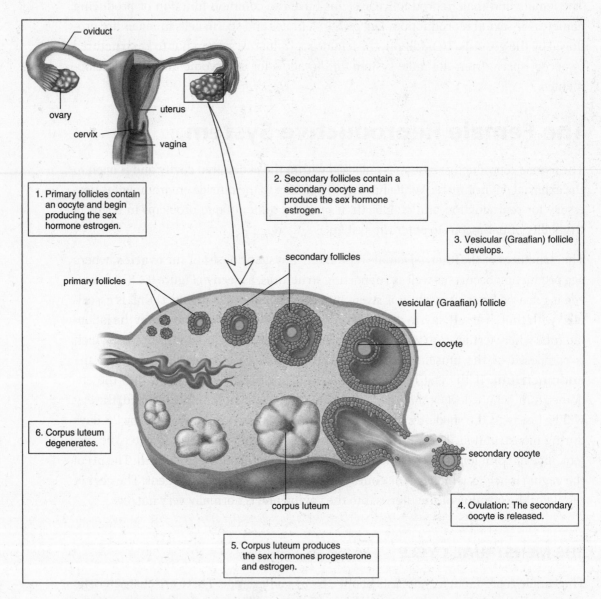

FIGURE 9.18: The female reproductive system. The ovaries release an egg into the fallopian tube during each reproductive cycle. Should the egg be fertilized, the resulting embryo implants in the uterus.

THE OVARIAN CYCLE

Eggs are produced through the ovarian cycle (also seen in Figure 9.19), whose timing must be carefully choreographed to the menstrual cycle. The ovarian cycle also lasts 28 days and consists of the following phases:

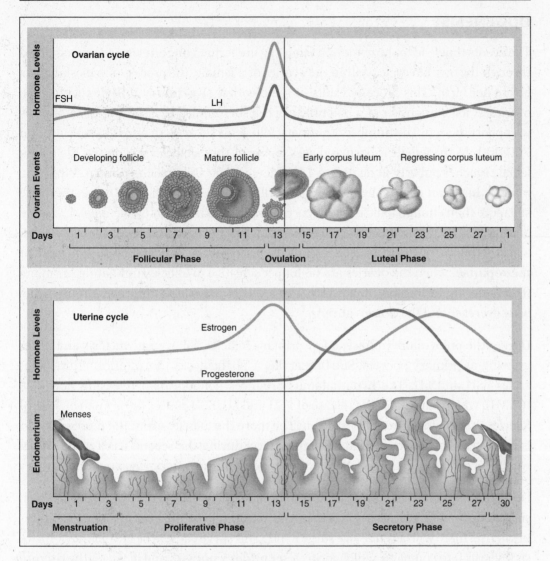

FIGURE 9.19: The female reproductive cycle. The control of the uterine cycle is achieved by estrogen and progesterone. The ovarian cycle is regulated primarily by FSH and LH.

➤ The **preovulatory** phase: This phase consists of the events prior to ovulation and lasts from days 1–13 of the cycle. This timing corresponds to menses and the proliferative phase of the menstrual cycle.

➤ **Ovulation**: The rupture of a follicle in the ovary and subsequent release of an egg to a fallopian tube constitutes ovulation. It occurs on day 14 of the cycle.

➤ The **postovulatory** phase: During this phase, the egg is released and may be fertilized. This phase lasts from days 15–28 and corresponds with the secretory phase of the menstrual cycle. Should fertilization occur, the embryo would implant into the endometrium during this phase. If fertilization has not occurred, the menstrual cycle restarts, causing the egg to be lost.

OOGENESIS

The events that lead to the ovulation of an egg are termed **oogenesis** and are regulated through the ovarian cycle. Within the ovaries of a female, the process of meiosis begins before her birth. This process results in the creation of **primary follicles** within the ovaries. A follicle consists of a potential egg cell surrounded by a shell of follicular cells to support the egg. The number of primary follicles is set at birth and is usually around 700,000. As the female is born and ages, many of these follicles will die. By the time a female reaches puberty at age 12 to 14, as few as 200,000 follicles remain. While the number has been drastically reduced and will continue to decline with age, there are still more than enough follicles to support the reproductive needs of a female, since only one egg will be released every 28 days. Until puberty begins, these follicles stay in an arrested phase of meiosis. The ability to perform the ovarian cycle will end at **menopause,** when the ovaries are no longer sensitive to follicle-stimulating hormone (FSH) and luteinizing hormone (LH). The levels of estrogen and progesterone in the body decrease and the ovaries atrophy.

During the preovulatory phase, a few primary follicles will resume meiosis and begin growing as primary oocytes. Starting at day 1 of the cycle, the anterior pituitary secretes FSH and LH. The hypothalamus produces gonadotropin releasing hormone (GnRH), which stimulates the release of FSH and LH. FSH causes the growth of several follicles that begin to produce estrogen. The more the follicles grow, the more estrogen is produced. This estrogen is at its highest level during the second week of the cycle, which corresponds to the rebuilding of the endometrium after menstruation.

During the second week of the cycle, the high levels of estrogen actually inhibit FSH, such that no more follicles begin to grow. As estrogen from the growing follicles continues to rise, there will be a massive surge in LH. This surge causes the first round of meiosis (meiosis I) to complete, which forms a **secondary oocyte,** and it causes the rupture of the follicle within the ovary. This is ovulation. It happens on day 14 of the cycle. The oocyte is released to the fallopian tubes and the remnants of the follicle remain in the ovary. If the oocyte is fertilized, meiosis II will occur, resulting in a mature egg (ovum). Only one mature egg is needed during ovulation, so the remaining three cells produced during meiosis are termed **polar bodies**. They are much smaller than the egg and will be degraded. If more than one egg is released on a given cycle, the potential exists for multiple fertilizations and multiple embryos, which results in fraternal twins or triplets.

The remains of the follicle in the ovary continue secreting estrogen and become the **corpus luteum,** which also secretes progesterone. The estrogen and progesterone will suppress FSH and LH so that no more eggs are released on this cycle. These hormones also keep the endometrium prepared to receive an embryo during the secretory phase (third and fourth weeks) of the menstrual cycle.

At the end of the fourth week of the cycle, if an embryo has not implanted into the endometrium, the cycle needs to restart. At this point, the corpus luteum degrades. Without the corpus luteum, the levels of estrogen and progesterone decline. The lack of these hormones, particularly progesterone, is the cause of menstruation, which can only occur when these levels are low. Further, the lack of estrogen and progesterone allows the pituitary gland to begin secreting FSH and LH again to begin the process of a new cycle.

Because estrogen and progesterone have the ability to suppress the actions of FSH and LH, they are the hormones of choice for use in birth control methods such as pills, patches, injections, rings, or implants. The use of synthetic estrogen and/or synthetic progesterone can be used to manipulate the ovaries into not ovulating, since FSH and LH are suppressed.

The Male Reproductive System

In contrast to the female system, the male reproductive system is not housed completely within the abdominal cavity. It is a closed system, as seen in Figure 9.20. The male gonads or **testes** produce sperm. The remaining reproductive structures serve as a means to transport sperm out of the body and into the female system.

Sperm begin their development in the **seminiferous tubules** of the testes where they are nourished by **Sertoli cells**. The testes are housed in the scrotum outside of the abdominal cavity, where the temperature is a few degrees cooler than body temperature.

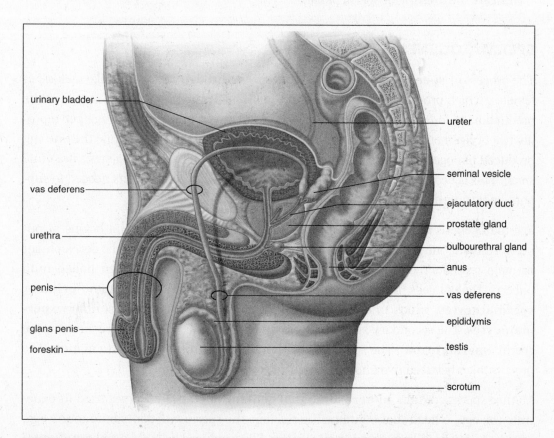

FIGURE 9.20: Sperm are produced in the testes of the male reproductive system. As sperm are released from the male system, secretions from a variety of glands are added to produce semen.

Oddly enough, sperm require a temperature cooler than normal body temperature to survive their development. As sperm develop in the testes, they move into the **epididymis** associated with each testis, which is also located in the scrotum. Once in the epididymis, the sperm acquire motility and are stored.

When ejaculation occurs, the sperm must be moved towards the male urethra. The sperm enter the **vas deferens,** which are tubes that move up into the abdominal cavity. From there, the two vas deferens merge into the **ejaculatory duct** and into the urethra. Recall that the urethra is also used for urine passage. When sperm are moving through, the urethra is unavailable to the bladder. Once the sperm are in the urethra, three types of glands add their secretions to the sperm as they pass by. This creates semen, which is a mixture of sperm and secretions. The urethra progresses through the length of the penis where it can be introduced into the female vagina.

The associated glands of the male reproductive system that provide secretions to semen are as follows:

➤ The **seminal vesicles** provide a fluid rich in nutrients to serve as an energy source for the sperm.
➤ The **prostate gland** wraps around the urethra and deposits a secretion that is alkaline, to balance the acidic environment of the vagina.
➤ The **bulbourethral glands** secrete a fluid prior to ejaculation that may serve to lubricate the urethra for sperm passage.

SPERMATOGENESIS

The process of **spermatogenesis** produces sperm through meiosis. Unlike meiosis in females, which produces one egg and three polar bodies, meiosis in men results in the production of four sperm cells. While women only need to release one egg per reproductive cycle, men need millions of sperm per fertilization attempt. While the one egg produced in oogenesis is quite large, the sperm produced in spermatogenesis are quite small. This is because the egg cell must contain additional components needed to support embryonic development.

Spermatogenesis requires the hormonal influence of testosterone and begins at puberty. Testosterone is secreted during embryonic development to cause the development of male reproductive structures, but testosterone development is then halted until puberty. Diploid cells in the testes called **spermatogonia** differentiate into **primary spermatocytes,** which undergo meiosis I, producing two haploid **secondary spermatocytes**. The secondary spermatocytes undergo meiosis II to produce four mature sperm (**spermatozoa**). The spermatozoa then move to the epididymis to mature. The process takes between two and three months to complete.

Mature sperm contain an **acrosome** that contains digestive enzymes used to penetrate the egg, a head that contains the nucleus the sperm will contribute to the egg, and the tail (a flagellum) that is propelled by ATP produced by large numbers of mitochondria.

Some of the same hormones that are used in the female reproductive system are also used to regulate spermatogenesis. GnRH from the hypothalamus allows for the secretion of LH from the anterior pituitary. LH causes the production of testosterone by cells in the testes. The secretion of GnRH from the hypothalamus also results in the release of FSH from the anterior pituitary. While testosterone is needed to stimulate spermatogenesis, FSH is also needed to make the potential sperm cells sensitive to testosterone. The levels of testosterone regulate sperm production in a manner that resembles a thermostat.

DEVELOPMENT

As the haploid nucleus of a sperm cell is contributed to an egg cell (also containing a haploid nucleus) during fertilization, the resulting cell is termed a **zygote**. The zygote begins cell division by mitosis, which produces a ball of identical cells—the **embryo**. In humans, the first eight weeks of development constitute embryonic development and all development after eight weeks constitutes fetal development. The human gestation period is 266 days. These nine months are divided into trimesters. Embryonic development is complete within the first trimester.

Fertilization

Sperm have the ability to survive about 48 hours in the female system, while an egg cell only survives about 24 hours. Sperm deposited prior to or right after ovulation are capable of fertilizing the egg, which should happen in the upper third of the fallopian tube. While 200 to 500 million sperm are typically released during ejaculation, only about 200 will make it to the egg cell. Secretions from the female system will change the membrane composition of the sperm near its acrosome. In this way, when the sperm bumps into the egg, the contents of its acrosome will be released due to membrane instability. This will allow the sperm to penetrate the **corona radiate** (outer layer) of the egg. Next the sperm must pass through the next layer of the egg, the **zona pellucida**. The first sperm to pass through the zona pellucida will pass its nucleus into the egg. This will cause a depolarization in the membrane of the egg, which will make it impenetrable to fertilization by other sperm. The nuclei of the egg and sperm fuse, creating the zygote.

Embryonic Development

About one day after fertilization, the zygote performs its first mitotic division, becoming an embryo. This initiates **cleavage,** which is the rapid cell division characteristic of early embryonic development. Within about four days, the embryo reaches the **morula** stage, in which it consists of a ball of cells. During early cleavage, the embryo may split into two, which results in identical twins. By about six days, the center of the embryo hollows out and becomes filled with fluid. The embryo is now termed a blastula or **blastocyst**. The outer cells of the blastocyst are the **trophoblast, which** will aid in implantation and the development of extraembryonic membranes and the placenta. The **inner cell**

mass of the blastocyst will continue development as the embryo. It is the source of embryonic stem cells, which have the ability to differentiate into any cell type. Implantation of the embryo begins about one week after fertilization and completes by the second week. The events of early embryonic development can be seen in Figure 9.21.

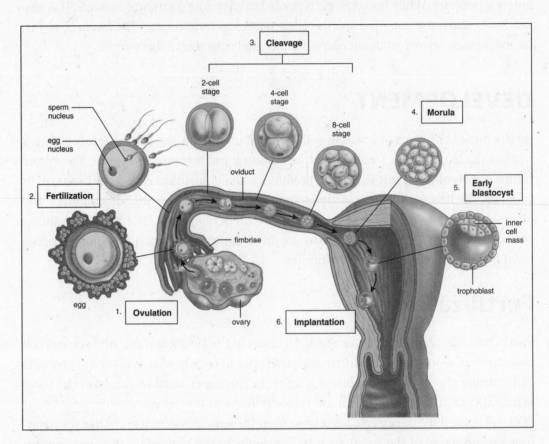

FIGURE 9.21: Early embryonic development. Fertilization occurs in the fallopian tube. The developing embryo moves down the tube to implant eventually in the endometrium of the uterus at the blastocyst stage of development.

The blastocyst produces a critical hormone that is important in the maintenance of pregnancy. Human chorionic gonadotropin (HCG) is the signal to the corpus luteum to not degrade. Normally, the degradation of the corpus luteum would cause a decline of estrogen and progesterone and would trigger menstruation. At this point in development, menstruation would mean a loss of the embryo, resulting in a spontaneous abortion. HCG ensures that the corpus luteum will continue to secrete estrogen and progesterone so that menstruation is delayed.

The next event of embryonic development is the gastrula stage. During **gastrulation**, three primary germ layers are formed as the cells in the embryo shift into layers. Once a cell enters a **germ layer**, its ability to differentiate into specific cell types is limited. The three germ layers and the fates of cells in these layers are as follows:

➤ **Ectoderm**: cells in this layer will express the genes needed to become skin cells and cells of the nervous system

➤ **Mesoderm**: cells in this layer will express the genes needed to become muscles, bones, and most internal organs

➤ **Endoderm**: cells in this layer will express the genes needed to become the lining of internal body cavities as well as the linings of the respiratory, digestive, urinary, and reproductive tracts

Once the germ layers are complete, **neuralization** begins the development of the nervous system. Mesoderm cells form the **notochord**. Ectoderm above the notochord starts to thicken and folds inward, forming neural folds that continue to deepen and fuse to produce a **neural tube** that will eventually develop into the central nervous system. At this point, a head and tail region have been established in the embryo.

As differentiation continues, certain cells can influence the gene expression of other cells in the process of **induction** via chemical messengers. Communication between cells is also used to establish positional information in the embryo, which is critical to the formation of internal organs as well as the limbs. **Homeobox genes** produce proteins that are essential for guiding the development of the shape of the embryo. The proteins produced by the homeoboxes are transcription factors that serve to turn on specific genes within cells at specific times.

Induction helps ensure that the right structures occur in the right places. An additional process that is necessary during embryonic development is **apoptosis** of certain cells. While it seems odd to talk about cell death during development, it is necessary. For example, the separation of fingers and toes is the result of apoptosis of the cells that at one time joined the structures.

The remainder of embryonic development deals with **organogenesis** and refining the shape of the embryo. Organ systems are developed on an as-needed basis with the most critical organs being produced first. By the fourth week, the heart is working and limbs are established. By the end of embryonic development (the eighth week), all major organs are established and most are functioning.

EXTRAEMBRYONIC MEMBRANES

While the embryo is in the process of implanting into the endometrium, four membranes will be formed outside of the embryo:

➤ The **amnion** surrounds the embryo in a fluid-filled sac that serves a protective function and provides cushioning for the embryo and fetus.

➤ The **allantois** is a membrane that will ultimately form the umbilical cord, which is the connection between the embryo and the placenta (the organ that will deliver nutrients and oxygen and remove carbon dioxide and wastes).

➤ The **yolk sac** is where the first blood cells develop. In other species, it serves as a source of nutrients.

➤ The **chorion** will eventually become the embryo's side of the placenta.

THE PLACENTA

The **placenta** develops from the chorion and grows in size during development. It provides nutrients and oxygen to the embryo and removes wastes. Recall that fetal hemoglobin has a greater affinity for oxygen than adult hemoglobin. The placenta produces HCG, estrogen, and progesterone to maintain the pregnancy. It also produces the hormone relaxin to release the ligaments that attach the pubic bones to provide more space in the birth canal. It takes about three months for the placenta to develop fully.

Fetal Development

Fetal development is primarily a refinement of the organ systems that are already established during embryonic development. The fetus enlarges and the organ systems are refined, so that they are all functioning or are capable of functioning at the end of gestation.

Birth

Labor is triggered by the hormone oxytocin, which is produced by the posterior pituitary gland. Oxytocin causes contractions of the uterus that intensify with time. Initially, the cervix must dilate, which can take hours. The amnion usually ruptures during the dilation stage. Once the cervix is dilated, contractions continue, leading to expulsion of the baby. After the baby is delivered, the umbilical cord is clamped and cut, which severs the connection to the placenta. Finally, the placenta is delivered at the end of labor.

Human Anatomy and Physiology

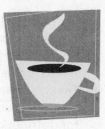

- ➤ The central nervous system consists of the brain and spinal cord, while the peripheral nervous system consists of nerves outside of the brain and spinal cord. The brain is divided into several distinct regions, as seen in Table 9.1.
- ➤ Neurons contain dendrites to receive messages from other cells, a cell body to process the message, an axon to convey an electrical impulse, and synaptic knobs to release chemical signals in the form of neurotransmitters to other cells.
  - ➤ Reflex actions can be processed through the spinal cord in a reflex arc, which consists of a sensory neuron, interneuron, and motor neuron.
- ➤ Muscles are used to support the body, regulate openings into the body, generate heat, and help blood move through veins. Muscle tissue can be smooth, skeletal, or cardiac.
  - ➤ The fibers of skeletal muscles are organized in sarcomeres.
- ➤ The skeletal system begins as cartilage in embryos, most of which is replaced by bone in the process of ossification.
  - ➤ Bone matrix is a major storage reserve for calcium and phosphates. Osteons are the structural unit of bone tissue.
- ➤ The major endocrine structures and hormones of the body can be reviewed in Table 9.2.
- ➤ Hormones are chemical messengers that travel via the blood to change the functioning of their target. Hormones come in two major classes: steroid and nonsteroid. Hormones are used to help the body maintain homeostasis, usually through negative feedback loops.
- ➤ Blood is a mixture of liquid plasma and formed elements. Red blood cells contain hemoglobin to transport O_2. White blood cells are involved with fighting infection through the immune system. Platelets are involved with blood clotting. Plasma carries water, gases, nutrients, wastes, ions, hormones and more.
- ➤ The cardiovascular system of humans consists of a four-chambered heart. The atria pump blood to the ventricles and the ventricles pump blood out of the heart.
  - ➤ The right side of the heart is associated with the pulmonary circuit (pumping to the lungs) and the left side of the heart is associated with the systemic circuit (pumping to the body).
  - ➤ The contractions of the heart are initiated by the SA node (pacemaker) that sends signals through the conducting system of the heart.
- ➤ The respiratory system is intimately connected with the circulatory system. The primary role of the respiratory system is to perform gas exchange to oxygenate blood coming from the right side (pulmonary circuit) of the heart.
  - ➤ Ventilation occurs as the result of differing pressures inside and outside the thoracic cavity. The rate of ventilation is controlled by the medulla in the brain, which monitors blood pH.

➤ The exchange of CO_2 is critical to pH maintenance. The conversion of CO_2 to carbonic acid to bicarbonate and hydrogen ions is a reversible reaction that is used to regulate pH.

➤ The role of the digestive system is to break down nutrients chemically to their monomer subunits. These nutrients then must be transported to the circulatory system for distribution to the cells of the body.

➤ The primary organs of excretion are the kidneys. The three nitrogenous waste products found in urine are urea, uric acid, and creatinine. The amount of water excreted has a direct influence on blood volume and pressure.

➤ The lymphatic system reclaims tissue fluid and returns it to the blood, delivers the end products of fat digestion to the blood, and fights infection via white blood cells.

➤ The immune system exists anywhere white blood cells are which includes the lymphatic system, the blood, and within tissues. The primary duty of the immune system is to destroy foreign cells, as well as self cells that are infected or cancerous.

   ➤ The nonspecific immune defenses are used to prevent foreign cells from entering the body or to quickly disable foreign cells that have entered. These defenses include physical and chemical barricades, defensive white blood cells, interferons, the complement system, inflammation, and fever.

   ➤ Specific defenses are used when the nonspecific defenses fail to destroy foreign invaders.

➤ Both the male and female reproductive systems are under hormonal control to produce gametes. The female system has the additional responsibility of housing embryonic and fetal development if fertilization occurs.

   ➤ The uterus performs the menstrual cycle on a 28-day cycle. The ovarian cycle regulates the release of eggs to synchronize with the menstrual cycle.

➤ During fertilization, one sperm penetrates the egg, which results in a diploid gamete. Embryonic development concludes after eight weeks and fetal development continues for the remainder of the gestation period. Fetal development consists of the growth and refinement of structures that were developed in embryonic development.

PART V
REVIEWING PCAT CHEMISTRY

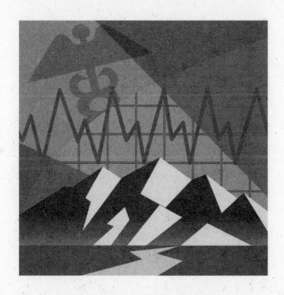

General Chemistry

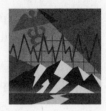

MATTER AND ITS CHANGES

Chemistry is defined as the science of matter. Matter is defined as anything that has mass and occupies space. The concept of matter may easily be visualized by considering the three states of matter: solid, liquid, and gas. You will be familiar with these states, and you can conclude that all the material that makes up our universe is matter, including air, steel, bricks, our bodies, dirt, wood, copper, gold, aluminum, water, and so on. Chemistry is concerned primarily with three aspects of matter:

1. The physical and chemical properties of matter
2. The physical and chemical changes that matter undergoes
3. The energy transfer associated with these changes

Properties of matter are divided into **physical properties,** such as color, electrical conductivity, shape, hardness, density, melting point, and ductility. These properties are further divided into quantitative (those with an associated number), such as a boiling point of 78.5°C or a density of 2.70 $^g/_{mL}$, and qualitative (having no associated number), such as color or ductility (that is, the ability to be drawn into a wire). **Chemical properties** are the possible chemical reactions that a substance undergoes, such as flammability or the ability of a metal to react with an acid to produce hydrogen gas.

Associated with physical and chemical properties are physical and chemical changes. **Physical changes** are changes in matter in which only the form changes while the chemical makeup remains intact. Changes of state such as boiling, freezing, melting, sublimation, and condensation are examples. In contrast, a **chemical change** (or **chemical reaction**) requires a change in chemical composition. An example of a chemical reaction is the combination of hydrogen gas and oxygen gas to form liquid water.

Chemistry involves three levels of description of matter:

➤ *Macroscopic*: processes that can be seen by the normal senses
➤ *Microscopic*: explanations of macroscopic observations in terms of atoms, molecules, and ions
➤ *Symbolic*: representing atoms, molecules, and ions with chemical symbols

    EXAMPLE: Formation of water

Macroscopic: Clear, colorless hydrogen and oxygen gases combine to form colorless liquid water.

Microscopic: Diatomic hydrogen molecules combine with diatomic oxygen molecules in a ratio of 2:1 (hydrogen: oxygen) to produce triatomic water molecules.

Symbolic (chemical symbols): $2H_2(g) + O_2(g) \longrightarrow 2 H_2O(l)$ (g) = gas and (l) = liquid

Symbolic (molecular structures):

The path from macroscopic observations to microscopic explanations aided by symbolic representation mirrors the steps of the scientific method. To have a good grasp of chemistry, you must be able to think on all three levels (macroscopic, microscopic, and symbolic), and be able to convert between the three representations.

Matter may be classified by the chemical composition of a sample. A broad division is between matter that has a fixed composition (**pure substances**), and matter that may have a variation in composition (**mixtures**). Mixtures may be either heterogeneous (clear phases can be seen by the eye or a microscope) or homogeneous (the matter consists of one continuous phase). Homogeneous mixtures are also called **solutions**. Heterogeneous mixtures may be separated into homogeneous mixtures by physical methods. A homogeneous mixture may be further separated into the pure substances that compose it by physical means. Pure substances come in two forms: elements and compounds. **Elements** cannot be broken down into simpler substances by chemical means. Elements consist of only one type of atom. **Compounds** are pure substances that can be separated into elements by chemical methods. Compounds contain two or more atoms combined in a fixed ratio. The figure below illustrates the relationships between the various classifications of matter.

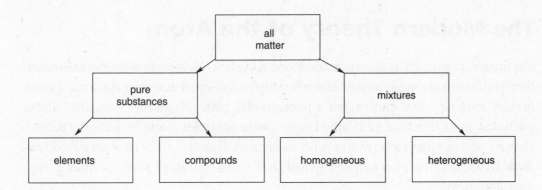

BASIC ATOMIC THEORY

In this section we will consider the basic structure and components of atoms using the nuclear atom model. Later, the model will be refined with respect to the location of the electrons.

The English chemist John Dalton first formulated the modern atomic theory by consolidating three macroscopic laws that had been established by several scientists.

➤ The **law of conservation of mass (**or **matter)**, which states that during a chemical reaction the total mass of the starting reactants equals the total mass of the products.
➤ The **law of definite composition** (or **proportions**), which states that a compound consists of two or more elements combined in a fixed ratio by mass.
➤ The **law of multiple proportions**, which states that if a pair of elements forms more than one compound, the combining masses of one of the elements with a fixed mass of the other element are in the ratio of small whole numbers.

Experiments with gases contributed to Dalton's theory. Dalton considered the data and concluded that the best explanation was that all matter is made of tiny, indivisible particles called atoms. The tenets of Dalton's atomic theory are summarized as follow:

1. All matter is composed of tiny indivisible particles called atoms.
2. Atoms of a given element are identical in all properties, and atoms of differing elements are different in some properties.
3. Compounds are atoms combined together in a fixed ratio of individual atoms.
4. Chemical reactions are the rearrangements of atoms to form different compounds in new fixed ratios of atoms.

The law of conservation of mass follows from the indivisibility of atoms. The laws of definite composition and multiple proportions result from the fixed combining ratios of different atoms of differing masses, which are observed macroscopically as fixed ratios of masses of elements. Inaccuracies have been found in each of Dalton's four points, but Dalton's theory provided a framework for experimental investigations supporting atomic theory in the nineteenth century, and led to modern atomic theory in the twentieth century.

The Modern Theory of the Atom

The modern theory of the atom was developed in the first thirty years of the twentieth century. The French physicist Antoine-Henri Becquerel discovered that some elements spontaneously emit rays that can expose a photographic plate. These rays are called **alpha particles** (particles with a +2 relative charge), **beta particles** (particles with a −1 relative charge), and **gamma rays** (energy with no charge). Together, these rays were called **radioactivity**, and this phenomenon hinted that atoms contained particles smaller than the whole atom.

The English physicist J. J. Thomson studied the rays generated from metal plates exposed to a current in an evacuated tube called a cathode ray tube. Thompson called the cathode rays **electrons**, and eventually it was shown that cathode rays and beta particles are identical. Thompson's experiment allowed the determination of the mass-to-charge ratio of the electron. The American physicist Robert Millikan determined the charge on the electron, and multiplying this charge by the mass-to-charge ratio yielded the mass of the electron which is 9.100×10^{-28} g. If the negative electron is part of a neutral atom, then there must also be a positive part.

The atom is composed mostly of empty space with the positive charge concentrated at the center, or nucleus. This nuclear atom is the currently accepted model for the atom, though it has been greatly refined. The positive particles at the center are called **protons**. Later, the nucleus was found also to contain **neutrons,** particles with a mass similar to the proton, but with no charge. Subatomic particles are summarized below.

Subatomic Particles				
Name	**Symbol**	**Relative Charge**	**Relative Mass**	**Location**
Proton	p^+ or p	+1	≈ 1 amu	Nucleus
Neutron	n^0 or n	0	≈ 1 amu	Nucleus
Electron	e^-	−1	1/1836 amu	Circulating outside the nucleus

Chemical processes do not affect the particles in the nucleus, but nuclear reactions or radioactivity can alter the number of nuclear particles.

To illustrate the size of atoms, consider the number of silver atoms that would span the diameter of a quarter. A quarter has a diameter of 24 mm. The diameter of a silver atom is 165 picometers. First, convert both measurements to meters.

$$24 \text{ mm} \times \frac{1 \text{ m}}{1000 \text{ mm}} = 0.024 \text{ m} \qquad 165 \text{ pm} \times \frac{1 \text{ m}}{10^{12} \text{ pm}} = 1.65 \times 10^{-10} \text{ m}.$$

Now divide the diameter of the atom into the diameter of the quarter:

$$\frac{0.024 \text{ m}}{\left(\dfrac{1.65 \times 10^{-10} \text{ m}}{\text{silver atom}} \right)} = 1.5 \times 10^{8} \text{ or } 150 \text{ million silver atoms.}$$

All atoms of the same element have the same number of protons. This number is called the element's **atomic number (Z)**. Carbon atoms have six protons. Gold atoms have 79 protons. The number of neutrons in the nucleus may vary. Atoms with different numbers of neutrons but identical numbers of protons are called **isotopes**. These atoms have a different mass but are chemically almost identical. The total number of protons and neutrons in the nucleus is called the **mass number (A)**. The much smaller electrons are insignificant in the mass of the atom. Each element has a corresponding one- or two-letter symbol. Carbon is C, nitrogen is N, gold is Au, and hydrogen is H. The atomic symbol of a particular isotope is written with the mass number (A) as a left superscript and the atomic number (Z) as a left subscript. For example, a carbon atom with 6 neutrons is $^{12}_{6}\text{C}$. The carbon isotope with eight neutrons is $^{14}_{6}\text{C}$.

The atomic number, Z, is redundant and is often omitted. The number of neutrons is $A - Z$. For ^{238}U, $Z = 92$ (92 p^{+}) and $A = 238$, so $238 - 92 = 146$ neutrons.

Each naturally occurring isotope makes up a specific fraction of the total atoms of that element called the relative abundance, usually given as a percentage. To convert a percentage to a fractional part, divide by 100. For boron, the two main isotopes are ^{11}B with a relative abundance of 80.09% and ^{10}B with a relative abundance of 19.91%. It is convenient to introduce a new unit that better matches the scale of atoms. The **amu (atomic mass unit)** is defined as $\frac{1}{12}$ of the mass of an atom of ^{12}C. 1 amu is close to the mass of a proton or a neutron.

To calculate the average atomic mass of an atom of a given element, use the following formula (frac. = fraction):

$$\text{Avg. atomic mass} = (\text{frac. of isotope 1}) \times (\text{mass of isotope 1}) + (\text{frac. of isotope 2})$$
$$\times (\text{mass of isotope 2}) + \ldots.$$

The sum will have as many terms as there are isotopes of the atom. For boron:

Atom	Abundance	Mass (amu)
^{10}B	19.91 %	10.012939
^{11}B	80.09 %	11.009305

$$\text{Avg. atomic mass} = (0.1991 \times 10.012939) + (0.8009 \times 11.009305) \text{ amu}$$
$$= 10.81 \text{ amu.}$$

Because the relative abundance of ^{11}B is greater than ^{10}B, the heavier element contributes a greater amount to the weighted average, which is closer to the mass of ^{11}B than to that of ^{10}B. Average atomic masses have been calculated from experimental data for most of the elements.

The Mole Concept

The amu is useful for individual atoms, but grams or kilograms are more practical units for a collection of atoms. A **mole** (abbreviated mol) is defined as the number of atoms in exactly 12 g of ^{12}C. This quantity is **Avogadro's number** (6.022×10^{23} particles/mol to four significant figures), and it should be memorized. One atom of ^{12}C has a mass of 12 amu. One mole of ^{12}C has a mass of exactly 12 g and contains $6.022 \times 10^{+23}$ ^{12}C atoms. The average atomic mass in amu is numerically equal to the mass in grams of one mole of a substance. Avogadro's number can be thought of as a conversion between the number of moles and the number of particles, which are usually atoms, ions, or molecules.

The mass in grams of one mole is called the **molar mass** (formerly called **molecular weight**). "Mass" is preferred because weight depends on gravity. The molar mass converts between grams of a substance and moles of a substance. An analogy is the way loose nails are normally sold in a hardware store. Nails are not counted individually but rather by weighing. If there are 1000 nails in a pound, 5 pounds of nails contain 5000 nails. Similarly, if there is 1 mole ($6.022 \times 10^{+23}$ atoms) of carbon in 12.01 g of carbon, $5 \times 12.01 \text{ g} = 60.06 \text{ g}$ of carbon would contain $5 \times 6.022 \times 10^{+23}$ atoms of carbon. Here are some examples using molar mass:

EXAMPLE: How many moles of gold are there in 200.0 g of gold (Au)?

$$200.0 \text{ g Au} \times \frac{1 \text{ mole Au}}{196.967 \text{ g Au}} = 1.015 \text{ mol Au}$$

EXAMPLE: How many g are needed to make 3.78 mol of sulfur?

$$3.78 \text{ mol S} \times \frac{32.07 \text{ g S}}{1 \text{ mol S}} = 121 \text{ g S}$$

EXAMPLE: How many individual copper atoms are in a piece of copper (Cu) of mass of 0.00246 g?

This calculation requires two steps: g Cu $\longrightarrow$ mol Cu $\longrightarrow$ Cu atoms

$$0.00246 \text{ g Cu} \times \frac{1 \text{ mole Cu}}{63.546 \text{ g Cu}} \times \frac{6.022 \times 10^{23} \text{ Cu atoms}}{1 \text{ mole Cu}} = 2.33 \times 10^{+19} \text{ Cu atoms}$$

The Periodic Table

The periodic table of the elements, first formulated by the Russian chemist Dmitri Mendeleev, is a powerful and useful tool that organizes a large amount of information in a compact document. With increasing atomic number, certain properties of the elements repeat in a periodic pattern. The patterns are not as exact as a sine wave or the phases of the moon, to take two examples, but patterns are clearly seen. Chemistry students must be familiar with parts of the periodic table. A periodic table is provided below. Periodic tables generally display the atomic number, the elemental symbol, and the average atomic mass for each element. For magnesium:

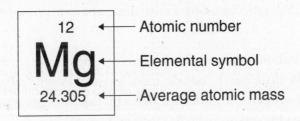

The shape and numbering scheme for a modern periodic table are shown in the figure below:

Periodic Table of the Elements

1	2	3	4	5	6	7	8	9	10	11	12	13	14	15	16	17	18
1 H 1.0079																	2 He 4.0026
3 Li 6.941	4 Be 9.0122											5 B 10.81	6 C 12.011	7 N 14.007	8 O 15.999	9 F 18.998	10 Ne 20.179
11 Na 22.989	12 Mg 24.305											13 Al 26.981	14 Si 28.086	15 P 30.974	16 S 32.06	17 Cl 35.453	18 Ar 39.948
19 K 39.098	20 Ca 40.08	21 Sc 44.956	22 Ti 47.88	23 V 50.941	24 Cr 51.996	25 Mn 54.938	26 Fe 55.847	27 Co 58.933	28 Ni 58.69	29 Cu 63.546	30 Zn 65.38	31 Ga 59.72	32 Ge 72.59	33 As 74.922	34 Se 78.96	35 Br 79.904	36 Kr 83.80
37 Rb 85.468	38 Sr 87.62	39 Y 88.906	40 Zr 91.22	41 Nb 92.905	42 Mo 95.94	43 Tc (98)	44 Ru 101.07	45 Rh 102.91	46 Pd 106.42	47 Ag 107.87	48 Cd 112.41	49 In 114.82	50 Sn 118.69	51 Sb 121.75	52 Te 127.60	53 I 126.90	54 Xe 131.29
55 Cs 132.91	56 Ba 137.33	57 * La 138.90	72 Hf 178.49	73 Ta 180.95	74 W 183.85	75 Re 186.21	76 Os 190.2	77 Ir 192.22	78 Pt 195.08	79 Au 196.97	80 Hg 200.59	81 Tl 204.38	82 Pb 207.2	83 Bi 208.98	84 Po (209)	85 At (210)	86 Rn (222)
87 Fr (223)	88 Ra 226.0	89 # Ac 227.03	104 Rf (261)	105 Db (262)	106 Sg (263)	107 Bh (262)	108 Hs (265)	109 Mt (266)	110 Uun (269)	111 Uuu (272)	112 Uub (277)						

		58 Ce 140.12	59 Pr 140.91	60 Nd 144.24	61 Pm (145)	62 Sm 150.36	63 Eu 151.96	64 Gd 157.25	65 Tb 158.92	66 Dy 162.50	67 Ho 164.93	68 Er 167.26	69 Tm 168.93	70 Yb 173.04	71 Lu 174.97
* Lanthanides															
# Actinides		90 Th 232.03	91 Pa 231.03	92 U 238.03	93 Np 237.05	94 Pu (244)	95 Am (243)	96 Cm (247)	97 Bk (247)	98 Cf (251)	99 Es (254)	100 Fm (257)	101 Md (257)	102 No (255)	103 Lr (256)

The rows of the table are called **periods** and are numbered from 1 to 7 from the top down. Columns in the table are called **groups** or **families**, and are numbered from 1 to 18.

A line on the table under the boxes for B, Si, As, Te, and At separates the **metals** (to the left) from the **nonmetals** (to the right). The majority of the elements are metals. Metals form cations (positively charged ions), are good conductors of heat and electricity, tend to be shiny, and can be drawn into wires. Nonmetals tend to be dull, poor conductors, and brittle. Several elements have properties that are borderline between metallic and nonmetallic. These elements (B, Si, Ge, As, Sb, and Te) are called **metalloids** or semi-metals. Note that these elements straddle the line mentioned above that separates metals and nonmetals.

The first two columns and the last six columns of the table include what are called the main group elements. Columns 3–12 are called the **transition metals**. The two rows separated from the main table beginning with Ce and Th are called the lanthanides and the actinides, respectively.

In addition to the divisions discussed above, there are four groups whose names you should know:

➤ Group 1, the **alkali metals**, includes the common metals sodium and potassium.
➤ Group 2, the **alkaline earth metals**, includes magnesium and calcium.
➤ Group 17, the **halogens,** includes fluorine, chlorine, and bromine.
➤ Group 18, the **noble gases,** includes neon and argon.

COMPOUNDS, MOLECULES, AND IONS

In this section we look in more detail at the types of possible compounds. Compounds are divided into two broad categories depending on the components that make up the sample. The two major classes of compounds are **covalent compounds,** which are formed by sharing electrons between atoms, and **ionic compounds,** which are made by transferring electrons from one atom to another. The covalent compounds are made up of collections of two or more atoms joined together in a unit called a **molecule**. Ionic compounds are made up of **ions,** which are charged particles.

In the chemical formula for a compound, the number of each type of atom present is shown by a subscript. If only one atom of a given element is present, the number 1 is omitted. Sometimes a group is placed in parentheses and given a subscript, for example, iron(II)nitrate, $Fe(NO_3)_2$, contains 1 Fe, 2 N, and 6 O.

You can determine whether a compound is covalent or ionic by looking at the formula.

Binary compounds (made of two elements):

➤ Two nonmetals: covalent; molecules (H_2O, SO_2, NCl_3, PF_3, P_4S_3, and SBr_2)
➤ A metal and a nonmetal: ionic; ions (MgO, NaBr, CaF_2, $FeCl_3$, and Na_2S)
➤ A metal and metal: metallic bonding (discussed later)

Compounds containing more than two elements:

➤ **Polyatomic ion** present: ionic; ions ($Ca(NO_3)_2$, NH_4Cl, $Fe_3(PO_4)_2$, and $K_2C_2O_4$)
➤ All nonmetal: may be a molecular **organic compound,** which must contain carbon and may contain hydrogen and other elements. Described in Chapter 11.

Naming Compounds

BINARY COVALENT COMPOUNDS

In naming binary covalent compounds, the leftmost element in the periodic table is named first and the rightmost element last. If the two elements are in the same group, the lower element is named first. The format for the name is:

prefix + first element name + prefix + second element root + -ide

The prefix indicates the number of atoms in the molecule. If there is only one atom of the first element, the mono- is excluded.

Prefix	mono-	di-	tri-	tetra-	penta-	hexa-
Number of Atoms	1	2	3	4	5	6

Examples:

CO	carbon monoxide		N_2O_4	dinitrogen tetraoxide
NO_2	nitrogen dioxide		P_4S_3	tetraphosphorus trisulfide
CF_4	carbon tetrafluoride		SF_6	sulfur hexafluoride

Several compounds do not adhere to this system and have longstanding common names.

H_2O	water	NH_3	ammonia	NO	nitric oxide

IONIC COMPOUNDS

In the process of forming a compound, if an atom gains one or more electrons, a negative ion or **anion** is formed. If an atom loses one or more electrons, a positive ion or **cation** is formed. Cations and anions are attracted to one another due to the opposite charges. The total number of cation positive charges must equal the total number of anion negative charges to make a neutral compound. The ions in an ionic crystal are arranged in a pattern like a three-dimensional checkerboard. A portion of the structure of sodium chloride is shown in the figure below (+ = cations, − = anions). Ions continue in the crystal up and down, right and left, and in front of and behind the page.

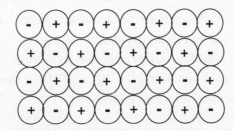

There is no molecule of sodium chloride in the structure. For ionic crystals, the smallest unit of the crystal that has the simplest whole number ratio of the ions is called the **formula unit**. Thus for sodium chloride, the formula unit consists of one sodium cation and one chloride anion.

For most of the main group elements, the charge formed by a monoatomic ion is related to the atom's position in the periodic table. Third period elements are illustrated below.

1	2	13	14	15	16	17	18
Na^+	Ca^{2+}	Al^{3+}	–	P^{3-}	O^{2-}	Cl^-	–

For the anions, the absolute value of the charge is the number of columns the element is to the left of the noble gases, Group 18. Group 14 elements tend to form covalent compounds instead of ionic compounds. (Sn and Pb may form ionic compounds with +2 or +4 charges.) Group 18, the noble gases, are not very reactive and do not form ions. The ions formed by transition metals are not so easily predicted, and some transition metals form ions of more than one charge (Fe^{2+} and Fe^{3+}).

Most of the more common polyatomic ions are anions, with the main exception being the ammonium ion, NH_4^+. Some of the more common polyatomic anions are NO_3^- (nitrate), SO_4^{2-} (sulfate), PO_4^{3-} (phosphate), OH^- (hydroxide), CO_3^{2-} (carbonate), and HCO_3^- (hydrogen carbonate).

Ionic compounds are made up of ions, and the compound must have no overall charge. The total positive charges are equal to the total negative charges. Examples are shown in the following table.

Cation Source	Anion Source	Cation	Anion	Formula
Calcium	Oxygen	Ca^{2+}	O^{2-}	CaO
Barium	Chlorine	Ba^{2+}	Cl^-	$BaCl_2$
Calcium	Nitrogen	Ca^{2+}	N^{3-}	Ca_3N_2
Iron (2+)	Chlorine	Fe^{2+}	Cl^-	$FeCl_2$
Iron (3+)	Chlorine	Fe^{3+}	Cl^-	$FeCl_3$
Calcium	Phosphate	Ca^{2+}	PO_4^{3-}	$Ca_3(PO_4)_2$
Ammonium	Nitrate	NH_4^+	NO_3^-	NH_4NO_3
Cobalt(2+)	Perchlorate	Co^{2+}	ClO_4^-	$Co(ClO_4)_2$

One way of obtaining the formula is to make the cation charge equal to the subscript on the anion, and making the subscript on the cation equal to the charge on the anion, ignoring the negative sign. For ionics, if a formula has a common factor in the subscripts, the common factor is divided out. Consider Ti^{4+} and O^{2-}. Crossing the charges gives Ti_2O_4. Dividing out the common factor of 2 gives TiO_2.

Ionic compounds are named simply by:

$$\text{cation name} + \text{anion name}$$

The name of monoatomic cations is the element name. The sodium atom, Na, and sodium cation, Na^+, are both called sodium. Anions are named by a combination of the root of the element name plus the suffix -ide. Sulfur, S, becomes S^{2-} sulfide, oxygen, O, becomes O^{2-} oxide, nitrogen, N, becomes N^{3-} nitride, and chlorine, Cl, becomes Cl^- chloride.

Formula	Name
NaCl	Sodium chloride
$CaCl_2$	Calcium chloride
K_2O	Potassium oxide
Na_3N	Sodium nitride
$AlBr_3$	Aluminum bromide

A Roman numeral in parentheses is used for cations with more than one possible charge.

Formula	Ions present	Name
$FeCl_2$	two Cl^- ions are balanced by one Fe^{2+} ion	Iron(II)chloride
CoS	one S^{2-} ion is balanced by one Co^{2+} ion	Cobalt(II)sulfide
Cr_2O_3	three O^{2-} ions are balanced by two Cr^{3+} ions	Chromium(III)oxide

With polyatomic ions, simply substitute the name of the polyatomic ion.

Formula	Name
$Ca(ClO_4)_2$	Calcium perchlorate
$Mg_3(PO_4)_2$	Magnesium phosphate
Rb_2SO_4	Rubidium sulfate
$(NH_4)_2C_2O_4$	Ammonium oxalate
$K_2Cr_2O_7$	Potassium dichromate
$Fe(NO_3)_3$	Iron(III)nitrate (Fe^{3+} balances 3 NO_3^- ions)
$CoSO_4$	Cobalt(II)sulfate (Co^{2+} balances one SO_4^{2-})
NH_4NO_2	Ammonium nitrite

Molar Mass of a Compound

The sum of the molar masses of the atoms in a formula gives a compound's molar mass.

H_2O: $(2 \times 1.008) + (1 \times 16.00)\ g = 18.02\ ^g/_{mol}\ H_2O$

C_2H_6O: $(2 \times 12.01) + (6 \times 1.008) + (1 \times 16.00)\ g = 46.07\ ^g/_{mol}\ C_2H_6O$

$$K_2CO_3: (2 \times 39.10) + (1 \times 12.01) + (3 \times 16.00) \text{ g} = 138.21 \text{ }^g/_{mol} K_2CO_3$$

$$Ca(NO_3)_2: (1 \times 40.08) + (2 \times 14.01) + (6 \times 16.00) \text{ g} = 164.10 \text{ }^g/_{mol} Ca(NO_3)_2$$

The same calculation done with the molar mass of elements can be used for compounds.

EXAMPLE: How many moles are there in 100.0 g of C_2H_6O?

$$100.0 \text{ g } C_2H_6O \times \frac{1 \text{ mol } C_2H_6O}{46.07 \text{g } C_2H_6O} = 2.171 \text{ mol } C_2H_6O$$

EXAMPLE: How many g are required to make 5.00 mol of K_2CO_3?

$$5.00 \text{ mol } K_2CO_3 \times \frac{138.21 \text{ g } K_2CO_3}{1 \text{ mol } K_2CO_3} = 691 \text{ g } K_2CO_3$$

EXAMPLE: How many oxygen atoms are there in 10.0 g of $Ca(NO_3)_2$?

This is a three-step process:

$$\text{g } Ca(NO_3)_2 \longrightarrow \text{mol } Ca(NO_3)_2 \longrightarrow \text{formula units } Ca(NO_3)_2 \longrightarrow \text{oxygen atoms}$$

$$10.0\text{g } Ca(NO_3)_2 \times \frac{1 \text{ mol } Ca(NO_3)_2}{164.10 \text{ g } Ca(NO_3)_2} \times \frac{6.022 \times 10^{23} \text{ formula units } Ca(NO_3)_2}{1 \text{ mol } Ca(NO_3)_2}$$

$$= 3.67 \times 10^{22} \text{ formula units } Ca(NO_3)_2$$

$$3.67 \times 10^{22} \text{ formula units } Ca(NO_3)_2 \times \frac{6 \text{ O atoms}}{1 \text{ formula unit } Ca(NO_3)_2}$$

$$= 2.20 \times 10^{23} \text{ O atoms}$$

Percent Composition and Determining Molecular Formulas

The percent composition is easily calculated from the formula of a compound. Ibuprofen, a common drug used in over-the-counter pain relievers, has the formula $C_{13}H_{18}O_2$. What is the percent composition by mass of each element in ibuprofen?

$$13 \times C = 13 \times 12.01 = 156.13 \text{ g C}$$
$$18 \times H = 18 \times 1.008 = 18.144 \text{ g H}$$
$$2 \times O = 2 \times 16.00 = \underline{32.00 \text{ g O}}$$
$$206.27 \text{ g total in one mole of ibuprofen}$$

$$\%C = \frac{156.13 \text{ g C}}{206.27 \text{ g total}} \times 100 = 75.692\% C$$

$$\% H = \frac{18.144\,g\,H}{206.27\,g\,total} \times 100 = 8.7962\%\,H$$

$$\% O = \frac{32.00\,g\,O}{206.27\,g\,total} \times 100 = \frac{15.51\%\,O}{100.00\,\%\,total}$$

Given the percent composition of a substance, determining the molecular formula is more difficult. Before demonstrating this calculation, the **empirical formula** must be defined. The molecular formula of a compound occasionally contains a common factor in the subscripts. Dividing out this factor yields the empirical formula.

Molecular formula	Empirical formula
C_2H_6	CH_3
$B_3N_3Cl_6$	$BNCl_2$
C_6H_6	CH
C_2H_6O	C_2H_6O

Formulas obtained from the percent composition are always the empirical formula; because the molecular formula is a multiple of the empirical formula, the ratio of the mass of the elements is the same and the percent composition will be the same.

EXAMPLE: A compound was analyzed and the percent composition by mass was found to be 49.41 % K, 20.26 % S, and 30.33 % O. Determine the empirical formula. A convenient amount to use for this problem is 100.0 g because the percents are numerically equal to the number of grams of each element. From the grams of each element, you can determine the number of moles of each element. The ratio of the moles is directly related to the ratio of the atoms in the formula.

$$49.41\,g\,K \times \frac{1\,mol\,K}{39.10\,g\,K} = 1.264\,mol\,K$$

$$20.26\,g\,S \times \frac{1\,mol\,S}{32.07\,g\,S} = 0.6317\,mol\,S$$

$$30.33\,g\,O \times \frac{1\,mol\,O}{16.00\,g\,O} = 1.896\,mol\,O$$

These moles are in the correct ratio, but a fraction of an atom is not possible.

$$K_{1.264}S_{0.6317}O_{1.896}$$

Divide each number of moles by the smallest number of moles to get a whole number.

$$K_{\frac{1.264}{0.6317}}S_{\frac{0.6317}{0.6317}}O_{\frac{1.896}{0.6317}} = K_{2.00}S_{1.000}O_{3.001} = K_2SO_3.$$

The numbers often will not end up being exactly whole numbers generally due to experimental errors. In this case the other numbers are very close to whole numbers.

Simple fractions that may occur in this type of calculation include:

$\frac{1}{2} = 0.500$ $\frac{1}{3} = 0.333$ $\frac{1}{4} = 0.250$ $\frac{1}{5} = 0.200$

$\frac{2}{3} = 0.667$ $\frac{2}{5} = 0.400$

$\frac{3}{4} = 0.750$ $\frac{3}{5} = 0.600$

$\frac{4}{5} = 0.800.$

These fractions may be removed from the formula by multiplying by a whole number.

CHEMICAL REACTIONS

A **chemical reaction** is a chemical change in which a set of chemical substances called **reactants** are transformed into a new set of chemical substances called **products**. A chemical reaction is represented symbolically by a **chemical equation**. In chemical equations, (s) = solid, (l) = liquid, (g) = gas, and (aq) = aqueous solution.

EXAMPLE: $CH_4(g) + 2O_2(g) \longrightarrow 2H_2O(l) + CO_2(g)$

The reactants are CH_4 and O_2, and the products are H_2O and CO_2. To make sure the equation is **balanced**, a number called a **coefficient** (in this case, 2) is placed in front of H_2O and O_2. That coefficient ensures that there is the same number of each type of atom in the reactants and in the products, as required by the law of conservation of mass.

Chemical reactions can be classified by the nature of the reactants and products.

➤ A **precipitation reaction** produces an insoluble compound called a **precipitate**.

EXAMPLE: Formation of a precipitate of barium sulfate

$Na_2SO_4(aq) + Ba(NO_3)_2(aq) \longrightarrow 2NaNO_3(aq) + BaSO_4(s)$

➤ A **neutralization reaction** is a reaction between a source of H^+, an **acid**, and a source of OH^-, a **base**, to form water and an ionic compound, a **salt**.

EXAMPLE: Reaction of HCl and NaOH

$HCl(aq) + NaOH(aq) \longrightarrow H_2O(l) + NaCl(aq)$

➤ An **oxidation-reduction reaction** is the transfer of electrons from one substance to another.

EXAMPLE: Magnesium transfers electrons to oxygen, yielding magnesium oxide.

$2Mg(s) + O_2(g) \longrightarrow 2\,MgO(s)$

Balancing Chemical Equations

Most equations can be balanced by trial and error. Equations are balanced by changing the coefficients. Never change the subscripts because this will change the compound or produce a nonexistent compound.

EXAMPLE: Balance the following equation:

$$Al(s) + Br_2(g) \longrightarrow AlBr_3(s)$$

Al is initially balanced. Balance Br atoms with a 3 in front of Br_2 and a 2 in front of $AlBr_3$. Rebalance the Al with a 2 in front of Al.

$$2Al(s) + 3Br_2(g) \longrightarrow 2AlBr_3(s)$$

A common type of equation that is balanced is the combustion of an organic compound.

EXAMPLE: Balance the following equation:

$$C_4H_{10}(g) + O_2(g) \longrightarrow H_2O(l) + CO_2(g)$$

Balance C with a 4 in front of CO_2. Balance H with a 5 in front of H_2O.

$$C_4H_{10}(g) + O_2(g) \longrightarrow 5H_2O(l) + 4CO_2(g)$$

Balancing the oxygen is tricky because three compounds have oxygen. There is an odd number of O atoms on the product side, but O_2 from the reactant side will always give an even number of O atoms. A method to get around this problem is to use a fractional number of O_2 molecules, $\frac{13}{2}$ in front of O_2 will balance the equation.

$$C_4H_{10}(g) + \frac{13}{2} O_2(g) \longrightarrow 5H_2O(l) + 4CO_2(g)$$

In general, a balanced equation has all whole-number coefficients. Double all coefficients to remove the fraction. Check the final equation.

$$2C_4H_{10}(g) + 13 O_2(g) \longrightarrow 10H_2O(l) + 8CO_2(g)$$

Consider the combustion of methane:

$$CH_4(g) + 2O_2(g) \longrightarrow 2H_2O(l) + CO_2(g)$$

The calculation of the relationships among the masses of reactants and products in a chemical reaction is called **stoichiometry**. **Molar ratios** are the ratios of the coefficients from the balanced equation. Examples of these molar ratios using the combustion of methane are $\dfrac{1 \text{ mol } CH_4}{2 \text{ mol } O_2}$, $\dfrac{2 \text{ mol } H_2O}{2 \text{ mol } O_2}$, or $\dfrac{1 \text{ mol } CH_4}{2 \text{ mol } H_2O}$. The reciprocal of each ratio is also valid. A molar ratio is a conversion factor for the moles of one substance to an equivalent number of moles for another substance in a given chemical reaction. Putting together the molar ratios and the molar mass, a path from grams of a component of the reaction, A, to the grams of any other component, B, can be drawn.

$$g \text{ of A} \longrightarrow \text{mol of A} \longrightarrow \text{mol of B} \longrightarrow g \text{ of B}$$

The first and last steps use the molar mass, and the middle step uses the molar ratio.

EXAMPLE:

$$N_2(g) + 3H_2(g) \longrightarrow 2NH_3(g)$$

If 46.8 g of H_2 (molar mass = 2.016 g/mol) is completely reacted with N_2, how many g of NH_3 (molar mass = 17.03 g/mol) will be formed?

$$g \text{ of } H_2 \longrightarrow \text{mol of } H_2 \longrightarrow \text{mol of } NH_3 \longrightarrow g \text{ of } NH_3$$

$$46.8 \text{ g } H_2 \times \frac{1 \text{ mol } H_2}{2.016 \text{ g } H_2} \times \frac{2 \text{ mol } NH_3}{3 \text{ mol } H_2} \times \frac{17.03 \text{ g } NH_3}{1 \text{ mol } NH_3} = 264 \text{ g } NH_3$$

This type of calculation can be carried out for any balanced equation.

Limiting Reactants

If there are two or more reactants in a chemical reaction, and the moles of the reactants are in the same ratio as the balanced equation, all the reactants will completely react. The other possibility is that one reactant is in limited supply, and there is not enough of that **limiting reactant** to completely consume the other reactants.

EXAMPLE:

$$4NH_3(g) + 5O_2(g) \longrightarrow 4NO(g) + 6H_2O(l)$$

A mixture of 4.0 mol of NH_3 can react completely with 5.0 mol of O_2 to produce products with no reactants left over. In this case, you would say the reactants are in a **stoichiometric ratio**. Consider the combination of 4.0 mol of NH_3 and 9.0 mol of O_2. In this case, the NH_3 would react with 5.0 mol of O_2 to form products, but after the 4.0 mol of NH_3 are reacted there is still $9.0 - 5.0 = 4.0$ mol of O_2 left over. The maximum amount of products formed is dependent on the limiting reactant, NH_3. The O_2 is in excess.

The maximum amount of product with a limiting reactant is determined by calculating the masses of products that are possible from the complete reaction of each reactant.

EXAMPLE: What is the maximum amount of H_2O formed from combustion of 25.0 g of C_3H_8 and 50.0 g of O_2? (Molar masses: $C_3H_8 = 44.09$ g/mol, $O_2 = 32.00$ g/mol, and $H_2O = 18.02$ g/mol)

$$C_3H_8(g) + 5O_2(g) \longrightarrow 3CO_2(g) + 4H_2O(l)$$

First, calculate the maximum amount of water formed from complete reaction of C_3H_8.

$$g \text{ of } C_3H_8 \longrightarrow \text{mol of } C_3H_8 \longrightarrow \text{mol of } H_2O \longrightarrow g \text{ of } H_2O$$

$$25.0 \text{ g } C_3H_8 \times \frac{1 \text{ mol } C_3H_8}{44.09 \text{ g } C_3H_8} \times \frac{4 \text{ mol } H_2O}{1 \text{ mol } C_3H_8} \times \frac{18.02 \text{ g } H_2O}{1 \text{ mol } H_2O} = 40.9 \text{ g } H_2O$$

Assuming all the O_2 reacts, the calculation is as follows:

$$\text{g of } O_2 \longrightarrow \text{mol of } O_2 \longrightarrow \text{mol of } H_2O \longrightarrow \text{g of } H_2O$$

$$50.0 \text{ g } O_2 \times \frac{1 \text{ mol } O_2}{32.00 \text{ g } O_2} \times \frac{4 \text{ mol } H_2O}{5 \text{ mol } O_2} \times \frac{18.02 \text{ g } H_2O}{1 \text{ mol } H_2O} = 22.5 \text{ g } H_2O$$

Complete reaction of the given O_2 produces 22.5 g of H_2O, which is less than the 40.9 g produced from complete reaction of the C_3H_8. The O_2 limits the reaction, and a maximum of 22.5 g of H_2O can form.

Percent Yield

Often reactions do not go to completion for many possible reasons. Sometimes reactions are not run long enough. Some reactions simply do not go to completion for energetic reasons. The efficiency of a reaction is measured by the **percent yield,** defined as:

$$\% \text{ yield} = \frac{\text{actual yield}}{\text{theoretical yield}} \times 100\%$$

EXAMPLE: 12.6 g of uranium (IV) oxide is reacted with excess hydrofluoric acid, yielding 13.1 g of uranium tetrafluoride. Calculate the percent yield. (Molar masses: $UO_2 = 270 \text{ g/mol}$, $UF_4 = 314 \text{ g/mol}$)

$$UO_2(s) + 4HF(g) \longrightarrow UF_4(g) + 2H_2O(l)$$

$$\text{g of } UO_2 \longrightarrow \text{mol of } UO_2 \longrightarrow \text{mol of } UF_4 \longrightarrow \text{g of } UF_4$$

Calculate the theoretical yield:

$$12.6 \text{ g } UO_2 \times \frac{1 \text{ mol } UO_2}{270 \text{ g } UO_2} \times \frac{1 \text{ mol } UF_4}{1 \text{ mol } UO_2} \times \frac{314 \text{ g } UF_4}{1 \text{ mol } UF_4} = 14.7 \text{ g } UF_4$$

$$\% \text{ yield} = \frac{13.1 \text{ g } UF_4}{14.7 \text{ g } UF_4} \times 100\% = 89.1\% \text{ yield}$$

Reactions in Aqueous Solution

The ions in solutions of ionic compounds allow the solutions to conduct electricity. Ionic substances that completely dissociate into ions are called **strong electrolytes.** Most soluble ionic compounds are strong electrolytes. Substances that only partially dissociate into ions are called **weak electrolytes.**

PRECIPITATION REACTIONS

In an ionic **precipitation reaction,** two solutions of ionic compounds are mixed, and an insoluble compound called a **precipitate** forms that settles out of the solution. You may predict if a precipitate will form by using a simple set of solubility rules for ionic compounds in aqueous solutions.

Solubility of Ionic Compounds

Compounds that are usually soluble

1. All salts of Group 1 cations, Li^+, Na^+, and K^+, and the ammonium ion, NH_4^+ are soluble.
2. All nitrates, NO_3^-, and acetates, CH_3COO^-, are soluble.
3. All chlorides, Cl^-, bromides, Br^-, and iodides, I^-, are soluble except when combined with Ag^+, Pb^{2+}, or Hg_2^{2+}
4. All sulfates, SO_4^{2-}, are soluble except when combined with Ca^{2+}, Sr^{2+}, Ba^{2+}, Pb^{2+}, Ag^+, or Hg_2^{2+}.

Compounds that are usually insoluble

5. All phosphates, PO_4^{3-}, carbonates, CO_3^{2-}, hydroxides, OH^-, and sulfides, S^{2-}, are insoluble except when combined with Group 1 cations or ammonium. $Ca(OH)_2$, $Sr(OH)_2$, and $Ba(OH)_2$ are also soluble.

Most of the rules concern anions. Only rule 1 focuses on the cations. To use these rules, first consider all ions that are in solution. Consider combinations of cations and anions and decide whether or not a precipitate will form.

> **EXAMPLE:** Predict whether a precipitate will form if barium nitrate is reacted with copper (II) sulfate.

$$Ba(NO_3)_2(aq) + CuSO_4(aq) \longrightarrow ?$$

The ions present in the reactant solutions that are formed by each soluble compound are:

$$Ba^{2+}(aq), \quad NO_3^-(aq), \quad Cu^{2+}(aq), \quad and \quad SO_4^{2-}(aq)$$

Consider the possible combinations of cations and anions. Ignore reactant combinations.

$$Ba^{2+} \quad and \quad SO_4^{2-} \quad \text{Precipitate according to rule 4.}$$

and

$$NO_3^- \quad and \quad Cu^{2+} \quad \text{Soluble according to rule 1.}$$

The formulas for the products are: Ba^{2+} and SO_4^{2-}: $BaSO_4$ and NO_3^- and Cu^{2+}: $Cu(NO_3)_2$. The balanced equation for this reaction, including the phases of the reactants and products, is as follows:

$$Ba(NO_3)_2(aq) + CuSO_4(aq) \longrightarrow BaSO_4(s) + Cu(NO_3)_2(aq)$$

The actual state of the species in solution is shown in the total or overall **ionic equation**. Soluble compounds are broken down into ions. Precipitates are left intact.

$$Ba^{2+}(aq) + 2NO_3^-(aq) + Cu^{2+}(aq) + SO_4^{2-}(aq) \longrightarrow BaSO_4(s) + Cu^{2+}(aq) + 2NO_3^-(aq)$$

The **net ionic equation** eliminates any species that are identical on the reactant and product side called **spectator ions**. In this case, eliminate Cu^{2+} and NO_3^-.

$$Ba^{2+}(aq) + SO_4^{2-}(aq) \longrightarrow BaSO_4(s)$$

Acids and Bases

Acids are defined as substances that dissolve in water to produce H^+ ions. An H^+ ion (a proton) is so small it does not actually exist independently in water but is associated tightly with a water molecule. A better representation is $H^+(aq)$ or even better $H_3O^+(aq)$, which is the **hydronium** ion. **Bases** are defined as substances that dissolve in water to produce OH^- (**hydroxide**) ions.

➤ Acids that dissociate 100 % are strong electrolytes and are termed **strong acids**. The six common strong acids are: HCl, HBr, HI, $HClO_4$, HNO_3, and H_2SO_4.
➤ Acids that only partially disassociate are weak electrolytes and are called **weak acids**. A large class of weak acids are organic compounds that contain the group -COOH. An example is the acid in vinegar, acetic acid, CH_3COOH. Other weak acids include HF, HCN, and H_3PO_4.
➤ **Strong bases** are strong electrolytes. Common strong bases are NaOH and KOH.
➤ **Weak bases** are weak electrolytes. Weak bases include ammonia, NH_3.

Ammonia produces OH^- ions by removing a proton from water according to the following reaction:

$$NH_3(aq) + H_2O(l) \longrightarrow NH_4^+(aq) + OH^-(aq)$$

Acids and bases react to produce an ionic solid (a salt) and water in a **neutralization reaction**.

$$HCl(aq) + NaOH(aq) \longrightarrow NaCl(aq) + HOH \text{ (or } H_2O) \text{ (l)}$$

The water is initially written as HOH to emphasize the reaction as an exchange reaction. The ionic equation and net ionic equation can be written for a neutralization reaction.

EXAMPLE: Consider the reaction between perchloric acid and potassium hydroxide:
$$HClO_4(aq) + KOH(aq) \longrightarrow KClO_4(aq) + H_2O \text{ (l)}$$

Ionic equation:

$$H^+(aq) + ClO_4^-(aq) + K^+(aq) + OH^-(aq) \longrightarrow K^+(aq) + ClO_4^-(aq) + H_2O(l)$$

Net ionic equation:
$$H^+(aq) + OH^-(aq) \longrightarrow H_2O(l)$$

Solution Stoichiometry

Reminder: 1 Liter = 1000 mL. This conversion factor will be used often with solutions.

Solutions consist of some **solute** that is dissolved in a **solvent**. Rather than weighing out a specific quantity of a substance, you use the concentration of a solution (the amount of solute per unit volume) and measure out a desired amount by volume. The most useful solution concentration unit for chemical reactions is **molarity (M)**, which is moles of solute per liter of solution. Note that this is per liter of solution, not per liter of solvent. Molarity is a conversion factor between the volume of solution and moles of solute.

EXAMPLE: If 50.51 g of $Ca(NO_3)_2$ (molar mass $= 164.1 ^g/_{mol}$) is dissolved in water and diluted to a final volume of 250.0 mL, what is the molarity of the solution?

$$g \, Ca(NO_3)_2 \longrightarrow mol \, Ca(NO_3)_2 \longrightarrow M \, of \, Ca(NO_3)_2 \, solution$$

$$50.51 \, g \, Ca(NO_3)_2 \times \frac{1 \, mol \, Ca(NO_3)_2}{164.1 \, g \, Ca(NO_3)_2} = 0.3078 \, mol \, Ca(NO_3$$

$$\frac{0.3078 \, mol \, Ca(NO_3)_2}{0.2500 \, L \, soln} = 1.231 \, M \, Ca(NO_3)_2$$

Note that each mole $Ca(NO_3)_2$ dissolves to form 1 mol Ca^{2+} and 2 mol of NO_3^- so the solution is 1.231 M Ca^{2+}, but is $2 \times 1.231 = 2.462$ M NO_3^-.

Once the molarity is known, a volume for a desired number of moles or the number of moles in a given volume may be calculated. For these calculations, molarity is most conveniently expressed by the unit mol/L where mol is for the solute and L is for the solution.

EXAMPLE: How many mL of 0.987 M NaOH solution will supply 0.345 mol of NaOH?

$$0.345 \, mol \, NaOH \times \frac{1 \, L \, soln}{0.987 \, mol \, NaOH} = 0.350 \, L \, or \, 350 \, mL \, of \, 0.987 \, M \, NaOH$$

EXAMPLE: How many mol of NaOH are there in 150.0 mL of 0.345 M NaOH?

$$0.1500 \, L \, soln \times \frac{0.345 \, mol \, NaOH}{1 \, L \, soln} = 0.0518 \, mol \, of \, NaOH$$

Another important use of molarity is for calculating a solution's concentration upon dilution. When solvent is added to a solution, the number of moles of solute does not change, only the volume. Dilution spreads a given amount of solute into a larger volume.

The molarity of the solution decreases upon dilution.

EXAMPLE: If 50.00 mL of 0.673 M $FeCl_2$ is mixed with 75.00 mL of water, what is the final concentration of the solution? (Final volume of solution is $50.00 + 75.00 \, mL = 125.00 \, mL$.)

$$V \, conc. \, solution \longrightarrow mol \, solute \longrightarrow M \, dilute \, solution$$

$$0.05000 \, L \, soln \times \frac{0.673 \, mol \, FeCl_2}{1 \, L \, soln} = 0.0337 \, mol \, of \, FeCl_2$$

$$\text{Molarity} = \frac{0.0337 \text{ mol FeCl}_2}{0.12500 \text{ L soln}} = 0.270 \text{ M FeCl}_2$$

Because the number of moles can be obtained from the molarity, stoichiometry calculations may be done using volumes and molarity in a manner similar to that using grams and the molar mass.

> **EXAMPLE:** How many mL of 0.235 M K_3PO_4 are needed to completely precipitate the calcium in 40.0 mL of 0.125 M $CaCl_2$?

$$2K_3PO_4(aq) + 3\,CaCl_2(aq) \longrightarrow Ca_3(PO_4)_2(s) + 6\,KCl(aq)$$
$$\text{V of CaCl}_2 \longrightarrow \text{mol of CaCl}_2 \longrightarrow \text{mol of K}_3PO_4 \longrightarrow \text{g of K}_3PO_4$$

$$0.0400 \text{ L soln} \times \frac{0.125 \text{ mol CaCl}_2}{1 \text{ L soln}} \times \frac{2 \text{ mol K}_3PO_4}{3 \text{ mol CaCl}_2} \times \frac{1 \text{ L soln}}{0.235 \text{ mol K}_3PO_4}$$

$$= 0.142 \text{ L or } 14.2 \text{ mL of } 0.235 \text{ M K}_3PO_4$$

In a **titration**, a solution of known concentration, the standard solution, is used to analyze other solutions of unknown concentrations. The **equivalence point** is reached when enough of the standard solution is added to completely react with the unknown.

> **EXAMPLE:** A 20.00 mL sample of HBr of unknown concentration required 29.63 mL of standard 0.9623 M NaOH to be neutralized. What is the molarity of the HBr solution?

$$HBr(aq) + NaOH(aq) \longrightarrow H_2O(l) + NaBr(aq)$$
$$\text{V of NaOH} \longrightarrow \text{mol of NaOH} \longrightarrow \text{mol of HBr} \longrightarrow \text{M of HBr}$$

$$0.02963 \text{ L NaOH} \times \frac{0.9623 \text{ mol NaOH}}{1 \text{ L soln}} \times \frac{1 \text{ mol HBr}}{1 \text{ mol NaOH}} \times \frac{1}{0.02000 \text{ L soln}}$$

$$= 1.426 \text{ M HBr}$$

Oxidation-Reduction Reactions

In an **oxidation-reduction reaction (redox** for short), electrons are transferred. The species gaining electrons is **reduced**, and the species losing electrons is **oxidized.**

> **EXAMPLE:** Formation of a metal oxide such as magnesium oxide is a redox reaction.
> $$2Mg(s) + O_2(g) \longrightarrow 2\,MgO(s)$$

In this reaction Mg loses 2 electrons and forms a 2+ ion, so Mg is oxidized. Simultaneously O gains two electrons and forms a 2- ion, so O is reduced.

The nature of the reaction is straightforward when ions are formed because the number of electrons lost or gained is clear. In other reactions, especially with molecular species, the transfer of electrons is not so apparent.

The **oxidation number** is a bookkeeping method used to assign electrons to atoms to allow determination of the change in the number of electrons associated with an atom. An increase in oxidation number is **oxidation**. A decrease in oxidation number is **reduction**. In order to assign an oxidation number to an atom, follow these rules:

Rules for Assigning an Oxidation Number

1. The oxidation number of an atom of an element in its elemental form is zero.
2. The oxidation number of a monoatomic ion is equal to the charge on the ion.
3. Flourine in compounds is assigned the oxidation number -1.
4. Oxygen in compounds is assigned the oxidation number -2 unless combined with fluorine. In the peroxide ion O_2^-, oxygen has an oxidation number of -1.
5. Hydrogen in compounds has an oxidation number of $+1$ except when combined with a metal, where it has an oxidation number of -1.
6. The oxidation number of other elements is determined by the fact that the sum of the oxidation numbers of all the atoms in a species is equal to the ionic charge. For neutral molecules or atoms the sum is zero.

Ionic examples:

NaCl: $Na^+ = +1$, $Cl^- = -1$ $\qquad\qquad$ Ca_3N_2: $Ca^{2+} = +2$, $N^{3-} = -3$

Examples using rule 6. Elemental symbols in parentheses represent an oxidation number

NO_2	$[(O) = -2]$	$(N) + 2(O) = 0$	$(N) = +4$
HCOOH	$[(O) = -2, (H) = +1]$	$2(H) + 2(O) + (C) = 0$	$(C) = +2$
PO_4^{3-}	$[(O) = -2]$	$(P) + 4(O) = -3$	$(P) = +5$
$C_2O_4^{2-}$	$[(O) = -2]$	$2(C) + 4(O) = -2$	$(C) = +3$

By looking at the change in oxidation number during the course of a reaction, you can determine which atom is oxidized or reduced.

$$2C_2H_6(g) + 7O_2(g) \longrightarrow 4CO_2(g) + 6H_2O(l)$$

Assigning oxidation numbers:

C_2H_6	$[(H) = +1]$	$2(C) + 6(H) = 0$	$(C) = -3$
O_2	$[(O) = 0]$		
CO_2	$[(O) = -2]$	$(C) + 2(O) = 0$	$(C) = +4$
H_2O	$[(O) = -2, (H) = +1]$		

Element	Reactant	Product	Change	Process
C	-3	$+4$	$+7$	oxidation
H	$+1$	$+1$	0	none
O	0	-2	-2	reduction

In terms of oxidation numbers, four carbon atoms lost seven electrons each for a total of 28 electrons transferred, and 14 oxygen atoms gained two electrons each for a total of

28 electrons accepted. Oxidation and reduction must occur together. The substance that brings about oxidation is called the **oxidizing agent** (in this example O_2), and the substance that causes reduction is called the **reducing agent** (in this case C_2H_6). The oxidation agent is reduced and the reducing agent is oxidized.

GASES

Gases are easier to study than solids or liquids because the molecules of gases are well separated from one another. In solids and liquids, the molecules are in contact. The equations that describe the behavior of gases are similar for all gases as long as the temperature is not too low or the pressure is not too high. Gases under these conditions are described as ideal gases.

One variable used in describing the state of a gas is **pressure**, which is defined as the force exerted per unit area. The most common unit of pressure is the **atmosphere** (atm), equivalent to the average pressure of the earth's atmosphere at sea level. Pressure is also measured by the length of a column of mercury that can be supported by the atmosphere in an inverted tube. A pressure of 1 atm can support a column of 760 mm mercury. A pressure of 1 mm of mercury is also called a torr. The equation 1 atm $=760$ torr $=760$ mm Hg is used often in working problems with gases. The official unit for pressure in the SI system is the Pascal $\left(Pa = \dfrac{N}{m^2} \right)$. The conversion factor from atm to kPa is 1 atm $=101.325$ kPa.

Temperature for gases must usually be given in Kelvin. The conversion from Celsius to Kelvin is $K = °C + 273.15$. For most purposes, $°C + 273$ is adequate.

The variables in the state of a gas—volume, pressure, etc.—are related in ways that are either direct variations or inverse variations or proportions.

➤ In a **direct variation**, an increase in one variable results in an increase in the other. If y varies directly with x, then, $y = ax$, where a is a constant.

➤ In an **inverse variation**, an increase in one variable results in a decrease in the other. If y varies inversely with x, then, $y = b/x$, where b is a constant. An inverse variation can also represented as $xy = b$.

The graph of a direct variation is shown below left, and the graph of an inverse variation is shown below right.

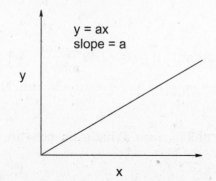

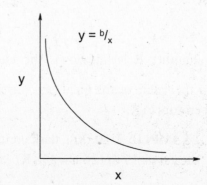

Three relationships discovered early in the study of gases are:

➤ **Boyle's Law:** Volume (V) varies inversely with pressure (P): $V = \text{constant}/P$ or $PV = \text{constant}$

➤ **Charles's Law:** Volume varies directly with absolute (Kelvin) temperature (T): $V = \text{constant} \times T$

➤ **Avogadro's Law:** Volume varies directly with moles (n) of gas: $V = \text{constant} \times n$

In each law above, variables not given in the equation are constant. For example, when using Boyle's Law, the temperature and number of moles of gas are constant.

You can rewrite these laws in a more convenient form by eliminating the constant of proportionality. For Boyle's Law, consider two states of a gas:

$$P_1 V_1 = \text{constant}$$
$$P_2 V_2 = \text{constant}$$
$$\text{so } P_1 V_1 = P_2 V_2$$

In a similar way, Charles's Law can be written as follows:

$$\frac{V_1}{T_1} = \frac{V_2}{T_2}$$

and Avogadro's Law becomes

$$\frac{V_1}{n_1} = \frac{V_2}{n_2}.$$

These relationships can be used to evaluate the effect on one variable when another changes.

EXAMPLE: A sample of 34.0 L of helium at 0 °C is heated to 75 °C. If the pressure and moles of helium are fixed, what is the new volume?

$$V_1 = 34.0 \text{ L}, V_2 = ?, T_1 = 0 + 273 = 273 \text{ K}, T_2 = 75 + 273 = 348 \text{ K}$$

$$\frac{V_1}{T_1} = \frac{V_2}{T_2} \rightarrow \frac{T_2 V_1}{T_1} = V_2 \longrightarrow \frac{(348 \text{ K})(34.0 \text{ L})}{(273 \text{ K})} = 43.3 \text{ L}$$

The three laws above can be combined into one general law called the **ideal gas law:**

$$PV = nRT$$

The quantity R is known as the ideal gas constant. $R = 0.08206 \frac{L \cdot atm}{mol \cdot K}$. When using this value of the ideal gas constant, volume must be in L, pressure in atm, and temperature in K.

EXAMPLE: A 10.00 L flask contains 1.00 mol of neon. What is the pressure of the gas at 25°C? (25°C = 298 K)

$$PV = nRT \longrightarrow P = \frac{nRT}{V} \longrightarrow P = \frac{(1.00 \text{ mol})\left(0.08206\dfrac{L \cdot atm}{mol \cdot K}\right)(298 \text{ K})}{(10.00 \text{ L})} = 2.45 \text{ atm}$$

The ideal gas law contains moles, so stoichiometry problems with gases are possible.

EXAMPLE: If 2.00 g of Mg (molar mass 24.305 $^g/_{mol}$) is reacted with excess hydrochloric acid, what volume of hydrogen gas is produced at 40°C at a pressure of 700 torr?

$$700 \text{ torr} \times \frac{1 \text{ atm}}{760 \text{ torr}} = 0.921 \text{ atm, and } 40°C + 273 = 313 \text{ K}$$

$$Mg(s) + 2HCl(g) \longrightarrow MgCl_2(aq) + H_2(g)$$

$$\text{g of Mg} \longrightarrow \text{mol of Mg} \longrightarrow \text{mol of } H_2 \longrightarrow V \text{ of } H_2$$

$$2.00 \text{ g Mg} \times \frac{1 \text{ mol Mg}}{24.305 \text{ g Mg}} \times \frac{1 \text{ mol } H_2}{1 \text{ mol Mg}} = 0.0823 \text{ mol } H_2$$

$$PV = nRT \longrightarrow V = \frac{nRT}{P} \longrightarrow V = \frac{(0.0823 \text{ mol})\left(0.08206\dfrac{L \cdot atm}{mol \cdot K}\right)(313 \text{ K})}{(0.921 \text{ atm})} = 2.30 \text{ atm}$$

Gases and Molar Masses

The number of moles of a substance is determined by dividing the mass of the substance, m, by the molar mass, $\mathcal{M}$ (a script M is used to prevent confusion with molarity). Substituting $^m/_{\mathcal{M}}$ for the number of mol, n, in the ideal gas law gives:

$$PV = \frac{m}{\mathcal{M}}RT \text{ , which can be rearranged to: } P\mathcal{M} = \frac{m}{V}RT$$

The quantity $\dfrac{m}{V}$ is simply the density, so the previous equation becomes

$$P\mathcal{M} = dRT.$$

This equation may be used to determine the molar mass of a gas.

Dalton's Law of Partial Pressures

In a mixture of gases, the gas molecules are well separated. There is little interaction between the molecules of the different gases. Each gas behaves as if it were in the container by itself. For each gas in a mixture, the **partial pressure**, P_x, of the gas is calculated as if the gas were the only gas present. **Dalton's law of partial pressures** states that the total pressure of a mixture of gases is the sum of the partial pressures of all the gases in the mixture.

$$P_{total} = P_1 + P_2 + P_3 + \ldots$$

Using the ideal gas law in the form $P = \dfrac{nRT}{V}$, and recognizing that all of the gases in the container are at the same temperature and volume, Dalton's law becomes:

$$P_{total} = P_1 + P_2 + P_3 + \ldots = \frac{n_1 RT}{V} + \frac{n_2 RT}{V} + \frac{n_3 RT}{V} + \ldots = (n_1 + n_2 + n_3 + \ldots)\left(\frac{RT}{V}\right)$$

The sum of the moles of gases in the mixture, $n_1 + n_2 + n_3 + \ldots$ is the total number of moles of gases present, n_{total}, so that $P_{total} = n_{total}\dfrac{RT}{V}$. Dalton's law is especially useful when a gas is collected over water. The collected gas will actually be a mixture of the gas and water from evaporation. $P_{gas} = P_{total} - P_{water}$, where P_{gas} is the pressure of the dry gas.

The **mole fraction**, χ, is defined as the moles of a substance divided by the total moles present in the system. The range of a mole fraction is $0.0 - 1.0$ and the total of all the mole fractions is 1.0.

$$\chi_1 = \frac{n_1}{n_{total}}$$

Dividing the equation for the partial pressure of a gas by the equation for the total pressure generates another expression for the mole fraction.

$$\frac{P_1}{P_{total}} = \frac{n_1\left(\dfrac{RT}{V}\right)}{(n_1 + n_2 + n_3 + \ldots)\left(\dfrac{RT}{V}\right)} \longrightarrow \frac{P_1}{P_{total}} = \frac{n_1}{n_1 + n_2 + n_3 + \ldots} = \chi_1 \longrightarrow P_1 = \chi_1 P_{total}$$

EXAMPLE: A mixture is prepared from $12.00\,g$ of O_2 and $36.00\,g$ of Ne. The total pressure of the mixture is 840 torr. What is the partial pressure of each gas?

$$12.00\,g\,O_2 \, \frac{1\text{ mole }O_2}{32.00\,g\,O_2} = 0.3750\text{ mol }O_2 \text{ and } 36.00\,g\,Ne\,\frac{1\text{ mole }Ne}{20.18\,g\,Ne} = 1.784\text{ mol }Ne$$

The total mol of the two gases is $0.3750 + 1.784 = 2.159$ mol.

$$\chi_{O_2} = \frac{0.375\text{ mol}}{2.159\text{ mol}} = 0.174 \text{ and } \chi_{Ne} = \frac{1784}{2.159} = 0.8263$$

$$P_{O_2} = \chi_{O_2} P_{total} = 0.174(840\text{ torr}) = 146\text{ torr} \text{ and}$$

$$P_{He} = \chi_{Ne} P_{total} = 0.8263(840\text{ torr}) = 694\text{ torr}$$

Kinetic Molecular Theory

In the discussion of gases above, the macroscopic properties of gases such as pressure, temperature, and volume were described. The behavior of gases is explained on the molecular level by the **kinetic molecular theory,** which has the following postulates:

➤ Particles of gases are separated from one another by large distances when compared to the size of the particles.

➤ Particles of a gas are in constant and random motion.

➤ When the particles of a gas collide with other particles or the sides of the container, no energy is lost, that is, the collisions are elastic.

➤ The particles exert neither repulsive nor attractive forces on one another.

➤ The average kinetic energy of gas particles is directly proportional to the absolute temperature in Kelvin.

The first four points are relatively clear and explain many of the properties of gases such as compressibility, pressure, and the similar behavior of different gases. The last point is important because it means that regardless of the gases involved, at the same temperature all gases have the same average kinetic energy. The last point can also be taken as a definition of temperature.

In a large sample of a gas such as oxygen there is a distribution of velocities. As the temperature increases, the speeds of the oxygen molecules shift to greater velocities and the distribution curve skews to higher velocities. A sample distribution of oxygen molecules at two temperatures is shown below. At the higher temperature the distribution broadens and flattens.

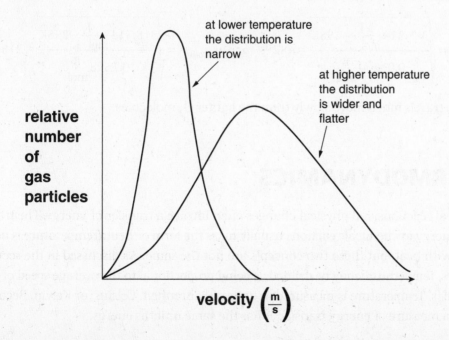

The average kinetic energy of an individual molecule of a gas is given by $\overline{KE} = \frac{1}{2}m\overline{u^2}$ where $\overline{u^2}$ is the average of the squares of the velocities of the molecules. The bar over a quantity indicates the average. The average kinetic energy of a mole of molecules is obtained by multiplying by Avogadro's number, N_A. The middle equation below simplifies to the rightmost equation because the mass of N_A molecules is the molar mass.

$$\overline{KE}_{molecule} = \frac{1}{2}m\overline{u^2} \longrightarrow \overline{KE}_{mole} = \frac{1}{2}(N_A m)\overline{u^2} \longrightarrow \overline{KE}_{mole} = \frac{1}{2}(\mathcal{M})\overline{u^2}$$

The kinetic molecular theory states that the average kinetic energy is proportional to the temperature in Kelvin. The constant of proportionality for one mole of gas is $\frac{3}{2}RT$.

$$\overline{KE}_{mole} = \frac{3}{2}RT$$

Combining the last two equations for $\overline{KE}_{mole}$ and solving for u_{rms} yields:

$$u_{rms} = \sqrt{\overline{u^2}} = \sqrt{\frac{3RT}{\mathcal{M}}}$$

In order to obtain the velocity in m/s, the gas constant must be $R = 8.314 \frac{J}{mol \cdot K}$ and the molar mass must be given in $^{kg}/_{mol}$. (Simply divide the molar mass in $^g/_{mol}$ by 1000.) The quantity u_{rms} is the **root mean square velocity,** which is an average velocity for a gas molecule. This quantity increases with temperature for a given gas. If two gases are compared at the same temperature, the velocity of the more massive gas will be smaller.

> **EXAMPLE:** Calculate the u_{rms} velocities of O_2 (molar mass $= 32.00\ ^g/_{mol}$) and Br_2 (molar mass $= 159.8\ ^g/_{mol}$) at 25°C.

$$u_{rms(O_2)} = \sqrt{\frac{3 \cdot 8.314 \frac{J}{mol \cdot K} 298K}{0.03200 \frac{g}{mol}}} = 482\ ^m/_s \quad \text{and} \quad u_{rms(Br_2)} = \sqrt{\frac{3 \cdot 8.314 \frac{J}{mol \cdot K} 298K}{0.1598 \frac{g}{mol}}} = 216\ ^m/_s$$

The Br_2 travels much more slowly than the lighter O_2 molecules.

THERMODYNAMICS

Chemical reactions and physical changes often involve a transfer of energy. The transfer of energy in chemical reactions usually takes the form of heat. Temperature is associated with heat, but these two concepts are not the same. As discussed in the section on gases, temperature may be defined as being proportional to the average speed of gas molecules. Temperature is measured in units of Fahrenheit, Celsius, or Kelvin. Because heat is a measure of energy transfer, it has the same units as energy.

In the SI system, the unit of energy is the **Joule**, $1 \ J = kg \dfrac{m^2}{s^2}$. **Thermodynamics**, as its name implies, is the study of the movement of heat. This section will discuss thermodynamics with respect to chemical reactions and physical changes such as melting or boiling.

Energy is defined as the ability to do work. **Work** is defined as a force acting on an object moving the object through some distance. Energy can take two basic forms:

➤ **Kinetic energy** is the energy of motion. It is determined by the formula KE = ½ mv², where KE is kinetic energy, m is the mass, and v is the velocity.

➤ **Potential energy** is energy due to position. Varieties of potential energy include solar, electrical, gravitational, and chemical. One form of potential energy is **chemical energy**, which is the energy stored in the bonds of molecules, such as the energy of a fuel like gasoline.

Two important concepts in thermodynamics are the system and the surroundings. The system is the part of the universe under study. The surroundings are everything else. For chemical reactions, the system is usually the compounds involved in a particular reaction.

The **first law of thermodynamics** states that the energy of the universe is fixed. This law is often called the law of conservation of energy. This law can be expressed mathematically as:

$$\Delta E_{univ} = \Delta E_{sys} + \Delta E_{surr} = 0 \text{ which implies } \Delta E_{sys} = -\Delta E_{surr},$$

where ΔE_{univ} is the energy change for the universe, ΔE_{sys} is the energy change for the system, and ΔE_{surr} is the energy change of the surroundings.

Energy lost by the system is gained by the surroundings and vice versa. The internal energy of the system can be described as the sum of the kinetic and potential energy contained in all the parts that make up the system. Changes in the energy of the system are the main concern of thermodynamics. The internal energy of the system may be changed in two ways: (1) by the flow of heat into or out of the system, or (2) by work done either to or by the system. This relationship is expressed in the following equation:

$$\Delta E = q + w$$

where q is the heat, and w is the work.

➤ If heat is added to (absorbed by) the system, the energy increases. This is called an **endothermic** process.

➤ If heat is lost (released) from the system, the energy decreases. This is called an **exothermic** process.

➤ Work done on the system causes an increase in the energy of the system.

➤ Work done by the system causes a decrease in the energy of the system.

In chemical systems, the main type of work is so-called PV or pressure-volume work. The change in energy of the system may be rewritten as follows:

$$\Delta E = q - \Delta PV$$

The negative sign is because $(+)\Delta V$ means $(-)W$.

Because most chemical reactions are carried out at constant pressure, the change in energy at constant pressure is:

$$\Delta E = q_p - P\Delta V$$

The subscript p refers to the heat transferred at constant pressure. One final rearrangement gives:

$$\Delta E + P\Delta V = q_p = \Delta H$$

Enthalpy, H, is the heat transferred at constant pressure. Enthalpy is one of the key properties in thermochemistry. To determine enthalpy, heat transferred at a constant pressure is measured. Volume changes do not have to be measured.

To measure a transfer of heat, we use the **specific heat capacity**, S (some books use C), which is the amount of heat needed to raise the temperature of 1 g of a substance

Substance	$S\left(\dfrac{J}{g \cdot ^\circ C}\right)$
$H_2O(l)$	4.184
Al(s)	0.900
C(diamond)	0.502
Fe(s)	0.444

by 1 K (or $^\circ$C). The specific heat capacities of some common substances are:

The equation used with the specific heat capacity is $q = mS\Delta T$ where q is heat, m is mass, and ΔT is the change in temperature.

> **EXAMPLE:** 1000 J of heat is added to 100.0 g of Fe(s) and Al(s) both at 25°C. What is the final temperature of each metal?

For Fe:	For Al:
$1000\,J = 100.0g\,(0.444\,^J/_{g \cdot ^\circ C})\Delta T$	$1000\,J = 100.0g\,(0.900\,^J/_{g \cdot ^\circ C})\,\Delta T$
$22.5^\circ = \Delta T$	$11.1^\circ C = \Delta T$
$T_f = T_i + \Delta T$	$T_f = T_i + \Delta T$
$T_f = 47.5^\circ C$	$T_f = 36.1^\circ C$

Notice that the same mass of both metals received the same amount of heat, but the one with the higher heat capacity increased less in temperature. Water has an unusually high heat capacity; this is important in regulating the temperature of living things, which are made up in large part of water.

Calorimetry

Calorimetry is the process of measuring heat. Even simple calorimeters such as the two coffee cups that are often used in chemistry labs can give good results.

Inside the calorimeter, a chemical reaction or a physical change such as the melting of ice takes place. The calorimeter contains water or, in the case of soluble reactants, a solution. The styrofoam cups and a cover prevent heat from escaping the calorimeter. The heat released (or absorbed) by the process under study will be transferred to the water (or solution) in the calorimeter. The heat gained or lost by the water or solution is equal and opposite in value to the heat released by the chemical or physical process. Heat transferred to the calorimeter is usually small and can be neglected.

The steps in calculating the q for a given process are:

$q = 0$ (total heat is zero because all the heat is held in the calorimeter)

$q = q_{rxn} + q_{soln}$ (q_{rxn} is the heat of the reaction of interest and q_{soln} the heat of the solution)

$q_{rxn} = -q_{soln}$ (combination of the first two equations)

$q_{rxn} = -(m_{soln}S_{soln}\Delta T_{soln})$ (using the definition of heat capacity).

q_{rxn} may be a physical process such as melting, dissolving, or simply a change in temperature of an object, or q_{rxn} may be a chemical reaction.

EXAMPLE: A 80.0 g piece of metal at 90.0°C is added to a calorimeter with 100.0 mL of water at 25°C. The final temperature of the water after the metal is added is 26.6°C. What is the heat capacity of the metal?

$q_{metal} = -q_{water}$

$m_{metal}S_{metal}\Delta T_{metal} = -(m_{water}S_{water}T_{water})$

$(80.0\,g)(S_{metal})(26.6 - 90.0°C) = -[(100.0\,g)(4.184\,J/g\cdot°c)(26.6 - 25.0°C)]$

$S_{metal}(-5072\,g\cdot°C) = -669.4\,J$

$$= 0.132\frac{J}{g\cdot°C}$$

EXAMPLE: A solution of 500.0 mL 2.00 M $Ba(NO_3)_2$ and 250.0 mL of 4.00 M Na_2SO_4 both at 25°C is mixed in a coffee cup calorimeter and $BaSO_4$ forms as a precipitate. The final temperature of the solution is 33.3°C. Assuming that negligible heat is transferred to the calorimeter, the density of the solution is 1.00 g/mL and the specific heat of the solution is 4.184 $J/g\cdot°c$, calculate the heat of this reaction and the enthalpy (heat per mole of reactant). Note that $0.500\,L \times \dfrac{2.00\,mol\,Ba(NO_3)_2}{1\,L\,soln} = 1.00$ mol $Ba(NO_3)_2$ and

$0.250\,L \times \dfrac{4.00\,mol\,Na_2SO_4}{1\,L\,soln} = 1.00$ mol Na_2SO_4, so there is a stoichiometric amount of each reactant.

$$Ba(NO_3)_2(aq) + Na_2SO_4(aq) \longrightarrow BaSO_4(s) + 2NaNO_3(aq)$$

$q_{rxn} = -(m_{soln1}S_{soln1}\Delta T_{soln1} + m_{soln2}S_{soln2}\Delta T_{soln2})$ (soln1 = $Ba(NO_3)_2$ and
soln2 = Na_2SO_4)

$= -[(500\,g)(4.184\,J/g\cdot°c)(33.3 - 25.0°C) + (250\,g)(4.184\,J/g\cdot°c)(33.3 - 25.0°C)]$

$= -(1.74 \times 10^4\,J + 8.68 \times 10^3\,J)$

$= -2.61 \times 10^4\,J$

The negative sign indicates that this is an exothermic reaction. Because 1.00 mol of Ba^{2+} and 1.00 mol of SO_4^{2-} reacted, $\Delta H = -2.61 \times 10^4$ J/1.00 mol or -2.61×10^4 J/mol or -26.1 kJ/mol.

Thermochemical Equations

Once the enthalpy is found, you can write a thermochemical equation. Below is the thermochemical equation for the burning of methane:

$$CH_4(g) + 2O_2(g) \longrightarrow CO_2(g) + 2H_2O(l) \quad \Delta H = -890 \text{ kJ/mol}$$

The enthalpy is for the number of moles in the balanced equation: 1 mol CH_4, 2 mol O_2, 1 mol CO_2, and 2 mol H_2O. The (−) sign means that the reaction is exothermic. Heat is released by the reaction, so heat is a product. Thus the equation can be rewritten:

$$CH_4(g) + 2O_2(g) \longrightarrow CO_2(g) + 2H_2O(l) + 890 \text{ kJ/mol}.$$

If the reaction is reversed, the equation becomes:

$$890 \text{ kJ/mol} + CO_2(g) + 2H_2O(l) \longrightarrow CH_4(g) + 2O_2(g).$$

For the reverse reaction, heat is a reactant and is absorbed during the course of the reaction, so $\Delta H = +890$ kJ/mol. If you reverse the reaction, you must reverse the sign of ΔH.

The equation may be multiplied by a number such as 3. This is equivalent to burning three times as much methane, so the heat is increased threefold.

$$3CH_4(g) + 6O_2(g) \longrightarrow 3CO_2(g) + 6H_2O(l) + 2670 \text{ kJ/mol}$$

When an equation is multiplied by some number, the ΔH of the equation must be multiplied by the same number.

If ΔH is considered a reactant or product, it may be used in stoichiometry problems:

> **EXAMPLE:** How much heat is released through the burning of 135.0 g of C_4H_{10}?
>
> $$2C_4H_{10}(g) + 13\ O_2(g) \longrightarrow 8CO_2(g) + 10\ H_2O(l) \quad \Delta H = -5762 \text{ kJ/mol}$$
>
> $$\text{g } C_4H_{10} \longrightarrow \text{mol } C_4H_{10} \longrightarrow \text{heat}$$
>
> $$135.0 \text{ g } C_4H_{10} \times \frac{1 \text{ mol } C_4H_{10}}{58.12 \text{ g } C_4H_{10}} \times \frac{5762 \text{ kJ}}{2 \text{ mol } C_4H_{10}} = 6692 \text{ kJ heat released}$$

The heat was divided by 2 because the balanced equation contains 2 moles of C_4H_{10}.

Hess's Law

Hess's Law states that if a series of reactions adds up to a total overall reaction, the enthalpy of the overall reaction is the sum of the enthalpies of the individual reactions.

The first three reactions below sum up to the fourth. The sum of the ΔH for the reactions is calculated as shown.

$$2\,N_2O_5(g) \longrightarrow 2\,N_2(g) + 5O_2(g) \qquad \Delta H_1 = +84\ kJ$$
$$2\,H_2O(l) \longrightarrow 2\,H_2(g) + O_2(g) \qquad \Delta H_2 = +572\ kJ$$
$$2\,N_2(g) + 2\,H_2(g) + 6\,O_2(g) \longrightarrow 4\,HNO_3(l) \qquad \Delta H_3 = -696\ kJ$$

$$2\,N_2O_5(g) + 2\,H_2O(l) \longrightarrow 4\,HNO_3(l) \qquad \Delta H_{tot} = \Delta H_1 + \Delta H_2 + \Delta H_3 = -40\ kJ$$

Hess's Law may be used to find the enthalpy of a target reaction that may actually be impossible to carry out.

EXAMPLE: Given the following set of reactions:

$$3C(s) + 4\,H_2(g) \longrightarrow C_3H_8(g) \qquad \Delta H_1 = -103.9\ kJ$$
$$C(s) + O_2(g) \longrightarrow CO_2(g) \qquad \Delta H_2 = -393.5\ kJ$$
$$2\,H_2(g) + O_2(g) \longrightarrow 2\,H_2O(l) \qquad \Delta H_3 = -571.6\ kJ$$

Calculate the enthalpy of the following reaction:

$$C_3H_8(g) + 5O_2(g) \longrightarrow 3CO_2(g) + 4\,H_2O(l) \qquad \Delta H = ?$$

The only place the reactant C_3H_8 appears is in reaction 1 on the products side, so the reaction and the enthalpy must be reversed. The reactant O_2 appears in two reactions, so it would be hard to balance. The products, CO_2 and H_2O, are in reaction 2 and 3, respectively, but each reaction must be multiplied by a number to obtain the desired number of molecules.

$-1 \times$ Rxn 1	$C_3H_8(g) \longrightarrow 3C(s) + 4\,H_2(g)$	$-1 \times \Delta H_1 = -(-103.9\ kJ) = +103.9\ kJ$
$3 \times$ Rxn 2	$3C(s) + 3O_2(g) \longrightarrow 3\,CO_2(g)$	$3 \times \Delta H_2 = 3(-393.5\ kJ) = -1180.5\ kJ$
$2 \times$ Rxn 3	$4\,H_2(g) + 2O_2(g) \longrightarrow 4\,H_2O(l)$	$2 \times \Delta H_3 = 2(-571.6\ kJ) = -1143.2\ kJ$

$$C_3H_8(g) + 5O_2(g) \longrightarrow 3CO_2(g) + 4\,H_2O(l) \qquad \Delta H_{tot} = -2219.8\ kJ$$

Hess's Law is useful, but it can be used only when suitable equations are known that add up to the desired equation. Enthalpy values may also be calculated using the **standard enthalpy of formation**, ΔH_f°, defined as the enthalpy for the formation of one mole of a substance from the elements in their standard states. Standard states for solids, liquids, and gases are the most stable form at 1 atm pressure and 25°C. Certain elements' standard state is molecular: H_2, N_2, O_2, F_2, Cl_2, P_4, Br_2, and I_2. Sulfur exists as S_8, but S is often used. The standard state of C is graphite. By definition, the standard enthalpy of formation of elements is zero. Some ΔH_f° reactions are shown below:

elements	$\longrightarrow$	1 mole
$H_2(g) + \tfrac{1}{2}\,O_2(g)$	$\longrightarrow$	$H_2O(l)$
$C(s) + 2Cl_2(g)$	$\longrightarrow$	$CCl_4(l)$
$H_2(g) + \tfrac{1}{8}\,S_8(s) + 2O_2(g)$	$\longrightarrow$	$H_2SO_4(l)$
$6C(s) + 6H_2(g) + 3O_2(g)$	$\longrightarrow$	$C_6H_{12}O_6(s)$

The ΔH can be calculated for any reaction in which ΔH_f° values of all reactants and products are known.

The formula for this calculation is:

$$\Delta H_{rxn} = \Sigma \, n_p \, \Delta H_f^\circ(\text{products}) - \Sigma \, n_r \, \Delta H_f^\circ(\text{reactants}).$$

(n_p and n_r are the number of moles of the products and reactants, respectively, in the balanced equation.)

EXAMPLE: Consider the following reaction:

$$2C_4H_{10}(g) + 13 \, O_2(g) \longrightarrow 8 \, CO_2(g) + 10 \, H_2O(g)$$
$$C_4H_{10}(g): \Delta H_f^\circ = -126.2 \text{ kJ/mol}$$
$$CO_2(g): \Delta H_f^\circ = -393.5 \text{ kJ/mol}$$
$$H_2O(g): \Delta H_f^\circ = -241.8 \text{ kJ/mol}$$

$$\begin{aligned}\Delta H_{rxn} &= [8 \, \Delta H_f^\circ(CO_2) + 10\Delta H_f^\circ(H_2O)] - [2\Delta H_f^\circ(C_4H_{10})] \text{ (Note: } O_2, \Delta H_f^\circ = 0)\\ &= [8(-393.5) + 10(-241.8)] - [2(-126.2)] \text{ kJ}\\ &= [-5566] - [-252.4] \text{ kJ} = -5313.6 \text{ kJ}\end{aligned}$$

DETAILED ATOMIC STRUCTURE

This section will describe the properties of matter, including the interaction between matter and electromagnetic radiation. Electromagnetic radiation is energy such as visible light, radio waves, X-rays, microwave radiation, and ultraviolet radiation. Electromagnetic radiation is characterized by oscillating periodic waves.

➤ The **wavelength** (λ) is the distance between successive crests or troughs in a wave. The units of wavelength are the units of length such as a meter.

➤ The **frequency** (ν) is the number of wavelengths passing a given point per second. The units of frequency are $\frac{1}{s}$ or equivalently Hertz (Hz).

All electromagnetic radiation travels at the speed of light, c, which is $2.998 \times 10^8 \, \text{m/s}$ in a vacuum. The frequency and wavelength of light are related by the equation:

$$\nu\lambda = c$$

EXAMPLE: A radio station has a frequency of 880 kHz. What is its wavelength? kHz means 10^3 Hz, so 880 kHz is $8.80 \times 10^{+5} \, \frac{1}{s}$.

$$\nu\lambda = c \longrightarrow (8.80 \times 10^{+5} \, \tfrac{1}{s}) \times (2.998 \times 10^8 \, \tfrac{m}{s}) \longrightarrow \lambda = 341 \text{ m}$$

Until about 1900, matter and energy were thought to have entirely different properties. Matter was believed to behave as discrete particles described by Newton's laws of motion and energy was believed to behave as continuous waves. In the first thirty years of the twentieth century, modern science showed that matter and energy can both behave with particlelike and wavelike properties. The German physicist Max Planck was able to explain the emission spectrum from a heated body by assuming that energy was not emitted in a continuous way but came in bundles of energy called quanta, dependent on the frequency.

$$E_q = h\nu$$

where E_q is the energy of the quantum, h is **Planck's constant** $(6.626 \times 10^{-34}\text{ J·s})$, and ν is the frequency of the light.

Albert Einstein used Planck's idea to explain the photoelectric effect. In the photoelectric effect, light shining on a metal electrode in a vacuum can eject electrons that travel through the vacuum to another electrode, completing an electrical circuit. Einstein proposed that particles of light called **photons** supplied the energy to eject the electrons. Einstein's work showed the dual nature of light.

During the 1800s, scientists studied emissions from gas-filled tubes that were subjected to an electrical discharge, such as a neon bulb. Unlike the emissions from heated objects, which give continuous spectra of all wavelengths, the emissions from the gas-filled tubes gave only a few lines, which were a function of the gas in the tube. These spectra are called **line emission spectra.** For hydrogen, in the region of visible light, the line spectrum contains only four prominent lines, at 656, 486, 434, and 410 nm $(1\text{ nm} = 1 \times 10^{-9}\text{ m})$. Because the spectra are a function of the material in the tube, scientists believed the spectra reflected something about the energy and structure of the atoms of the gas in the tube. A formula was derived by the Swedish physicist Johannes Rydberg for the reciprocal of the wavelength of the lines in the emission spectrum of hydrogen:

$$\frac{1}{\lambda} = 10{,}967{,}758 \text{ m}^{-1}\left(\frac{1}{n_1^2} - \frac{1}{n_2^2}\right)$$

where n_1 and n_2 are integers with $n_1 < n_2$.

Bohr Model

The Bohr model of the hydrogen atom was the first explanation for the line spectra. The Danish physicist Niels Bohr assumed that in hydrogen, the electron travels around the hydrogen nucleus, a proton, in circular orbits similar to the solar system. Bohr assumed that the energy of the electron in an orbit was quantized, or restricted to specific energy levels labeled with quantum numbers, n. The values for n are integers beginning with 1. The lowest energy level, $n = 1$, has the smallest radius. The radius of the orbit for the next higher energy level, $n = 2$, is larger. A sketch of the Bohr model and the associated energy levels is shown on the following page.

Bohr calculated that the energy of a given level in the hydrogen atom is:

$$E_n = -2.179 \times 10^{-18} \text{ J}\left(\frac{1}{n^2}\right).$$

The energy is negative because the energy of a completely separated proton and electron was defined by Bohr to be zero. The energy of the transition between orbits is easily calculated. If the initial orbital is labeled n_i and the final orbit n_f, the energy of the transition between levels is shown on the next page under the Bohr model:

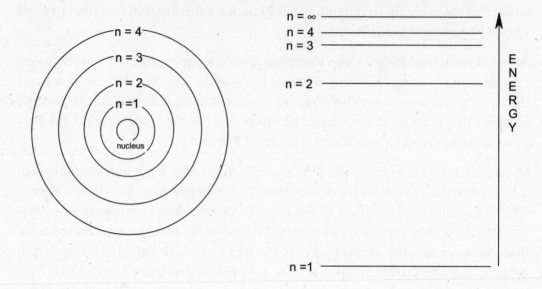

$$\Delta E = -2.179 \times 10^{-18} \text{ J} \left(\frac{1}{n_f^2}\right) - \left[-2.179 \times 10^{-18} \text{ J} \left(\frac{1}{n_i^2}\right)\right]$$

or

$$\Delta E = -2.179 \times 10^{-18} \text{ J} \left(\frac{1}{n_f^2} - \frac{1}{n_i^2}\right).$$

For the transition between $n_i = 4$ to $n_f = 2$,

$$\Delta E = -2.179 \times 10^{-18} \text{ J} \left(\frac{1}{4} - \frac{1}{16}\right)$$

$$\Delta E = -2.179 \times 10^{-18} \text{ J} (0.1875) = -4.086 \times 10^{-19} \text{ J}.$$

The negative sign indicates that energy is leaving the atom; that is, the process is exothermic. Bohr postulated that this photon is emitted by the atom with an energy equivalent to the energy difference of the two orbits. If the transition were reversed, the ΔE would be positive, indicating an endothermic process in which a photon is absorbed by the atom.

The frequency of the photon associated with the transition described above may be calculated from $\Delta E = h\nu$ or $\nu = {}^E/_h$. (The negative sign in the energy is ignored because it simply gives the direction of energy flow. A frequency is a positive number.)

$$\frac{4.086 \times 10^{-19} \text{ J}}{6.626 \times 10^{-34} \text{ J} \cdot \text{s}} = 6.1667 \times 10^{14} \, {}^{1}\!/_{s}$$

The wavelength of light is determined using the relation $\nu\lambda = c$ in the form $\lambda = {}^c/_\nu$.

$$\lambda = \frac{2.998 \times 10^8 \; \frac{m}{s}}{6.1667 \times 10^{14} \frac{1}{s}}. = 4.86 \times 10^{-7} \; m \; or \; 486 \, nm.$$

Note that this calculated value corresponds to one of the wavelengths in the line emission spectra of hydrogen. Through theoretical means, Bohr had derived the experimental value for this wavelength and other wavelengths from the emission spectrum of hydrogen.

Bohr attempted to extend his model to atoms with more than one proton. The model did not work for any other atoms. Attempts to refine the model did not work. The energies were correct, but there was something fundamentally wrong with Bohr's model.

The Quantum Atom

The problem with Bohr's model was that it did not account for a fundamental property of the electron. In 1924, after Bohr's model was established, the French physicist Louis de Broglie thought that if light can behave both as a particle and as a wave, then matter might behave both as a particle and as a wave with a **de Broglie wavelength** given by:

$$\lambda = \frac{h}{mv}$$

where m is the mass of the particle and v is the particle's velocity.

The de Broglie wavelength is negligible for everyday objects such as baseballs and trucks, but the size of the de Broglie wavelength of an electron is close to the size of an atom. The wavelength of matter was confirmed experimentally by the diffraction of electrons by aluminum foil.

The **quantum mechanical model** of the atom replaced Bohr's model. It was developed separately by German physicist Werner Heisenberg and the Austrian physicist Erwin Schrödinger. Schrödinger developed an equation based on de Broglie's wavelength and the basic wave equation from physics. The solutions to his equation are called wave functions or orbitals, to distinguish them from Bohr's orbits. Electrons are described by the probability of finding the electron at a point in space called **electron density** by chemists. Regions with high probabilities of finding an electron have larger electron densities.

Quantum Numbers

Each solution to Schrödinger's equation is labeled by three integers. These integers are called **quantum numbers**—n, ℓ, and m_ℓ. Schrodinger's equation restricts the values of these quantum numbers. A fourth quantum number, m_s, is due to the spin of the electron.

The **principal quantum number, n**, is restricted to positive integer values starting with 1. In other words, its possible values are 1, 2, 3, 4, 5, 6, etc. The value of n primarily determines the energy of the electron. The lower the value of n, the lower the energy, and the closer the electron is to the nucleus.

The **azimuthal quantum number** (or angular momentum quantum number), ℓ, is restricted by the value of n to values from 0 and increases by one until n−1 is reached.

Principal	Possible ℓ values
1	0
2	0, 1
3	0, 1, 2
4	0, 1, 2, 3
5	0, 1, 2, 3, 4
etc.	

The azimuthal quantum number determines the shape of the orbital. Each number corresponds to a letter that names an orbital.

ℓvalue	0	1	2	3	4	5
Name	s	p	d	f	g	h

The **magnetic quantum number, m_ℓ**, is restricted by the value of ℓ to integers beginning at $-\ell$ and increasing by 1 until $+\ell$ is reached, and m_ℓ determines an orbital's orientation in space.

ℓ value	Possible m_ℓ values
0(s)	0
1(p)	−1,0,1
2(d)	−2,−1,0,1,2
3(f)	−3,−2,−1,0,1,2,3
etc.	

From the table above, you can see that for any given value of n, there is one ns orbital, three np orbitals, five nd orbitals, seven nf orbitals, etc.

The **spin quantum number, m_s**, is restricted to values of $+\frac{1}{2}$ and $-\frac{1}{2}$.

The orbitals have shapes that are determined by the quantum number ℓ. All s orbitals are spherical and centered on the nucleus. As n increases, the size of the sphere increases. (1s<2s<3s<4s<5s etc.) All p orbitals are dumbbell-shaped, and on each n level the three p orbitals are oriented in three mutually perpendicular directions along the x, y, and z axes respectively. As with the s orbital, size increases with increasing n value. Four of the d orbitals have a similar shape, usually described as a cloverleaf; one has a different shape. Representations of the shapes of s and p orbitals are shown below.

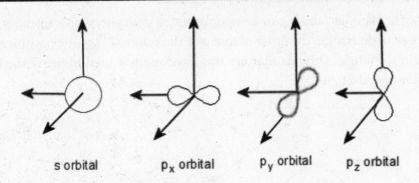

s orbital p_x orbital p_y orbital p_z orbital

Electron Configurations

The atoms of the elements in the periodic table may be built up one by one by placing electrons in the lowest available orbital. Several rules must be followed.

➤ The **Pauli exclusion principle** states that no two electrons in an atom may have all four quantum numbers of identical value. If the first three quantum numbers are identical, the only possibilities for the fourth quantum number, m_s, are $+\frac{1}{2}$ or $-\frac{1}{2}$. This means that an orbital can have at most two electrons and if there are two electrons in an orbital, the electrons must have opposite values for m_s. When two electrons occupy one orbital with m_s values of $+\frac{1}{2}$ and $-\frac{1}{2}$, the spins are said to be paired. If two electrons are in separate orbitals with the same value for m_s, the spins are said to be parallel.

➤ **Hund's rule** states that if a set of orbitals with equivalent energy is not completely filled, electrons will fill the orbitals to give a maximum number of half-filled orbitals with parallel spins. For example, if electrons are added to an unfilled 3p level (three orbitals), an electron will be placed in each orbital with parallel spins before any electron is paired up.

The energies of the orbitals are a function of both n and ℓ. For a given value of n, the energies of the orbitals in a multielectron atom are in the order $ns < np < nd < nf <$ etc. For lower values of n, the orbitals are well separated in energy. As n increases, the orbitals from different values of n begin to overlap. A diagram of the relative energies of the lowest energy levels for a representative multielectron atom is shown below.

___ 5p ___ ___ ___		___ ___ ___ ___ ___
5s ___ ___ ___		4d
4s 4p ___ ___ ___		___ ___ ___ ___ ___
3s 3p ___ ___		3d
2s 2p ___ ___ ___		
1s		

The energy levels order above can be approximated with the simple memory device shown below to determine the order of filling of the orbitals. First the possible orbitals are listed in a triangle. Orbitals that are not listed are not used in filling the known atoms in the periodic table.

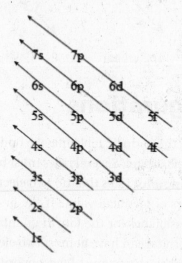

The order of filling may be traced by drawing diagonal lines slanting from the lower right to the upper left, as shown in the diagram. The resulting order $1s \rightarrow 2s \rightarrow 2p \rightarrow 3s \rightarrow 3p \rightarrow 4s \rightarrow 3d \rightarrow 4p \rightarrow 5s \rightarrow 4d \rightarrow 5p \rightarrow 6s \rightarrow 4f \rightarrow 5d \rightarrow 6p \rightarrow 7s \rightarrow 5f \rightarrow 6d \rightarrow 7p$ will be adequate for most atoms, with a few exceptions. The periodic table itself may also be used to determine the filling order.

The electron configuration for an element lists the orbitals that contain electrons and the number of electrons in each orbital. There are several ways to represent the electron configuration. Line diagrams use lines to represent the orbitals and arrows to represent the electron spin. An up arrow corresponds to $m_s = +\frac{1}{2}$ and a down arrow corresponds to $m_s = -\frac{1}{2}$. The *aufbau* (German for "to build up") approach is generally used. Hydrogen is first with one electron and one proton. Successive elements are "created" by adding one proton to the nucleus and one electron to the next lowest available orbital, following Hund's rule when necessary. The number in parentheses is the atomic number = number of electrons. Below are line diagrams for the first 10 elements.

H (1) $\uparrow$
       1s

He(2) $\uparrow\downarrow$
       1s

Li(3) $\uparrow\downarrow$ $\uparrow$
       1s   2s

Be(4) $\uparrow\downarrow$ $\uparrow\downarrow$
       1s   2s

B(5) $\uparrow\downarrow$ $\uparrow\downarrow$ $\uparrow$ __
       1s   2s   2p

C(6)   ↑↓   ↑↓   ↑   ↑   ___   (Separate orbitals due to Hund's Rule)
       1s   2s   2p

N(7)   ↑↓   ↑↓   ↑   ↑   ↑
       1s   2s   2p

O(8)   ↑↓   ↑↓   ↑↓ ↑   ↑
       1s   2s   2p

F(9)   ↑↓   ↑↓   ↑↓ ↑↓ ↑
       1s   2s   2p

Ne(10) ↑↓   ↑↓   ↑↓ ↑↓ ↑↓
       1s   2s   2p

Line diagrams become cumbersome as the number of electrons increases. Orbitals may be represented as a number-letter combination. The number of electrons in an orbital is represented as a superscript. The ten electronic configurations above may be rewritten as:

H $1s^1$ (Pronounced "one s one")
He $1s^2$
Li $1s^2 2s^1$
Be $1s^2 2s^2$
B $1s^2 2s^2 2p^1$
C $1s^2 2s^2 2p^2$
N $1s^2 2s^2 2p^3$
O $1s^2 2s^2 2p^4$
F $1s^2 2s^2 2p^5$
Ne $1s^2 2s^2 2p^6 = [Ne]$

Because the electrons in neon will also be present in all following atoms, the electron configurations for each noble gas may be abbreviated as shown above. This abbreviation will also be used in the following electron configurations for the next eight elements.

Na $[Ne]3s^1$
Mg $[Ne]3s^2$
Al $[Ne]3s^2 3p^1$
Si $[Ne]3s^2 3p^2$
P $[Ne]3s^2 3p^3$
S $[Ne]3s^2 3p^4$
Cl $[Ne]3s^2 3p^5$
Ar $[Ne]3s^2 3p^6 = [Ar]$

The next 18 elements will fill the $4s(2e^-)$, $3d(10e^-)$, and $4p(6e^-)$ orbitals.

A more common problem is to write the electron configuration of a given element.

EXAMPLE: What is the electron configuration of Pt?

Pt has 78 electrons. Fill the orbitals in order until 78 electrons are placed in orbitals.

$$Pt - 1s^2 2s^2 2p^6 3s^2 3p^6 4s^2 3d^{10} 4p^6 5s^2 4d^{10} 5p^6 6s^2 \, 4f^{14} \, 5d^8$$

When the Russian chemist Dmitri Mendeleev prepared the original periodic table, he placed elements in groups by their chemical properties before the electron had ever been discovered. The modern view of the periodic table recognizes that the elements are in groups because they have similar electron configurations. The shape of the periodic table can now be understood:

➤ **The first two columns** (groups 1 and 2) are where the s orbitals are being filled.
➤ **The last six columns** (groups 13–18) are where the p orbitals are being filled.
➤ **The ten columns in the middle** (groups 3–12) are where the d orbitals are being filled.
➤ **The two rows at the bottom** of the table (the lanthanide and actinide series) are elements where the f orbitals are being filled.

The electron configurations of the alkali metals are generalized as $[NG]ns^1$ where $[NG]$ is the electron configuration of the preceding noble gas. The electron configurations of the alkali metal cations are those of each immediately preceding noble gas, for example, $Na^+ = [Ne]$.

Electron configurations of the noble gases are called **core electrons**. These electrons are especially stable and do not normally take part in chemical reactions. A filled set of d electrons is unreactive and considered part of the core. Electrons that are not contained in the core electrons are called **valence electrons**. Valence electrons are the chemically reactive electrons. Each alkali metal has one valence electron (the ns^1 electron).

The valence electron configuration is a function of the group in the periodic table. The valence electron configurations for each of the main group elements are:

Group	1	2	13	14	15	16	17	18
e^- configuration	ns^1	ns^2	ns^2np^1	ns^2np^2	ns^2np^3	ns^2np^4	ns^2np^5	ns^2np^6
number of valence e^-	1	2	3	4	5	6	7	8

Electron Configuration of Ions

Main group elements gain or lose electrons to achieve the electron configuration of the closest noble gas. For the third period of the periodic table:

Atom		Ion	
Na	$[Ne]3s^1$	Na^+	$[Ne]$
Mg	$[Ne]3s^2$	Mg^{2+}	$[Ne]$
Al	$[Ne]3s^2 3p^1$	Al^{3+}	$[Ne]$
Si	$[Ne]3s^2 3p^2$	usually forms covalent compounds	
P	$[Ne]3s^2 3p^3$	P^{3-}	$[Ne]3s^2 3p^6 = [Ar]$
S	$[Ne]3s^2 3p^4$	S^{2-}	$[Ne]3s^2 3p^6 = [Ar]$
Cl	$[Ne]3s^2 3p^5$	Cl^-	$[Ne]3s^2 3p^6 = [Ar]$

Transition metal cations are different. The last electron that goes into a transition metal is a d electron. When ions form, the energy levels change in such a way that the $(n+1)s$ electrons are lost before the nd electrons. In the case of Fe^{3+}:

Fe $[Ar]4s^2 3d^6$ Fe^{3+} $[Ar]3d^5$

First the two 4s electrons are lost. Next one 3d electron is removed. For most of the transition metal cations the electron configuration will be $[NG]nd^x$.

Each electron has a spin and functions as a tiny magnet. When two electrons are paired in an orbital, the two spins cancel each other out.

➤ Species with all electrons paired are **diamagnetic** and are repelled by a magnetic field.

➤ Species with unpaired electrons are **paramagnetic** and are attracted to a magnetic field.

> **EXAMPLE:** Which of the following atoms or ions are paramagnetic? Note: all the electrons in a noble gas configuration are paired.

N   Fe   Be S^{2-}

The appropriate electron configurations are:

N   [He] ↑↓   ↑   ↑   ↑   three unpaired electrons
          2s   2p   paramagnetic

Fe   [Ar] ↑↓   ↑↓ ↑   ↑   ↑   ↑   four unpaired electrons
          4s   3d   paramagnetic

Be   [He] ↑↓   zero unpaired electrons
          2s   diamagnetic

S^{2-} [Ar]   zero unpaired electrons
                                                diamagnetic

All the electron configurations discussed above are the most stable or **ground state** configurations for each atom or ion. If the correct amount of energy is supplied, an atom may enter an **excited state** with electrons in higher energy orbitals than the ground state. For example, the ground state and two excited states for an Fe atom are:

Fe $[Ar]4s^2 3d^6$ (ground state)
Fe $[Ar]4s^2 3d^5 4p^1$ (excited state)
Fe $[Ar]4s^0 3d^6 4p^2$ (excited state)

Atoms in excited states are not stable and will return to the ground state with a release of energy in the form of heat or light.

Periodic Properties

Certain physical properties show periodic behavior when plotted against the atomic number; in other words, there is a repeating rise and fall in the values. The periodicity is not exact like a sine wave, but the trends are relatively clear and useful for predicting some chemical and physical behaviors of the elements.

ATOMIC RADIUS

Atomic radius is a measure of the size of an atom. The atomic radius is usually defined as one-half the distance between two atomic nuclei, which assumes that the atoms are spherical and are in physical contact with each other. The trend in atomic radii for main group elements is that the radii increase in size going down a column and the radii decrease in size going across a period from left to right. The increase as you go down a period is easily explained because the outermost electron is in an orbital with a larger value of n, meaning a bigger orbital.

$$Li < Na < K < Rb < Cs \text{ because}$$
$$2s < 3s < 4s < 5s < 6s$$

There is a large jump in radius between a noble gas and the following alkali metal because the alkali metal introduces a new principal quantum number.

> **EXAMPLE:** Ar $[Ne]3s^23p^6$ has a radius of 98 pm (1 pm $= 10^{-12}$ m). K $[Ar]4s^1$ has a radius that is over twice this big, 227 pm, because the last electron added to K is in the 4s orbital.

For ions, the radii of cations of the same charge show a regular increase when going down a column. The same is true of anions of the same charge when going down a column. Both of these effects are due to the increasing size of the orbitals.

$$Li^+ (90 \text{ pm}) < Na^+ (116 \text{ pm}) < K^+ (153 \text{ pm}) < Rb^+ (166 \text{ pm}) < Cs^+ (181 \text{ pm})$$
$$F^- (119 \text{ pm}) < Cl^- (167 \text{ pm}) < Br^- (182 \text{ pm}) < I^- (206 \text{ pm})$$

If you compare the radius of an ion to the radius of the atom from which that ion is derived, the cations are smaller than the parent atom because there is an excess of protons in the cation that can pull the electrons closer. Anions are larger than the parent atom because there is an excess of electrons over protons.

$Na^+ (116 \text{ pm}) < Na (186 \text{ pm})$ $\qquad\qquad$ $Cl^- (167 \text{ pm}) > Cl (100 \text{ pm})$

11 p$^+$	11 p$^+$	17 p$^+$	17 p$^+$
10 e$^-$	11 e$^-$	18 e$^-$	17 e$^-$
[Ne]	[Ne]3s^1	[Ar]	[Ne]3s^{2}3p^5

These effects are most prominent in highly charged ions. For example, B^{3+} (25 pm) is less than one-third the size of a B atom (85 pm).

Comparisons across a period are not valid because in a given period, both cations and anions are formed. A more apt comparison is that of **isoelectronic** ions, which are ions with the same number of electrons. For example, consider these ions which all have the electron configuration of [Ne].

Ion	Al^{3+}	<	Mg^{2+}	<	Na^+	<	F^-	<	O^{2-}	<	N^{3-}
p+	13		12		11		9		8		7
e−	10		10		10		10		10		10
radius (pm)	68		86		116		119		126		132

If an element forms more than one cation, the cation with the higher charge will be smaller. Lead can form either a 2+ or a 4+ cation.

$$Pb^{4+} \, (92 \text{ pm}) < Pb^{2+} \, (133 \text{ pm})$$
$$82 \text{ p}^+ \qquad 82 \text{ p}^+$$
$$78 \text{ e}^- \qquad 80 \text{ e}^-$$

IONIZATION ENERGY

Ionization energy (IE) is defined as the energy required to remove an electron from an atom in the gas phase. Removing the first electron is the first ionization energy. Removing a second electron is the second ionization energy, and so on as long as there are electrons to remove.

$$Mg(g) \rightarrow Mg^+(g) + e^- \qquad \Delta E = \text{1st ionization energy} = 737 \text{ kJ/mol}$$
$$Mg^+(g) \rightarrow Mg^{2+}(g) + e^- \qquad \Delta E = \text{2nd ionization energy} = 1451 \text{ kJ/mol}$$
$$Mg^{2+}(g) \rightarrow Mg^{3+}(g) + e^- \qquad \Delta E = \text{3rd ionization energy} = 7732 \text{ kJ/mol}$$

The ionization energies increase in value as electrons are removed because as the positive charge increases, it becomes harder to remove a negatively charged electron. If a core electron is removed, there will be a large increase in the ionization energy. This is demonstrated for Mg. The second ionization energy is approximately double the first, but the third ionization energy is over five times as large as the second. Mg^{2+} has the electron configuration [Ne]. The third electron is removed from the neon core electrons.

In going down a group of the periodic table, the trend is that the first ionization energy decreases. This makes sense because the outer electrons are farther away from the nucleus in the elements lower in the table, and those electrons would be expected to be relatively easy to remove. As you go across the table from left to right, the general trend is for the first ionization energy to increase. There are some exceptions to this general trend that can be explained by considering the electron configuration of the elements.

ELECTRON AFFINITY

Electron affinity is defined as the energy change when an electron is added to an atom in the gas phase.

$$Cl(g) + e^- \longrightarrow Cl^-(g) \quad \Delta E = \text{Electron affinity} = -349 \text{ kJ/mol}$$

The electron affinity for Cl has a large negative value due to the fact that adding an electron is a favorable process because a noble gas configuration is formed. The halogens each form a noble gas electron configuration upon adding an electron, so atoms of each of these elements have large negative electron affinities. The trends in electron affinities are not as regular as those for atomic radii or first ionization energy. The electron affinities for noble gases are (+) because when an electron is added, the stable noble gas configuration is broken, an unfavorable process.

ELECTRONEGATIVITY

Electronegativity is an important periodic property that is used to understand bonding. Electronegativitiy is defined as the power of an atom in a compound to draw electrons to itself. Electronegativity tends to increase as you go up a group and as you cross a period from left to right. Electronegativity will be used extensively in the discussion of chemical bonding.

CHEMICAL BONDING

There are three main types of chemical bonding.
➤ **Ionic bonding** occurs when electrons are transferred between atoms.
➤ **Covalent bonding** occurs when atoms share electrons between bonded atoms.
➤ In **metallic bonding**, fixed metal cations are surrounded by freely moving electrons.

Metallic bonding is important only for metals and a few compounds. Metals conduct electricity. Conduction occurs when charged particles can move through a continuous circuit. In the case of metals, the current is carried by freely moving electrons. Bonding in metals is described as metal cations in fixed positions surrounded by electrons that can move freely through the solid. Some chemists describe this as cations in a sea of electrons. This bonding explains many of the properties of metals discussed later.

Classifying Bond Types Based on Formulas

You can classify the type of bonding in different substances by considering the chemical formula of the substance. Study the following table:

Bonding Type from Formulas
➤ Single element in the formula

1. Metal element—metallic bonding
2. Nonmetal element—covalent bonding (except noble gases = no bonding)
3. Metalloid element—covalent or metallic bonding depending on the element and structure

➤ Two elements in the formula (binary compound)

1. Metal and metal—metallic bonding
2. Metal and nonmetal—ionic bonding
3. Nonmetal and nonmetal—covalent bonding

➤ More than two elements in the formula

1. Polyatomic ion present—ionic bonding
2. All nonmetals, no polyatomic ion—covalent bonding

Most nonmetal elements exist as covalently bonded discrete molecules such as O_2, N_2, P_4, S_8, C_{60}, and Cl_2. Some nonmetals exist as network solids. These substances can be best described as giant molecules that are covalently bonded, forming one-, two-, or three-dimensional continuous networks. Examples of nonmetal elements that exist as network solids are Si, C(diamond), C(graphite), and As.

Polyatomic ions are covalently bonded within the ion, but they form ionic compounds with ions of opposite charge.

Examples:

Formula	Type of element(s)	Bonding
Fe	one metal	metallic
Si	one metalloid	covalent
Br_2	one nonmetal	covalent
Ne	nonmetal (noble gas)	no covalent bonding
KBr	metal + nonmetal	ionic
CO_2	nonmetal + nonmetal	covalent
$MgBr_2$	metal + nonmetal	ionic
$NaNO_3$	polyatomic ion (NO_3^-)	ionic
NH_4NO_3	polyatomic ion(s) (NH_4^+, NO_3^-)	ionic
NH_4Cl	polyatomic ion (NH_4^+)	ionic
$C_6H_{12}O_6$	nonmetals (no polyatomic ions)	covalent

Ionic Bonding

Ionic bonding is the electrical attraction between the positively charged cations and the negatively charged anions. The strength of an ionic bond is measured by the **lattice energy,** which is the energy released when gaseous ions condense into the ionic solid. The strength of an ionic bond depends on two main factors:

➤ Higher-charged ions form stronger ionic bonds.
➤ Smaller ions form stronger bonds due to the closer approach of the ions.

> **EXAMPLE:** Magnesium oxide, MgO, has a lattice energy more than four times greater than that of NaF because the ions in MgO are 2+ and 2− and the ions in NaF are 1+ and 1−. MgO has a shorter interionic distance, allowing closer interaction of the ions. Both factors strengthen the electrical attraction between ions in MgO, as compared to NaF.

Covalent Bonds and Lewis Structures

The American physicist Gilbert Newton Lewis first postulated that atoms share electrons so as to achieve a noble gas configuration, and that the electrons in molecules arrange into pairs of electrons. These pairs may be shared between two atoms (a bond pair) or belong to a single atom (a lone pair). Simple electron dot structures to indicate the distribution of electrons are called **Lewis structures** to honor Lewis's theory.

A simple Lewis structure for hydrogen shows a pair of shared electrons between two hydrogen atoms, H:H. These shared pairs of electrons are generally represented by a line standing for the two electrons forming the bond, H-H. Each hydrogen atom achieves the noble gas configuration of [He] by allowing the shared pair to count for both atoms.

A more complicated example is the Lewis structure of F_2. F has seven valence electrons. Two F atoms can contribute one electron each to the bond pair between the atoms. This gives both F atoms an octet or [Ne] configuration.

$$\ddot{\ddot{F}}\cdot + \cdot\ddot{\ddot{F}}: \longrightarrow :\ddot{\ddot{F}}-\ddot{\ddot{F}}:$$

RULES FOR CONSTRUCTING LEWIS STRUCTURES

<u>Basic Rules</u>
Step 1: Sum up the number of valence electrons contributed by each atom in the molecule or ion. The group number is equivalent to the number of valence electrons or the number of valence electrons +10. For anions, add an electron for each negative charge. For cations, subtract an electron for each positive charge.

A notation	1	2	13	14	15	16	17	18
2nd Period	Li	Be	B	C	N	O	F	Ne
Valence e⁻	1	2	3	4	5	6	7	8

Step 2: Write the skeletal structure of the molecule or ion. Most structures have a single atom in the middle, which will be the least electronegative atom.

Step 3: Using two valence electrons, form a bond from the central to the outer atoms.

Step 4: Hydrogen is satisfied with two electrons giving it a [He] electron configuration. For other elements, the octet rule applies. The **octet rule** states that an atom is most stable if there are eight electrons from the lone pairs and bond pairs surrounding the atom. Put lone pairs on the outer atoms first and if electrons are left over, place lone pairs on the central atom. Do not use more electrons than the initial total.

Step 5: Check that each nonhydrogen atom obeys the octet rule. If an atom has less than an octet, it may be necessary to convert a lone pair on an adjacent atom into a bond pair. This creates a four-electron double bond. Triple bonds are also possible.

Additional Rules

1. Do not violate the octet rule for C, N, O, and F. (There are a few exceptions to this rule. For example, NO_2 has an odd number of electrons and N will only have seven e^- around it.)

2. Be and B may have less than an octet because they are not very electronegative. There are structures of Be and B that follow the octet rule, but do not move an electron from a very electronegative atom to Be or B just to meet the octet rule.

3. Elements in the third period of the periodic table or below (such as P, S, Cl, and Br) may exceed the octet rule. Only exceed the octet rule if necessary or if a more reasonable formal charge results. (Formal charge is described later.)

4. Some structures have more than one "central" atom. In these cases, apply the above rules to each atomic center.

Examples: All of the following structures follow the octet rule. The initial structures for SO_4^{2-} and ClO_2^- will be modified later to give more reasonable formal charges.

	CH_4	NH_3	SO_4^{2-}	NH_4^+	ClO_2^-
	$1C = 4e^-$	$1N = 5e^-$	$1S = 6e^-$	$1N = 5e^-$	$1Cl = 7e^-$
	$4H = 4e^-$	$3H = 3e^-$	$4O = 24e^-$	$4H = 4e^-$	$2O = 12e^-$
			$2- = 2e^-$	$1+ = -1e^-$	$1- = 1e^-$
	$8e^-$	$8e^-$	$32e^-$	$8e^-$	$20e^-$

	CH_4	NH_3	SO_4^{2-}	NH_4^+	ClO_2^-
Bonds to central atom	H–C–H with H above and below	H–N–H with H below	O–S–O with O above and below	H–N–H with H above and below	O–Cl–O
e- left	0	2	24	0	16
	done			done	
Lone pairs on outer atoms		H–N–H with H below	:O–S–O: structure		:O–Cl–O:
e- left		2	0		4
			done		
Lone pairs on central atom and final structures	final CH_4	final NH_3	$[SO_4]^{2-}$	$[NH_4]^+$	$[ClO_2]^-$

In the final structures, ions are bracketed, with the overall charge indicated outside the brackets. After all the electrons are added, check all nonhydrogen atoms for octets.

The next three examples require formation of multiple bonds.

	NO_3^-	SO_2	N_2
	$1N = 5e^-$	$1S = 6e^-$	$2N = 10e^-$
	$3O = 18e^-$	$2O = 12e^-$	
	$\underline{1- = 1e^-}$	$\underline{}$	
	$24e^-$	$18e^-$	

Bonds to central atom	O—N—O
	    |
	    O
		O—S—O	N—N

e- left	18	14	8

Lone pairs on outer atoms	:Ö—N—Ö:
	    |
	   :Ö:
		:Ö—S—Ö:	:N̈—N̈:

e- left	0 done	2	0 done
Lone pairs on central atom		:Ö—S̈—Ö:	
e- left		0 done	

All electrons have been used, but the central atoms do not have octets. Lone pairs on the outer atoms are used to make double bonds in NO_3^- and SO_2 and a triple bond in N_2.

Final structures	$\left[\begin{array}{c}:O{=}N{-}\ddot{O}: \\ \quad\quad\| \\ \quad :\ddot{O}: \end{array}\right]^-$	:Ö=S̈—Ö:	:N≡N:

Resonance

In NO_3^- there are three choices for the oxygen atom to which the double bond is drawn. In SO_2 there are two choices. This choice is arbitrary. The three possible structures for a nitrate ion are shown below.

$$\left[\begin{array}{c}\ddot{O}{=}N{-}\ddot{O}: \\ \quad\| \\ :\ddot{O}: \end{array}\right]^- \longleftrightarrow \left[\begin{array}{c}:\ddot{O}{-}N{-}\ddot{O}: \\ \quad\| \\ :\ddot{O}: \end{array}\right]^- \longleftrightarrow \left[\begin{array}{c}:\ddot{O}{-}N{=}\ddot{O} \\ \quad\| \\ :\ddot{O}: \end{array}\right]^-$$

Each structure has two single bonds to O and one double bond to O. Structures such as these, which differ only by the distribution of electrons, are called **resonance structures**. The double-bond electrons are said to be delocalized over three atoms. A quantum chemical effect of delocalizing electrons throughout the molecule is that the structure is more stable than similar structures without resonance. The actual structure of NO_3^- is an average of all three structures called a **resonance hybrid.** Resonance "smears" the two electrons of the double bond throughout the molecule, making each N-O bond equivalent and effectively 1 and 1/3 bonds. The structure below attempts to represent the delocalization.

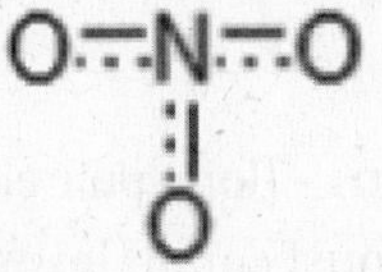

Structures That Violate the Octet Rule

Some examples of Be and B compounds are shown below. The first two on the left have less than an octet, but the two on the right have an octet for Be or B.

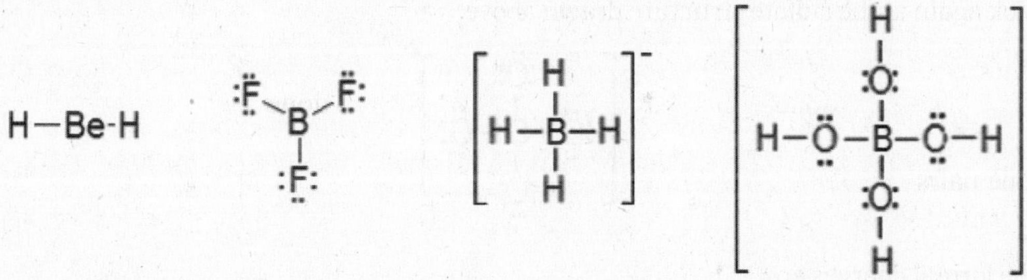

Some examples of **hypervalent species** (having more than an octet) are SF_4, PCl_5, XeF_4, and $BrCl_3$. The Lewis structures of these species can be constructed following the rules outlined above. Xenon tetrafluoride is an example of a noble gas compound. The heavier noble gases Kr and Xe can form compounds with more reactive elements like oxygen and fluorine. The three lone pairs on each F and Cl have been omitted for clarity.

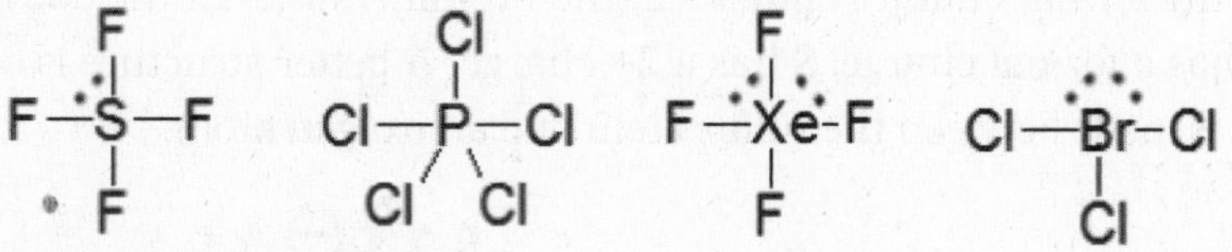

Formal Charge

There are three equivalent resonance structures for a nitrate ion. The energies of these three structures are equivalent and contribute equally to the total structure of the molecule. Some species such as the cyanate ion, OCN^-, have nonequivalent resonance structures. Three resonance structures for cyanate are:

$$[\ddot{\text{O}}\!-\!\text{C}\!\equiv\!\text{N}\!:]^- \longleftrightarrow [\ddot{\text{O}}\!=\!\text{C}\!=\!\ddot{\text{N}}]^- \longleftrightarrow [:\!\text{O}\!\equiv\!\text{C}\!-\!\ddot{\text{N}}\!:]^-$$

The energies of these three structures are different. Assigning **formal charges** is a way of measuring the number of electrons associated with a given atom in a compound relative to the number of valence electrons in the uncombined atom. Lone pair electrons belong to the atom on which they reside. Bond pair atoms are split equally between the two atoms sharing the bond.

Rules for Assigning Formal Charge

1. Formal charge = valence electrons − [lone pair electrons + $\frac{1}{2}$ (bond pair electrons)]
2. The sum of the formal charges must equal the overall charge. For neutral molecules the overall charge is zero.
3. If several structures exist, the best structures are those with the fewest formal charges and with any negative charges on the more electronegative atoms. Charges of 2+ or higher on a single atom or 2− or lower on a single atom are unreasonable if there are resonance structures with charges closer to zero.

Look again at the sulfate structure drawn above.

$$\left[\begin{array}{c}\ddot{\text{O}}\\ | \\ :\ddot{\text{O}}\!-\!\text{S}\!-\!\ddot{\text{O}}: \\ | \\ \ddot{\text{O}}:\end{array}\right]^{2-}$$

The formal charges are:

$S = 6 - (0 + \frac{1}{2}(8)) = +2$
$O = 6 - (6 + \frac{1}{2}(2)) = -1$

Formal charges are indicated on structures with the formal charge next to the atom. The sum of the formal charges equals −2, the overall charge. In the above structure, every atom has a formal charge. S has a 2+ charge. A better structure is obtained if a double bond is made between the sulfur atom and an oxygen atom.

$S = 6 - (0 + \frac{1}{2}(10)) = +1$
$O\ (A) = 6 - (4 + \frac{1}{2}(4)) = 0$
$O(B) = 6 - (6 + \frac{1}{2}(2)) = -1$

One less atom has a formal charge, and S is +1. A second double bond gives:

$S = 6 - (0 + \frac{1}{2}(12)) = 0$
$O(A) = 6 - (4 + \frac{1}{2}(4)) = 0$
$O(B) = 6 - (6 + \frac{1}{2}(2)) = -1$

For a -2 ion, two atoms each with a -1 charge is the best possible structure you can draw. The addition of double bonds also allows for resonance structures, which adds stability that more than makes up for violating the octet rule.

Assign formal charges to the cyanate ion to determine the best structure:

$O = 6 - (6 + \frac{1}{2}(2)) = -1$ $O = 6 - (4 + \frac{1}{2}(4)) = 0$ $O = 6 - (2 + \frac{1}{2}(6)) = +1$
$C = 4 - (0 + \frac{1}{2}(8)) = 0$ $C = 4 - (0 + \frac{1}{2}(8)) = 0$ $C = 4 - (0 + \frac{1}{2}(8)) = 0$
$N = 5 - (2 + \frac{1}{2}(6)) = 0$ $N = 5 - (4 + \frac{1}{2}(4)) = -1$ $N = 5 - (6 + \frac{1}{2}(2)) = -2$

The right structure is least stable because it has two atoms with formal charge, one of which is 2−. The center and left structures differ in that the −1 charge is either on N or O. The O atom is more electronegative than N, so the best structure is the one on the left.

Valence Shell Electron Pair Repulsion (VSEPR) and Molecular Shape

A Lewis structure simply gives the correct distribution of electrons and bonded atoms, but does not describe the molecular geometry. A simple way to determine the shape is the **Valence Shell Electron Pair Repulsion (VSEPR)** model, in which electrons are distributed to minimize repulsions between pairs of electrons on the center atom.

Assigning a VSEPR Shape

Step 1. Obtain a valid Lewis structure.
Step 2. Assign effective electron pairs to the bonds and lone pairs about the central atom. An effective pair of electrons is defined as either:

1. A lone pair (2 electrons)
2. A single bond pair (2 electrons)
3. A double bond (4 electrons)
4. A triple bond (6 electrons)

Another possible name used for an effective electron pair is the steric number. Electrons in multiple bonds occupy the same region in space, so these electrons (for VSEPR purposes) are counted as effectively a single electron pair.

Step 3. Count the number of effective electron pairs about an atom. These electrons will be arranged in geometries according to the table below. The central atom is A and the attached atoms are B in the molecular structures. Atoms in the plane of the page are shown with a regular line. Atoms above the plane of the page are shown with a wedged line. Atoms that are behind the plane of the page are shown with a dashed wedge.

The effect of lone pairs can be seen in the structures of CH_4, NH_3, and H_2O, which have a tetrahedral arrangement of effective electron pairs. Removing the lone pairs yields the molecular shape. The bond angle is reduced because the relative sizes of the effective electron pairs about the central atom are:

lone pair > triple bond > double bond > single bond.

e$^-$ pair distribution

Effective Electron Pairs	Geometry	Structure	Angles	Examples
2	Linear	B—A—B	180°	CO_2, OCN^-
3	Trigonal Planar		120°	NO_3^-, BF_3, SO_3
4	Tetrahedral		109.5°	CH_4, SO_4^{2-}, XeO_4
5	Trigonal Bipyramidal		120°, 180°, 90°	PF_5, SF_5^+
6	Octahedral		180°, 90°	SF_6, BrF_6^-

Shape and
H-X-H angle

Tetrahedral	Trigonal Pyramidal	Bent
109.5°	107°	105.5°

The most common shapes encountered when applying the VSEPR method are shown in the table below.

Lone Pairs on the Central Atom

Here are a few examples of Lewis structures and the predicted molecular shapes. The three lone pairs on each external F and Cl have been omitted for clarity. Note that the Lewis structures may not necessarily be a good indicator of the actual shape.

Effective e⁻ pairs	6	3	3
Lonepairs	2	0	1
Shape	square planar	trigonal planar	bent

Effective e⁻ pairs	5	5	4
Lonepairs	2	0	0
Shape	T-shaped	trigonal bipyramidal	tetrahedral

Polarity of Molecules

Once the shape of a molecule is known, the polarity of the molecule may be determined. A molecule is **polar** if there is a separation between the center of the positive charge and the center of the negative charge. Polar molecules have a **permanent dipole**, which points in the direction from the center of positive charge toward the center of negative charge. The polarity can be determined by considering the sum of the bond polarities.

The polarity of the bond is determined by the difference in electronegativities of the atoms in the bond:

➤ A difference of 0.0–0.5 is considered a nonpolar covalent bond.

➤ A difference of 0.5–2.0 is considered a polar covalent bond.

➤ A difference of 2.0 or greater is considered an ionic bond.

These numbers are estimates for the boundary between the bond types.

Bond polarity is due to unequal sharing of electrons. The more electronegative atom develops less than a full negative charge, indicated by a δ^-. The less electronegative atom develops less than a full positive charge, indicated by a δ^+. The bond polarity can be represented by a bond vector from the less electronegative to the more electronegative atom that is proportional to the difference in electronegativity. Bond polarity should not be confused with molecular polarity, which applies to the entire molecule. The bond vector for HF is shown below. With only one bond, the bond vector is also the dipole.

The electronegativities of selected elements are given below for use in determining bond polarity and molecular polarity. When considering the difference in electronegativity, the absolute value of the difference is used.

H=2.1,	C=2.5	N=3.0	O=3.5	F=4.0
Li=0.9	Si=1.8	P=2.1	S=2.5	Cl=3.0

EXAMPLE: Classify the bond polarity of the following bonds: Li-F, C-H, C-O, P-S, C-F, O-H, and N-Cl.

Elements	1st	2nd	Difference	Type
Li-F	0.9	4.0	3.1	ionic
C-H	2.5	2.1	0.4	nonpolar covalent
C-O	2.5	3.5	1.0	polar covalent
P-S	2.1	2.5	0.4	nonpolar covalent
C-F	2.5	4.0	1.5	polar covalent
O-H	3.5	2.1	1.4	polar covalent
N-Cl	3.0	3.0	0.0	nonpolar covalent

To determine whether a molecule is polar, obtain a valid VSEPR structure. Draw bond vectors in space along the bonds for each polar bond in the molecule.

➤ If there are no vectors because all the bonds are nonpolar, the molecule is nonpolar.

➤ If there are polar bonds, add the vectors in space. If the vectors cancel out, the molecule is nonpolar. If the vectors do not cancel out, the molecule is polar and the dipole is in the direction of the vector sum.

➤ There are a limited number of ways that bond vectors can interact. The following vector combinations will cancel out:

1. Two equivalent vectors at 180°, such as in CO_2
2. Three equivalent vectors at 120°, such as in SO_3
3. Four equivalent vectors at 109.5°, such as in CH_4

The molecular shape and partial charges are shown on the left (lone pair electrons except those on the central atom are omitted), and the bond vectors are shown on the right for some nonpolar molecules.

XeF_4 is square planar and the two pairs of Xe-F bonds at 180° cancel out in pairs.

PF_5 has two P-F bond vectors at 180° that cancel each other out. There are also three bond vectors at 120° that cancel out.

Below are some examples of polar molecules. Lone pairs except those on the central atom have been omitted.

NH_3 is trigonal pyramidal because of the lone pair on nitrogen. The bond vectors point towards the nitrogen. The net result of the three N-H bonds is a dipole pointing away from the nitrogen, on the side opposite the hydrogens. This molecule is polar.

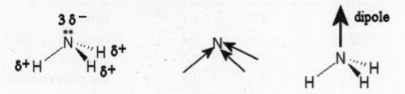

SF_4 has a seesaw shape. The two S-F vectors at 180° (A and B) cancel each other out, but the two at 120° (C and D) are not canceled, and the molecule is polar.

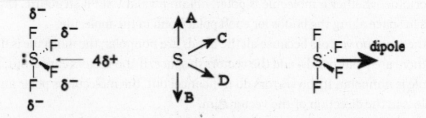

Bond Energies

Average bond energies (BE) have been tabulated for a large number of bonds. These bond energies will not be exact for a specific compound, but can be used for estimating enthalpy changes. Enthalpy of a reaction may be estimated by the formula:

$$\Delta H_{rxn(estimate)} = \Sigma \, BE(\text{bonds broken}) - \Sigma \, BE(\text{bonds formed})$$

Energy is required to break bonds. Energy is released when bonds form. The value obtained from this calculation is not as exact as would be obtained from calculations using ΔH values.

EXAMPLE: Consider the combustion of methane with the associated bond energies:

$$CH_4(g) + 2O_2(g) \longrightarrow 2H_2O(g) + CO_2(g)$$

Bond energies (in kJ): C-H (416), O=O (498), C=O (803), O-H (467)

$$\Delta H_{rxn}(\text{estimate}) = 4(C-H) + 2(O=O) - [4(O-H) + 2(C=O)]$$
$$= [4(416) + 2(498)] - [2(803) + 4(467)] \, kJ$$
$$= 2660 - 3474 \, kJ$$
$$= -814 \, kJ/mol$$

Calculation of this value from ΔH_f gives −801 kJ, so the estimate has a 1.6 % error.

SOLIDS AND LIQUIDS

Interparticle or Intermolecular Forces

All gases, if at low enough pressure and high enough temperature, behave in a similar fashion regardless of the composition of the gas. The much larger relative volumes of gases mean that gas particles (atoms or molecules) are well separated from one another. In solids and liquids, the particles are in contact. In liquids the particles can move freely about. In solids the particles vibrate about fixed positions. The behavior of solids and liquids depends upon the forces involved in the interactions of the particles.

There are three types of intermolecular forces (interatomic for noble gases) present in solids and liquids:

➤ Nonpolar molecules and isolated atoms interact through **London dispersion forces** (also called van der Waals forces).

➤ Polar molecules interact through **dipole-dipole forces**.

➤ Certain molecules that contain hydrogen bound to the more electronegative elements (O, N, and F) interact with especially strong dipole-dipole interactions called **hydrogen bonds**.

London dispersion forces arise from a temporary asymmetric distribution of electrons in a molecule or atom. The random motion of electrons in a nonpolar species occasionally creates an **instantaneous dipole,** which is a temporary separation of positive and negative charge. Another instantaneous dipole will be induced in an adjacent molecule, creating a weak electrical attraction. London forces are the weakest intermolecular forces. The importance of London forces depends on how easily the electron cloud about the atom in a molecule can be deformed. This property is called **polarizability**. Polarizability increases as the total number of electrons and size of the atoms in the molecule increase. London forces increase with molar mass for molecules or atoms of similar structure and size. London forces are present in all matter, but they are important only if stronger interactions are not possible.

Polar molecules have permanent dipoles. Each molecule has a separation of positive charge from negative charge. In polar solids or liquids, the positive end of one molecule will interact through electrical attraction with the negative part of an adjacent molecule.

If hydrogen is bound to a highly electronegative atom such as nitrogen, oxygen, or fluorine, the hydrogen develops a slight positive charge. The positive hydrogen atom will be strongly attracted to the lone pair of highly electronegative atoms creating a **hydrogen bond**, which is an especially strong dipole-dipole interaction. Hydrogen-bonded compounds tend to have unusually high boiling points when compared to substances of similar molar masses that do not take part in hydrogen bonding. Hydrogen bonds are also important in water and in biological molecules such as proteins, DNA, and carbohydrates. Some examples of hydrogen bonds formed by water and urea are shown below as dotted lines.

The relative strengths of interparticle forces are:

hydrogen bonds > dipole-dipole forces > London dispersion forces

Liquids

Liquids can best be described as consisting of molecules in contact with one another but able to move randomly through the bulk of the liquid. Liquids have short-range order, but long-range disorder. Several physical properties are used to characterize liquids.

Viscosity is the resistance of a liquid to flow. Viscosity is high for substances with stronger intermolecular forces. The viscosity of gasoline is less than that of water, which is in turn less that that of honey due to the strong hydrogen bonding in water.

The internal molecules of a liquid interact evenly in all directions with the other molecules of the liquid. Molecules on the surface interact with other molecules on the surface and within the liquid. Because there are no molecules above surface molecules, the uneven forces tend to draw surface molecules into the bulk of the liquid. The energy required to increase the surface area of a liquid is called the **surface tension**. The stronger the intermolecular forces, the higher the surface tension. Insects such as water bugs can be supported on the surface of water because of its high surface tension.

In a small-diameter tube made of a substance to which a liquid is attracted (such as water in a thin glass tube), the liquid will tend to be drawn into the tube until the force of gravity stops the rise of the liquid. This tendency for water to rise in a thin tube is called **capillary action**. Capillary action is important in plants to draw water into the leaves against gravity.

Phase Changes

At any given temperature a fraction of the molecules will have sufficient energy to escape from the liquid phase to the gas phase. In an open container with a constant temperature the entire liquid will evaporate. In a closed container, at first molecules will leave the liquid faster than gaseous molecules return to the liquid. Over time the rate of molecules going from the liquid to the gas phase will equal the rate of gaseous molecules returning to the liquid. This is a dynamic **equilibrium** state. Both processes continue, but there will be no net change in the number of gas molecules above the liquid. The pressure of the vapor above the liquid is called the equilibrium **vapor pressure**. The vapor pressure increases with temperature, but the increase is not linear. Vapor pressure decreases with increasing intermolecular forces. A sample vapor pressure curve versus temperature is shown below for two liquids.

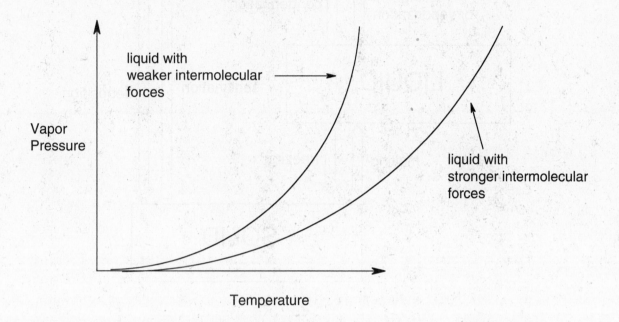

When the vapor pressure reaches the external atmospheric pressure, molecules form bubbles, the process called **boiling**. The temperature at which the boiling occurs at 1 atm pressure is called the **normal boiling point.**

Boiling is an example of a **phase change** in which a substance in one of the three states of matter converts to one of the other states of matter. Types of phase changes:

➤ For most substances, if you start with the substance in the solid state and increase the temperature, the substance will **melt** to a liquid.
➤ Then if you increase the temperature still further, the substance will **boil** or vaporize to a gas.
➤ If you cool down a gas, it will **condense** to a liquid.
➤ If you cool the liquid, it will **freeze** into a solid.

Direct conversion from a solid to a gas is called **sublimation** and its reverse is called **deposition**. Each of these phase changes has enthalpy associated with the change. Phase change enthalpies are listed for water below. For each reaction the change assumes 1 mole of substance. If any of these processes are reversed, the enthalpy must be multiplied by -1.

$H_2O(s) \rightarrow H_2O(l)\ \Delta H_{fusion}$

$H_2O(l) \rightarrow H_2O(g)\ \Delta H_{vaporization}$

$H_2O(s) \rightarrow H_2O(g)\ \Delta H_{sublimation}$ (This process occurs at pressures below 4.5 mm Hg.)

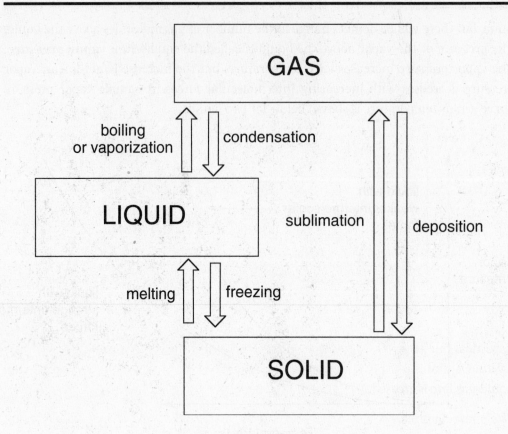

All of the energy added during the phase change goes into the transition from one phase to another, so the temperature remains fixed during the phase change.

The heat required to melt a substance is always less than the heat required to vaporize the substance. That is because melting simply breaks down the order of the solid without breaking the intermolecular forces, but boiling requires completely breaking the intermolecular forces to separate the molecules from one another.

Pure substances will show different boiling and melting points at different pressures. These data can be used to construct a **phase diagram** that shows what phase is stable for a given combination of pressure and temperature. A generic phase diagram is shown below. The lines between the regions represent the combination of pressure and temperature where phase transitions occur. Phase transitions at 1 atm pressure are the **normal melting point** (solid to liquid), **normal boiling point** (liquid to gas), and **normal sublimation point** (solid to gas, not shown in this diagram). The point at which the three phases meet is called the **triple point**. This is the only combination of temperature and pressure where solid, liquid, and gas can be in equilibrium. The termination of the vapor-liquid line is called the **critical point**. At temperatures above the critical point, no amount of applied pressure can liquefy the gas. A substance in this region is called a **supercritical fluid**.

A horizontal line ($A \rightarrow B$) traces the changes that occur if the temperature changes at a fixed pressure. A substance beginning at **A** as a solid melts as the temperature reaches the solid-liquid line and boils when the temperature reaches the liquid-gas line.

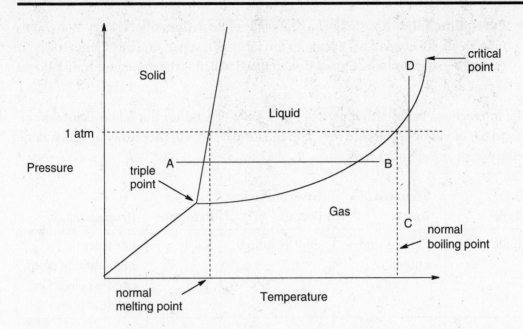

A vertical line (**C → D**) represents changes in temperature at a constant pressure. A substance that is a gas at C will convert to a liquid as the pressure is increased and the liquid-gas line is crossed.

The phase diagram above is typical of most substances that exist in only three phases. In most substances, the solid-liquid line has a positive slope. Water is unusual in that the solid phase is less dense than the liquid phase. This is why ice floats. A phase diagram for water is shown below.

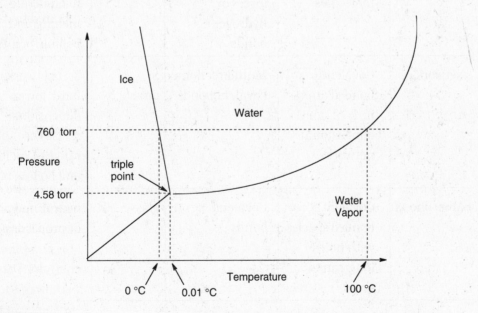

Solids

➤ **Amorphous solids** have no long-range order, but short-range order may be possible. Glass is an example of an amorphous solid. A good description of an amorphous solid is that it is a supercooled liquid.

➤ **Crystalline solids** have long-range periodic order in three dimensions. Many common solids are crystalline. Examples are table salt, sugar, and most ionic solids. A crystalline solid is characterized by a unit cell which is the minimum translational repeat unit.

The interactions between the particles of a solid depend on the solid's composition. Properties of various solids are shown in the table below. All the entries are crystalline solids except amorphous solids.

Type	Structural Units	Interparticle Forces	Example	Properties
Ionic	Cations and anions	Ionic bonding	NaCl	hard, brittle, high melting point, conduct electricity in liquid phase
Metallic	Metal cations surrounded by electrons	Metallic bonding	Fe	malleable, ductile, conduct electricity, low to high melting and boiling points
Molecular	Covalently bonded discrete molecules	London dispersion dipole-dipole forces or hydrogen bonds	Ar CO H_2O	soft, poor conductors of heat and electricity, low to moderate melting and boiling points
Network	Covalently bonded atoms in 1-, 2-, or 3-dimensional networks	Multidirectional covalent bonds	Si quartz	3-D networks, hard, lower dimensional species are softer, range of melting and boiling points
Amorphous	Covalent bonded species with no long-range order	Covalent bonds	glass	wide range of properties

SOLUTIONS

Solution is another name for a homogeneous mixture, or a mixture with only one phase. The phase of a solution may be a gas such as air, which is a mixture of nitrogen, oxygen, and other gases; a liquid such as sugar water; or a solid such as 14-carat gold, which is a mixture of 14 parts gold and 10 parts other metals. The component of a solution that is present in the greater amount is called the **solvent**. The component or components that are present in a lesser amount are called **solutes**. The phase of the solution is usually the same phase as the solvent.

Solutions form if the interactions between solute and solvent are stronger than the sum of the interactions between solute-solute or solvent-solvent. The forces between particles in solutions are similar to those in pure solids and pure liquids. One new type of interparticle force is possible in solutions. This force is an **ion-dipole** interaction, in which an ion interacts with polar molecules in an electrical attraction. The ion-dipole interaction between water and ions in an NaCl solution is shown below.

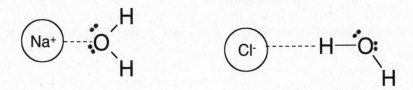

It has been found that substances with similar interparticle forces will be soluble in each other. For example, organic substances that can form hydrogen bonds such as ethyl alcohol, CH_3-CH_2-OH, or acetic acid, CH_3COOH, are readily soluble in water. Substances with only London dispersion forces are soluble in each other. For example, grease, a mixture of long chain hydrocarbons (CH_3-$(CH_2)_x$-CH_3, where x=from about 10 to 20) with only nonpolar C-C and C-H bonds, dissolves in octane, C_8H_{18}, one of the major components of gasoline. The generalizations of this paragraph are often summarized in the simple statement "like dissolves like." Hydrocarbon oils (only London forces) do not dissolve in water (hydrogen bonding forces).

Factors Affecting Solubility

The concentration of solutions can be described qualitatively as **concentrated** (more solute dissolved) or **dilute** (less solute dissolved). A solution with the maximum amount of a solute that can dissolve in a given amount of solvent under a given set of conditions is **saturated**. A **supersaturated** solution is an unstable state in which more solute is dissolved than in a saturated solution. If crystals start to form in a supersaturated solution, the solute precipitates until the solution becomes saturated.

Solubility and temperature:

➤ Solid and liquid solutes: solubility increases with increasing temperature, with some exceptions

➤ Gaseous solutes: solubility generally decreases with increasing temperature

Solubility and pressure:

➤ Solid and liquid solutes: changes in pressure have little effect

➤ Gaseous solutes: solubility increases with increasing partial pressure of the gas according to **Henry's law**: $s_{gas} = k_H P_{gas}$ (where s_{gas} is the solubility of the gas, k_H is the

Henry's law constant, and P_{gas} is the partial pressure of the solute gas above the solution)

Concentration Units

The concentration of a solution is measured quantitatively by several units. Each unit is generally an amount of solute per amount of solution or solvent. The definitions of the various concentration units are given below.

$$\text{Mass fraction} = \frac{\text{mass of solute}}{\text{mass of solution}}$$

$$\text{Mass percent (mass \%)} = \frac{\text{mass of solute}}{\text{mass of solution}} \times 100\% \text{ (often called weight percent)}$$

For very small amounts of solute such as pollutants, parts per million or parts per billion are used.

$$\text{Parts per million (ppm)} = \frac{\text{mass of solute}}{\text{mass of solution}} \times 10^6$$

$$\text{Parts per billion (ppb)} = \frac{\text{mass of solute}}{\text{mass of solution}} \times 10^9$$

1 L of water has a mass of $1000\,g$, and $1\,mg = 0.001\,g$. For $1\,mg$ solute the ratio of solute to solvent is $0.001\,g/1000\,g = 10^6$, so 1 ppm is approximately $1\,mg$ of solute per L of solution. Similarly $0.001\,mg$ of solute per liter of solution is approximately 1 ppb.

$$\text{Molarity (M)} = \frac{\text{mol of solute}}{\text{L of solution}}$$

$$\text{Molality (m)} = \frac{\text{mol of solute}}{\text{kg of solvent}}$$

$$\text{Mole Fraction}(\chi) = \frac{\text{mol of solute}}{\text{total moles in system}}$$

Conversion between units is often necessary.

> **EXAMPLE**: Calculate the mass percent, molarity, molality, and mole fraction of a solution prepared by mixing $210\,g$ of water with $90.0\,g$ of H_2SO_4. The density of the solution is $1.22\,g/mL$.

First you must determine the values of the quantities needed for the calculations.

The solution has a total mass of $210 + 90.0 = 300\,g$.

The solution has a volume of $300\,g \times {}^{1mL}/_{1.22\,g} = 246\,mL$.

The molar mass of water is $18.02\,g/mol$.

The molar mass of H_2SO_4 is 98.09 g/mol.

$$\text{The solution contains } 210.0 \text{ g } H_2O \times \frac{1 \text{ mol } H_2O}{18.02 \text{ g } H_2O} = 11.7 \text{ mol } H_2O.$$

$$\text{The solution contains } 90.0 \text{ g } H_2SO_4 \times \frac{1 \text{ mol } H_2SO_4}{98.09 \text{ g } H_2SO_4} = 0.918 \text{ mol } H_2SO_4.$$

$$\text{Mass percent (mass \%)} = \frac{90.0 \text{ g } H_2SO_4}{300 \text{ g soln}} \times 100\% = 30.0\% \text{ } H_2SO_4$$

$$\text{Molarity (M)} = \frac{0.918 \text{ mol } H_2SO_4}{0.246 \text{ L soln}} = 3.73 \text{ M } H_2SO_4$$

$$\text{Molality (m)} = \frac{0.918 \text{ mol } H_2SO_4}{0.210 \text{ kg } H_2O} = 4.37 \text{ m } H_2SO_4$$

$$\text{Mole Fraction } (\chi) = \frac{0.918 \text{ mol } H_2SO_4}{0.918 \text{ mol } H_2SO_4 + 11.7 \text{ mol } H_2O} = 0.0728$$

Colligative Properties

Several physical properties of solutions differ from those of the pure solvent. Those properties that depend only upon the number of particles in solution and not the identity of the solute are called **colligative properties**. When compared to the pure solvent, solutions have:

➤ Lower vapor pressures
➤ Lower freezing points
➤ Higher boiling points
➤ Osmotic pressures

The lower vapor pressure of solutions is given by **Raoult's law**:

$$P_{soln} = \chi_{solvent} P_{solvent}$$

where P_{soln} is the vapor pressure of the solution, $\chi_{solvent}$ is the mole fraction of solvent (not solute), and $P_{solvent}$ is the vapor pressure of the pure solvent. If the solute is also volatile, the vapor pressure is the combination of the vapor pressure of both components. The equation becomes:

$$P_{soln} = \chi_{solvent1} P_{solvent1} + \chi_{solvent2} P_{solvent2}.$$

The freezing point depression of solutions is given by:

$$\Delta T_{fp} = K_{fp} m$$

where ΔT_{fp} is the freezing point depression, K_{fp} is the freezing point depression constant, and m is the molality of the solute. K_{fp} is dependent on the solvent (for water it is $1.86°$ C/m).

The boiling point elevation of solutions is given by a similar expression:

$$\Delta T_{bp} = K_{bp} m$$

where ΔT_{bp} is the boiling point elevation, K_{bp} is the boiling point elevation constant, and m is the molality of the solute. K_{bp} is dependent on the solvent (for water it is 0.51°C/m).

A fourth colligative property is osmotic pressure. A semipermeable membrane is a barrier that allows flow of solvent but not solute. If there is a difference in concentration of a solute across a semipermeable membrane, the solvent flows in a direction to equalize the concentrations on the two sides of the membrane. In the example shown below, the solution within the membrane is placed into a more dilute solution or pure solvent.

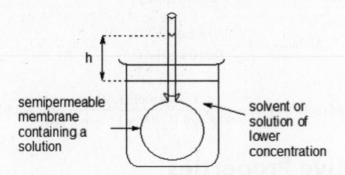

Solvent flows into the membrane to equalize the concentrations. The flow continues until the pressure from the weight of the solution that has risen in the tube balances with the osmotic pressure of the solution. **Osmotic pressure** is the pressure required to prevent the flow of the solvent into the membrane. It is given by:

$$\Pi = MRT$$

where Π is the osmotic pressure (atm), M is the molarity of the solute, R is the gas constant $\left(0.08026\dfrac{L \cdot atm}{mol \cdot k}\right)$, and T is the Kelvin temperature.

COLLIGATIVE PROPERTIES OF IONIC COMPOUNDS

Because ionic compounds break down into ions in water, the colligative property equations must be multiplied by the **van't Hoff factor, i,** which is an experimental measure of the moles of particles in solution per mole of solute dissolved. Theoretically, sodium chloride has a van't Hoff factor of 2, but due to ion pairing the experimental value is less.

A 0.10 m NaCl solution will have a lower vapor pressure, lower freezing point, higher boiling point, and greater osmotic pressure than a 0.10 m solution of sucrose, a molecular solid.

COLLIGATIVE PROPERTIES AND MOLAR MASS

Colligative properties may be used to determine the molar mass of a substance.

EXAMPLE: *p*-dichlorobenzene freezes at 53.1°C, and its K_{fp} has a value of 7.10°C kg/mol. A solution of 1.90 g of a new drug in 12.5 g of *p*-dichlorobenzene freezes at 47.1°C. What is the molar mass of the drug according to these data?

$$\Delta T_{fp} \longrightarrow m \longrightarrow \text{mol solute} \longrightarrow \text{molar mass}$$

$$\Delta T_{fp} = 53.1 - 47.1°C = 6.0°C$$

$$\Delta T_{fp} = K_{fp}m, \text{ so } m = \frac{\Delta T_{fp}}{K_{fp}}$$

$$m = \frac{6.0°C}{7.10\left(\dfrac{°C \text{ kg}}{\text{mol}}\right)} = 0.85 \frac{\text{mol}}{\text{kg}}$$

$$m = \frac{\text{mol solute}}{\text{kg solvent}} \text{ so } m \times \text{kg solvent} = \text{mol solute}$$

$$0.85 \frac{\text{mol}}{\text{kg}} \times 0.0125 \text{ kg} = 0.011 \text{ mol}$$

$$\text{Molar mass} = \frac{\text{g}}{\text{mol}} = \frac{1.90 \text{ g}}{0.011 \text{ mol}} = 1.7 \times 10^2 \text{ g/mol}$$

KINETICS

Some chemical reactions are fast, such as the burning of iron powder in a sparkler. Some reactions are slow, such as the rusting of an iron gate. Both reactions are oxidation of iron to oxides or related compounds, but the form of the iron determines the speed at which it combines with oxygen. A rise in temperature speeds up a chemical reaction, such as the rate at which milk sours. The study of the rates of reactions is called **kinetics**.

In basic physics, the velocity or rate of an object is defined as the distance traveled per unit time, $d = r \times t$. In the study of the rates of chemical reactions, the distance is replaced by concentration, and rates are given in units of concentration per unit time such as molar per second or molar per minute. The rate of a reaction depends upon what concentration is being measured. For a sample reaction given below,

$$aA + bB \rightarrow cC + dD$$

the rate is defined with respect to the disappearance of a reactant, $\text{Rate} = -\dfrac{\Delta[A]}{\Delta t}$, or the appearance of a product, $\text{Rate} = +\dfrac{\Delta[D]}{\Delta t}$. ([A] = Molar concentration of A).

The change for reactants is negative; for products, it is positive. The relationships of the reaction rates are related to the balanced equation. The mathematical relationships are:

$$\text{Rate} = -\left(\frac{1}{a}\right)\frac{\Delta[A]}{\Delta t} = -\left(\frac{1}{b}\right)\frac{\Delta[B]}{\Delta t} = +\left(\frac{1}{c}\right)\frac{\Delta[C]}{\Delta t} = +\left(\frac{1}{d}\right)\frac{\Delta[D]}{\Delta t}.$$

EXAMPLE: Consider the formation of ammonia.

$$N_2(g) + 3H_2(g) \rightarrow 2NH_3(g)$$

Using the sample equation, the relative rates for N_2 and NH_3 are:

$$-\left(\frac{1}{1}\right)\frac{\Delta[N_2]}{\Delta t} = +\left(\frac{1}{2}\right)\frac{\Delta[NH_3]}{\Delta t} \quad \text{or} -2\frac{\Delta[N_2]}{\Delta t} = +\frac{\Delta[NH_3]}{\Delta t}.$$

Ammonia is being formed at twice the rate that nitrogen is disappearing.

The kinetics of chemical reactions are generally studied early in the course of the reaction when the concentration of products is small. Under these conditions the reverse reaction is negligible, and the rate of reactions is given by a **rate law**:

$$\text{Rate} = k[A]^x[B]^y$$

where k is a rate constant that is fixed for a given reaction at a given temperature. The exponent x is the **order** of the reaction in A (y is the order of the reaction in B). Most chemical reactants have orders equal to 0, 1, or 2. During the reaction, the concentration of the reactants decreases and thus the rate decreases. Increasing the concentration of a substance in the rate law increases the rate of a reaction.

Determining the Order of a Reaction

The order of the reaction may be determined by a technique called the **method of initial rates**. A reaction is run with variations in the concentrations of the reactants. In some reactions the concentration of one reactant is held constant.

$$2NO(g) + Cl_2(g) \rightarrow 2NOCl(g)$$

The initial rate is for the disappearance of Cl_2. $\text{Rate} = -\dfrac{\Delta[Cl_2]}{\Delta t}$

Exp	[NO]	[Cl$_2$]	Initial Rate (M/s)
1	0.020	0.010	8.27×10^{-5}
2	0.020	0.020	1.65×10^{-4}
3	0.020	0.040	3.31×10^{-4}
4	0.040	0.020	6.60×10^{-4}

For this reaction the rate law is of the form

$$\text{Rate} = k[NO]^x[Cl_2]^y.$$

The concentrations were picked so that the concentration of one reactant doubles and one remains fixed. Dividing the rate law for reaction 2 by the rate law for reaction 1 gives:

$$\frac{Rate_2 = k[NO]_2^x[Cl_2]_2^y}{Rate_1 = k[NO]_1^x[Cl_2]_1^y} \Rightarrow \frac{1.65\times10^{-4} = k[0.020]^x[0.020]^y}{8.27\times10^{-5} = k[0.020]^x[0.010]^y}$$

$$\Rightarrow 1.995 = 2^y$$

The k and the [NO] terms cancel out leaving the ratio of 2 for the concentration of Cl_2. The simplified equation determines $y = 1$. Note that the ratio of the rates is not exactly 2 because of experimental errors. In a similar manner you can determine x from experiments 4 and 2. The value of $x = 2$.

The rate law is Rate $= k[NO]^2[Cl_2]$. The order of the reaction is not related to the coefficients of the balanced equation and must be determined experimentally.

Once you have the rate law, the value of k may be obtained from any of the experiments. From experiment 3:

$$Rate = k[NO]^2[Cl_2]$$

$$3.31\times10^{-4}\ M/s = k(0.020\ M)^2(0.040\ M)^2 \rightarrow k = 20.7\frac{1}{M^2 s}.$$

The units of k will depend on the overall order of the reaction.

1st order: $\frac{1}{time}$, 2nd order: $\frac{1}{M\times time}$; and 3rd order (as in this example): $\frac{1}{M^2\times time}$.

Integrated Rate Law

The **integrated rate law** gives the concentration as a function of time. Derivation of the integrated rate law requires calculus, so the results will simply be stated. Two cases will be considered for a single reactant producing product: the first order and second order.

$$A \rightarrow products$$

For a first-order reaction, the rate law is rate $= k[A]$. Integrating this equation gives:

$$\ln[A]_t = -kt + \ln[A]_o$$

where $[A]_t$ is the concentration at time t, $[A]_o$ is the concentration at time 0, k is the rate constant, and t is the time.

An equivalent representation is $[A]_t = [A]_o e^{-kt}$. Either form may be used. The first form is convenient for plotting an equation because it is in the form $y = mx + b$, so a plot of $\ln[A]_t$ as y and t as x will have slope of $-k$ and a y intercept of $\ln[A]_o$. The second form is probably easier for calculations.

A convenient quantity to use for a first order reaction is the **half life ($t_{1/2}$)**, which is defined as the time required for the initial concentration of a reaction to be reduced by one half. Half life for a first order reaction is easily obtained. The concentration at $t_{1/2}$ is one half the initial concentration: $[A]_{t_{1/2}} = \frac{1}{2}[A]_o$. Substituting in the integrated rate law equation:

$\ln\left(\dfrac{[A]_0}{2}\right) = -kt_{1/2} + \ln[A]_0$. Rearranging the equation gives: $\ln\left(\dfrac{[A]_0}{2}\right) - \ln[A]_0 = -kt_{1/2}$

Using one of the laws of logarithms, the equation can be solved for the half-life:

$$\frac{\ln 2}{k} = t_{1/2}\ln(2) = 0.693, \text{ so } \frac{0.693}{k} = t_{1/2}.$$

The half-life of the decomposition of SO_2Cl_2 with a k of 2.83×10^{-3} $1/\text{min}$ is:

$$\frac{0.693}{2.83 \times 10^{-3}\left(\dfrac{1}{\text{min}}\right)} = 245 \text{ min.}$$

The half-life is independent of the concentration (this is true only for a first-order reaction). The half-life remains constant during the course of the reaction. The percent remaining as a function of number of half-lives is given in the table below:

Number of half-lives elapsed	Percentage remaining
0	100
1	50
2	25
3	12.5
4	6.25
5	3.13
etc.	

This table allows you to estimate the fraction left by the number of half-lives that have elapsed. For example, what percentage of SO_2Cl_2 remains after 600 min of reaction? Two half-lives is $2 \times 245 = 490$ min and three half-lives is $3 \times 245 = 785$ min. Because 600 min of the reaction is between 490 and 735 min, the percentage remaining is between 12.5 and 25 %.

A second-order rate law has the form $\text{rate} = k[A]^2$. Integrating the rate law for this reaction gives:

$$\frac{1}{[A]_t} = kt + \frac{1}{[A]_0}.$$

For a second-order reaction, a plot of $\dfrac{1}{[A]_t}$ as y and t as x will have slope of $+k$ and a

y intercept of $\dfrac{1}{[A]_0}$. The half-life of a second-order reaction can also be derived by

substituting $\dfrac{[A]_0}{2}$ for $[A]_t$:

$$\frac{1}{\left(\dfrac{[A]_0}{2}\right)} = kt_{1/2} + \frac{1}{[A]_0} \quad \text{Solving for } t_{1/2} \text{ gives} = \frac{1}{[A]_0 k} = t_{1/2}$$

The half-life depends on the initial concentration. Because the concentration decreases over the course of a reaction, the half-life of a second-order reaction increases with time.

The Effect of Temperature on k

The rates of chemical reactions are explained by collision theory, which is an extension of the kinetic molecular theory first discussed in the description of gases. Reactants will be successfully converted to products when the reactant molecules collide with sufficient energy and with the correct orientation. These two factors are incorporated into the **Arrhenius equation,** which gives the value of the rate constant as a function of the temperature:

$$k = Ae^{-\left(\frac{E_a}{RT}\right)},$$

where k is the rate constant, A is the frequency factor (a measure of the frequency of molecular collisions and the fraction with proper orientations), E_a is the activation energy (the minimum energy required for successful reaction to occur), R is the gas constant, and T is the Kelvin temperature.

Note: This equation indicates that as the temperature increases, the rate constant increases. The reverse is true for the activation energy. As the activation energy increases, the rate constant decreases and the reaction rate slows down.

Catalysts

Catalysts are substances that speed up the rate of a reaction but are not consumed during the reaction. Catalysts are used to make industrial preparations more efficient. Catalytic converters on automobiles convert exhaust gases to less toxic substances. Enzymes are natural catalysts that accelerate important biological reactions. For example, proteases in the stomach reduce the time required to break down proteins. Catalysts work by lowering the activation energy of reaction. The lower activation energy increases the value of the rate constant. Catalysts have no effect on the energies of the reactants or products, so the energy or enthalpy change of the reaction does not change. The concentrations at equilibrium (discussed below) are also not affected by a catalyst.

EQUILIBRIUM

If a reaction goes on long enough, the concentration of products will increase and the reverse reaction will begin to occur. Eventually the rates of the forward and reverse reactions will become equal. The concentration of reactants and products will not change, even though both the forward and reverse reactions continue to occur. When forward and reverse rates of a reaction are equal, the reaction is at **equilibrium**. Equilibrium is dynamic. Because both reactions are occurring, equilibrium reactions are written with a double arrow.

The equilibrium is characterized by the **equilibrium constant, K**. A capital K is used to distinguish this constant from the kinetic rate constant. For a gas phase reaction:

$$aA(g) + bB(g) \rightleftharpoons cC(g) + dD(g).$$

The equilibrium constant K_c is given by:

$$K_c = \frac{[C]^c [D]^d}{[A]^a [B]^b}.$$

All the concentrations are at equilibrium. The equilibrium expression may be written directly from the balanced equation. The units for K are usually ignored.

> **EXAMPLE:** Consider an equilibrium obtained by introducing H_2, I_2, and HI into a 5.00 L flask at 825 K. At equilibrium, the flask contains 7.500 mol of HI, 1.875 mol of H_2, and 0.261 mol I_2. Calculate the equilibrium constant.

The balanced equation is:

$$H_2(g) + I_2(g) \rightleftharpoons 2\,HI(g).$$

The concentrations at equilibrium are:

$$[HI] = \frac{7.500 \text{ mol HI}}{5.00 \text{ L}} = 1.50 \text{ M HI}$$

$$[H_2] = \frac{1.875 \text{ mol } H_2}{5.00 \text{ L}} = 0.375 \text{ M } H_2$$

$$[I_2] = \frac{0.261 \text{ mol } I_2}{5.00 \text{ L}} = 0.0522 \text{ M } I_2.$$

The equilibrium constant is:

$$K_e = \frac{[HI]^2}{[H_2][I_2]} = \frac{(1.50)^2}{(0.0522)(0.375)} = 115.$$

Pressures are usually easier to measure for gases, so a different equilibrium constant may be used, K_p. This constant has the same form as the regular equilibrium constant expression (which may be distinguished as K_c), except pressures are used.

$$K_p = \frac{(P_{HI})^2}{(P_{H2})(P_{I2})}$$

Unless otherwise indicated, K means K_c. K_c and K_p will differ in number except when the number of gas molecules in the reactants equals the number of gas molecules in the products.

Because the concentration of pure solids and liquids is fixed at a given temperature and pressure, these values are incorporated into K. Pure solids and liquids are left out of the equilibrium constant expression.

The value of K indicates the relative amounts of products and reactants at equilibrium:

➤ $K > 1$: mostly products present at equilibrium
➤ $K = 1$: both reactants and products present at equilibrium
➤ $K < 1$: mostly reactants present at equilibrium

If an equation is altered, the form of the equilibrium constant expression is also changed.

EXAMPLE: Consider the reaction for the formation of HI discussed earlier.

$$H_2(g) + I_2(g) \rightleftharpoons 2HI(g)$$

The reverse of the equation is:

$$2HI(g) \rightleftharpoons H_2(g) + I_2(g).$$

The equilibrium constant expression for the reverse reaction is:

$$K_{rev} = \frac{[H_2][I_2]}{[HI]^2}.$$

Clearly, $K_{rev} = \dfrac{1}{K_{for}}$. If a reaction is reversed, take the reciprocal of K.

You may also multiply or divide a reaction by a number that changes the values of the exponents in the equilibrium constant expression.

EXAMPLE: You can multiply the original equation by 3.

$$3H_2(g) + 3I_2(g) \rightleftharpoons 6HI(g)$$

The corresponding equilibrium constant expression is:

$$K_{3x} = \frac{[HI]^6}{[H_2]^3[I_2]^3}.$$

So $K_{3x} = (K_{for})^3$. If a reaction is multiplied by a number, then K is raised to that number.

Equations may also be combined.

EXAMPLE:

Rxn 1	$2SO_2(g) \rightleftharpoons 2S(s) + 2O_2(g)$	
Rxn 2	$2S(s) + 3O_2(g) \rightleftharpoons 2SO_3(g)$	
Sum	$2SO_2(g) + O_2(g) \rightleftharpoons 2SO_3(g)$	

Multiplying $K_1 \times K_2$ gives:

$$\frac{[O_2]^2}{[SO_2]^2} \times \frac{[SO_3]^2}{[O_2]^3} = \frac{[SO_3]^2}{[SO_2]^2[O_2]} = K_{sum}.$$

$$\underbrace{}_{K_1} \quad \underbrace{}_{K_2}$$

If a series of reactions adds up to a total reaction, the equilibrium constant for the sum reaction is the product of the equilibrium constants of the reactions that make up the sum.

Reaction Quotient

The **reaction quotient (Q)** has the same form as the equilibrium constant expression except that the concentrations used are the initial concentrations. For example:

$$aA + bB \rightleftharpoons cC + dD.$$

The reaction quotient is given by:

$$Q = \frac{[C]_o^c[D]_o^d}{[A]_o^a[B]_o^b}.$$

The reaction quotient may be used to predict in which direction a reaction will proceed.
➤ $Q = K$: at equilibrium, no shift
➤ $Q > K$: too much of the products, shift to the reactants (left)
➤ $Q < K$: too little of the products, shift to the products (right)

EXAMPLE:
$K = 115$ at $825\,K$ for the reaction:
$H_2(g) + I_2(g) \rightleftharpoons 2\,HI(g)$
if $[HI]_o = 2.00$ M, $[H_2]_o = 0.125$ M, and $[I_2]_o = 0.150$ M

Determine the direction the reaction will shift.

$$Q = \frac{[HI]_o^2}{[H_2]_o[I_2]_o} = \frac{(2.00)^2}{(0.125)(0.150)} = 213 > K = 115$$

Q is greater than K, so the reaction shifts to the left to decrease the products and increase the reactants until $Q = K$.

Le Châtelier's Principle

The reaction quotient is also useful for predicting in which direction a reaction at equilibrium will shift if the conditions are altered. The general rule used to predict these changes is called **Le Châtelier's Principle**. It states that a system at equilibrium that is changed so it is no longer at equilibrium will respond in a way that counteracts the change. A summary of important possible changes to equilibrium is given below.

Change	Counteraction	Shift direction
Reduce products	Increase products	Forward (right or to products)
Increase products	Reduce products	Reverse (left or to reactants)
Reduce reactants	Increase reactants	Reverse
Increase reactants	Decrease reactants	Forward
Increase temperature	Decrease heat	Forward for endothermic Reverse for exothermic
Decrease temperature	Increase heat	Reverse for endothermic Forward for exothermic
Increase pressure or Decrease volume	Reduce pressure	To the side with fewer gas molecules
Decrease pressure or Increase volume	Increase pressure	To the side with more gas molecules

Each of these entries can be justified by calculating Q after the given change to predict the direction the reaction will shift. For the temperature changes, consider that heat is a reactant in an endothermic reaction, and heat is a product in an exothermic reaction.

> **EXAMPLE:** Consider the formation of ammonia written as a thermochemical equation ($\Delta H = -92.2$ kJ):

$$N_2(g) + 3H_2(g) \rightleftharpoons 2NH_3(g) + 92.2 \text{ kJ.}$$

➤ If H_2 is added, the reaction will shift to the right to decrease the added H_2.
➤ If the temperature is increased, the reverse reaction will run to absorb the heat (shift left).
➤ If the volume is doubled, this lowers the pressure, and the system shifts to the left to increase the pressure by generating more gas molecules.

Acid-Base Equilibrium

In the Arrhenius definition, acids form H^+ ions in water, and bases produce OH^- in water. A more general description is the **Brønsted-Lowry** theory of acids and bases, in which acids are defined as proton (H^+) donors, and bases are defined as proton acceptors.

➤ A substance that is a Brønsted-Lowry acid must have a hydrogen atom in its formula. Not all hydrogen atoms are acidic; for example hydrogen atoms bound to carbon are generally not acidic.
➤ A substance that is a Brønsted-Lowry base must have a lone pair of electrons to accept the proton.

> **EXAMPLE:** A Brønsted-Lowry acid-base reaction is the ionization of HCl in water.
> $$HCl(aq) + H_2O(l) \rightarrow Cl^-(aq) + H_3O^+(aq)$$
> acid   base

The proton on HCl is donated to water, forming the hydronium ion, H_3O^+. This reaction goes nearly to completion, so the reaction is not written as an equilibrium. Acids that ionize nearly 100% such as HCl are **strong acids**. There are six common strong acids: HCl, HBr, HI, HNO_3, H_2SO_4, and $HClO_4$.

Other acids that do not ionize 100 percent are called **weak acids**. An example is acetic acid.

$$CH_3COOH(aq) + H_2O(l) \rightleftharpoons CH_3COO^-(aq) + H_3O^+(aq)$$
$$\text{acid} \qquad\qquad \text{base}$$

In a 1 M solution of acetic acid, only 4 out of every 1000 molecules ionize.

Ammonia functions as a **weak base** in water because it abstracts a proton from water leaving the hydroxide ion.

$$NH_3(aq) + H_2O(l) \rightleftharpoons NH_4^+(aq) + OH^-(aq)$$
$$\text{base} \quad\ \text{acid}$$

The reverses of the three equations above are also acid-base reactions. The reverse reactions involve a proton transfer back to the original acid.

EXAMPLE: This is illustrated in the acid-base reaction of HF, a weak acid.

$$HF(aq) + H_2O(l) \rightleftharpoons F^-(aq) + H_3O^+(aq)$$
$$\text{Acid} \quad\ \text{Base} \quad\ \ \text{Base} \quad\ \text{Acid}$$

Conjugate acid-base pairs are an acid and a related base that differs by one proton lost in the acid-base transfer. The conjugate base has a charge that is one less than the conjugate acid. The greater the tendency of an acid to donate a proton, the stronger the acid will be. An abbreviated table of relative acid strengths is shown below.

Acids	Conjugate Bases	Acid Strength
HCl	Cl^-	Strong
HNO_3	NO_3^-	Strong
H_3O^+	H_2O	Hydronium Ion
H_3PO_4	$H_2PO_4^-$	Weak Acids
HF	F^-	Weak
HNO_2	NO_2^-	Weak
CH_3COOH	CH_3COO^-	Weak
NH_4^+	NH_3	Weak
HCN	CN^-	Weak
H_2O	OH^-	Water
OH^-	O^{2-}	Very Weak
H	H^-	Very Weak

In the acid column, acid strength increases from the bottom to the top. In the base column, base strength increases from top to bottom. If an acid has a strong tendency to donate its proton, the conjugate base of this acid will have little affinity for protons. So the stronger the acid, the weaker the conjugate base will be.

The relative strengths of the acids can be used to predict which side of an acid-base equilibrium will be favored.

$$H_3PO_4(aq) + CH_3COO^-(aq) \rightleftharpoons H_2PO_4^-(aq) + CH_3COOH(aq)$$

H_3PO_4 is a stronger acid than CH_3COOH, so this equilibrium will favor the right side. This reaction may be thought of as a competition for the proton. The stronger base (in this case CH_3COO^-) is the conjugate of the weakest acid. In the competition for the proton, CH_3COO^- beats $H_2PO_4^-$ and the right side is favored. The acid base equilibria will always favor the side with the weakest acid and weakest base pair.

A larger number of weak acids contain the **carboxylic acid group** (-COOH). Acetic acid and citric acid (below) are examples.

A large number of weak bases are derivatives of ammonia called **amines** in which the H atoms have been replaced by carbon-containing groups, such as methyl amine,

CH_3NH_2, and trimethyl amine, $(CH_3)_3N$. The lone pair on the nitrogen atom of these molecules accepts a proton.

In the table of relative acid and base strengths, water appears both as an acid and as a base. Such substances are called **amphiprotic**. The **autoionization** of water is an acid-base reaction between two water molecules.

$$H_2O(l) + H_2O(l) \rightleftharpoons OH^-(aq) + H_3O^+(aq) \quad K_w = [H_3O^+][OH^-] \text{ (at 25 °C, } K_w = 10^{-14})$$

Note that the small value of K_w means that the concentration of water does not change significantly, so it is omitted from the equilibrium constant expression.

An equal number of hydronium ions and hydroxide ions are formed by the ionization of water ($[H_3O^+]=[OH^-]$), which means $[H_3O^+]^2 = 1.0 \times 10^{-14}$. Taking the square root of both sides gives $[H_3O^+] = 1.0 \times 10^{-7} = [OH^-]$.

Aqueous solutions are either:

➤ neutral if $[H_3O^+] = [OH^-]$
➤ acidic if $[H_3O^+] > [OH^-]$
➤ basic if $[H_3O^+] < [OH^-]$

The product of $[H_3O^+][OH^-]$ must be 10^{-14}, so as $[H_3O^+]$ increases $[OH^-]$ will decrease and vice versa.

$[H_3O^+]$	$[OH^-]$	solution
10^{-1}	10^{-13}	acidic
10^{-5}	10^{-9}	acidic
10^{-7}	10^{-7}	neutral
10^{-10}	10^{-4}	basic
10^{-12}	10^{-2}	basic

pH

The concentrations of H_3O^+ and OH^- tend to involve large negative exponents. Before pocket calculators, these numbers were cumbersome, so a more convenient quantity was defined by taking the negative logarithm of the H_3O^+ concentration. This is the **pH scale**. The term pH stands for "power of H," with H meaning H^+ or more correctly H_3O^+.

$$pH = -\log[H_3O^+], \quad \text{sometimes written} \quad -\log[H^+]$$

It should always be understood that $H^+(aq)$ is a shorthand for $H_3O^+(aq)$.

Aqueous solutions can be categorized as:

			example	pH
➤	$pH < 7$	$[H_3O^+] > [OH^-]$	acidic $[H_3O^+] = 10^{-3} > [OH^-] = 10^{-11}M$	3
➤	$pH = 7$	$[H_3O^+] = [OH^-]$	neutral $[H_3O^+] = 10^{-7} = [OH^-] = 10^{-7}M$	7
➤	$pH > 7$	$[H_3O^+] < [OH^-]$	basic $[H_3O^+] = 10^{-9} < [OH^-] = 10^{-5}M$	9

pH is often measured by pH paper, which has dyes that change color with changes in pH or by a meter. For pH values that are not even powers of ten, it is useful to bracket the pH value. For example, if $[H_3O^+] = 2.0 \times 10^{-4}$ the concentration is between 10^{-4} and 10^{-3}. The pH will be between 4.0 and 3.0, but closer to 4.0. (actual value, $pH = -\log(2.0 \times 10^{-4}) = 3.7$)

Acid Dissociation Constant, K_a

The equation for the ionization of an acid has a corresponding equilibrium constant called the **acid dissociation constant, K_a**. For a generic acid HA, the K_a equation is:

$$HA(aq) + H_2O(l) \rightleftharpoons H_3O^+(aq) + A^-(aq)$$

The equilibrium constant expression which omits the solvent water is:

$$K_a = \frac{[H_3O^+][A^-]}{[HA]}.$$

Likewise, the equation for the ionization of a base may be written with a corresponding equilibrium constant called the **base dissociation constant, K_b**.

For a generic base B, the K_b equation is:

$$B(aq) + H_2O(l) \rightleftharpoons BH^+(aq) + OH^-(aq).$$

The equilibrium constant expression which omits the solvent water is:

$$K_b = \frac{[BH^+][OH^-]}{[B]}.$$

K_a and K_b values vary over a wide range (from less than 10^{-20} to much greater than 1.0) depending on the relative strength of the acid or base. Some values illustrating the wide range are listed below. The numerical values confirm the reciprocal nature of the strengths of conjugate acid-base pairs.

Acid	K_a	Conjugate base	K_b
HCl	Very large	Cl^-	Very small
HF	7.2×10^{-4}	F^-	1.4×10^{-11}
CH_3COOH	1.8×10^{-5}	CH_3COO^-	5.6×10^{-10}
$Al(H_2O)_6^{3+}$	7.9×10^{-6}	$Al(H_2O)_5(OH)^{2+}$	1.3×10^{-9}
HCN	4.0×10^{-10}	CN^-	2.5×10^{-5}
H_2O	1.0×10^{-14}	OH^-	1.0
H_2	Very small	H^-	Very large

Some acids have more than one acidic proton. For example, H_2SO_3 is a diprotic acid:

$$H_2SO_3(aq) + H_2O(l) \rightleftharpoons H_3O^+(aq) + HSO_3^-(aq) \quad K_{a1} = 1.2 \times 10^{-2}$$
$$HSO_3^-(aq) + H_2O(l) \rightleftharpoons H_3O^+(aq) + SO_3^{2-}(aq) \quad K_{a2} = 6.2 \times 10^{-8}.$$

Successive ionization constants decrease in value ($K_{a1} > K_{a2} > K_{a3} >$ etc.). HSO_3^- is about a 10^5 times weaker acid than H_2SO_3. Removal of the second proton is always more difficult because the second proton is taken from a species with one more overall negative charge.

For an acid HA, the conjugate base is A^-, and the K_b equation and equilibrium constant expression are:

$$A^-(aq) + H_2O(l) \rightleftharpoons HA(aq) + OH^-(aq)$$

and

$$K_b = \frac{[HA][OH^-]}{[A^-]}.$$

By multiplying $K_a \times K_b$ an important result is obtained.

$$K_a \times K_b = \frac{[H_3O^+][A^-]}{[HA]} \times \frac{[HA][OH^-]}{[A^-]} = [H_3O^+][OH^-] = K_w$$

pH of Acid or Base Solutions

STRONG ACIDS

Because strong acids ionize 100%, $[H_3O^+] = [HA]_o$, and $pH = -\log[HA]_o$. A 0.015 M HNO_3 solution has $[H_3O^+] = 0.015$ M and $pH = -\log(0.015) = 1.82$.

STRONG BASES

Strong bases such as sodium hydroxide ionize 100%, so $[OH^-] = [NaOH]_o$. A 0.00034 M NaOH solution has a hydroxide concentration $[OH^-] = 0.00034$ M.

$$[H_3O^+] = \frac{K_w}{[OH^-]} = \frac{1 \times 10^{-14}}{[0.00034]} = 2.9 \times 10^{-11}. \text{ The pH} = -\log(2.9 \text{ X } 10^{-11}) = 10.54$$

The pOH is defined in a way analogous to pH; $pOH = -\log[OH^-]$. The quantities pH and pOH are related through K_w. Taking the $-\log$ of the K_w equilibrium expression gives:

$$-\log(K_w) = -\log([H_3O^+][OH^-]) \rightarrow 14.00 = pH + pOH.$$

The pH of the NaOH solution could be calculated using pOH.

$$pOH = -\log(0.00034) = 3.46 \rightarrow pH = 14.00 - 3.46 = 10.54$$

Weak Acids

Weak acids do not ionize 100 percent. The concentration $[H_3O^+]$ and the pH depend upon the percent ionization.

EXAMPLE: Consider a 2.00 M solution of an acid, HA, which ionizes 1%. Consider the process in two steps. The concentrations of interest can be recorded in a table.

$$HA(aq) + H_2O(l) \rightleftharpoons A^-(aq) + H_3O^+(aq)$$

Initial	2.00 M	0 M	0 M
Change	−0.02 M	+0.02 M	+0.02 M
Equilibrium	1.98 M	0.02 M	0.02 M

The corresponding K_a would be:

$$K_a = \frac{[H_3O^+][A^-]}{[HA]} = \frac{[0.02][0.02]}{[1.98]} = 2 \times 10^{-4}.$$

The pH in this example is $pH = -\log(0.02) = 1.7$.

You can also calculate pH from K_a and $[HA]_o$.

EXAMPLE: Determine the pH of a 0.50 M solution of HF ($K_a = 7.2 \times 10^{-4}$). A table is used with x representing the changes in concentration.

$$HF(aq) + H_2O(l) \rightleftharpoons F^-(aq) + H_3O^+(aq)$$

Initial	0.50 M	0 M	0 M
Change	−x M	+x M	+x M
Equilibrium	0.50−x M	x M	x M

The K_a expression is:

$$K_a = \frac{[H_3O^+][F^-]}{[HF]} = 7.2 \times 10^{-4} = \frac{(x)(x)}{(0.50 - x)} = \frac{x^2}{(0.50 - x)}$$

This equation is a quadratic equation. K_a is small, x will be very small, and $0.50 - x \approx 0.50$. This is justified only if x is 5% or less of $[HF]_o$. The simplified equation is:

$$7.2 \times 10^{-4} = \frac{x^2}{(0.50)} \rightarrow 3.6 \times 10^{-4} = x^2 \rightarrow \sqrt{3.6 \times 10^{-4}} = x \rightarrow 0.019\,M = x$$

$$pH = -\log(0.019) = 1.72.$$

The percent ionization is $\dfrac{0.019}{0.50} \times 100\% = 3.8\% < 5\%$ so simplification is justified.

WEAK BASES

Weak base problems are similar to weak acid problems except for the K_b equation and equilibrium constant expression, K_b. The OH^- concentration can be found using a table similar to that used in the previous example. pOH is calculated and converted to pH.

Salts

Salt is another name for ionic compound. A salt thus consists of a cation and an anion. Reaction of an acid with a base produces a salt and water. The acid-base properties of the salt formed will depend upon the nature of the acid or base that formed the salt. There are four possibilities.

Cation source	Anion source	Acidity, equilibrium	Salt
Strong base (NaOH)	Strong acid (HNO_3)	Neutral	$NaNO_3$
Strong base (NaOH)	Weak acid (HF)	Basic, K_b of F^-	NaF
Weak base (NH_3)	Strong acid (HCl)	Acidic, K_a of NH_4^+	NH_4Cl
Weak base (NH_3)	Weak acid (HF)	Acidic or Basic, depends on larger of K_a of NH_4^+ or K_b of F^-	NH_4F

Neither the cation nor the anion of a salt formed by a strong acid and a strong base has any acidity or basicity. These ions do not affect the pH. Anions from weak acids are conjugate bases, and these species will tend to make the solution basic by the following K_b reaction illustrated for F^- from NaF:

$$F^-(aq) + H_2O(l) \rightleftharpoons HF(aq) + OH^-(aq)$$

The $K_b = \dfrac{K_w}{K_a(HF)} = \dfrac{1.0 \times 10^{-14}}{7.2 \times 10^{-4}} = 1.4 \times 10^{-11}$. HF is a relatively strong weak acid, and F^- is a very weak base.

Lewis Acids and Bases

Certain reactions behave in a similar fashion to the acid-base reactions described above but do not involve the transfer of a proton. Consider the two following reactions.

$$NH_3(aq) + H_2O(l) \rightleftharpoons NH_4^+(aq) + OH^-(aq)$$
$$NH_3(g) + BF_3(g) \rightleftharpoons H_3N\text{-}BF_3(g)$$

In both reactions, the lone electron pair of ammonia is reacting with an electron-poor species (H^+ in the first reaction and BF_3 in the second reaction) to form a new bond (N-H in the first and N-B in the second). The second reaction can be classified as an acid-base reaction if the definition of acids and bases is expanded to the Lewis theory.

➤ A **Lewis base** is defined as an electron pair donor.
➤ A **Lewis acid** is defined as an electron pair acceptor.

Lewis acids are electron-poor species such as H^+, highly charged transition metal ions such as Fe^{2+}, Ni^{2+}, and Co^{3+}; molecular oxides such as NO_2, SO_2, and CO_2; and certain electron-deficient compounds of elements such as Be, Al, or B. Lewis bases must by definition contain unshared pairs of electrons such as NH_3, H_2O, and Cl^-.

Buffers

Solutions that are mixtures containing appreciable amounts of both a weak acid and its conjugate base are called **buffers**. A weak acid will dissociate into hydronium and its conjugate base to an extent determined by the value of K_a.

$$HA(aq) + H_2O(l) \rightleftharpoons H_3O^+(aq) + A^-(aq)$$

Now consider the dissociation into a solution of low pH. This solution already contains H_3O^+ ions. The equilibrium is still governed by K_a, but it will take less dissociation to reach the value of K_a because the $[H_3O^+]$ is initially nonzero. This suppression of the dissociation is called the **common ion effect**. The common ion in this case is H_3O^+, but it could just as well have been the conjugate base of the acid A^-.

Buffer solutions resist changes in pH when strong acids or strong bases are added. This is especially important in biological systems because most biological molecules function best in a narrow pH range and do not tolerate large changes in pH well.

The pH of a buffer can be calculated through the **Henderson-Hasselbalch equation**:

$$pH = pK_a + \log\frac{[A^-]}{[HA]}$$

where $pK_a = -\log K_a$. The pH is a function of the pK_a which is fixed and the ratio of the conjugate base to the weak acid.

   EXAMPLE: Consider a solution that has the following concentrations: $[HF] = 1.5$ M and $[F^-] = 0.50$M. What is the pH of this solution?

The K_a of HF is 7.2×10^{-4} so $pK_a = -\log(7.2 \times 10^{-4}) = 3.14$. According to the Henderson-Hasselbalch equation, the pH of the buffer would be:

$$pH = 3.14 + \log\frac{[0.50]}{[1.5]} = 3.14 + \log(0.33) = 3.14 + (-0.48) = 2.66.$$

Now consider a solution that has the composition $[HF] = [F^-] = 1.5$ M:

$$pH = 3.14 + \log\frac{[1.5]}{[1.5]} = 3.14 + \log(1) = 3.14 + (0) = 3.14.$$

So

➤ If $[A^-] = [HA]$, $pH = pK_a$
➤ If $[A^-] > [HA]$, $pH > pK_a$
➤ If $[A^-] < [HA]$, $pH < pK_a$

A buffer resists pH changes by reacting with the added strong acid or base to remove either species from the system. In the case of a HF/F$^-$ buffer, the added strong base reacts with HF to form F$^-$.

$$HF(aq) + OH^-(aq) \rightleftharpoons F^-(aq) + H_2O(l).$$

This will increase F$^-$ and decrease the HF in the buffer, so the solution is more basic, but the change will not be as large as if the added OH$^-$ remained in solution.

Added strong acid will react with F$^-$ to form HF.

$$F^-(aq) + H_3O^+(aq) \rightarrow HF(aq) + H_2O(l)$$

The solution becomes more acidic, but the change will be small.

Buffers are most effective when the concentrations of weak acid and conjugate base are much greater than the concentration of the strong acid or base added to the buffer, and when the ratio of conjugate base to weak acid is between 0.1 and 10. The last condition means that a buffer has an effective range of $pK_a \pm 1.0$ pH units.

Solubility Equilibria

The equilibrium equation for sparingly soluble solids where M is a cation and A is the anion is

$$M_xA_y(s) \rightleftharpoons x[M^{y+}](aq) + y[A^{x-}](aq).$$

The resulting equilibrium expression is

$$K_{sp} = [M^{y+}]^x[A^{x-}]^y.$$

K_{sp} is called the **solubility product constant**. Some examples of K_{sp} equations, K_{sp} expressions, and numerical values are:

$$AgCl(s) \rightleftharpoons Ag^+(aq) + Cl^-(aq) \qquad K_{sp} = [Ag^+][Cl^-] = 1.8 \times 10^{-10}$$
$$PbCl_2(s) \rightleftharpoons Pb^{2+}(aq) + 2Cl^-(aq) \qquad K_{sp} = [Pb^{2+}][Cl^-]^2 = 1.7 \times 10^{-5}$$
$$Ag_2SO_4(s) \rightleftharpoons 2\,Ag^+(aq) + SO_4^{2-}(aq) \qquad K_{sp} = [Ag^+]^2[SO_4^{2-}] = 1.2 \times 10^{-5}$$
$$Cu_3(AsO_4)_2 \rightleftharpoons 3Cu^{2+}(aq) + 2AsO_4^{3-} \qquad K_{sp} = [Cu^{2+}]^3[AsO_4^{3-}]^2 = 7.6 \times 10^{-36}$$

Solubility is usually given in terms of g of solute per 100 g of water. Assuming that the density of the solution is very close to 1.00 g/mL, which is not unreasonable for slightly soluble salts. The K_{sp} may be determined through simple calculations.

> **EXAMPLE:** 0.123 g of $SrCrO_4$ (molar mass = 203.62 $^g/_{mol}$) dissolves in 100 g of water to produce a saturated solution. Find the K_{sp} for this substance.

The appropriate equilibrium is:

$$SrCrO_4(s) \rightleftharpoons Sr^{2+}(aq) + CrO_4^{2-}(aq) \text{ and } K_{sp} = [Sr^{2+}][CrO_4^{2-}]$$

$$0.123 \text{ g } SrCrO_4 \times \frac{1 \text{ mol } SrCrO_4}{203.62 \text{ g } SrCrO_4} = 0.000604 \text{ mol } SrCrO_4.$$

A solution of 100 g would have a volume of 100 mL or 0.100 L.

$$\text{The molarity of } SrCrO_4 = \frac{0.000604 \text{ mol } SrCrO_4}{0.100 \text{ L}} = 0.00604 \text{ M } SrCrO_4.$$

Because one mole of each ion is formed from each mol of $SrCrO_4$, $[Sr^{2+}] = [CrO_4^2]$ = 0.00604 M. (For other salts in which more than one ion forms per mole of solute, the molarity of that ion must be doubled, tripled, etc. depending on how many ions form per mol of solute.) You may now substitute ion concentrations into the K_{sp} expression:

$$K_{sp} = [Sr^{2+}][CrO_4^{2-}] = (0.00604)(0.00604) = 3.65 \text{ X } 10^{-5}.$$

SOME FACTORS AFFECTING SOLUBILITY EQUILIBRIA

CaF_2 is less soluble in solutions that contain either Ca^{2+} or F^- than in pure water, due to the common ion effect. If the anion of the solid is a Brønsted-Lowry base, it will be more soluble in an acid solution because the base will react with water to form the conjugate acid; this reduces the concentration of the anion, allowing more salt to dissolve.

> **EXAMPLE:** Consider CaF_2 dissolving in an acidic solution.

$$CaF_2(aq) \rightleftharpoons Ca^{2+}(aq) + 2F^-(aq)$$

If the solution is acidic, H_3O^+ will reduce the F^- concentration by the reaction:

$$F^-(aq) + H_3O^+(aq) \rightleftharpoons HF(aq) + H_2O(l).$$

Removing F^- allows more CaF_2 to dissolve to restore the equilibrium.

ENTROPY AND FREE ENERGY

Many chemical reactions start as soon as the reactants are brought together and continue until one or both reactants are used up. Other reactions require energy input for the reaction to occur.

➤ Reactions with large equilibrium constants are **product-favored** (or **spontaneous) reactions.**

➤ Reactions with small equilibrium constants are called **reactant-favored** (or **nonspontaneous) reactions.**

It has been observed that reactions that lead to dispersal of energy tend to be product favored. Energy can also be dispersed if the volume of a system increases. This is especially true for gases. There are two main factors that control the dispersal of energy:

➤ An exothermic reaction transfers heat to the surroundings, thus dispersing energy over a wider number of particles. Most product-favored reactions are exothermic.

➤ Some endothermic processes are product favored. In these reactions spreading out of matter increases disorder. This increase in disorder is measured by a quantity called **entropy, S.**

Certain qualitative generalizations can be made about entropy:

$$S(solid) < S(liquid) \ll S(gas).$$

Gases often dominate entropy because the volumes of gases are about 1000 times greater than those of solids and liquids. Reactions that increase the number of gas molecules have large entropy changes. The following have large positive entropy changes:

$$H_2O(l) \longrightarrow H_2O(g)$$
$$N_2O_4(g) \longrightarrow 2NO_2(g)$$
$$2NH_3(g) \longrightarrow 3H_2(g) + N_2(g).$$

➤ For solid and liquid solutes, the entropy of the pure substance is less than the entropy of the mixture:

$$S(solute) + S(solvent) < S(solution).$$

➤ For gaseous solutes dissolving in a liquid solvent, the opposite is true, because the volume is greatly decreased.

$$S(solute) + S(solvent) > S(solution)$$

➤ In general, the entropy of mixtures is greater than the entropy of pure substances.

➤ The more complicated a molecule is, the greater the entropy, because there are many more possible arrangements of the molecule.

Each substance has an entropy of formation, S_f°, similar to an enthalpy of formation ΔH_f°. Because the entropy of a perfect crystal of a substance at 0 K is defined as zero, even elements have entropies of formation values at temperatures greater than 0 K. Mathematically, the equation for the entropy of a reaction is analogous to that for ΔH_{rxn}°:

$$\Delta S_{rxn}^\circ = \Sigma n_p S_f^\circ(products) - \Sigma n_r S_f^\circ(reactants)$$

EXAMPLE: For the following species in the gas phase at 25 °C:

$$S_f^\circ(NH_3) = 192.5 \frac{J}{mol\,K}, \quad S_f^\circ(H_2) = 130.7 \frac{J}{mol\,K}, \text{ and } S_f^\circ(N_2) = 191.6 \frac{J}{mol\,K}.$$

$$2NH_3(g) \leftrightharpoons 3H_2(g) + N_2(g)$$

$$S_{rxn}^\circ = \left[3 \times S_f^\circ(H_2) + S_f^\circ(N_2)\right] - \left[2 \times S_f^\circ(NH_3)\right]$$

$$= [3(130.7) + (191.6)] - [2(192.5)] \frac{J}{mol\,K}$$

$$= [583.7] - [385] = +198.7 \frac{J}{mol\,K}$$

Note that the entropy change is (+) as would be expected with an increase in the number of gas molecules.

The Second Law and Free Energy

The **Second Law of Thermodynamics** states that the total entropy of the universe is increasing. In other words, things are continuously becoming more disordered. The change in entropy for the universe is:

$$\Delta S_{universe} = \Delta S_{system} + \Delta S_{surrounddings}.$$

$\Delta S_{surroundings} = -\dfrac{\Delta H_{rxn}}{T}$, and the second law equation becomes:

$$\Delta S_{universe} = \Delta S_{rxn} - \frac{\Delta H_{rxn}}{T}.$$

This equation allows calculation of $\Delta S_{universe}$ from two quantities associated with the reaction of interest, ΔH_{rxn} and ΔS_{rxn}.

A simpler quantity ΔG can be defined by multiplying this equation by $-T$, and rearranging which gives:

$$-T\Delta S_{universe} = \Delta H_{rxn} - T\Delta S_{rxn} = \Delta G_{sys}.$$

The quantity ΔG is called the **Gibbs free energy**. Note that it will have units of J/mol or kJ/mol just like enthalpy. Because T is always positive, ΔG and $\Delta S_{universe}$ have opposite signs.

Sign of ΔH_{sys}	Sign of ΔS_{sys}	Sign of ΔG_{sys}	Product favored?
(−)	(+)	(−)	yes
(−)	(−)	(−) at low T, (+) at high T	at low T
(+)	(+)	(+) at low T, (−) at high T	at high T
(+)	(−)	(+)	no

In the first entry, both ΔH and ΔS favor the reaction. The opposite is true for the last entry. In the second entry, ΔH is favorable and ΔS is not. At low temperature, ΔH dominates, and at higher temperature, ΔS dominates.

The standard free energy of formation is analogous to ΔH_f° (ΔG_f° of elements $=0$).

EXAMPLE: It is important to note that ΔH_{rxr}° is usually given in $\dfrac{kJ}{mol}$ and ΔS_{rxn}° is given in $\dfrac{J}{mol\,K}$. To convert both energy units in kJ, divide ΔS_{rxn}° by 1000.

For the breakdown of NH_3 to H_2 and N_2 at 298 K ($\Delta H_{rxn}^\circ = 92.2\,kJ/mol$):

$$\Delta G_{rxn}^\circ = \Delta H_{rxn}^\circ - T\Delta S_{rxn}^\circ$$

$$= +92.2\frac{kJ}{mol} - (298\,K)\left(+0.1987\frac{kJ}{mol\,K}\right) = +92.2 - 59.2\frac{kJ}{mol}$$

$$= +33\frac{kJ}{mol}.$$

In this case, ΔH is unfavorable, but ΔS is favorable. At 298 K, the favorable effects of entropy are not large enough to overcome the unfavorable enthalpy. If the temperature is raised, the contribution of entropy becomes more important. At 500 K:

$$\Delta G_{rxn}^\circ = \Delta H_{rxn}^\circ - T\Delta S_{rxn}^\circ$$

$$= +92.2\,kJ/mol - (500\,K)\left(+0.1987\frac{kJ}{mol\,K}\right) = +92.2 - 99.4\frac{kJ}{mol} = -7.2\frac{kJ}{mol}.$$

If the ΔG_f° for all species in a reaction are known, the following equation may be used:

$$\Delta G_{rxn}^\circ = \Sigma n_p \Delta G_f^\circ(products) - \Sigma n_r \Delta G_f^\circ(reactants).$$

EXAMPLE:

$$H_2(g) + CO_2(g) \rightleftharpoons H_2O(\ell) + CO(g).$$

Substance	ΔG_f° value $\left(\dfrac{kJ}{mol}\right)$
H_2	0 (by definition)
CO_2	−394.4
H_2O	−237.1
CO	−137.2

$$\Delta G_{rxn}^\circ = \left[\Delta G_f^\circ(H_2O) + \Delta G_f^\circ(CO)\right] - \left[\Delta G_f^\circ(CO_2)\right]$$

$$= [(-237.1) + (-137.2)] - [(-394.4)]\frac{kJ}{mol}$$

$$= [-374.3] - [-394.4] = +20.1\frac{kJ}{mol}\ (\text{reactant favored}).$$

Hess's Law applies to ΔG_{rxn}° values. If a series of reactions add up to a total reaction, the ΔG_{rxn}° for the total reactions is the sum of the ΔG_{rxn}° of the individual reactions.

$$2S\,(s)+2O_2(g) \rightleftharpoons 2SO_2\,(g) \qquad \Delta G_{rxn1}^{\circ} = -600.4\,kJ/mol$$

$$\underline{2SO_2\,(g)+O_2\,(g) \rightleftharpoons 2SO_3\,(g)} \qquad \Delta G_{rxn2}^{\circ} = \underline{-141.6}\,kJ/mol$$

$$2S(s)+3O_2(g) \rightleftharpoons 2SO_3(g)\;\Delta G_{total}^{\circ} = -600.4 + (-141.6)\frac{kJ}{mol} = -742/\frac{kJ}{mol} = (product\ favored)$$

To calculate the free energy, ΔG, for systems not at standard conditions, use the following equation:

$$\Delta G = \Delta G_{rxn}^{\circ} + RT\ln Q$$

where R is the gas constant $8.314\,\dfrac{J}{mol\,K}$, T is temperature in K, and Q is the reaction quotient which has the same form as K with initial concentrations.

ΔG_{rxr}° is related to the equilibrium constant. For a reaction with $\Delta G = (-)$, spontaneous or product favored, the reaction tends to shift to the products $(K>Q)$. For a reaction with $\Delta G = (+)$, non spontaneous or reactant favored, the reaction tends to shift to the reactants $(K<Q)$. For a reaction with $\Delta G = 0$, there is no tendency to shift to either products or reactants $(K=Q)$. This is a definition of equilibrium. So if $\Delta G = 0$, $Q = K$. Substitute into the equation for ΔG with concentration changes:

$$\Delta G = \Delta G_{rxn}^{\circ} + RT\ln Q \text{ at equilibrium } \Delta G = 0 \text{ and } Q = K$$

$$\Delta G_{rxn}^{\circ} = -RT\ln K, \text{ which may be rearranged to } K = e^{-\frac{\Delta G_{rxn}^{\circ}}{RT}}$$

ELECTROCHEMISTRY

Electrochemical Potentials

In an oxidation-reduction reaction that is product favored, electrons are transferred as soon as the reactants are mixed. If the half reactions are separated, the electrons can flow through a salt bridge that uses ions to carry the current through a salt bridge. This current may be used to do electrical work. Such a setup is called an **electrochemical** or **galvanic cell**. An example is shown below. Many other arrangements are possible.

Metal or other material is often used to connect the external circuit to the two half cells. These connectors are called electrodes. The electrode for the oxidation cell is the **anode**,

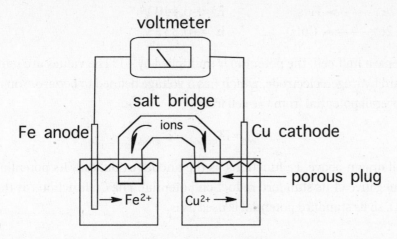

and the one for the reduction cell is the **cathode**. Sometimes an unreactive metal like platinum may be used as an electrode. In the above cell the anode (oxidation reaction) is:

$$Fe(s) \longrightarrow Fe^{2+}(aq) + 2e^-$$

and the cathode (reduction reaction) is:

$$Cu^{2+}(aq) + 2e^- \longrightarrow Cu(s).$$

Electrons flow from the iron anode, where Fe^{2+} ions go into solution, through the wire to the copper cathode, where Cu^{2+} ions are reduced and deposited as Cu on the cathode. At the same time, ions move through the salt bridge to keep the charges balanced. The electrochemical cell is often represented by the notation:

$$anode \mid solution\ species \parallel solution\ species \mid cathode.$$

The double line represents the salt bridge. For the above cell this representation is:

$$Fe(s) \mid Fe^{2+}(aq) \parallel Cu^{2+}(aq) \mid Cu(s).$$

A voltage arises when there is a difference in electrical potential. Electrons move from regions of high electrical potential to regions of low electrical potential. A positive voltage for an electrochemical cell means there is a tendency for the reaction to proceed in the direction as written. A negative voltage means the reaction has a strong tendency to proceed in the reverse direction.

Charge is measured in **Coulombs (C)**. An electron has a charge of 1.602×10^{-19} C. A **volt (V)** is defined as one Joule of work done when one Coulomb of charge moves through a potential of one volt.

$$1\,V = \frac{1\,J}{1\,C} \ \text{ or } \ 1\,J = 1\,V \times 1\,C$$

The **standard reduction potential (E°)** is defined as the voltage of an electrochemical cell written as a reduction reaction. For example, for iron and copper the standard reduction potentials are:

$$\text{Fe}^{2+}(aq) + 2e^- \longrightarrow \text{Fe}(s) \qquad E° = -0.440 \text{ V}$$
$$\text{Cu}^{2+}(aq) + 2e^- \longrightarrow \text{Cu}(s) \qquad E° = +0.337 \text{ V}.$$

If you reverse a half cell, the potential is multiplied by -1. The values are referenced to the standard hydrogen electrode, which has a voltage defined to be zero. You can determine the overall potential from the cell from

$$E°_{cell} = E°_{Cathode} - E°_{anode}.$$

For the cell drawn above, Fe functions as the anode (oxidation). Its potential must be made the negative of its standard reduction potential. The Cu functions as the cathode (reduction), so its standard potential is used as is.

$$E°_{cell} = E°_{Cu} - E°_{Fe} = (+0.337 \text{ V}) - (-0.440 \text{ V}) = +0.777 \text{ V}$$

$$\text{Fe}(s) \longrightarrow \text{Fe}^{2+}(aq) + 2e^- \qquad E° = +0.440 \text{ V} \ (-1 \times E° \ (\text{Fe}^{2+} \longrightarrow \text{Fe}))$$
$$\underline{\text{Cu}^{2+}(aq) + 2e^- \longrightarrow \text{Cu}(s) \qquad E° = +0.337 \text{ V} \ (+1 \times E° \ (\text{Cu}^{2+} \longrightarrow \text{Cu}))}$$
$$\text{Fe}(s) + \text{Cu}^{2+}(aq) \longrightarrow \text{Fe}^{2+}(aq) + \text{Cu}(s) \ E° = +0.777 \text{ V}$$

EXAMPLE: Here is another example of $E°_{cell}$ from half reactions.

$$\text{MnO}_4^-(aq) + 8\text{H}^+(aq) + 5e^- \longrightarrow \text{Mn}^{2+}(aq) + 4 \text{ H}_2\text{O}(l) \qquad E°_{cathode} = +1.510 \text{ V}$$
$$\underline{5\text{Fe}^{2+}(aq) \longrightarrow 5\text{Fe}^{3+}(aq) + 5e^- \qquad -E°_{anode} = -0.771 \text{ V}}$$
$$\text{MnO}_4^-(aq) + 8\text{H}^+(aq) + 5\text{Fe}^{2+}(aq) \longrightarrow \text{Mn}^{2+}(aq) + 5\text{Fe}^{3+}(aq) + 4\text{H}_2\text{O}(l) \qquad +0.739 \text{ V}$$

When calculating $E°_{cell}$ values, **never multiply the $E°_{cell}$ values by the number that the half reaction was multiplied by to balance the equation.** Voltage is defined as $1V = \dfrac{1J}{1C}$. When you multiply the charge by 5, you also multiply the energy by 5, and the ratio (the voltage) is still the same value.

The Relationships between $E°_{cell}$, $\Delta G°$, and K

The standard cell potential is a measure of the direction of an oxidation-reduction reaction. It has been found that the relationship between $\Delta G°$ and $E°_{cell}$ is:

$$\Delta G° = -nFE°_{cell},$$

where n is the number of moles of electrons transferred in the oxidation-reduction reaction and F is Faraday's constant. $F = 96500 \text{ C/mol } e^-$. The $(-)$ sign is necessary because $\Delta G°$ is negative and $E°_{cell}$ is positive for a product-favored reaction.

EXAMPLE: Consider the following oxidation-reduction reaction. Recall that the $5e^-$ are transferred in this reaction.

$$\text{MnO}_4^-(aq) + 8\text{H}_3\text{O}^+(aq) + 5\text{Fe}^{2+}(aq) \rightleftharpoons \text{Mn}^{2+}(aq) + 12 \text{ H}_2\text{O}(l) + \text{Fe}^{3+}(aq) \ E°_{cell} = +0.739 \text{ V}$$

You can calculate $\Delta G°$ using the relationship:

$$\Delta G° = -nFE°_{cell}$$

$$= -\frac{5 \text{ mol e}^-}{\text{mol}} \times \frac{96500 \text{ C}}{1 \text{ mol e}^-} \times \frac{0.739 \text{ J}}{1 \text{ C}} \times \frac{1 \text{ kJ}}{1000 \text{ J}} = -357 \frac{\text{kJ}}{\text{mol}}.$$

The mol in the denominator of the first term means per mole of the reactants and products (1 mol MnO_4^-(aq), 8 mol H_3O^+(aq), etc.).

The standard free energy, $\Delta G°$, has been related to the equilibrium constant, K, and the standard electrochemical cell potential, $E°_{cell}$. These two relationships may be combined to relate K and $E°_{cell}$:

$$\Delta G° = -nFE°_{cell} \text{ and } \Delta G° = -RT\ln K.$$

Equating these two equations and solving for $E°_{cell}$ gives

$$E°_{cell} = \frac{RT}{nF}\ln K.$$

R, T, and F are constants. If their values are substituted into the above equation, the equation simplifies to:

$$E°_{cell} = \frac{0.0257 \text{ V}}{n}\ln K \text{ or in base 10 logarithms, } E°_{cell} = \frac{0.0592 \text{ V}}{n}\log K.$$

Cell potential under nonstandard conditions may be calculated according to the **Nernst equation**:

$$E_{cell} = E°_{cell} - \frac{0.0592 \text{ V}}{n}\log Q.$$

A summary of the relationships between values of $E°_{cell}$, $\Delta G°$, and K and the favored side of the equation is shown in the table below.

K	DG°	$E°_{cell}$	Side favored
K >> 1	$\Delta G° < 0$	$E°_{cell} > 0$	Product favored
K ≈ 1	$\Delta G° = 0$	$E°_{cell} = 0$	Neither
K << 1	$\Delta G° > 0$	$E°_{cell} < 0$	Reactant favored

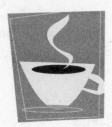

CRAM SESSION

Important Terms You Should Know

acid
acid dissociation constant (K$_a$)
alkaline earth metals
alkali metals
amphiprotic
Amu
anion
anode
atmosphere (atm)
atom
atomic number (Z)
atomic radius
autoionization
average atomic mass
average bond energy
Avogadro's Law
azmuthal quantum number (λ)

balanced equation
base
Bohr's model
boiling point
boiling point elevation
bond pair
Boyle's law
Brønsted-Lowry theory
Buffer

calorimetry
capillary action
catalyst
cathode

cation
Charles's law
chemical equation
chemical reaction
coefficient
colligative property
common ion
compound
conjugate acid
Coulomb (C)
core electron
covalent
critical point

de Broglie wavelength
diamagnetic
dipole
dipole-dipole forces

electrochemistry
electrolyte
electron
electron affinity
electron configuration
electronegativity
element
emission spectra
empirical formula
endothermic
energy level
enthalpy (H)
enthalpy of fusion
enthalpy of vaporization

entropy (S)
equilibrium
equilibrium constant (K)
excited state
exothermic

formal charge
free energy (G)
freezing point depression
frequency (ν)

ground state
group

half life
halogens
Henry's law
Hess's law
Hund's rule
hydrogen bond

ideal gas law
integrated rate law
ion
ion-dipole forces
ionic
ionic radii
ionization energy
isotope
Kelvin (K)
kinetic energy
kinetic molecular theory
kinetics

Le Châtelier's
  Principle
Lewis acid/base
Lewis structure
limiting reactant
London dispersion
  forces
lone pair

magnetic quantum
  number (m_l)
mass number (A)
mass percent (mass %)
melting point
metal
metallic bonding
metalloid
method of initial rates
mixture
molality (m)
molarity (M)
molar mass
molar ratio
mole
molecule
mole fraction

neutralization
neutron
noble gases
nonmetal

orbit
osmotic pressure (Π)
oxidation
oxidation number

paired spins
paramagnetic
partial pressure

Pauli exclusion
  principle
percent composition
percent yield
period
Periodic Table
pH
phase change
photon
Planck's constant (h)
polar
polarizable
polyatomic ion
potential energy
precipitate
pressure
principal quantum
  number (n)
product favored
proton
pure substance

quantum mechanics
quantum number

Raoult's law
rate constant (k)
reactant favored
reaction order
reaction quotient
reduction
resonance
root mean square
  velocity (u_{rms})

salt bridge
saturated solution
solubility product
  constant
solute

solution
solvent
s, p, d, f orbitals
specific heat (S)
speed of light (c)
spin quantum
  number (m_s)
standard enthalpy
  offormation
  ($\Delta H°_f$)
standard reduction
  potential (E°)
standard state
stoichiometry
strong acid
strong base
strong electrolyte
sublimation point
surface tension

thermochemical
  equation
thermodynamics
titration
triple point

uncertainty
  principle

valence electron
van't Hoff factor
  (i)
vapor pressure
viscosity
volt
VSEPR

wavelength (λ)
weak acid
weak electrolyte

Important Equations You Should Know

Avogadro's number $= 6.022 \times 10^{+23}$ particles/mol

$$\% \text{ yield} = \frac{\text{actual yield}}{\text{theoretical yield}} \times 100\%$$

$$\text{Molarity (M)} = \frac{\text{moles of solute}}{\text{Liters of soution}} \quad \text{and} \quad M \times V = \text{mol}$$

$$P_1V_1 = P_2V_2 \qquad \frac{V_1}{T_1} = \frac{V_2}{T_2} \qquad \frac{V_1}{n_1} = \frac{V_2}{n_2} \qquad PV = nRT$$

$$P\mathcal{M} = \frac{m}{V}RT \qquad P_{total} = P_1 + P_2 + P_3 + \ldots \qquad \chi_1 = \frac{n_1}{n_{total}}$$

$$u_{rms} = \sqrt{\overline{u^2}} = \sqrt{\frac{3RT}{\mathcal{M}}}$$

$$q = mS\Delta T \qquad q_{rxn} = -(m_{soln}S_{soln}\Delta T_{soln})$$

$$\Delta H_{rxn} = \Sigma\, n_p\, \Delta H^\circ_f \text{ (products)} - \Sigma\, n_r\, \Delta H^\circ_f \text{ (reactants)}$$

$$\nu\lambda = E q = h \times \nu \quad \Delta E = -2.179 \times 10^{-18}\left(\frac{1}{n_f^2} - \frac{1}{n_i^2}\right)$$

Formal charge $=$ Valence electrons $-$ [Lone pair electrons $+ \frac{1}{2}$ (Bond pair electrons)]

$$\Delta H_{rxn(estimate)} = \Sigma\, BE\text{(bonds broken)} - \Sigma\, BE \text{ (bonds formed)}$$

$$s_{gas} = k_H P_{gas}$$

$$\text{Mass fraction} = \frac{\text{mass of solute}}{\text{mass of solution}}$$

$$\text{Mass percent (mass \%)} = \frac{\text{mass of solute}}{\text{mass of solution}} \times 100\%$$

$$\text{Parts per million (ppm)} = \frac{\text{mass of solute}}{\text{mass of solution}} \times 10^6$$

$$\text{Parts per billion (ppb)} = \frac{\text{mass of solute}}{\text{mass of solution}} \times 10^9$$

Molality $(m) = \dfrac{\text{mol of solute}}{\text{kg of solvent}}$

$P_{soln} = \chi_{solvent1}\, P_{solvent}$ $\qquad \Delta T_f = K_f m$ $\qquad\qquad \Delta T_b = K_b m$ $\qquad\qquad \Pi = MRT$

1st order reaction $\qquad\qquad \ln[A]_t = -kt + \ln[A]_\circ$ $\qquad \dfrac{0.693}{k} = t_{1/2}$

2nd order reaction $\qquad\qquad \dfrac{1}{[A]_t} = kt + \dfrac{1}{[A]_o}$ $\qquad \dfrac{1}{[A]_o K} = t_{1/2}$

$k = Ae^{-\left(\frac{E_a}{RT}\right)}$

$aA(g) + bB(g) \rightleftharpoons cC(g) + dD(g)$ $\qquad\qquad K = \dfrac{[C]^c[D]^d}{[A]^a[B]^b}$

$pH = -\log[H_3O^+]$ or sometimes written $-\log[H^+]$

$HA(aq) + H_2O(l) \rightleftharpoons H_3O^+(aq) + A^-(aq)$ $\qquad K_a = \dfrac{[H_3O^+][A^-]}{[HA]}$

$B(aq) + H_2O(l) \rightleftharpoons BH^+(aq) + OH^-(aq)$ $\qquad K_b = \dfrac{[BH^+][OH^-]}{[B]}$

$K_a \times K_b = K_w$

$pH = pK_a + \log\dfrac{[A^-]}{[HA]}$

$M_xA_y(s) \rightleftharpoons x[M^{y+}](aq) + y[A^{x-}](aq)$ $\qquad\qquad K_{sp} = [M^{y+}]^x[A^{x-}]^y$

$\Delta S^\circ_{rxn} = \Sigma n_p\, S^\circ_f(\text{products}) - \Sigma n_r S^\circ_f(\text{reactants})$

$\Delta G_{sys} = \Delta H_{rxn} - T\Delta S_{rxn}$ $\qquad \Delta G = \Delta G^\circ_{rxn} + RT\ln Q$ $\qquad \Delta G^\circ_{rxn} = -RT\ln K$ $\quad$ or $\quad K = e^{-\frac{\Delta G_{rxn}}{RT}}$

$E^\circ_{cell} = E^\circ_{Cathode} - E^\circ_{anode}$

$\Delta G^\circ = -nFE^\circ_{cell}$ $\qquad E_{cell} = E^\circ_{cell} - \dfrac{0.0592V}{n}\log Q$ $\qquad E^\circ_{cell} = \dfrac{RT}{nF}\ln K$

CHAPTER 11

Organic Chemistry

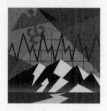

> **Read This Chapter to Learn About:**
> ➤ Structure
> ➤ Reactivity
> ➤ Separation and Purification
> ➤ Characterization

PART I. STRUCTURE
BONDING

Chemical bonds conventionally fall into one of two categories: ionic and covalent. When the electronegativity difference between the atoms is quite small, the electron density is equitably distributed along the internuclear axis, and it reaches a maximum at the midpoint of the bond. Such a bond is said to be purely covalent. On the other hand, when the two nuclei have widely divergent electronegativities, the electron density is not "shared" at all: two ionic species are formed and the electron density approaches zero along the internuclear axis at the edge of the ionic radius. Polar covalent bonds result from an uneven sharing of electron density, a situation that sets up a permanent dipole along the bond axis. The O-H and C-F bonds are examples of polar covalent bonds. Such bonds are stronger than one would expect, because the covalent attraction is augmented by the Coulombic forces set up by the dipole.

With respect to global connectivity, the Lewis dot diagram represents a simple but powerful device. These diagrams are built up by considering the valence electrons brought to the table by each atom and forming bonds by intuitively combining unpaired electrons. For example, formaldehyde (H_2CO) is constructed in Figure 11.1.

There are two types of electron pairs in the molecule above: (1) shared pairs (or bonds), which are represented by lines (each line representing two shared electrons), and (2)

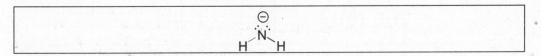

Step 1: draw atoms with
valence electrons

Step 2: form bonds by
combining unpaired electrons

Step 3: draw shared pairs as
single lines, lone pairs as dots

FIGURE 11.1: Lewis structure for formaldehyde

lone pairs, which are depicted using two dots. When calculating formal charges, assign to a given atom all of its lone pair electrons and half of each shared pair; then compare the sum to the number of valence electrons normally carried. For example, consider the amide anion (Figure 11.2). The nitrogen atom is surrounded by two lone pairs (nitrogen "owns" all four) and two shared pairs (nitrogen "owns" only one in each pair), giving a total of six electrons assigned to nitrogen. Compared to the five valence electrons normally carried by nitrogen, this represents an excess of one electron; therefore, a formal charge of −1 is given to the nitrogen atom.

FIGURE 11.2: Lewis structure for the amide anion

Often molecules can be represented by multiple Lewis structures. These are known as **resonance forms**, and while all reasonable candidates tell us something about the nature of the molecule in question, some resonance structures are more significant contributors than others. In making such an assessment, the following guidelines are helpful:

A. Rules of Charge Separation
   1. All things being equal, structures should have minimal charge separation.
   2. Any charge separation should be guided by electronegativity trends.

B. Octet Rules
   1. Little octet rule: all things being equal, each atom should have an octet.
   2. Big octet rule: no row 2 element can accommodate more than 8 electrons.

Of all these, only the big octet rule is inviolable. Structures that break the first three rules are less desirable—those that break the last one are unreasonable and unsupportable. However, even when one structure satisfies all the "rules," other resonance forms may need to be considered to predict the properties of a molecule.

butadiene

LCAO	Schematic	Nodes	Popul'n	Frontier
$+\varphi_1-\varphi_2+\varphi_3-\varphi_4$		3	———	
$+\varphi_1-\varphi_2-\varphi_3+\varphi_4$		2	———	LUMO
$+\varphi_1+\varphi_2-\varphi_3-\varphi_4$		1	$\Updownarrow$	HOMO
$+\varphi_1+\varphi_2+\varphi_3+\varphi_4$		0	$\Updownarrow$	

Table 11.1. Π molecular orbitals for butadiene

Double bonds are formed by the interaction of two adjacent p orbitals. Similarly, extended π systems develop when three or more adjacent p orbitals are present, as is the case with butadiene (Table 11.1). Such double bonds are said to be *conjugated*, a term that stems from their tendency to undergo reactions as an interconnected system, rather than as isolated double bonds.

Molecules with multiple double bonds are more stable if those bonds are arranged in alternating arrays, so that extended π systems can be formed. For example, 1,3-pentadiene is more stable than 1,4-pentadiene. In the former case, the double bonds are said to be conjugated. A similar (but weaker) effect can arise from the interaction of p-orbitals with adjacent σ bonds. For example, the methyl cation is not a very stable species, owing to the empty p orbital on carbon and the resulting violation of the octet rule. However, the ethyl cation is a bit more stable, because the C-H sigma bond on the methyl group can spill a bit of electron density into the empty p orbital, thereby stabilizing the cationic center (Figure 11.3). This is an effect known as hyperconjugation, and while the sharing of electron density is not nearly as effective here as in true conjugation, it is still responsible for the following stability trend in carbocations and radicals: methyl < primary < secondary < tertiary.

Aromaticity is a special form of conjugation that confers particular stability to compounds, and it arises only from systems possessing a cyclic, contiguous, and coplanar array of p orbitals (Figure 11.4). But this arrangement can also result in antiaromaticity, whereby molecules are less stable than expected. The difference between aromatic-

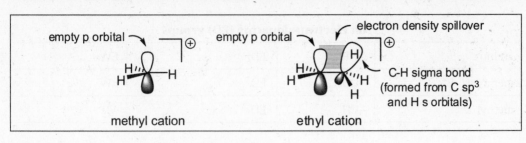

FIGURE 11.3:   Hyperconjugation in the ethyl cation

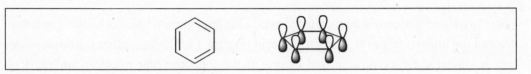

FIGURE 11.4:   Contiguous P orbitals in benzene

ity and antiaromaticity lies in the number of π-electrons housed in the cyclic array. This can be predicted using Hückel's Rule, which states that systems having $4n$ π electrons (4, 8, 12 electrons, etc.) tend to be antiaromatic, and those having $(4n+2)$ π electrons (2, 6, 10 electrons, etc.) tend to be aromatic.

Electronic systems can be strongly impacted by substituents, which are generally designated either electron withdrawing (EW) or electron donating (ED). There are two components of electron-withdrawing and electron-donating behavior: resonance and induction. As the term suggests, the resonance effect can be represented by electron-pushing arrows to give different resonance forms. This effect may be weak or strong, but it can exert influence over very large distances through extended π-systems. The inductive effect stems primarily from electronegativity; it can be quite strong, but its influence is local—the magnitude drops off sharply as distance from the functional group increases. Table 11.2 summarizes these effects for some common functional groups. In most cases the inductive and resonance effects work in concert, while in some instances they are at odds.

Table 11.2. Some common ED and EW groups			
functional group	**formula**	**resonance effect**	**inductive effect**
Net electron-withdrawing (EW) groups			
acetyl	$-COCH_3$	EW	EW
carbomethoxy	$-CO_2CH_3$	EW	EW
chloro	$-Cl$	ED	EW
cyano	$-CN$	EW	EW
nitro	$-NO_2$	EW	EW
phenylsulfonyl	$-SO_2Ph$	EW	EW

Net electron-donating (ED) groups			
amino	$-NH_2$	ED	EW
methoxy	$-OCH_3$	ED	EW
methyl	$-CH_3$	ED	ED

SHAPE

There are three frequently encountered central-atom geometries in organic chemistry: digonal (or linear), trigonal, and tetrahedral (Figure 11.5). Each atom within a molecule is almost always characterized by one of these geometries, the chief hallmark of which is the associated bond angle: 180° for linear arrays, 120° for trigonal planar centers, and 109.5° for tetrahedral arrangements. One classical approach to rationalize these geometries is through hybridization of atomic orbitals, as shown in Figure 11.6.

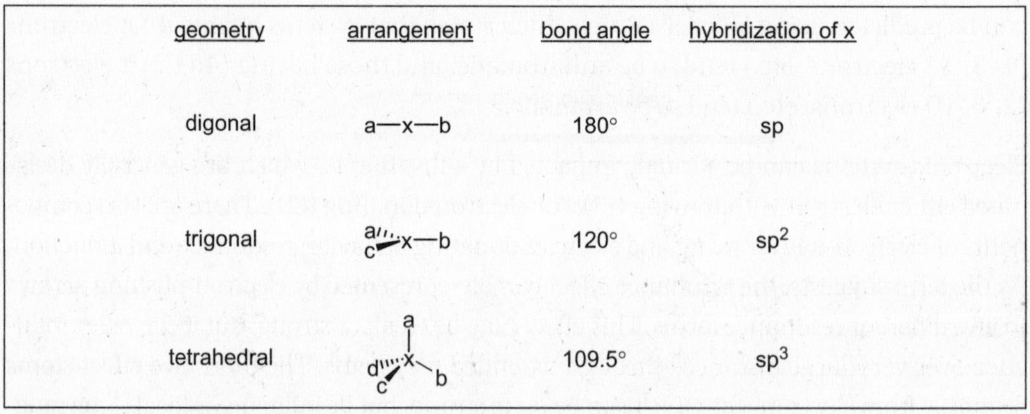

geometry	arrangement	bond angle	hybridization of x
digonal	a—x—b	180°	sp
trigonal	a c⟍x—b	120°	sp^2
tetrahedral	a d⟍x⟍b c	109.5°	sp^3

FIGURE 11.5: Common central atom geometries in organic chemistry

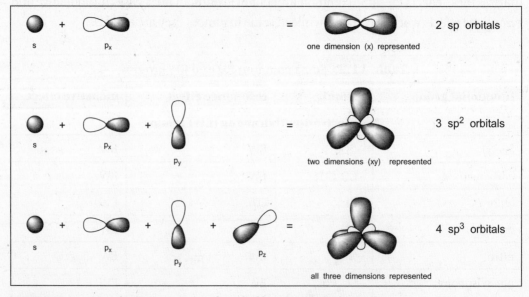

FIGURE 11.6: Central atom geometry as described by orbital hybridization

In cases where a tetrahedral center is surrounded by four uniquely different groups, the center is said to be asymmetric, or chiral. Molecules containing asymmetric centers (chiral centers, or stereocenters) are themselves usually chiral, and therefore exist in two enantiomeric forms, which are nonsuperimposible mirror images (Figure 11.7). Enantiomers are identical in almost all physical properties with one notable exception. A chiral compound rotates plane-polarized light that passes through it, a phenomenon known as optical rotation. Its enantiomer rotates plane-polarized light to the same degree, but in the opposite direction. Racemic mixtures, which contain exactly equal amounts of enantiomers, do not exhibit optical activity.

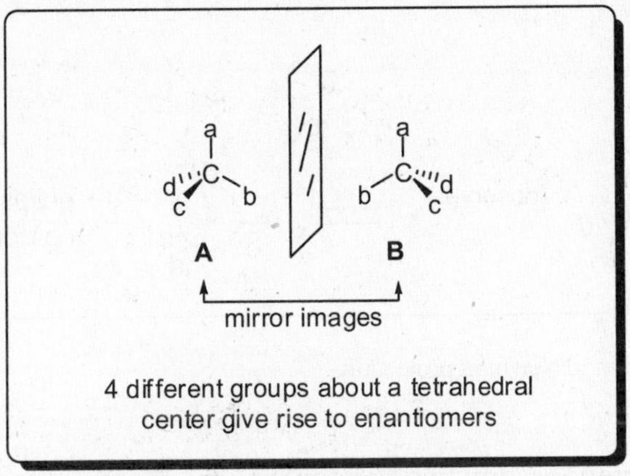

FIGURE 11.7: Tetrahedral centers and enantiomerism

Compounds with more than one chiral center can form diastereomers, as is the case with the naturally occurring sugar D-ribose (Figure 11.8). Since there are three chiral centers, the total number of unique permutations is $2^3 = 8$. D-Ribose represents one such permutation, and the enantiomer of D-ribose is L-ribose. Notice that *each and every chiral center is inverted*—this is true for any set of enantiomers. Thus, L-ribose accounts for one stereoisomer of D-ribose, but there are six others—all of them diastereomers of D-ribose. Thus, a diastereomer is a stereoisomer in which one or more, *but not all*, chiral centers have been inverted.

Once connectivity has been established, molecular conformation must be considered, and this can be examined in several ways. For example, the sawhorse projection

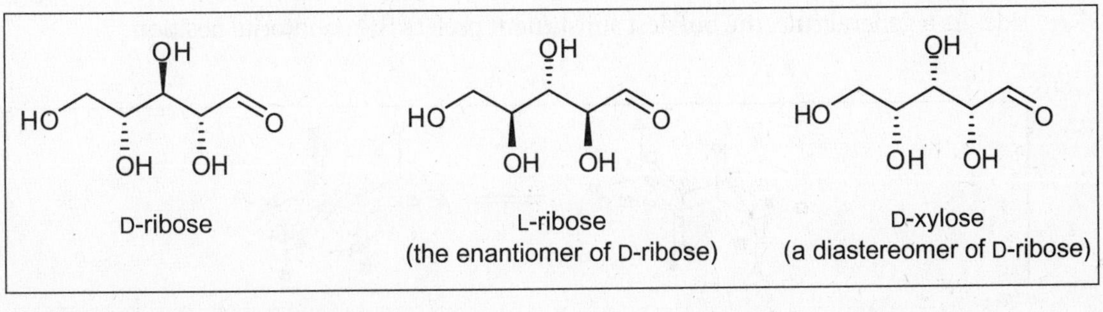

FIGURE 11.8: Enantiomers vs. diastereomers

(Figure 11.9) views the molecule from the side, whereas a Newman projection looks at the molecule along a carbon-carbon bond (indicated by the observer's eye). Newman projections are useful for examining the difference between staggered and eclipsed conformations.

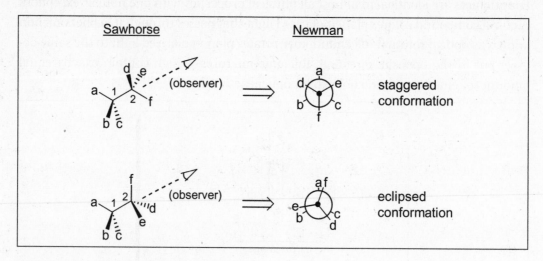

FIGURE 11.9: Sawhorse and Newman projections

In staggered conformations, any two substituents are characterized by one of two relationships. Substituents are **gauche** with respect to each other if they are side by side. In the illustration, there are six gauche relationships: a-e, e-c, c-f, f-b, b-d, and d-a. The other relationship is **antiperiplanar,** in which case the two substituents are as far away as possible from each other. In eclipsed conformations, there is only one type of relationship between substituents, namely eclipsed. It should come as no surprise that eclipsed conformations are of higher energy than staggered conformations. By the same token, staggered conformations that place large groups in a gauche arrangement are of higher energy than those that have those groups antiperiplanar with respect to each other.

Cyclic molecules are less flexible than than open-chain analogs, and they can adopt far fewer conformations. For example, the most stable arrangement in cyclohexane is the so-called chair conformation (Figure 11.10), in which substituents can adopt one of two attitudes: axial (shown as triangles in the left chair) or equatorial (shown as squares)—every chair conformation has six of each type. Note that a chair flip interchanges axial and equatorial substituents, so that all of the triangles become equatorial on the right side. As a general rule, the bulkiest substituent prefers the equatorial position.

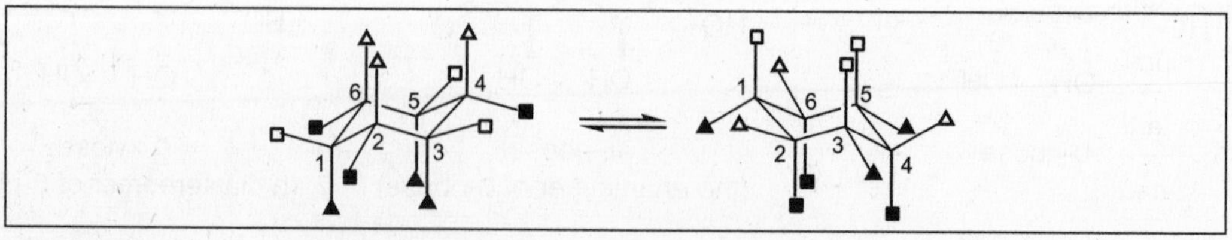

FIGURE 11.10: The chair flip of cyclohexane

Cyclic molecules can experience bond angle strain and torsional strain. The former is caused by a deviation from the ideal sp^3 bond angle (109.5°). This is worst for the three-membered ring, and almost nil for five- and six-membered rings. Torsional strain, on the other hand, derives from the torque on individual bonds from eclipsed substituents trying to get out of each other's way. Again, this is most pronounced in cyclopropane, and all the other cycloalkanes twist in ways to minimize or eliminate this strain. In general, ring strain decreases according to the trend: $3 > 4 \gg 5 > 6$.

NOMENCLATURE

Straight-chain hydrocarbons are named according to the number of carbons in the chain (Table 11.3). If used as a substituent, the names are modified by changing the suffix "-ane" to "-yl"; thus, a two-carbon alkane is ethane, but a two-carbon substituent is ethyl. In the event of branched hydrocarbons, rules established by IUPAC (International Union of Pure and Applied Chemists) dictate that the longest possible chain be used as the main chain, then all remaining carbons constitute substituents. If two different chains of equal length can be identified, then the one giving the greatest number of substituents should be chosen.

When molecules contain functional groups, then the parent chain is defined as the longest possible carbon chain which contains the highest priority functional group (Table 11.4). Once that parent chain is identified, then all other functionalities become substituents (modifiers). For example, consider the two compounds in Figure 11.11. Both contain the hydroxy (-OH) functional group, but in the left it defines the parent chain. Therefore, the "-ol" form is used, and the compound is named "propan-2-ol." However, the right compound has both the hydroxy and the carbonyl functional

Table 11.3. Simple alkanes		
name	no. of carbons	formula
Methane	1	CH_4
Ethane	2	CH_3CH_3
Propane	3	$CH_3CH_2CH_3$
Butane	4	$CH_3(CH_2)_2CH_3$
Pentane	5	$CH_3(CH_2)_3CH_3$
Hexane	6	$CH_3(CH_2)_4CH_3$
Heptane	7	$CH_3(CH_2)_5CH_3$
Octane	8	$CH_3(CH_2)_6CH_3$
Nonane	9	$CH_3(CH_2)_7CH_3$
Decane	10	$CH_3(CH_2)_8CH_3$

Table 11.4. IUPAC Priorities of the functional groups			
Functional group	**Formula**	**As parent**	**As modifier**
carboxylate ester	R-CO$_2$R'	alkyl –oate	–
carboxylic acid	R-CO$_2$H	–oic acid	carboxy–
acyl halide	R-COX (Cl, Br, I)	–oyl halide	–
amide	R-CONH$_2$	–amide	–
nitrile	R-CN	–nitrile	cyano–
aldehyde	R-COH	–al	oxo–
ketone	R-C(O)-R'	–one	oxo–
alcohol	–OH	–ol	hydroxy–
amine	–NH$_2$	–amine	–amino
ether	R–OR'	(only used as modifiers)	alkoxy–
nitro	R–NO$_2$		nitro–
halide	R–X (F, Cl, Br, I)		halo– (e.g., chloro–)

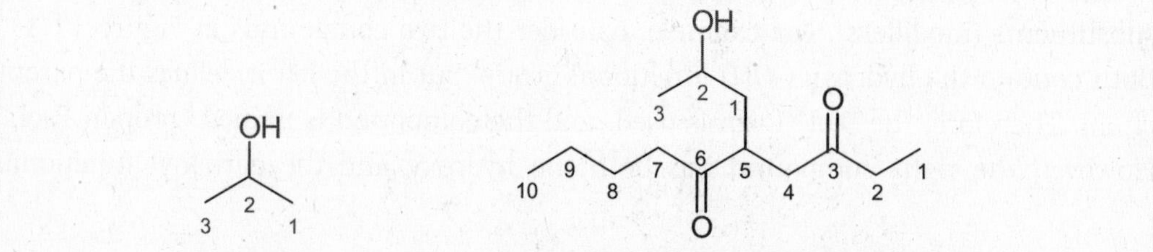

propan-2-ol   5-(2-hydroxypropyl)decan-3,6-dione

FIGURE 11.11: Functional groups in the main chain and as substituent

groups. Since the carbonyl has the higher IUPAC priority, it defines the parent chain; the hydroxy group thus serves only as a modifier, and the "-ol" suffix is not used.

There are also IUPAC rules governing the nomenclature of stereoisomers, or absolute stereochemistry. Since any chiral carbon is surrounded by four different groups, the first order of business is to prioritize the substituents according to the IUPAC convention known as the Cahn-Ingold-Prelog (CIP) rules. The algorithm for CIP prioritization is as follows:

1. Examine each atom connected directly to the chiral center (we shall call these the "field atoms"); rank according to atomic number (high atomic number has priority).
2. In the event of a field atom tie, examine the substituents connected to the field atoms.
   a) Field atoms with higher-atomic-number substituents have priority.
   b) If substituent atomic number is tied, then field atoms with more substituents have priority.

For the purposes of prioritization, double and triple bonds are expanded—that is, a double bond to oxygen is assumed to be two oxygen substituents. If two or more field atoms remain in a tie, then the contest continues on the next atom out for each center, following the path of highest priority.

The next step is to orient the molecule so that the lowest-priority field atom (d) is going directly away from us, as is shown on the right side of Figure 11.12. Viewing this projection, we observe whether the progression of a → b → c occurs in a clockwise or counterclockwise sense. If clockwise, the enantiomer is labeled *R* (from the Latin *rectus*, proper); if counterclockwise, *S* (Latin *sinistrorsus*, to the left).

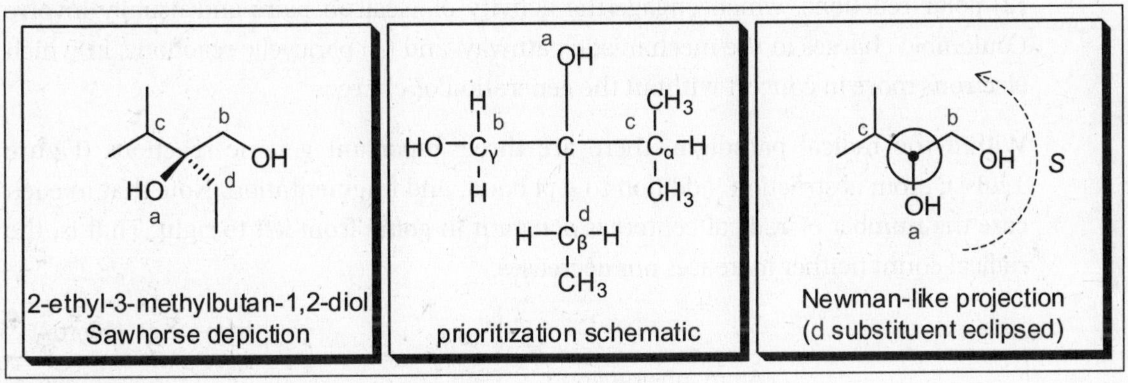

**2-ethyl-3-methylbutan-1,2-diol
Sawhorse depiction**

prioritization schematic

**Newman-like projection
(d substituent eclipsed)**

FIGURE 11.12: R/S Designation using CIP rules

The stereochemistry of double bonds is also specified using CIP priorities. In this protocol, each double bond is virtually rent in two and the substituents on each side are prioritized according to the CIP rules described above (Figure 11.13, inset). If the two high-priority substituents (a) are pointing in the same direction, the double bond is specified as Z (from

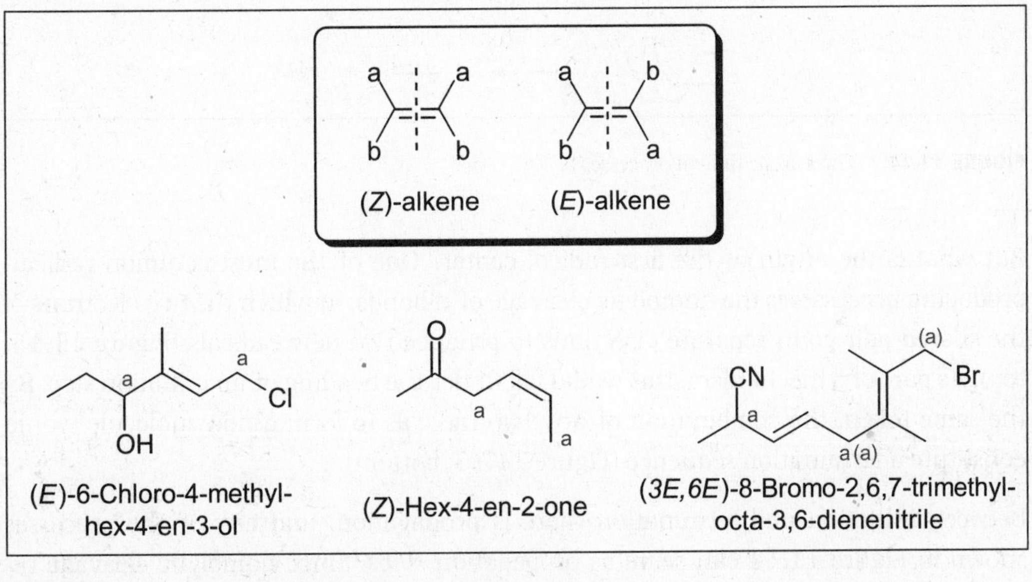

(Z)-alkene   **(E)-alkene**

**(E)-6-Chloro-4-methyl-
hex-4-en-3-ol**

(Z)-Hex-4-en-2-one

**(3E,6E)-8-Bromo-2,6,7-trimethyl-
octa-3,6-dienenitrile**

FIGURE 11.13: Stereochemistry of alkenes using CIP (E/Z)

the German, *zusammen*, or together); if they point in opposite directions, the double bond is designated *E* (German *entgegen*, or across from). Adding this stereochemical information to the chemical name proceeds exactly as described for *R/S* designation.

PART II. REACTIVITY
OVERVIEW OF REACTION MECHANISMS

Generally speaking, mechanistic steps fall into three broad categories: (1) radical reactions, which involve species with unpaired electrons and the motion of single electrons, (2) polar reactions, which engage the activity of electron pairs and usually involve Coulombic charges in the mechanistic pathway, and (3) pericyclic reactions, in which electrons move in concert without the generation of charge.

Within the radical paradigm, there are three important generic reactions (Figure 11.14): atom abstraction, addition to a pi bond, and fragmentation. Note that in each case the number of radical centers is constant in going from left to right. That is, the radical count neither increases nor decreases.

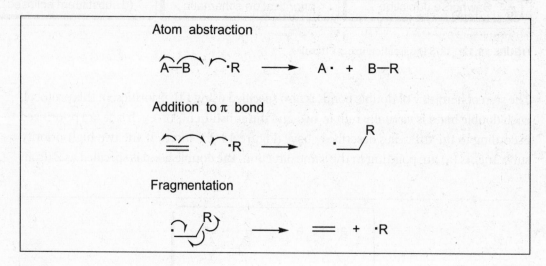

FIGURE 11.14:   Three basic radical processes

But what is the origin of the first radical center? One of the most common radical-producing processes is the homolytic cleavage of σ bonds, in which the two electrons of the shared pair go in separate directions to produce two new radicals (Figure 11.15, top). As part of a mechanism, this would fall under the heading of an initiation step. By the same token, the combination of any two radicals to form a new molecule would constitute a termination sequence (Figure 11.15, bottom).

Between initiation and termination there is propagation, and any of the processes shown in Figure 11.14 can serve as propagation steps. Since homolytic cleavage requires quite a bit of energy, if we relied on the stoichiometric generation of radicals

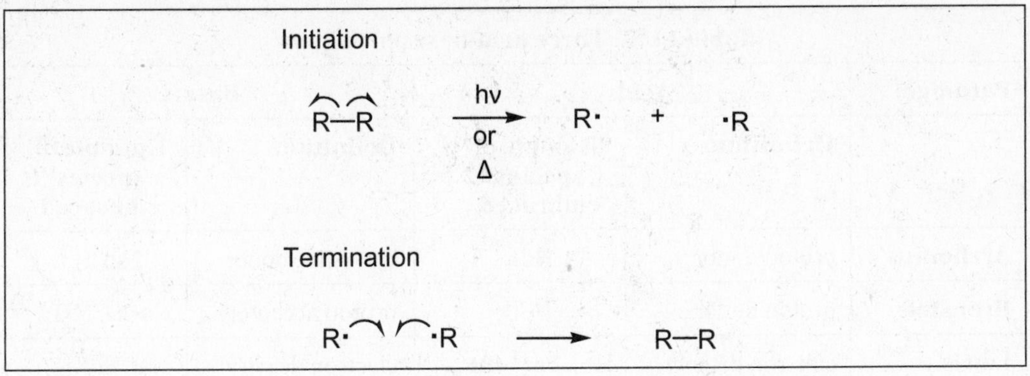

FIGURE 11.15: Radical initiation and termination

through this process, then the rate would be so slow as to be synthetically useless. Instead, once a single radical is formed, it can engage in a series of self-sustaining propagation steps to generate new compounds. This is nicely illustrated with the radical bromination of methane (Figure 11.16). The initiation step involves the homolytic cleavage of molecular bromine into two bromine radicals. In principle, this step (at a costly 46 kcal/mol) must only occur once. Afterwards, the bromine radical attacks methane, engaging in hydrogen atom abstraction to form hydrobromic acid and methyl radical (Step 1). The methyl radical, in turn, attacks molecular bromine (present in stoichiometric quantity), which suffers bromine atom abstraction and produces methyl bromide and regenerates bromine radical (Step 2). Notice that each of the propagation steps consumes stoichiometric reactant and generates stoichiometric product.

Turning our attention to polar chemistry, the most common representative of this class is the proton transfer, otherwise known as acid-base reactions. There are three general

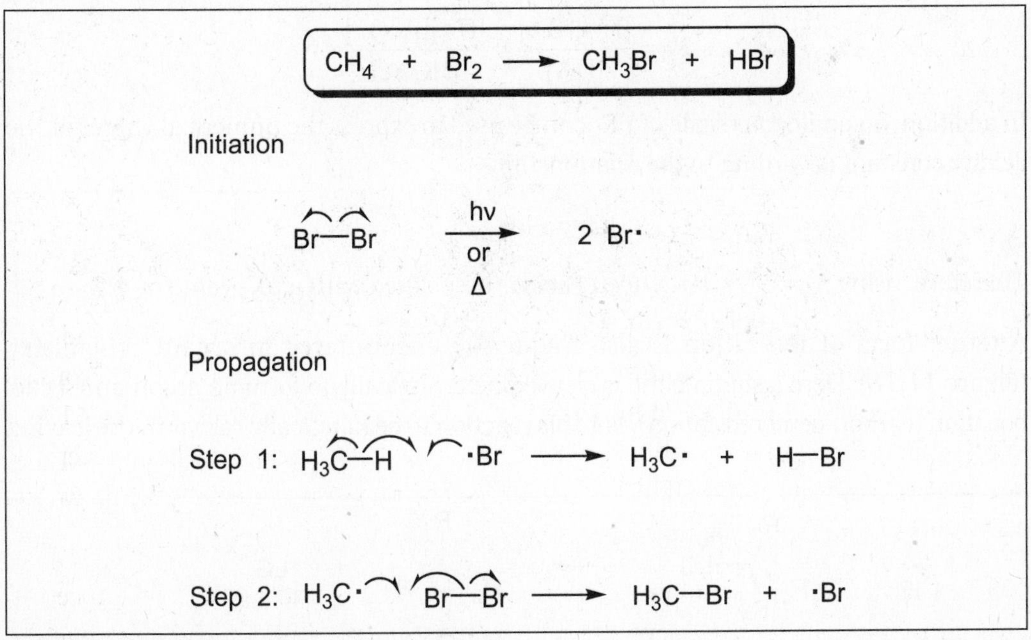

FIGURE 11.16: Radical bromination of methane

Table 11.5. Three acid-base paradigms				
Paradigm	**Acid**		**Base**	
	Definition	**Example of species embraced**	**Definition**	**Example of species embraced**
Arrhenius	proton donor	HCl	hydroxide donor	NaOH
Brønsted	proton donor	HCl	proton acceptor	NaOH, **NH₃**
Lewis	electron density acceptor	HCl, **Fe³⁺**, **BF₃**	electron density donor	NaOH, NH₃

paradigms of acid-base chemistry, as shown in Table 11.5. We will use the Lewis acid-base concept as a workhorse for understanding much of the mechanistic underpinnings of polar chemistry. However, proton transfer is best treated using the Brønsted notion of acids and bases. For example, we can represent the experimentally derived equilibrium constant for the ionization of acetic acid (AcOH) as shown in Figure 11.17, where the equilibrium constant bears the special designation of **acidity constant** (K_a).

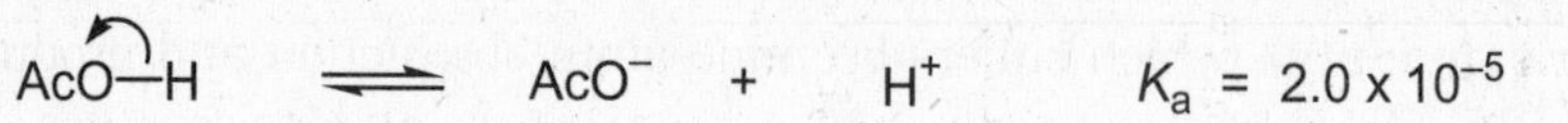

$$AcO-H \rightleftharpoons AcO^- + H^+ \qquad K_a = 2.0 \times 10^{-5}$$

FIGURE 11.17: The ionization of acetic acid

We can also express the acidity constant in terms of the chemical species involved, which has the generic form

$$Ka = \frac{[H^+][A^-]}{[HA]} = \frac{[H^+][AcO^-]}{[HOAc]}.$$

In addition, an analogous scale of pK_a can be used to express the numerical values of the acidity constant according to the relationship

$$pK_a = -\log_{10}(K_a).$$

Therefore, using $K_a = 2.0 \times 10^{-5}$, acetic acid is associated with a pK_a value of 4.7.

Another form of ionization is also frequently encountered in organic chemistry (Figure 11.18). Here a sigma bond is cleaved heterolytically to form an anion and a carbocation (carbon-centered cation). For this reaction to be kinetically relevant, the leaving

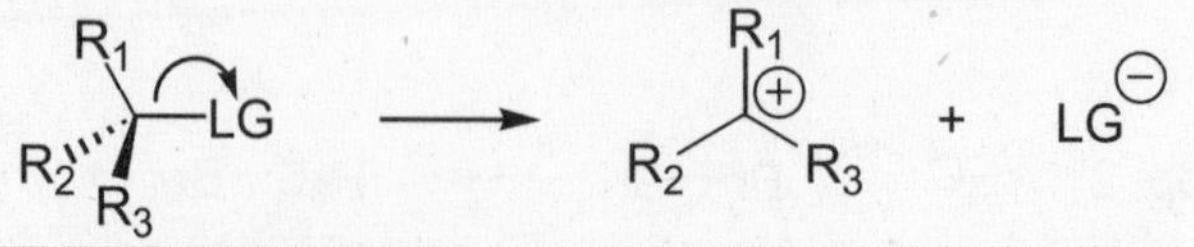

FIGURE 11.18: Unimolecular ionization

group (LG) must provide a very stable anion, and the carbocation must be secondary, tertiary, or otherwise stabilized (for example, allylic or benzylic). Good leaving groups (such as chloride or water) are generally species with strong conjugate acids (HCl and hydronium, respectively). Once a carbocation has been formed, it can suffer subsequent capture by a nucleophile to form a new bond. In principle, any species that would be classified as a Lewis base is a potential nucleophile, since a nucleophile is also a source of electron density.

When ionization is followed by nucleophilic capture, an overall process known as unimolecular substitution (S_N1) occurs. An illustrative example is the solvolysis reaction, in which solvent molecules act as the nucleophilic species. Thus, when 2-bromobutane is dissolved in methanol, ionization ensues to form a secondary carbocation which is captured by solvent to give (after proton loss) 2-methoxybutane (Figure 11.19). Note that even though optically pure (S)-2-bromobutane is used, the product is obtained as a racemic mixture.

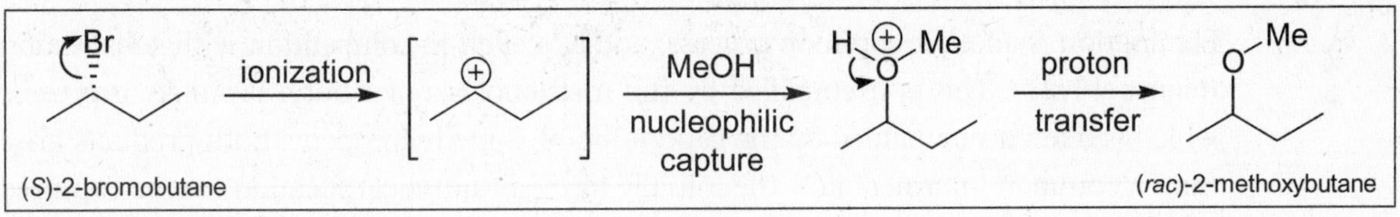

FIGURE 11.19: The S_N1 mechanism

Another characteristic of this mechanism—as the name implies—is the unimolecular nature of its kinetics. In other words, the rate of the reaction is dependent only upon the concentration of the substrate, according to the rate law

$$rate = k[2\text{-bromobutane}].$$

Since ionization involves breaking a bond, it is the most demanding step energetically. It is therefore the slowest, or rate-determining step. Furthermore, since this step involves only the substrate, it is the only component of the overall rate law.

When the nucleophile is strong enough, substitution can take place directly, without the need for prior ionization. For example, treatment of 2-bromobutane with sodium cyanide leads to direct displacement in one step via an S_N2 mechanism (Figure 11.20). One significant outcome of the S_N2 mechanism is that stereochemical information is preserved. This is due to the so-called backside attack of the nucleophile, which

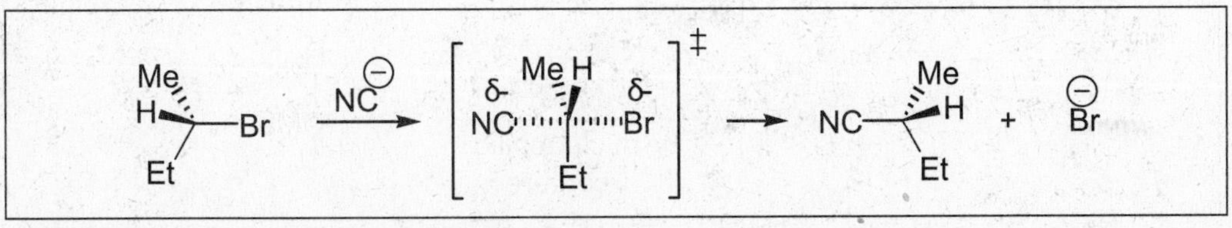

FIGURE 11.20:   Inversion of stereochemistry in S_N2

approaches the electrophile from the side opposite the leaving group, leading to a trigonal bipyramidal transition state.

The S_N2 reaction proceeds by a concerted mechanism, unlike the stepwise S_N1 sequence. Thus, there is a single activation energy that governs the kinetics of the process. Since the transition state involves both the substrate and the nucleophile, the rate law must also include terms for both species, as follows:

$$rate = k[2\text{-bromobutane}][NaCN].$$

For this reason, S_N2 reactions are particularly sensitive to concentration effects—a twofold dilution of each reagent results in a fourfold decrease in rate. Aside from concentration, the rate of the S_N2 reaction also depends upon the nature of the two species involved. Since the backside attack is sterically demanding, S_N2 reactivity drops off as substitution about the electrophilic center increases. Therefore, primary centers react faster than secondary, and tertiary centers are generally unreactive towards S_N2 displacement.

Elimination is another common process, and it is often in competition with substitution (Figure 11.21). This is exemplified by the methanolysis of *t*-butyl bromide, a process which is often accompanied by the generation of 2-methylpropene. Both products arise from a common intermediate—the initially formed *t*-butyl carbocation can be captured by methanol to give the corresponding ether (S_N1 product), or it can suffer direct proton loss to form a double bond. The combination of ionization followed by proton loss constitutes the E1 mechanism. Like the S_N1 mechanism, it is stepwise and it is encountered only when a relatively stable carbocation can be formed.

With stronger bases another eliminative pathway becomes feasible, namely bimolecular elimination (E2). This is a concerted process in which the base removes a β-proton as the leaving group leaves. Like the S_N2 reaction, the E2 has a single transition state involving both the base and the substrate; therefore, the observed kinetics are second order and the rate is dependent upon the concentration of both species (Figure 11.22). Note that as the reaction progresses, two molecules give rise to three molecules, an entropically very favorable result. Therefore, like the E1 mechanism, bimolecular elimina-

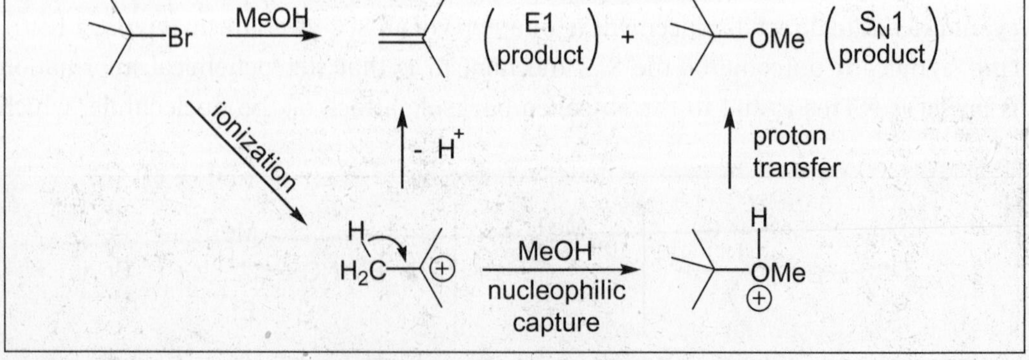

FIGURE 11.21: Competition between E1 and S_N1 mechanisms

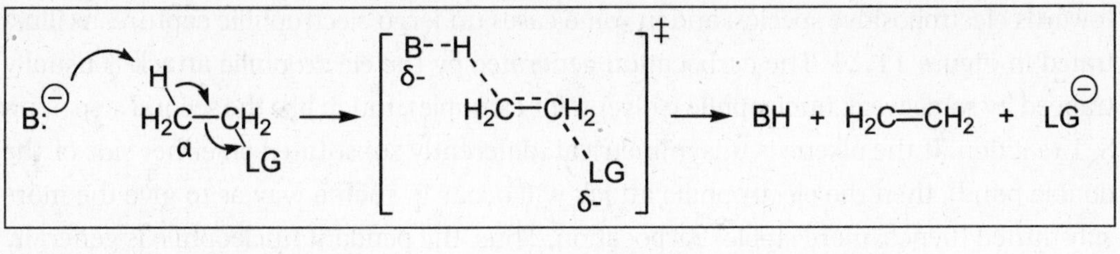

FIGURE 11.22:   The E2 mechanism

tion is made much more spontaneous with increasing temperature. Moreover, E2 elim-
inations tend to be practically irreversible.

So far we have discussed nucleophilic attack at an sp^3-hybridized electrophilic center
bearing a leaving group. However, we can imagine another way to push electrons to
form a stabilized anionic charge. Figure 11.23 shows two such possibilities. In the first,
a nucleophile adds to an electron-deficient double bond in such a way as to place the
anionic center adjacent to the stabilizing electron-withdrawing group. This type of
reaction is often called conjugate addition, since the stabilizing group is usually a π
system in conjugation with the double bond. It is also the basis for nucleophilic aromatic substitution. The other common mode of addition onto an sp^2 center is by nucleophilic attack onto a carbonyl carbon (Figure 11.23, bottom). This provides, after
aqueous workup, an alcohol—and various modes of carbonyl addition are frequently
used for the synthesis of complex alcohols.

In the absence of electron-withdrawing groups, alkenes are actually somewhat nucleophilic. The π electron density is somewhat far removed from the Coulombic tether of the
nuclei. It seems intuitively supportable, then, to posit that the π bond might be polarized

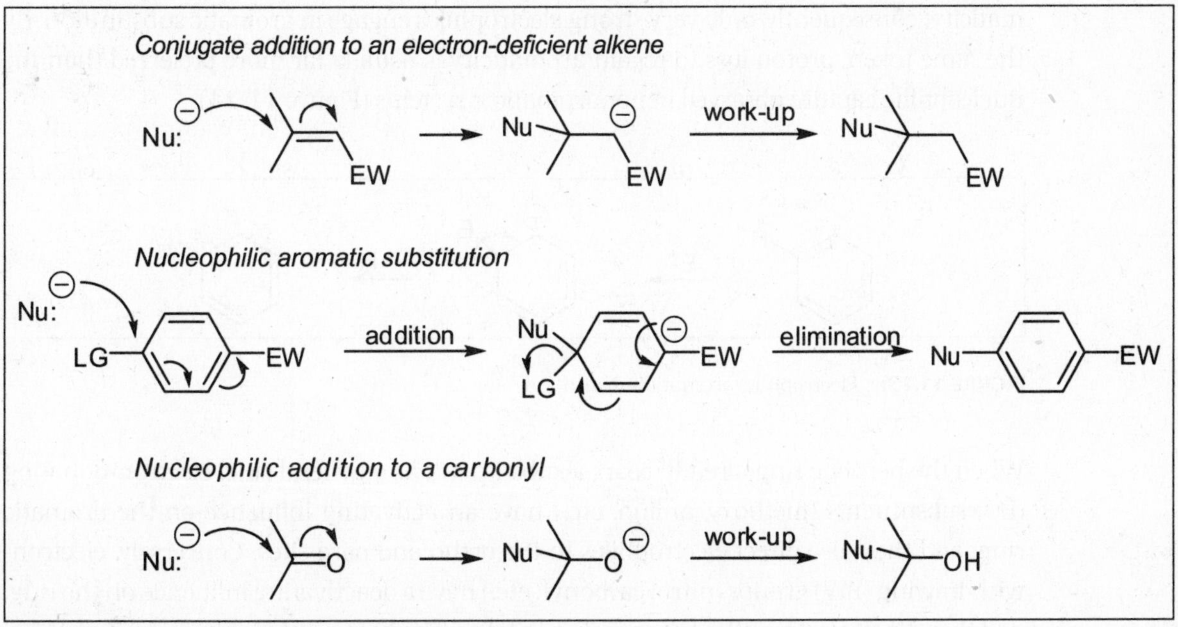

FIGURE 11.23:   Nucleophilic attack at an sp^2 carbon

towards electropositive species, and in some cases undergo electrophilic capture, as illustrated in Figure 11.24. The carbocation generated by the electrophilic attack is usually trapped by some weak nucleophile (solvent, for example), much like the second step of an S_N1 reaction. If the alkene is unsymmetrical (differently substituted on either side of the double bond), then the electrophilic attack will occur in such a way as to give the more substituted (hence, more stable) carbocation. Thus, the pendant nucleophile is generally found at the more substituted position. This regiochemical outcome is said to follow the Markovnikov rule, and the more substituted product is dubbed the Markovnikov product.

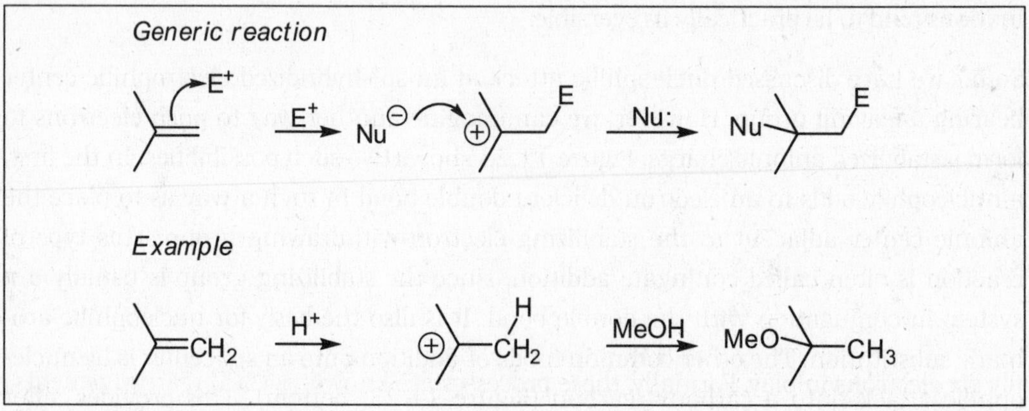

FIGURE 11.24: Electrophilic attack of an alkene

This mode of reactivity is also enormously important in aromatic chemistry. As shown in Figure 11.25, an aromatic ring can capture an electrophile to form a doubly allylic carbocationic intermediate, which quenches the positive charge by loss of a proton to form a new aromatic species. The first step is energetically challenging, since it destroys aromaticity; consequently, only very strong electrophiles engage in aromatic substitution. By the same token, proton loss to regain aromaticity is usually far more preferred than the nucleophilic capture observed in nonaromatic π systems (Figure 11.24).

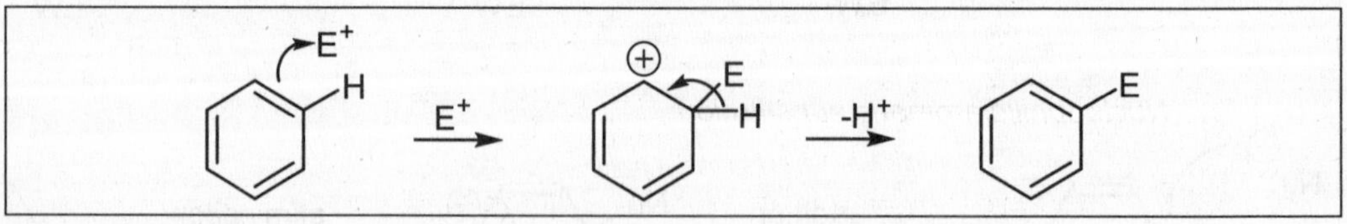

FIGURE 11.25: Electrophilic aromatic substitution

When the benzene ring already bears a substituent, as a general rule, electron-donating (ED) substituents (methoxy, amino, etc.) have an activating influence on the aromatic ring, and they also direct electrophiles to the ortho and para sites. Conversely, electron-withdrawing (EW) groups (nitro, carbonyl, etc.) have a deactivating influence on the ring, and they direct electrophiles to the meta positions. The halogens exhibit unique behavior: they are deactivating, but ortho/para directing (Table 11.6).

Table 11.6. Substituent effects on electrophilic aromatic substitution	
Electron-donating (ED) groups	**Electron-withdrawing (EW) groups**
activating *o,p-directing* −NR$_2$ (amino, amido) −OR (alkoxy, hydroxy) −R (alkyl)	*deactivating* *m-directing* −NO$_2$ (nitro) −CO$_2$R (esters, acids) −C(O)R (ketones, aldehydes) −SO$_3$H (sulfo) −CN (cyano)
Halogens	
deactivating *o,p-directing* −F, −Cl, −Br, −I	

Finally, we consider the pericyclic reactions, to which the sigmatropic rearrangements belong. Figure 11.26 illustrates one example, known as the Cope rearrangement. At face value, a σ bond has moved from the right side to the left—however, there are actually six electrons in play. Formally, these processes are known as [3,3] rearrangements, because there is a three-atom array walking across a three-atom array. Atoms other than carbon are also fair game. For example, oxygen can replace one of the sp^3 carbons in what is known as the Claisen rearrangement (Figure 11.27). Unlike the Cope, which

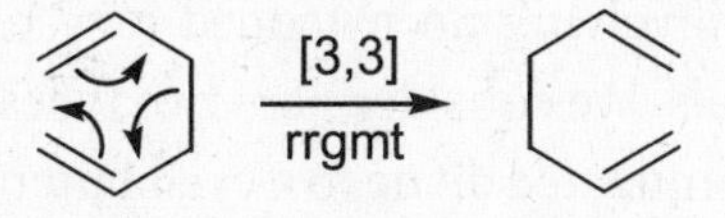

FIGURE 11.26: The Cope rearrangement

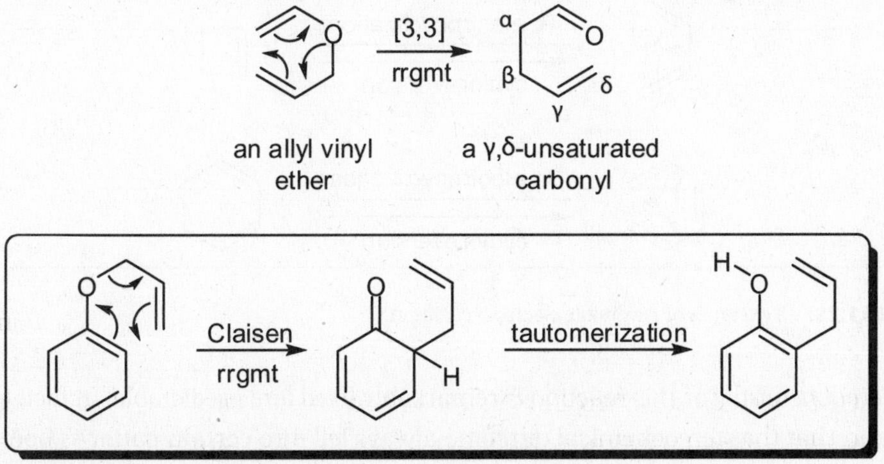

FIGURE 11.27: The Claisen rearrangement

converts a diene to another diene, the Claisen actually provides different functionality. Thus, we start with an allyl vinyl ether, and the rearrangement results in a γ, δ-unsaturated carbonyl compound. In the case of allyl phenyl ethers, the initially formed rearrangement product tautomerizes to restore aromaticity.

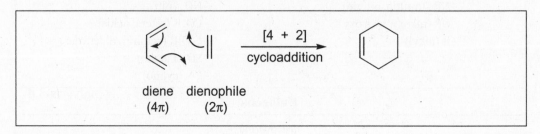

FIGURE 11.28: The prototypical Diels-Alder reaction

Two types of pericyclic reactions are particularly important for their ring-forming capabilities. One is the Diels-Alder reaction, also known as the [4+2] cycloaddition. Here the formal nomenclature is not based on the number of atoms involved, but the number of electrons. Thus, a 4π component (called the diene) and a 2π component (called the dienophile) come together to form a cyclohexene, as shown in Figure 11.28. Again, we can see that the reaction involves the concerted motion of six electrons—this is important, because the transition state has considerable aromatic character, an outcome that provides for a particularly low activation barrier.

Another way to produce cyclic molecules from acyclic precursors is through electrocyclization. This is a process involving an extended π system, and could encompass a rather large array of p orbitals. We consider here two types: 4π and 6π. The overall process is the conversion of a conjugated diene to a cyclobutene (4π) or a conjugated triene to a cyclohexatriene (6π), as shown in Figure 11.29. Both are best considered equilibrium reactions, and the reverse process is known as a cycloreversion.

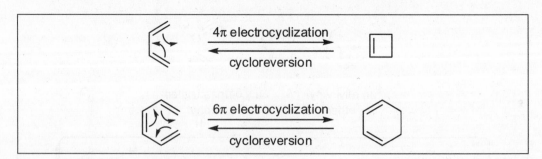

FIGURE 11.29: Two types of reversible electrocyclization

The stereochemistry of this reaction is remarkably fixed and predictable. In fact, the observation that the stereochemical outcome always fell into certain patterns opened up many of the applications of molecular orbital (MO) theory that we use today (and also earned a Nobel prize for Fukui and Hoffmann in 1981). For example, if *trans,trans*-2,4-

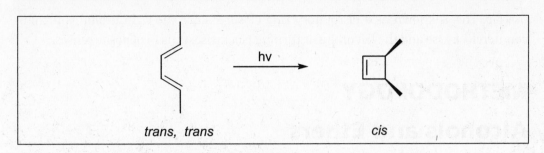

FIGURE 11.30: The stereochemical outcome of photochemical 4π electrocyclization

hexadiene (Figure 11.30) is subjected to photochemical conditions, only *cis*-3,4-dimethylbutadiene is formed.

An examination of molecular orbital theory provides some insight (Figure 11.31). Light promotes an electron into the lowest unoccupied molecular orbital (LUMO) thus converting it to a singly occupied molecular orbital (SOMO), which now controls the course of the reaction. If we superimpose the SOMO onto a depiction of the diene (inset), we see that the two end lobes must turn in towards each other to enjoy constructive orbital

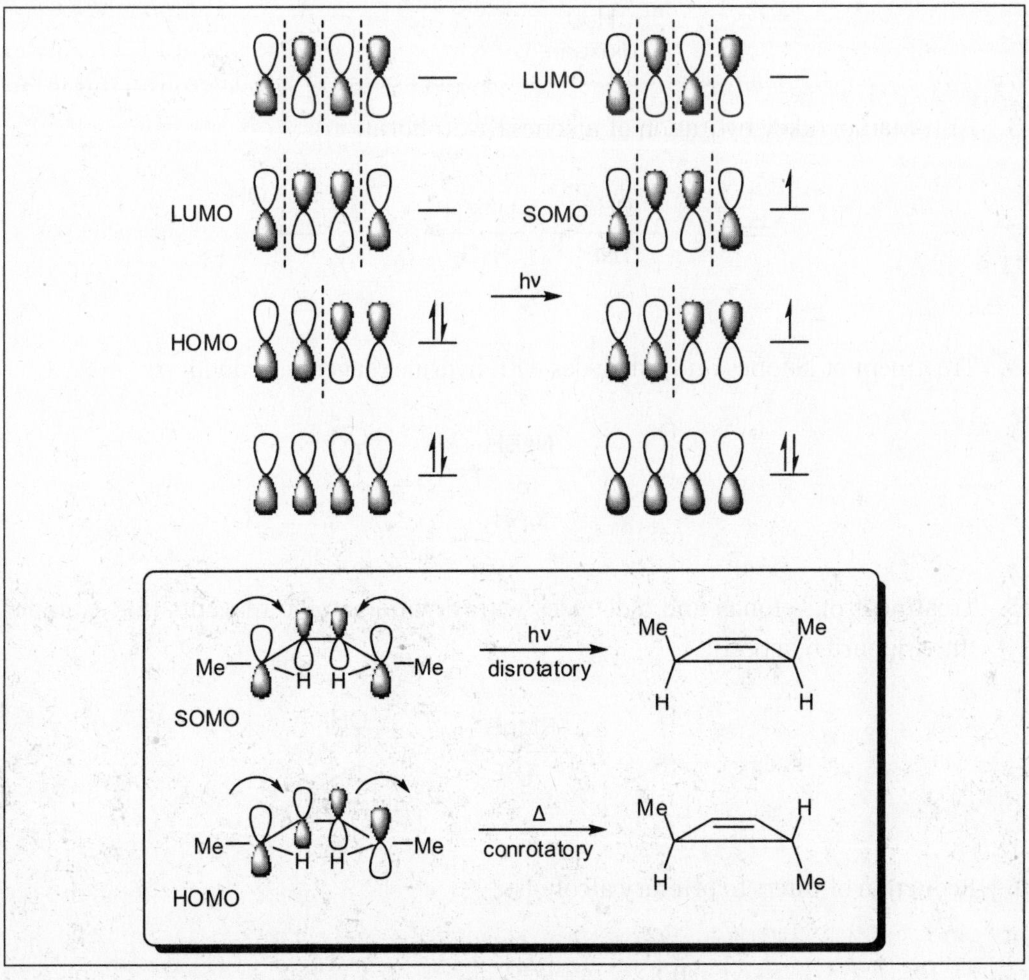

FIGURE 11.31: The molecular orbital underpinnings of electrocyclization

overlap. This is known as a disrotatory ring closure, since the right orbital is turning counterclockwise and the left orbital is turning clockwise, thus in opposite senses.

METHODOLOGY

Alcohols and Ethers

PREPARATION OF ALCOHOLS

1. Simple Markovnikov hydration of alkenes (acid-catalyzed hydration):

2. Oxymercuriation-demercuriation (also results in Markovnikov hydration):

3. Anti-Markovnikov hydration of alkenes (hydroboration):

4. Treatment of ketones and aldehydes with hydride reagents (reduction):

5. Treatment of ketones and aldehydes with organometallic reagents (for example, the Grignard reaction):

6. Reduction of esters to primary alcohols:

7. S_N2 reaction of hydroxide with alkyl halides, tosylates, or mesylates (works best with primary substrates):

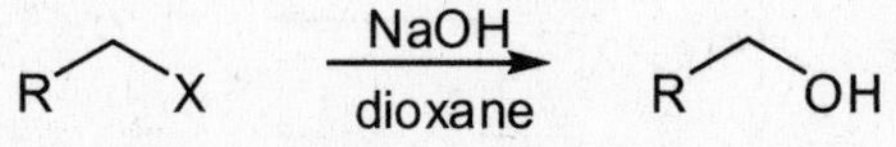

X = Br, Cl, I, OTs, OMs

8. Nucleophilic ring opening of epoxides with nucleophiles:

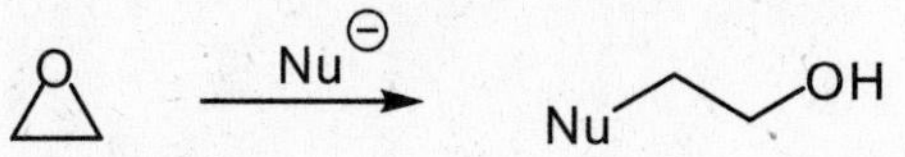

REACTIONS OF ALCOHOLS

1. Jones oxidation of secondary alcohols to ketones:

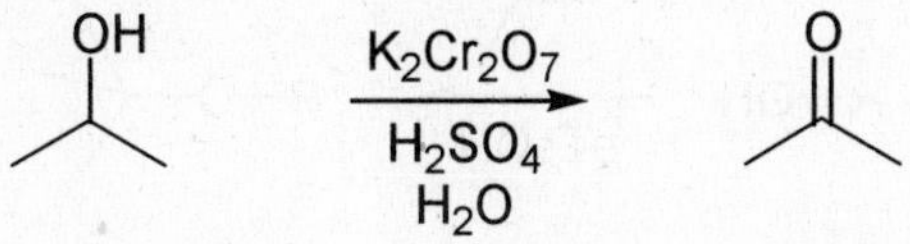

2. Jones oxidation of primary alcohols to carboxylic acids:

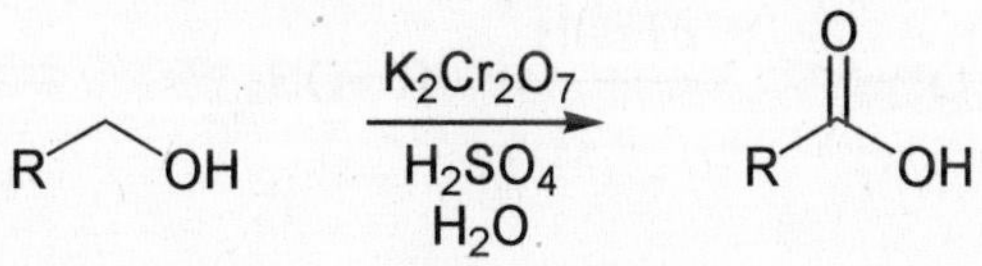

3. PCC oxidation of primary alcohols to aldehydes:

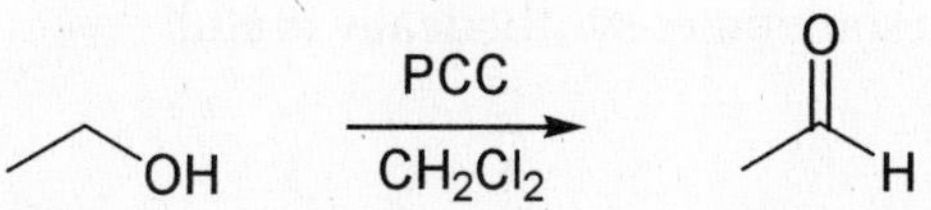

4. Conversion to the corresponding halides or tosylates (good leaving groups):

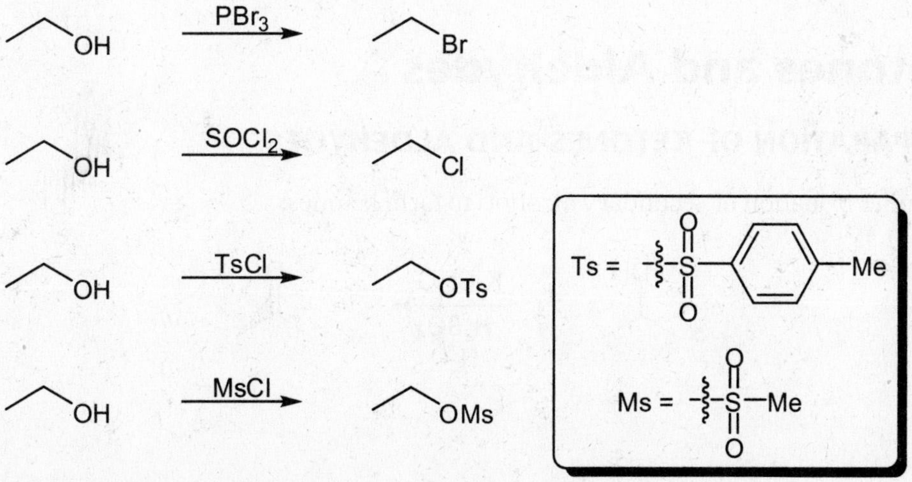

5. Acid-catalyzed dehydration:

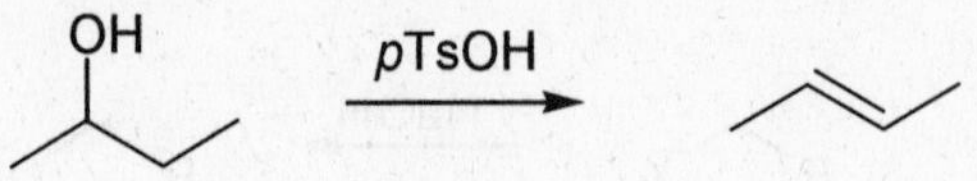

6. Reaction with acyl chlorides to form esters:

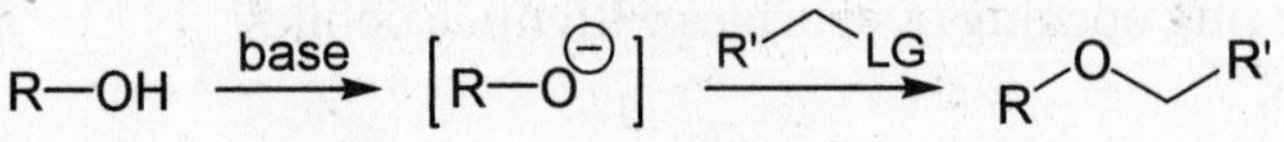

PREPARATION OF ETHERS

1. The alkylation of alkoxide anions (Williamson ether synthesis):

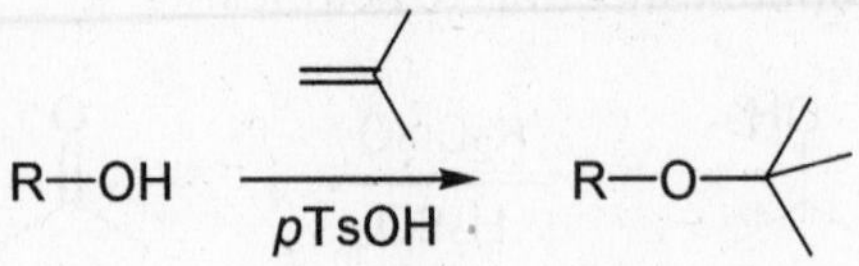

2. The acid-catalyzed addition of alcohols across alkenes:

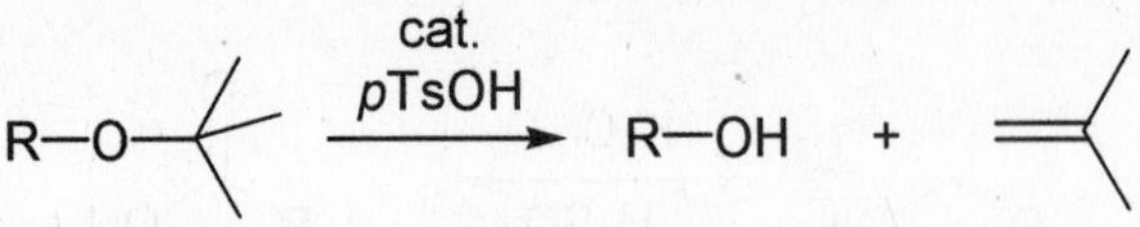

REACTIONS OF ETHERS

Ethers tend to be relatively inert. However, the acid-catalyzed elimination of tertiary ethers to form alkenes is sometimes synthetically useful:

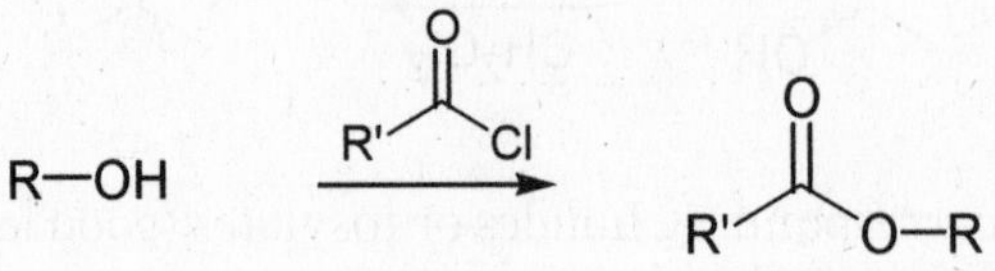

Ketones and Aldehydes

PREPARATION OF KETONES AND ALDEHYDES

1. Jones oxidation of secondary alcohols to form ketones:

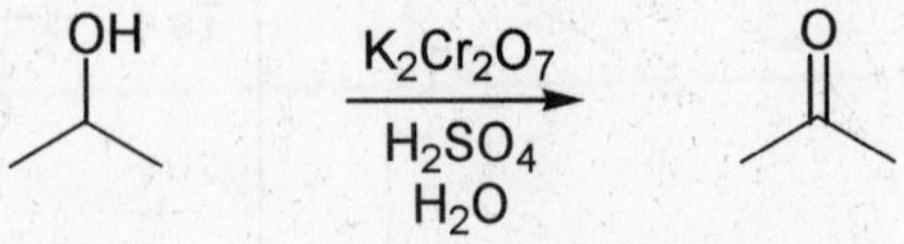

2. PCC oxidation of primary alcohols to form aldehydes:

3. Selective oxidation of benzylic alcohols with manganese dioxide (most other alcohols are unaffected):

4. Ozonolysis of alkenes to form carbonyls:

5. Oxidative cleavage of vic-diols with periodic acid:

6. Reduction of acyl chlorides to aldehydes using lithium tri(*t*-butoxy)aluminum hydride:

7. DIBAL reduction of esters to aldehydes:

8. DIBAL reduction of nitriles to aldehydes:

9. Markovnikov hydration of terminal alkynes to methyl ketones:

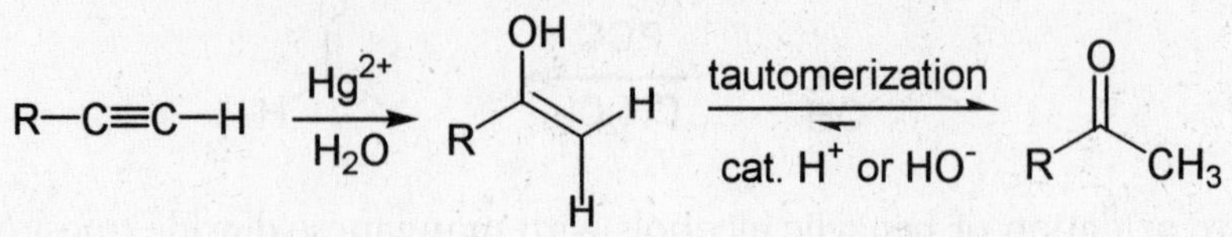

10. Anti-Markovnikov hydration of terminal alkynes to aldehydes:

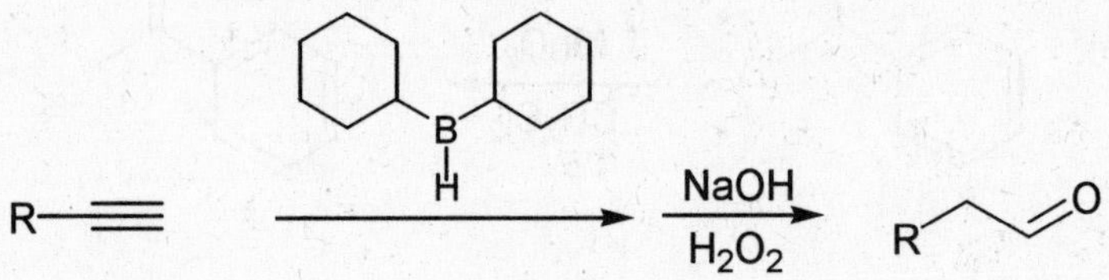

REACTIONS OF KETONES AND ALDEHYDES

1. Hydride reduction to alcohols:

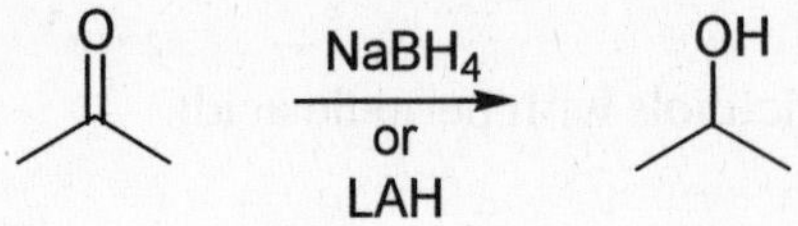

2. Nucleophilic addition of organometallics (Grignard reaction):

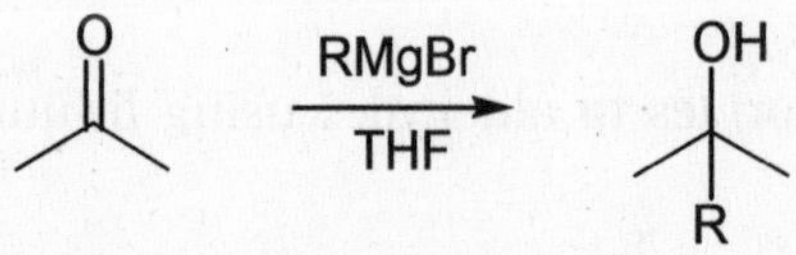

3. Conversion to alkenes with phosphonium ylides (Wittig reaction):

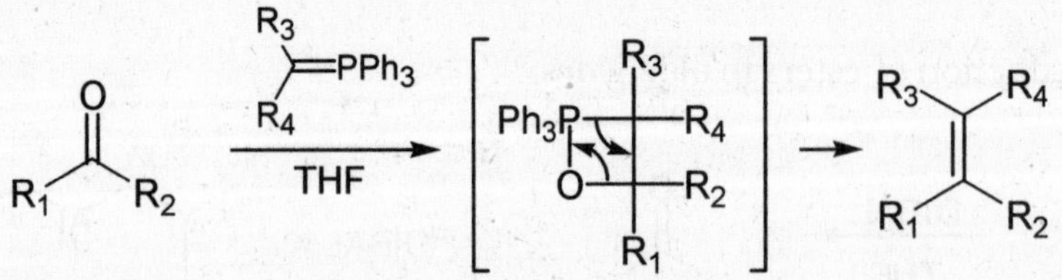

4. Acid-catalyzed formation of acetals:

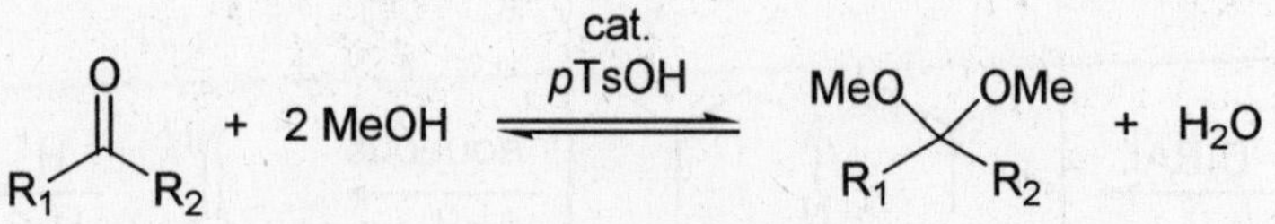

5. Condensation with primary amines to form imines:

6. Condensation with secondary amines to form enamines:

7. Reaction with amines in the presence of sodium cyanoborohydride to form amines (reductive amination):

8. Alkylation of enolate carbanions:

9. Condensation with other carbonyl compounds (aldol condensation):

10. Addition onto electron-deficient alkenes (conjugate addition):

11. Tandem conjugate addition/aldol condensation (Robinson annulation):

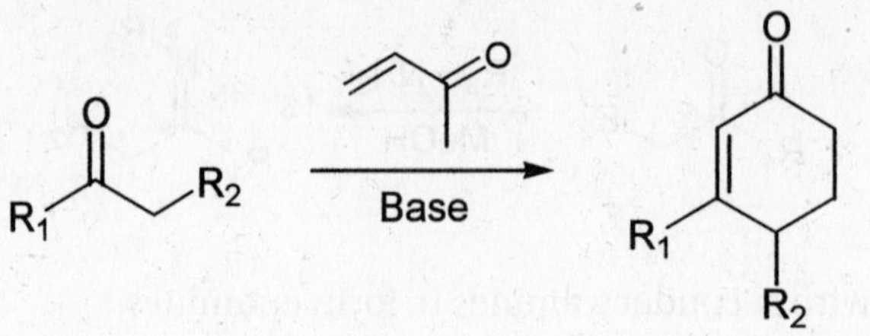

12. Conversion to esters by action of *m*-chloroperbenzoic acid (Baeyer-Villiger oxidation):

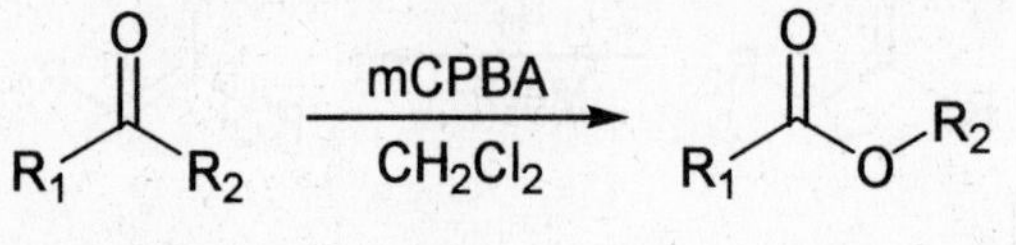

Alkenes and Alkynes

PREPARATION OF ALKENES

1. Acid-catalyzed dehydration of alcohols (E1 elimination):

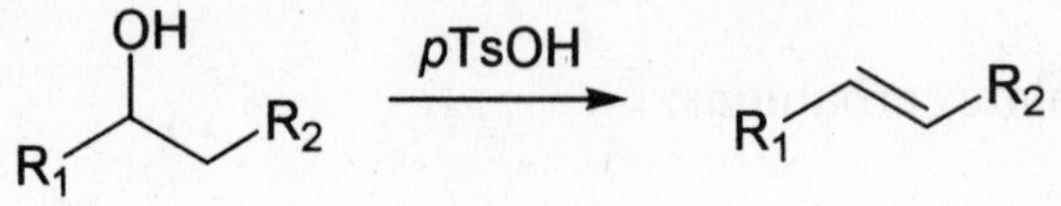

2. Base-catalyzed elimination (E2 elimination):

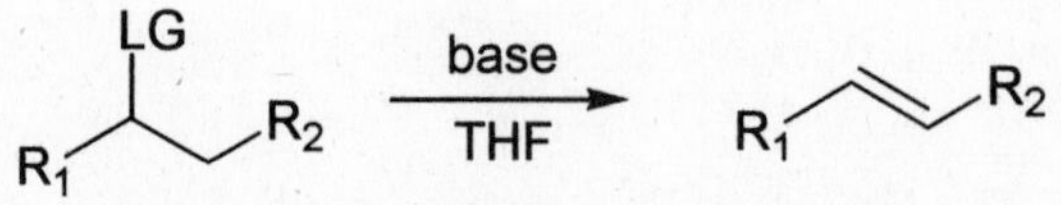

3. Reaction of carbonyl compounds with phosphonium ylides (Wittig reaction):

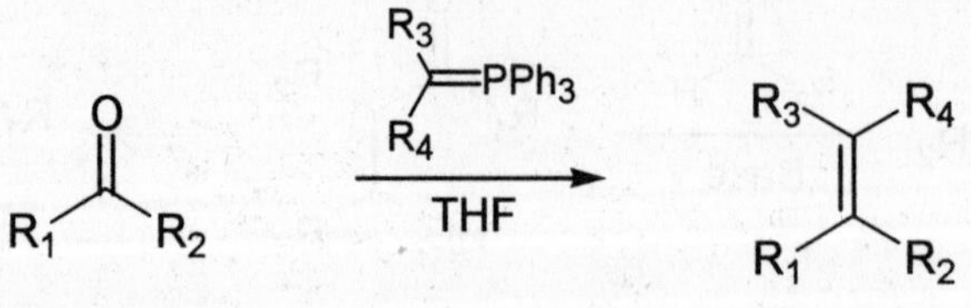

4. Conversion of alkynes to cis-alkenes using catalytic hydrogenation:

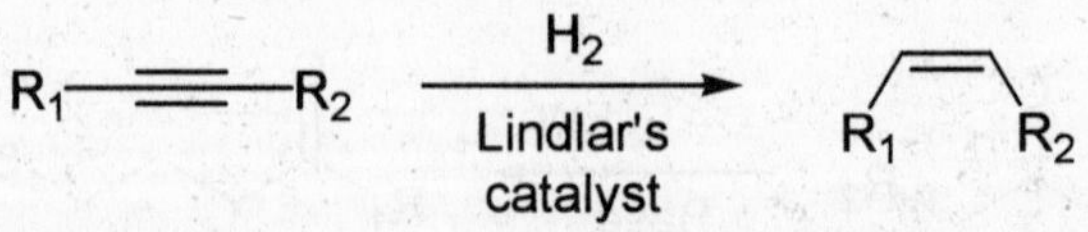

5. Conversion of alkynes to trans-alkenes using dissolving metal reduction:

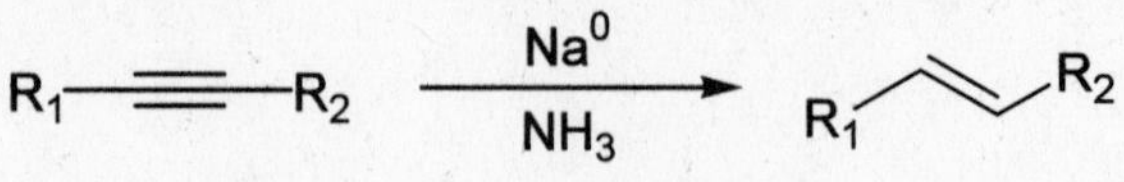

6. Conversion of amines to alkenes through the Hofmann elimination:

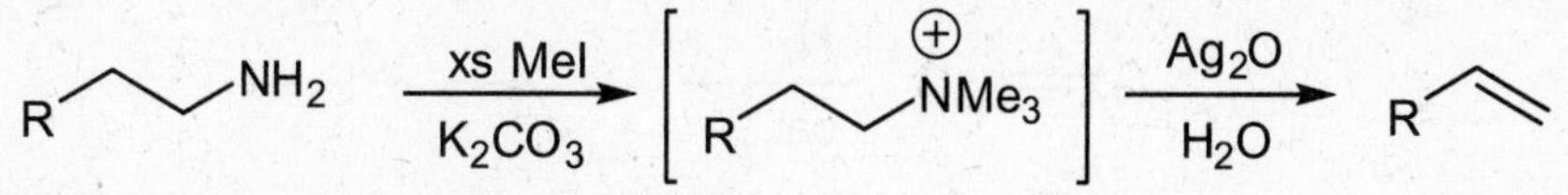

REACTIONS OF ALKENES

1. Acid-catalyzed Markovnikov hydration to form alcohols:

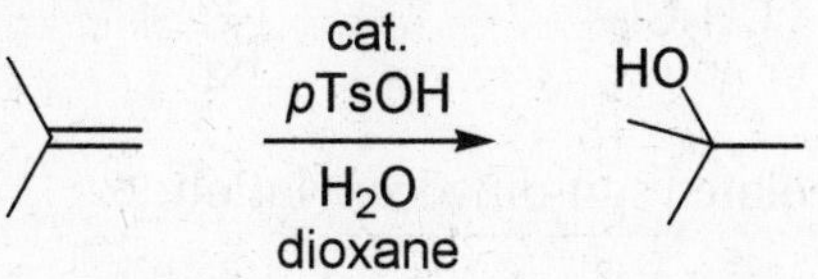

2. Mercury-catalyzed Markovnikov hydration (oxymercuriation/demercuriation):

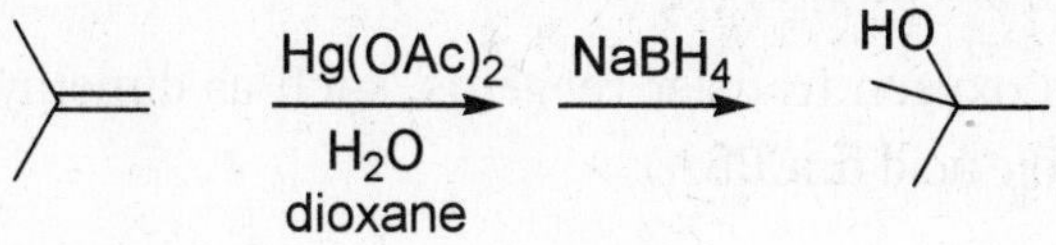

3. Anti-Markovnikov hydration (hydroboration):

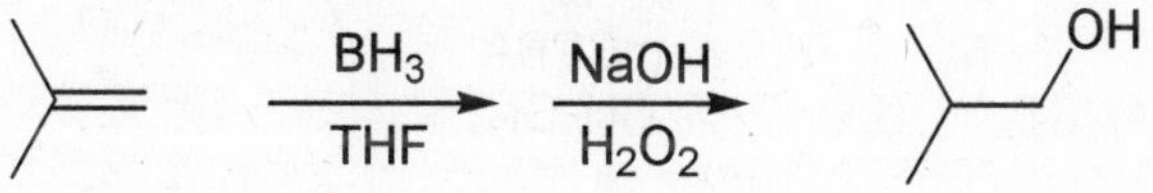

4. Markovnikov hydrobromination:

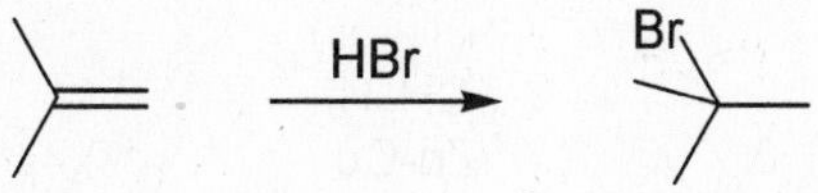

5. Anti-Markovnikov hydrobromination in the presence of radical initiators:

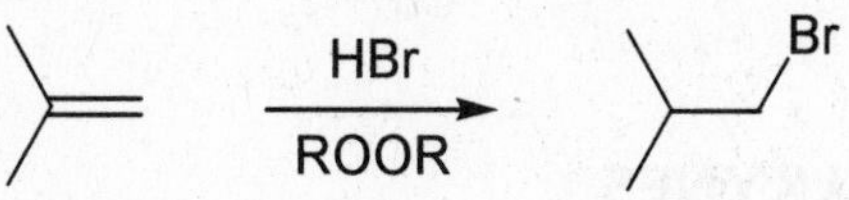

6. Dibromination with bromine in an inert solvent:

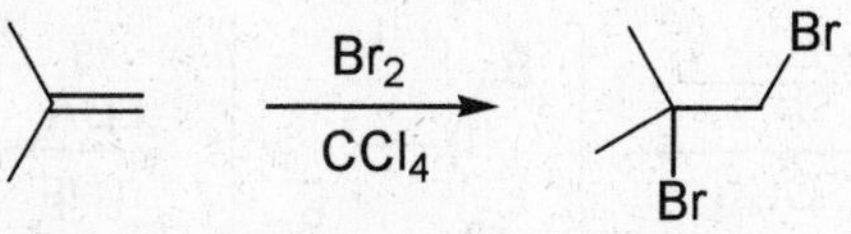

7. Formation of bromohydrins by reaction with bromine in the presence of water:

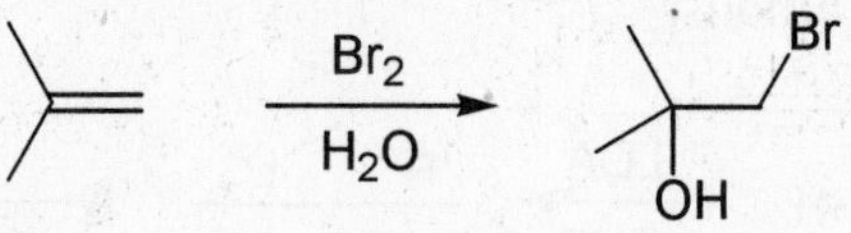

8. Catalytic hydrogenation to form alkenes:

$$\xrightarrow[\text{cat.}]{\text{H}_2}$$

9. Ozonolysis with reductive work-up to form carbonyl compounds:

$$\xrightarrow[\text{CH}_2\text{Cl}_2]{\text{O}_3} \quad \xrightarrow{\text{Me}_2\text{S}}$$

10. Osmium tetroxide-mediated syn-dihydroxylation:

$$\xrightarrow[\text{H}_2\text{O}_2]{\text{OsO}_4}$$

11. Epoxidation with oxygen transfer reagents, such as dimethyldioxirane (DMD) or m-chloroperbenzoic acid (mCPBA):

$$\xrightarrow[\substack{\text{mCPBA} \\ \text{CH}_2\text{Cl}_2}]{\substack{\text{DMD /} \\ \text{acetone} \\ \text{or}}}$$

12. Cyclopropanation using carbene precursors, such as diazomethane or diiodomethane and zinc/copper couple (Simmons-Smith reaction):

$$\xrightarrow[\substack{\text{CH}_2\text{N}_2 \\ \text{Cu}^0}]{\substack{\text{CH}_2\text{I}_2 \\ \text{Zn-Cu} \\ \text{or}}}$$

PREPARATION OF ALKYNES

1. Conversion of alkenes to alkynes by dibromination followed by double elimination:

$$\xrightarrow[\text{CCl}_4]{\text{Br}_2} \qquad \xrightarrow[\text{THF}]{\substack{\text{xs} \\ \text{LDA}}}$$

2. Alkylation of alkynyl anions:

$$\xrightarrow[\text{THF}]{\text{LDA}} \qquad \xrightarrow{\text{R}' \diagup \text{LG}}$$

REACTIONS OF ALKYNES

1. Markovnikov hydration of terminal alkynes to form methyl ketones:

$$R-\!\!\!\equiv\!\!\! \quad \xrightarrow[\substack{H_2O \\ dioxane}]{HgSO_4} \quad R \overset{O}{\underset{}{\diagup}} Me$$

2. Anti-Markovnikov hydration of terminal alkynes to form aldehydes:

$$R-\!\!\!\equiv\!\!\! \quad \xrightarrow{\qquad} \quad \xrightarrow[H_2O_2]{NaOH} \quad R\diagdown\!\!\diagup\!\!\!\overset{O}{\diagup}$$

3. Reduction of internal alkynes to cis-alkenes by hydrogenation using Lindlar's catalyst:

$$R_1-\!\!\!\equiv\!\!\!-R_2 \quad \xrightarrow[\substack{Lindlar's \\ catalyst}]{H_2} \quad \underset{R_1 \quad R_2}{\diagup\!=\!\diagdown}$$

4. Reduction of internal alkynes to trans-alkenes by (dissolving metal reduction):

$$R_1-\!\!\!\equiv\!\!\!-R_2 \quad \xrightarrow[NH_3]{Na^0} \quad \underset{R_1}{\diagup}\!\!=\!\!\underset{R_2}{\diagdown}$$

Carboxylic Acid Derivatives

PREPARATION OF CARBOXYLIC ACIDS

1. Jones oxidation of primary alcohols or aldehydes:

$$R\diagdown\!\!\diagup OH \quad \xrightarrow[\substack{H_2SO_4 \\ H_2O}]{K_2Cr_2O_7} \quad R\overset{O}{\underset{}{\diagup}} OH$$

$$R\overset{O}{\underset{}{\diagup}} H \quad \xrightarrow[\substack{H_2SO_4 \\ H_2O}]{K_2Cr_2O_7} \quad R\overset{O}{\underset{}{\diagup}} OH$$

2. Base-catalyzed hydrolysis of esters (saponification):

$$R\overset{O}{\underset{}{\diagup}} OR' \quad \xrightarrow[H_2O]{KOH} \quad R\overset{O}{\underset{}{\diagup}} OK \quad \xrightarrow[work\text{-}up]{acidic} \quad R\overset{O}{\underset{}{\diagup}} OH$$

3. Acid-catalyzed hydrolysis of nitriles:

$$R-C\equiv N \xrightarrow[\text{H}_2\text{O}]{\text{H}_2\text{SO}_4} R\text{—C(=O)—OH}$$

4. Action of Grignard reagents on carbon dioxide:

$$R-Br \xrightarrow[\text{THF}]{\text{Mg}^0} R-MgBr \xrightarrow{\text{CO}_2} R\text{—C(=O)—OH}$$

REACTIONS OF CARBOXYLIC ACIDS

1. Conversion to acyl chlorides using thionyl chloride or oxalyl chloride:

$$R\text{—C(=O)—OH} \xrightarrow[\substack{\text{Cl—C(=O)—C(=O)—Cl} \\ \text{cat. DMF}}]{\substack{\text{SOCl}_2 \\ \text{or}}} R\text{—C(=O)—Cl}$$

2. Reduction to alcohols using lithium aluminum hydride:

$$R\text{—C(=O)—OH} \xrightarrow[\text{THF}]{\text{LAH}} R\text{—CH}_2\text{—OH}$$

3. Acid-catalyzed esterification in an alcohol solvent:

$$R\text{—C(=O)—OH} \xrightarrow[\text{cat. H}^+]{\text{R'—OH}} R\text{—C(=O)—O—R'}$$

PREPARATION OF CARBOXYLATE ESTERS

1. Acid-catalyzed esterification in an alcohol solvent:

$$R\text{—C(=O)—OH} \xrightarrow[\text{cat. H}^+]{\text{R'—OH}} R\text{—C(=O)—O—R'}$$

2. Reaction of alcohols with acyl halides:

$$R\text{—C(=O)—Cl} \xrightarrow{\text{R'—OH}} R\text{—C(=O)—O—R'}$$

3. Reaction of carboxylic acids with diazomethane to form methyl esters:

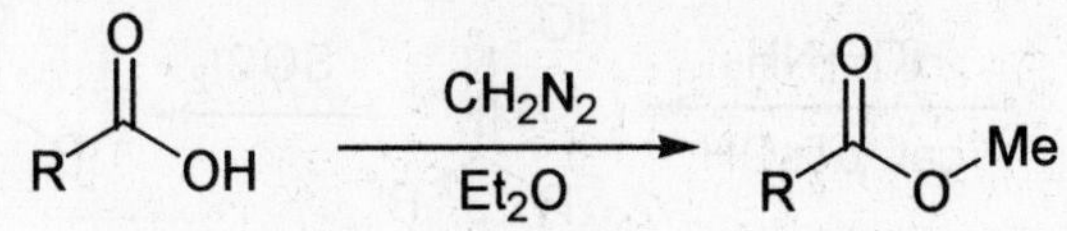

REACTIONS OF CARBOXYLATE ESTERS

1. Base-catalyzed hydrolysis (saponification):

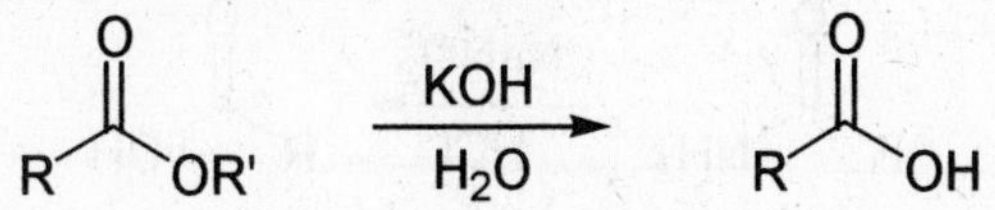

2. Transesterification under acidic or basic conditions:

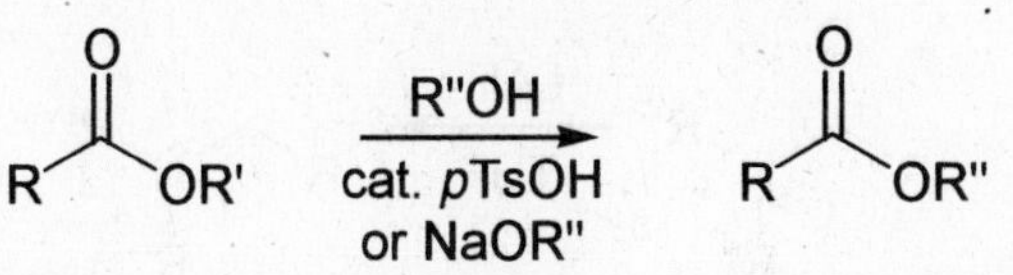

3. Reduction to primary alcohols using lithium aluminum hydride:

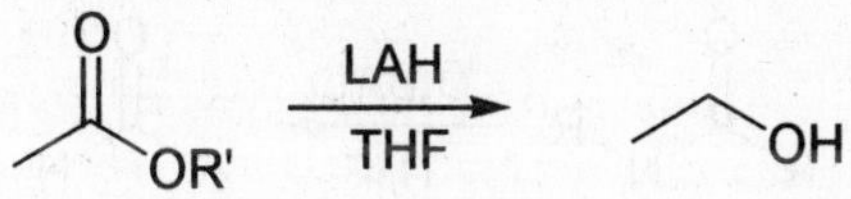

4. Reduction to aldehydes using diisobutylaluminum hydride (DIBAL):

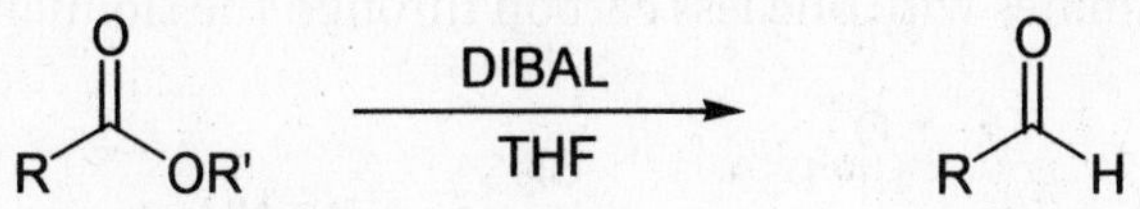

PREPARATION OF AMIDES

1. Reaction of amines with acyl halides:

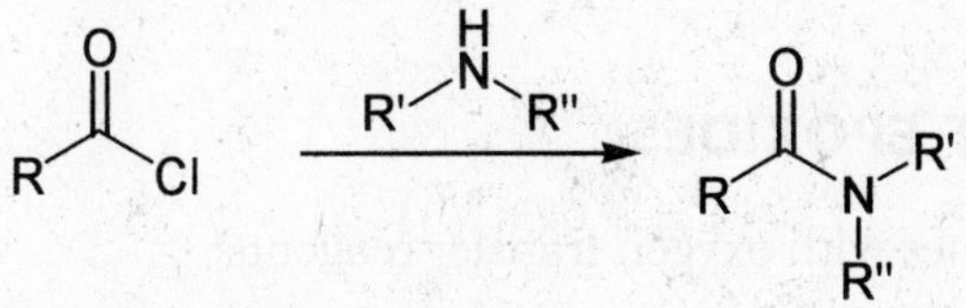

2. Reaction of amines with leaving groups:

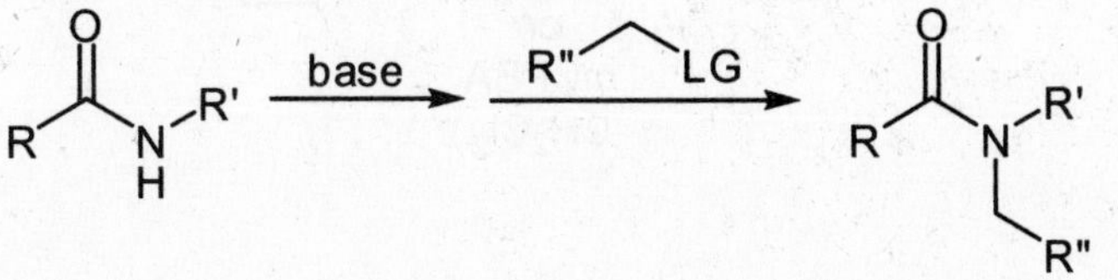

3. Conversion of ketones to hydroxylamines, followed by Beckmann rearrangement:

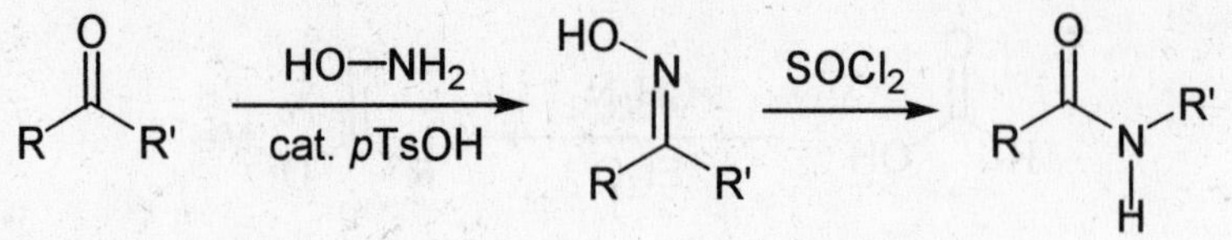

REACTIONS OF AMIDES

1. Conversion to carboxylic acids by diazotization and hydrolysis:

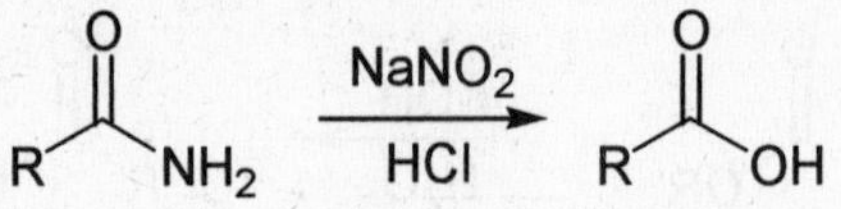

2. Reduction with lithium aluminum hydride to form amines:

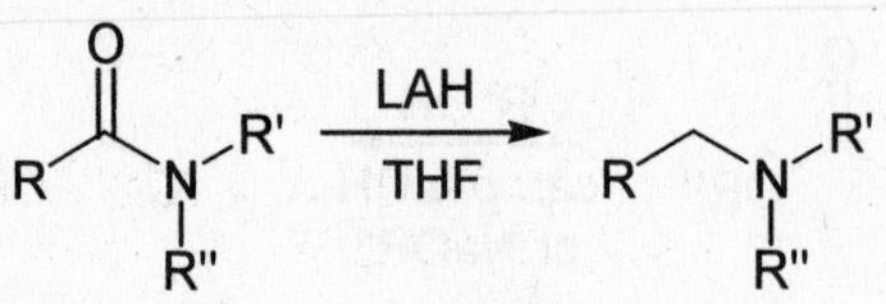

3. Reduction with diisobutylaluminum hydride (DIBAL) to form aldehydes:

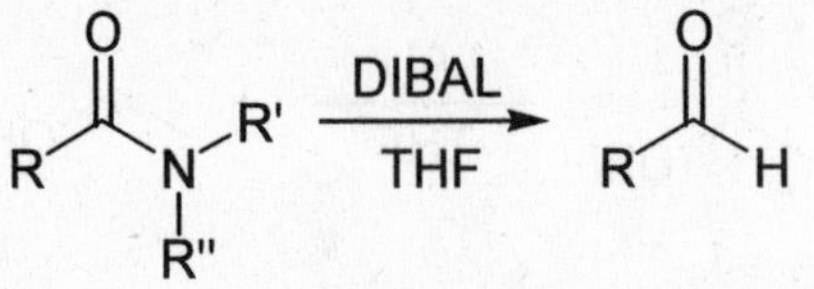

4. Conversion to amines with one less carbon through the Hofmann rearrangement:

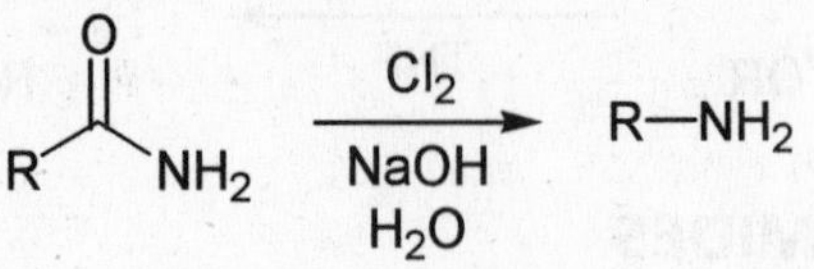

Epoxides

PREPARATION OF EPOXIDES

1. Oxidation of alkenes with oxygen transfer reagents:

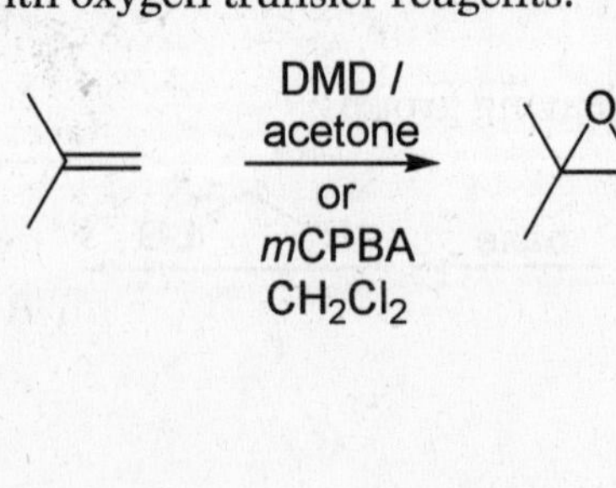

2. Base-catalyzed ring closure of halohydrins:

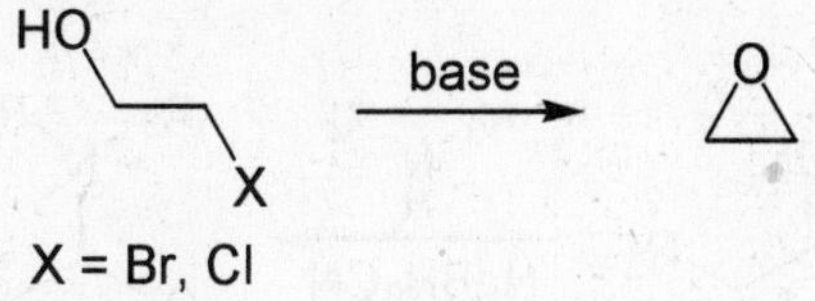

X = Br, Cl

REACTIONS OF EPOXIDES

1. Base-catalyzed nucleophilic ring-opening at the less hindered carbon:

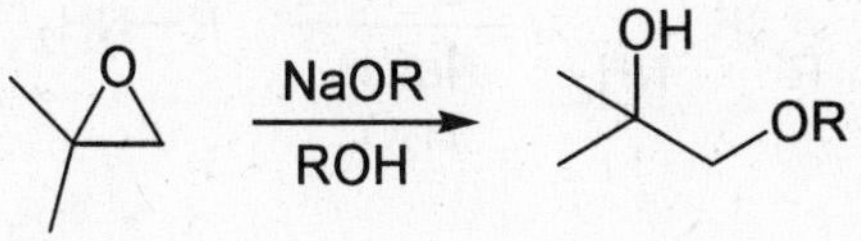

2. Acid-catalyzed nucleophilic ring-opening at the more substituted site:

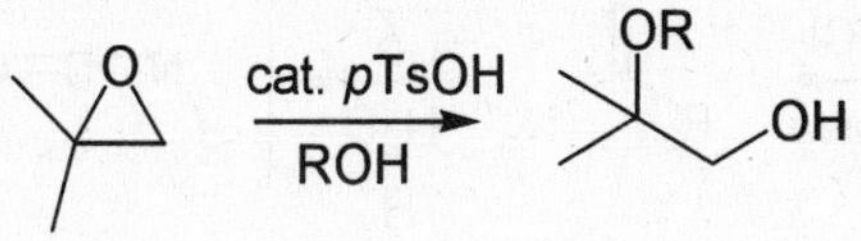

Amines

PREPARATION OF AMINES

1. Using phthalimide (the Gabriel synthesis):

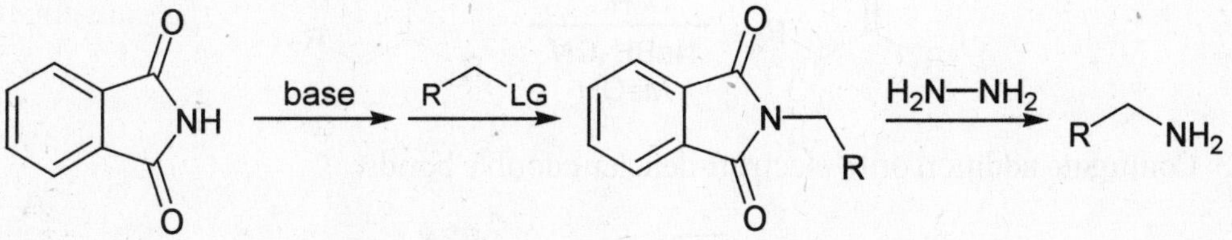

2. Direct alkylation of amide anions:

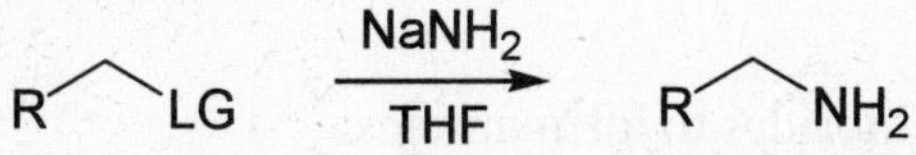

3. Reaction of azide anion with electrophiles, followed by reduction (the Staudinger reaction):

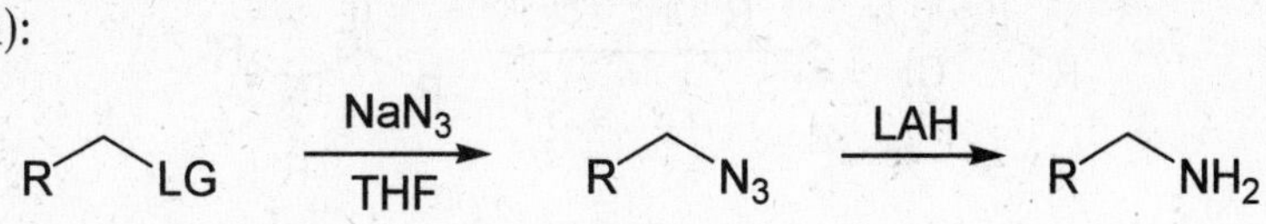

4. Reduction of carboxamides using lithium aluminum hydride:

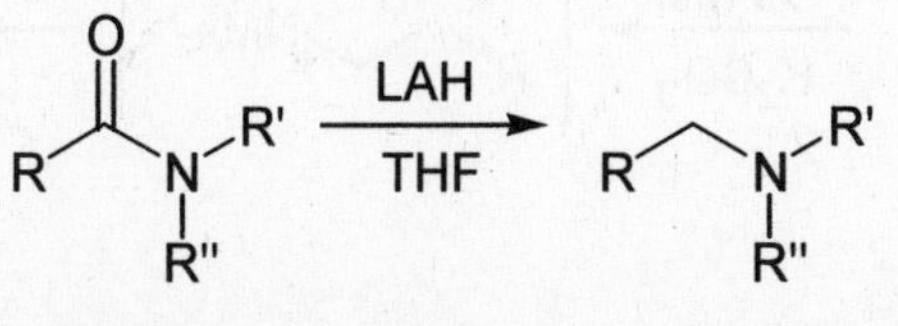

5. Reaction of ketones with amines in the presence of sodium cyanoborohydride (reductive amination):

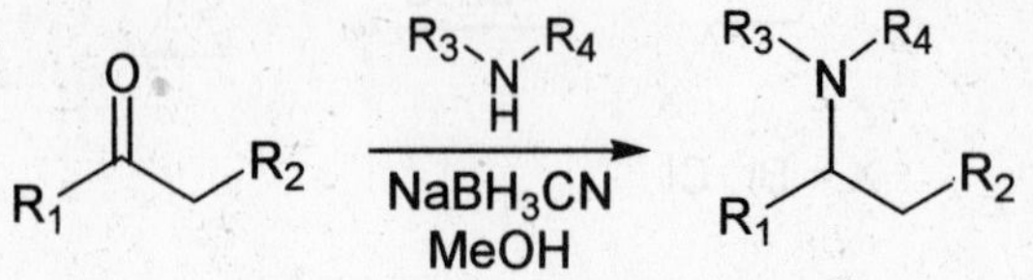

6. From carboxamides via the Hofmann rearrangement:

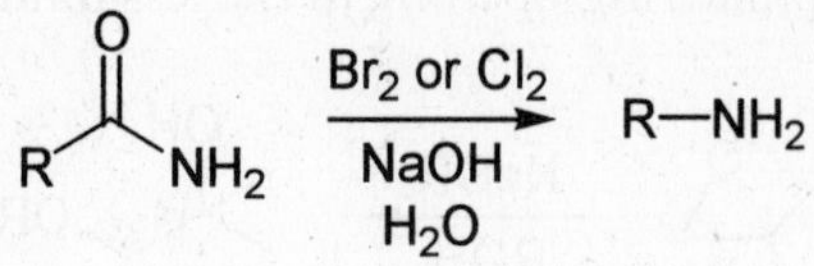

7. From carboxylic acids via the Curtius rearrangement:

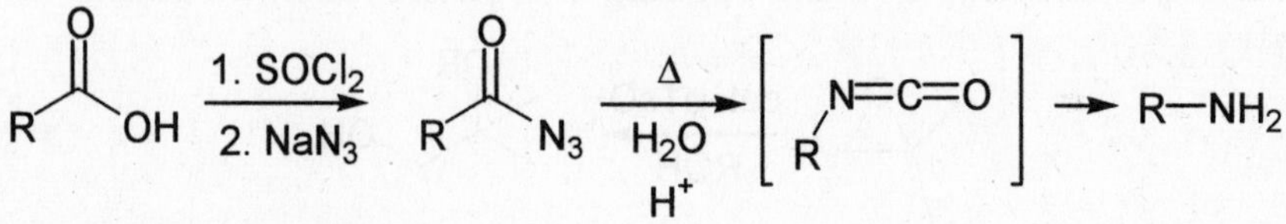

REACTIONS OF AMINES

1. Reaction with ketones in the presence of sodium cyanoborohydride (reductive amination):

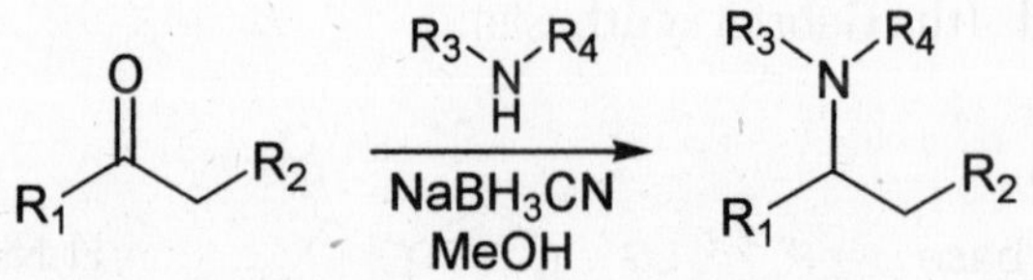

2. Conjugate addition onto electron-deficient double bonds:

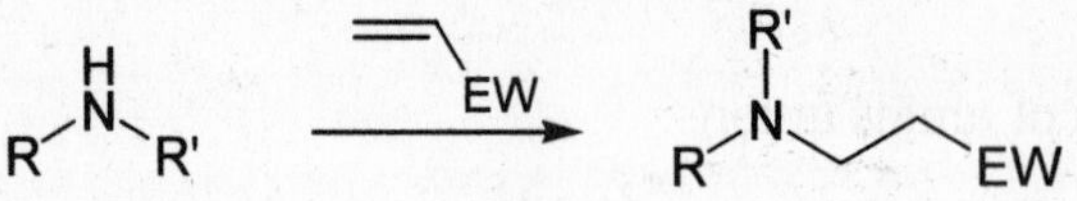

3. Reaction with acyl chlorides to form amides:

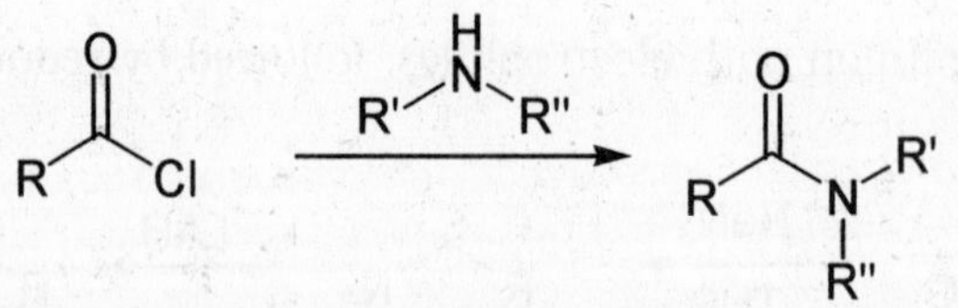

4. Conversion to alkenes via Hofmann elimination:

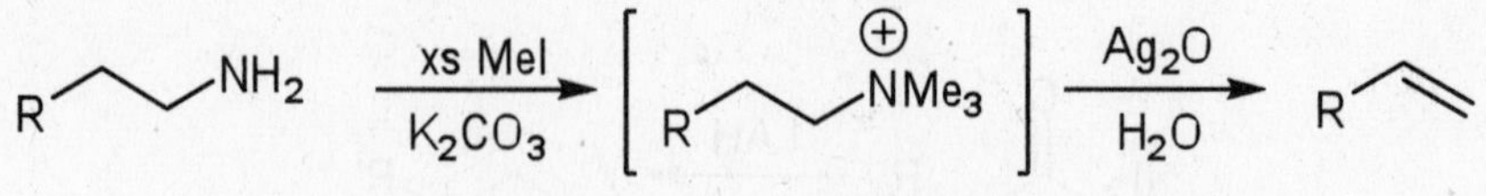

5. Reaction with primary amines to form imines:

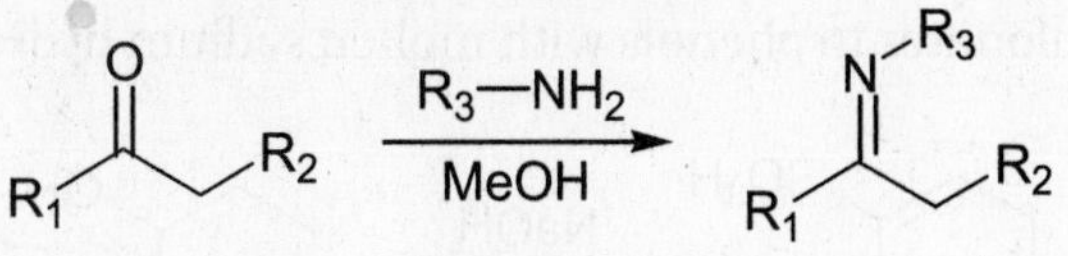

6. Reaction with secondary amines to form enamines:

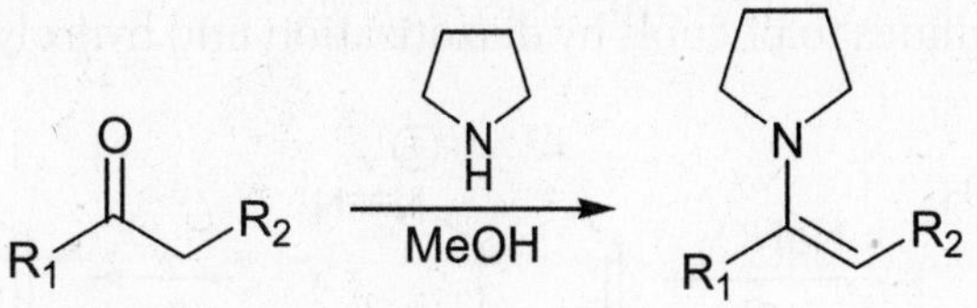

Aromatic Chemistry

FUNCTIONALIZATION OF BENZENE

1. Nitration:

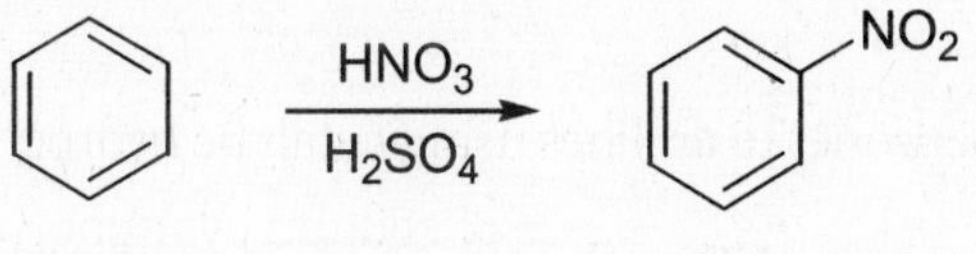

2. Sulfonation:

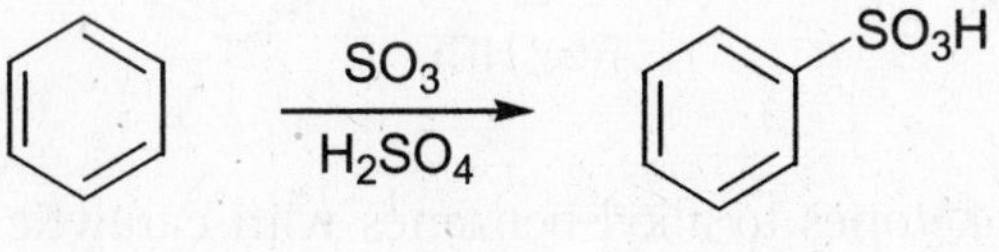

3. Halogenation:

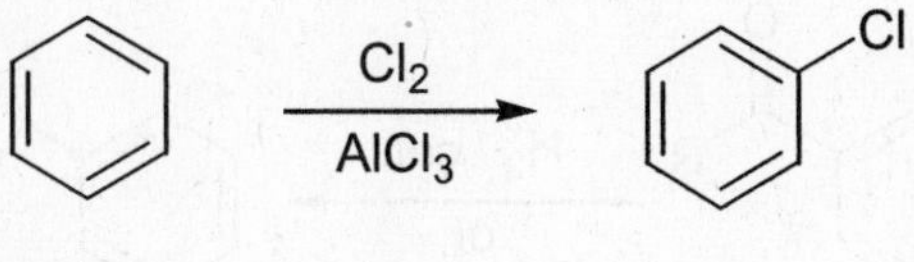

4. Friedel-Crafts alkylation:

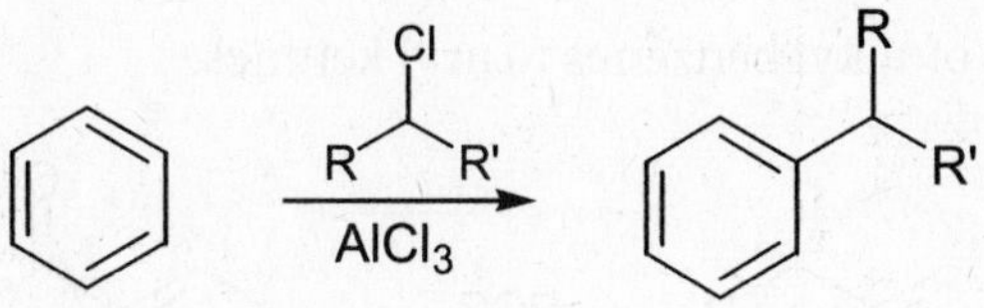

5. Friedel-Crafts acylation:

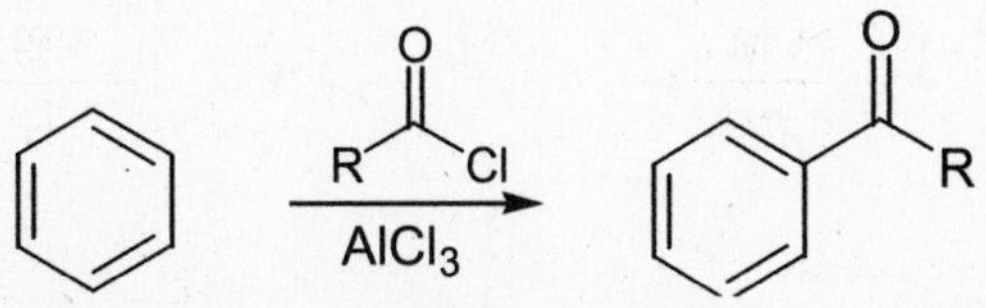

FUNCTIONAL GROUP TRANSFORMATIONS

1. Conversion of sulfonates to phenols with molten sodium hydroxide (fusion):

2. Conversion of anilines to phenols by diazotization and hydrolysis:

3. Nucleophilic aromatic substitution onto electron-deficient aryl halides:

4. Reduction of nitrobenzenes to anilines using catalytic hydrogenation or iron in HCl:

5. Reduction of aryl ketones to alkyl benzenes with catalytic hydrogenation or the action of zinc amalgam in HCl (the Clemmensen reduction):

6. Benzylic oxidation of alkyl benzenes to aryl ketones:

PART III. SEPARATION AND PURIFICATION

EXTRACTION

The basis of extraction techniques is the "like dissolves like" rule. Water typically dissolves inorganic salts (such as lithium chloride) and other ionized species, while organic solvents (ethyl acetate, methylene chloride, diethyl ether, etc.) dissolve neutral organic molecules. However, some compounds (e.g., alcohols) exhibit solubility in both media. Therefore, it is important to remember that this method of separation relies on partitioning—that is, the preferential dissolution of a species into one solvent over another. For example, 2-pentanol is somewhat soluble in water (about $17\,\text{g}/100\,\text{mL}\,H_2O$), but infinitely soluble in diethyl ether. Thus, 2-pentanol can be preferentially partitioned into ether.

One of the most common uses of extraction is during aqueous workup as a way to remove inorganic materials from the desired organic product. On a practical note, workup is usually carried out using two immiscible solvents—that is, in a biphasic system. If a reaction has been carried out in THF, dioxane, or methanol, then, it is generally desirable to remove those solvents by evaporation before workup, because they have high solubilities in both aqueous and organic phases, and can set up single-phase systems (that is, nothing to separate) or emulsions. Typical extraction solvents include ethyl acetate, hexane, chloroform, methylene chloride, and diethyl ether. All of these form crisp delineations between phases.

While extractions are usually carried out with a neutral aqueous phase, sometimes pH modulation can be used to advantage. For example, a mixture of naphthalenesulfonic acid and naphthalene can be separated by washing with bicarbonate, in which case the sulfonic acid is deprotonated and partitioned into the aqueous phase. Similarly, a mixture of naphthalene and quinoline can be separated by an acid wash

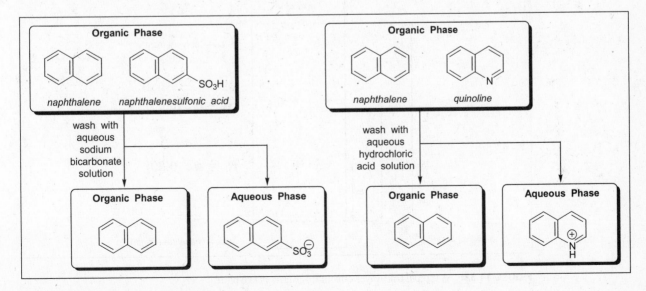

FIGURE 11.32: Two pH-controlled extractions

(Figure 11.32), taking advantage of the basic nature of the heterocyclic nitrogen (pK_a 9.5). If it is necessary to isolate the quinoline, it is neutralized with bicarbonate and extracted back into an organic solvent.

CHROMATOGRAPHY

Chromatography represents the most versatile separation technique readily available to the organic chemist. Conceptually, the technique is very simple—there are two components: a stationary phase (usually silica or cellulose) and a mobile phase (usually a solvent system). Any two compounds usually have different partitioning characteristics between the stationary and mobile phases. Since the mobile phase is moving (thus the name), then the more time a compound spends in that phase, the farther it will travel.

Chromatographic techniques fall into one of two categories: analytical and preparative. Analytical techniques are used to follow the course of reactions and determine purity of products. These methods include gas chromatography (GC), high-performance liquid chromatography (HPLC), and thin-layer chromatography (TLC). Sample sizes for these procedures are usually quite small, from microgram to milligram quantities. In some cases, the chromatographic method is coupled to another analytical instrument, such as a mass spectrometer or NMR spectrometer, so that the components that elute can be easily identified. Preparative methods are used to purify larger quantities of a compound for further use.

By far the most common chromatographic technique used in the laboratory is TLC. Figure 11.33 depicts a typical TLC plate developed in a 1:1 mixture of ethyl acetate and hexane, which exhibits two well-separated components. The spots can be characterized

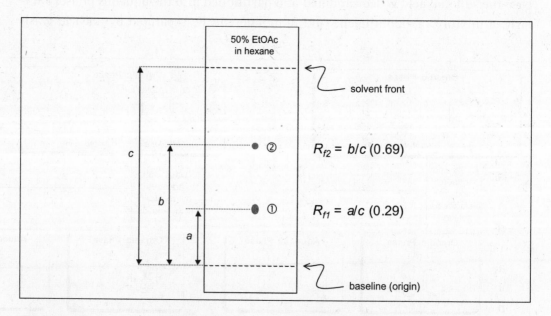

FIGURE 11.33: A typical thin-layer chromatography (TLC) plate

by their R_f value, which is defined as the distance traveled from the origin divided by the distance traveled by the mobile phase. Generally speaking, the slower-moving component (R_f 0.29) is either larger, more polar, or both. If we wanted a larger R_f value, we could boost the solvent polarity by increasing the proportion of ethyl acetate in the mobile phase. Conversely, more hexane would result in lower-running spots.

DISTILLATION AND SUBLIMATION

If chromatography is the most versatile separation method in the laboratory, it might be argued that distillation is the most common. This technique is used very frequently for purifying solvents and reagents before use. When volatile components are being removed from nonvolatile impurities, the method of *simple distillation* is employed (Figure 11.34). In this familiar protocol, a liquid is heated to the boil, forcing vapor into a water-cooled condensor, where it is converted back to liquid and is conveyed by gravity to a receiving flask.

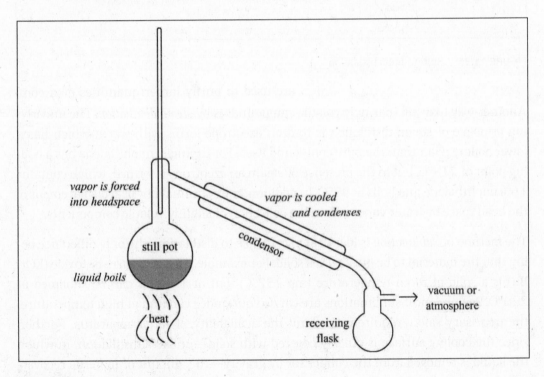

FIGURE 11.34: Simple distillation

When separating two liquids with similar boiling points—or substances that tend to form azeotropes—*fractional distillation* is used. In this method, a connector with large surface area (such as a Vigreux column) is inserted between the still pot and the distillation head. The purpose of this intervening portion is to provide greater surface area upon which the vapor can condense and revolatilize, leading to greater efficiency of separation. In more sophisticated apparatus, the Vigreux column and condensor are separated by an automated valve which opens intermittently, thus precisely controlling the rate of distillation.

For compounds with limited volatility, the technique of *bulb-to-bulb distillation* (Figure 11.35) is sometimes successful. In this distillation, the liquid never truly boils—that is to say, the vapor pressure of the compound does not reach the local pressure of the environment. Instead, the sample is placed in a flask (or bulb) and subjected to high vacuum and heat, which sets up a vapor pressure adequate to equilibrate through a passage to another bulb, which is cooled with air, water, or dry ice.

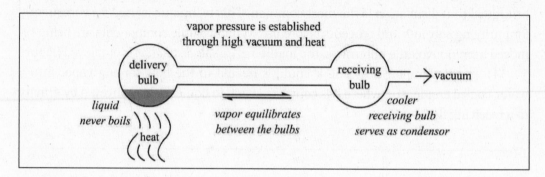

FIGURE 11.35: Bulb-to-bulb distillation

Another way to distill sparingly volatile compounds is by *steam distillation*. The underlying principle of steam distillation is that an azeotrope forms with water, which has a lower boiling point than the pure compound itself. For example, naphthalene has a boiling point of 218°C, but in the presence of steam an azeotrope is formed, which contains 16% naphthalene and boils at 99°C. In addition, the continual physical displacement of the head space by water vapor aids in the collection of slightly volatile components.

The method of *sublimation* is identical in principle to distillation, the only difference being that the material to be purified is a solid. For example, potassium *tert*-butoxide (KOt-Bu) is a solid at room temperature (mp 257°C), but at 1 torr it can be sublimed at 220°C. Because most sublimations are carried out under vacuum at high temperature, the necessary safety requirements limit the availability of large apparatus. Further, since the cooling surface is quickly covered with solid—unlike a distillation, in which the liquid is removed from the condensor by gravity—the amount of material recoverable from a single sublimation tends to be small.

RECRYSTALLIZATION

Chromatography is the most versatile method of purification, and distillation the most common, but recrystallization is the most elegant. Unfortunately, it is also the hardest to master and the most poorly comprehended by the beginning experimentalist. In essence, the principle is quite simple: coax one compound out of solution while leaving any impurities or byproducts dissolved, then separate the newly formed crystals from the solution.

Consider a 10 g sample of a substance (Compound A) which is contaminated with a 5% impurity (Compound B). Another way to express this is to say that we have a mixture of 9.5 g Compound A and 0.5 g Compound B. For the sake of discussion, let us say that both compounds happen to have the same solubility characteristics in methanol: 20 g/L at room temperature and 400 g/L at the boiling point of methanol. Therefore, 25 mL of boiling methanol should be sufficient to completely dissolve the sample, since it would have the capacity to dissolve 10 g of each substance (400 g/L × 0.025 L = 10 g). After the solution has cooled to room temperature, however, the methanol can only hold 0.5 g in solution (20 g/L × 0.025 L = 0.5 g). Inasmuch as 0.5 g of each compound remains dissolved, 9.0 g of Compound A and *none* of Compound B should be present as a precipitate. Thus, by simple filtration of this mixture Compound A can be obtained in pure form and 95% recovery (9.0 g recovered / 9.5 g originally = 0.95).

With this example in mind, it is easy to see that recrystallization works best if the sample is already relatively pure. Since Compound B is present in comparatively small amounts, its concentration is significantly lower than that of Compound A. In fact, paradoxically, we can sometimes remove a *less soluble component* by this method if it is present in small enough quantity. However, if we were presented with a 1:1 mixture of the compounds described above, the situation would not have been so straightforward.

PART IV. CHARACTERIZATION

OVERVIEW

The process of characterization is facilitated by several powerful analytical protocols. We will examine five of the more frequently encountered techniques, which can be divided into two broad categories. For example, Table 11.7 summarizes three nondestructive analytical methods based on absorption spectroscopy—that is, the interaction of light with matter. There are also two destructive methods (Table 11.8) that are still workhorses of structure determination—and while the sample is sacrificed for the analysis, the methods only require milligram quantities.

Table 11.7. Methods of nondestructive electromagnetic spectroscopy			
Method	**Transition observed**	**Absorption range**	**Provides information about**
UV-Vis	electronic	200–800 nm	extended π systems
IR	vibrational	600–4,000 cm^{-1}	functional groups
NMR	nuclear spin flip	25–1,000 MHz (instrument-dependent)	skeletal framework and 3-dimensional arrangement of atoms

Table 11.8. Two important destructive analytical techniques		
Method	**Principle**	**Provides information about**
Combustion analysis	samples undergo perfect combustion in excess O_2; combustion products are quantified	molecular composition
Mass spectrometry	samples are ionized and accelerated through a magnetic field; fragments are separated based on mass/charge ratio	molecular weight and structure

COMBUSTION ANALYSIS

Combustion analysis data are presented as weight percent of each given element, as shown in the boxed area of Figure 11.36. To be useful, though, these data must be converted to a mole ratio of elements. The first thing to recognize here is that the weight percent values for carbon, hydrogen, and nitrogen do not add up to 100%. Given the practical considerations above, we shall assume the balance is made up by oxygen (in this case, 12.58%), unless we have evidence from alternative analyses that other elements are present. Next, since we must leverage the mass quantities into molar ratios, a third column is introduced containing the atomic weights of all elements involved. Dividing the weight percent by the atomic weight gives a modified value designated χ, or molar contribution (fourth column), which has no particular meaning on its own; however, if we divide each χ value by the sum of all the χ values, we can express the elemental abundance as a mole percent value (fifth column). The final step is to find the molar ratio—the best way to approach this is to divide all mole percent values by the smallest value. For example, carbon is present in 31.80 mol% and nitrogen is present in 4.54 mol%; dividing 31.80 by 4.54, we can say that the molar ratio of carbon to nitrogen is 7.00:1.00 (sixth column).

work-up of analytical data

	Element	wt%	at. wt.	χ	mol%	mol ratio
provided by analysis	C	**66.10**	12.011	5.503	31.80	7.00
	H	**10.31**	1.0079	10.229	59.11	13.02
	N	**11.01**	14.007	0.786	4.54	1.00
	O	12.58	15.999	0.786	4.54	1.00
	Total	100.00		17.305	100.00	

FIGURE 11.36: Treatment of combustion analysis data

The empirical formula already can tell us much about the structure of the molecule, aside from the obvious benefit of knowing the identity and ratio of elements on board. One useful feature we can extract from the elemental data is the degree of unsaturation (DoU), also known as the index of hydrogen deficiency (IHD). Each double bond or ring in a compound confers one degree of unsaturation (Figure 11.37). For example, benzene has four degrees of unsaturation—one for the ring, and one for each double bond in the ring.

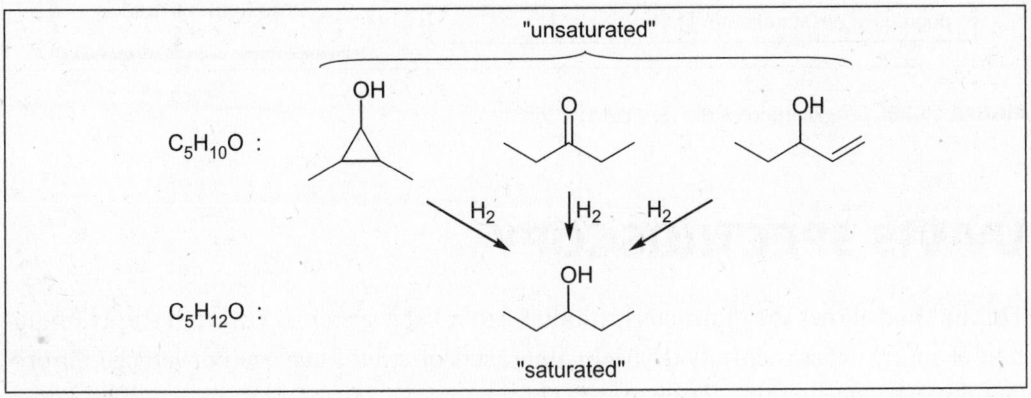

FIGURE 11.37: Saturated and unsaturated compounds

When presented with a molecular formula, the following method is useful in determining the degree of unsaturation:

1. Calculate the hydrogen count for the corresponding saturated molecule:
   a) Number of hydrogens = 2(number of carbons) + 2
   b) Oxygen (or any divalent species) has no effect on this count.
   c) For every nitrogen (or any trivalent species) add 1.
   d) For every halogen (or any monovalent species) subtract 1.

2. Compare the actual hydrogen count to the saturated hydrogen count:
   a) Divide the difference by 2 to get the DoU.
   b) If the difference is an odd number, recheck the math in step 1.

Applying these guidelines to an example, let us consider the empirical formula $C_5H_7N_2OCl$ (Figure 11.38). Since the formula has five carbons, we would predict twelve (2n + 2) hydrogen atoms for a simple hydrocarbon. The presence of oxygen has no effect on this value, but we adjust the hydrogen count up by two on account of the two nitrogen atoms, and then down by one because of the monovalent chlorine. The adjusted saturation count for hydrogen is thus thirteen. The empirical formula has only seven, for a difference of six—dividing this value by two gives three degrees of unsaturation. With this in hand, we can limit our consideration to those molecules that exhibit the proper degree of unsaturation—one such example is shown in the inset.

DoU Calculation for $C_5H_7N_2OCl$	
"normal" saturation count	12
modification for oxygen	0
modification for nitrogen	+2
modification for chlorine	−1
adjusted saturation count	13
actual hydrogen count	7
Δ between actual and saturated	6
degrees of unsaturation (Δ Π 2)	3

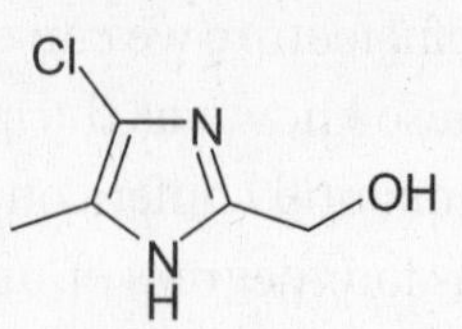

one of many structures
consistent with the
empirical formula

FIGURE 11.38: Application of the DoU calculation

UV-VIS SPECTROSCOPY

This method allows the characterization of extended π systems. Through the examination of many experimentally derived values, sets of rules have been developed for predicting the wavelength of maximum absorbance (λ_{max}) for various substrates as a function of structure, work carried out primarily by Woodward, Fieser, and Nielsen. A brief summary of these rules is presented in Table 11.9. While not immediately intuitive, they are straighforward to apply once the framework is understood, and they are very powerful predictive tools.

Table 11.9. Abbreviated rules for predicting λ_{max} for UV-Vis absorptions

		dienes	enones and enals				benzophenones, benzaldehydes, and benzoic acids		
base chromophore									
base absorbance λ_{max} (nm)		214	202	215		245 208 (R=H)	246 250 (R=H)		230
modifications to the base absorbance									
substituents	position	all	α	β	γ	δ	o	m	p
	-R	5	10	12	18	18	3	3	10
	-OR	6	35	30	17	31	7	7	25
	-Br	5	25	30	25	25	2	2	15
	-Cl	5	15	12	12	12	0	0	10
	-NR$_2$	60		95			20	20	85
π system architecture	double bond extending conjugation	+ 30 nm							
	exocyclic character of a double bond	+ 5 nm					not typically relevant		
	homoannular diene component	+ 39 nm							

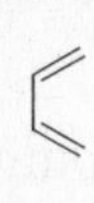

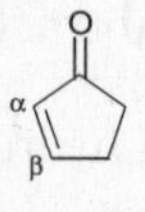

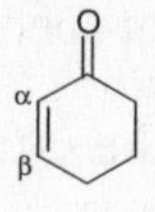

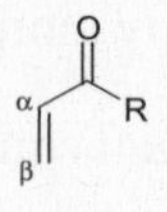

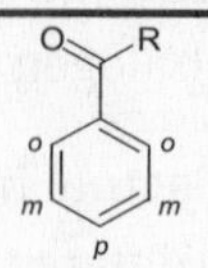

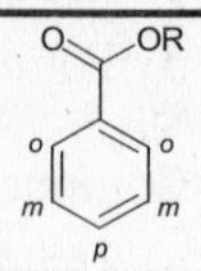

Two specialized terminologies also deserve mention. First, a *homoannular diene* refers to any two double bonds that are incorporated into the same ring. Therefore, 1,3-cyclohexadiene would be considered a homoannular diene, but cyclohex-2-enone would not, since only one double bond is incorporated into the ring itself. For every instance of a homoannular component, we add 39 nm to the base absorbance. Second, even though the etymology of an exocyclic double bond means "outside the ring," it is best thought of as a double bond that terminates in a ring. Each time this occurs, we add 5 nm to the base absorbance.

To get some practice in applying these rules, consider the tricyclic enone shown in Figure 11.39. We choose the base absorption of 215 (six-membered-ring enone) and tack on three double bonds to extend the conjugation (30 nm each for 90 nm total). We have thus established the domain of the chromophore (shown in red). It is often helpful to highlight the chromophore for accounting purposes, even by darkening in with a pencil. Examination of the chromophore thus reveals that ring C houses one homoannular diene component, so we add 39 nm to the ledger. Careful scrutiny also reveals two occurrences of exocyclic double bonds: both the α, β and the $\varepsilon\zeta$ olefins terminate in ring B. We add 5 nm for each occurrence.

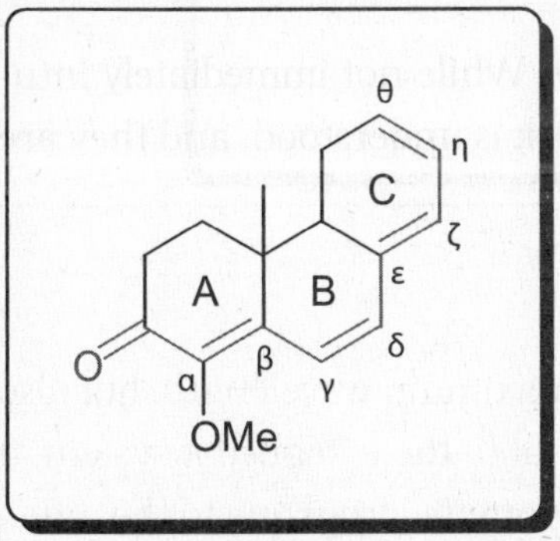

Base chromophore (6-ring enone)	215
3 x double bond extensions	+ 90
homoannular diene (in ring C)	+ 39
2 x exocyclic double bonds	+ 10
α -alkoxy substituent	+ 35
β -alkyl substituent	+ 12
ε -alkyl substituent (same as γ)	+ 18
θ -alkyl substituent (same as γ)	+ 18
Predicted λ_{max}	437

FIGURE 11.39: Example in the application of predictive UV-Vis rules

The accounting of substituents is sometimes tricky, particularly for cyclic molecules. First, we must recognize that the substituent connected to the carbonyl group is already accounted for, so we do not double-count it. We start instead with the methoxy substituent in the α-position, which adds 35 nm to the chromophore. The rest of the substituents are dealt with in the same manner. To help sort out what are bona fide substituents, imagine the chromophore (red portion) is a hallway we could walk through—how many doorways would we see and in what positions? Thus, starting from the carbonyl, we would see a door to our right at the α-position, one on our left at the β-position, another left door at ε, and finally a left door at θ. For accounting purposes, it matters not that there are substituents attached to those substituents (it also is inconsequential whether the "doors" are on the right or left—it simply helps us visualize the virtual corridor).

The intensity of the absorbance can also be diagnostic. For example, in the tricyclic enone above we would expect to see at least two bands in the UV-Vis spectrum. The absorbance calculated in Figure 11.39 corresponds to the $\pi \rightarrow \pi^*$ transition from the HOMO to the LUMO. However, the lone pair electrons on oxygen can also undergo excitation. Since they are technically not connected to the extended π system, they are neither bonding nor antibonding; therefore, they are considered nonbonding (n) electrons. The absorption is thus designated an $n \rightarrow \pi^*$ transition (Figure 11.40). Because the energy gap is smaller, this absorption occurs at higher wavelengths than the $\pi \rightarrow \pi^*$ transitions.

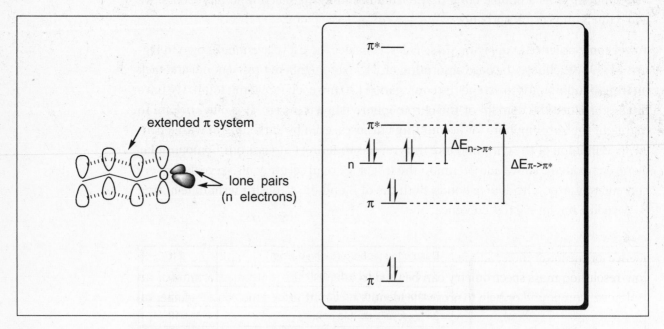

FIGURE 11.40: Two possible electronic transitions in enones

The two types of excitation events differ not only in the maximum wavelength, but also in intensity. Since the lone pairs are essentially orthogonal to the extended π system, it would seem difficult to imagine how electrons could be promoted from one to the other. Indeed, these $n \rightarrow \pi^*$ events are known as symmetry-forbidden electronic transitions. Like so many other forbidden things, they still happen, but the quantum efficiency is much lower; therefore, the intensity of the absorption is considerably weaker than the $\pi \rightarrow \pi^*$absorption.

MASS SPECTROMETRY

Mass spectrometry is based on the principle of differentiating molecules by accelerating charged species through a strong magnetic field or across a voltage potential, in which behavior is dictated by the charge-to-mass ratio of the ions. The classical method for ion generation is known as EI, or electron impact. Here a sample is bombarded with very high-energy electrons, which transfer energy into the molecules, much as photons of visible light induce the formation of an excited state in UV-Vis spectroscopy. However, these excited species are so energetic that the only way to relax is by releasing an electron, thereby forming a radical cation, as shown in Figure 11.41. This species is known as the molecular ion.

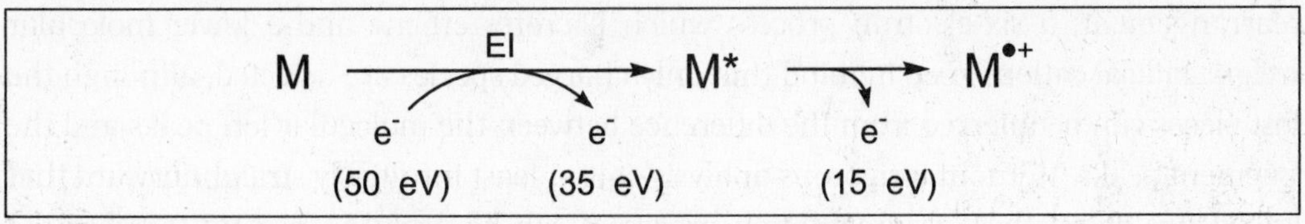

FIGURE 11.41: Formation of a molecular ion by electron impact (EI)

Once formed, these ions are accelerated through some differentiating field. The classical approach for differentiation is to pass the beam of charged particles through a magnetic field, which refracts the ions based on their charge to mass ratios and velocities. If we assume that only one electron is lost (that is, the charge of all species is +1), then the time of flight can be directly correlated to mass—thus, the name "mass spectrometry."

Indeed, some of the most useful information from this technique derives from the mass of the molecular ion. For example, while combustion analysis gives information about the atomic ratios within a molecule, it does not provide a definitive value for the molecular weight. In other words, a compound with molecular formula $C_6H_{12}O$ would give the same elemental analysis results as a $C_{12}H_{24}O_2$ compound. However, mass spectrometry can provide this missing information: a molecular ion peak at 200 amu is very strong evidence for the latter molecular formula. Thus the combination of elemental analysis and low-resolution mass spectrometry can be used to establish the molecular formula of an unknown compound or help to prove the identity of a synthesized molecule—elemental analysis provides the ratio of elements and mass spectrometry fixes the total weight.

Moreover, the very decomposition processes that diminish the molecular ion peak can themselves provide important structural information about the substrate. As one example, radical cations derived from ketones undergo fragmentation in the vicinity of the carbonyl. Figure 11.42 shows two such processes for 2-methylhexan-3-one. The first involves σ bond cleavage, in which the isopropyl radical and an acyl cation are formed from the initial radical cation. The molecular ion can also undergo the McLafferty

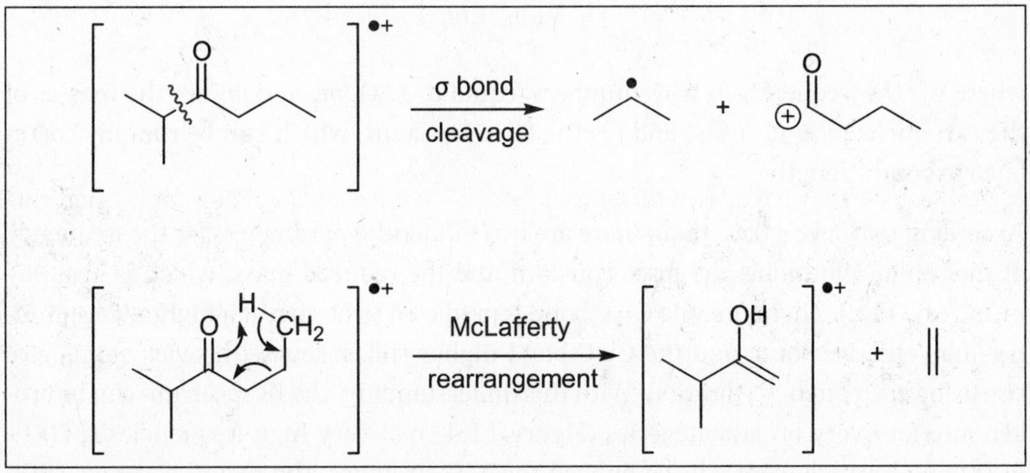

FIGURE 11.42: Two fragmentation processes for 2-methylhexan-3-one radical cation

rearrangement, a six-electron process which liberates ethene and a lower molecular weight radical cation. Keep in mind that only charged species are detected, although the lost pieces can be inferred from the difference between the molecular ion peaks and the fragment peaks. Without a rigorous analysis, it is at least intuitively straightforward that knowledge about these fragmentation processes can be useful in piecing together the structure of the original compound. Indeed, the painstaking interpretation of fragmentation patterns was once *de rigeur* for structure proof; however, the increasingly powerful (and more convenient) technique of NMR has provided an alternative source of structural knowledge available previously only from MS data.

Another very diagnostic feature in mass spectroscopy is the isotopic fingerprint left by bromine and chlorine. Unlike, carbon, hydrogen, nitrogen, and oxygen, which have one overwhelmingly predominant isotope (^{1}H, 99.98%; ^{12}C, 98.93%; ^{14}N, 99.62%; ^{16}O, 99.76%), bromine has two almost equally abundant natural isotopes (^{79}Br, 50.51%; ^{81}Br, 49.49%), and chlorine has a roughly 3:1 ratio of isomers in nature (^{35}Cl, 75.47%; ^{37}Cl, 24.53%). The practical result of this phenomenon is that molecules containing chlorine or bromine leave characteristic M+2 patterns in a ratio of 1:1 or 3:1, depending upon which halogen is present.

INFRARED SPECTROSCOPY

Just like the electronic transitions, movement among vibrational energy levels is quantized and can be studied through spectrophotometric methods. For most vibrational excitations, absorption occurs in the infrared region of the spectrum. Although governed by quantum considerations, many vibrational modes can be modeled using classical physics. For example, a stretching vibration between two nuclei can be characterized using Hooke's Law, which predicts that the frequency of an absorbance is given by the relationship

$$\bar{v} = k \sqrt{\dfrac{f}{\left(\dfrac{m_1 m_2}{m_1 + m_2}\right)}}$$

where $\bar{v}$ is the frequency in wavenumbers (equal to $1/\lambda$), m_1 and m_2 are the masses of the two nuclei in amu units, and f is the force constant, which can be roughly correlated to bond strength.

According to Hooke's Law, then, there are two influential parameters for the frequency of molecular vibrations: the force constant and the reduced mass, which is given by $m_1 m_2 / (m_1 + m_2)$. Therefore, the C=C bond is predicted to absorb at a higher wavenumber than the C-C bond, and the C≡C bond higher still. Likewise, heavier atoms give rise to lower-frequency vibration. With this understanding, the IR spectrum can be broken into four very broad categories (Figure 11.43): at very high frequencies (2500 – 4000 cm^{-1}) we see what can be dubbed the X-H stretches; the region between 1900 and 2500 cm^{-1} is home to the triple bonds; the region between 1500 and 1900 cm^{-1}

houses many of the doubly bonded species, including alkene and carbonyl stretches; and the portion of the spectrum bounded by 400 and 1500 cm⁻¹ is known as the fingerprint region.

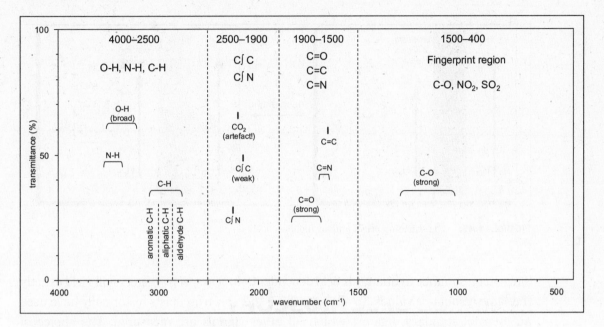

FIGURE 11.43:   Overview of infrared absorbance ranges

PROTON NMR SPECTROSCOPY

When nuclei are placed in a strong magnetic field, the spin states become nondegenerate; nuclei in the lower-energy spin state can then be promoted to the next level by the absorption of electromagnetic radiation of the appropriate energy, as depicted in Figure 11.44.

In a local environment in which the electron cloud has been impoverished (by the inductive effect of an electronegative atom, for example), the nucleus is shielded less and

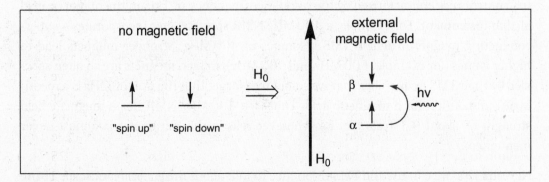

FIGURE 11.44:   The splitting of degenerate nuclear spin states

thus experiences a stronger "effective" magnetic field (H_{eff}) (Figure 11.45). Consequently, the energy splitting is enhanced and the resonance occurs at correspondingly higher frequency. This phenomenon of higher-frequency absorbances in electron-poor regions is known as deshielding.

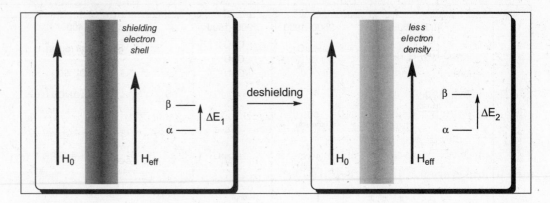

FIGURE 11.45: The shielding effect and deshielding

Since the resonance frequency is field dependent, no two spectrometers will yield exactly the same resonance values. To alleviate this issue, spectroscopists historically have used an internal standard, against which all other signals are measured. The choice of tetramethylsilane (TMS, Figure 11.46) as an NMR standard was driven by a few practical considerations. First, it is thermally stable and liquid at room temperature; second, it has twelve protons that are identical, so the intensity of absorption is high; and finally, the protons in TMS are quite shielded (silicon is not particularly electronegative), so almost all other proton resonances we observe occur at higher frequencies relative to TMS.

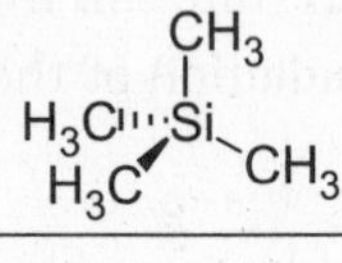

$$H_3C\overset{\displaystyle CH_3}{\underset{\displaystyle H_3C}{\cdots Si \cdots}} CH_3$$

FIGURE 11.46: The NMR standard, tetramethylsilane (TMS)

Instruments are characterized by the resonance frequency of TMS in the magnetic field of that instrument. For example, a 400 MHz NMR spectrometer incorporates a superconducting magnet in which TMS resonates at 400 MHz. Stronger magnets lead to higher values (for example, 600 MHz and 900 MHz); in fact, magnets are so often specified by their TMS frequencies that we sometimes forget that the unit of MHz is a meaningless dimension for a magnetic field. That is, a 400 MHz NMR has a magnetic field strength of about 9.3 Tesla, yet for whatever reason this parameter is almost never mentioned.

Nevertheless, we can use the TMS resonance to talk about the general landscape of the NMR spectrum. Figure 11.47 shows a typical measurement domain for a 400 MHz spectrometer, which is bounded on the right by the resonance frequency of TMS (400,000,000 Hz). The range through which most organic molecules absorb extends to about 400,004,000 Hz, or 4000 Hz relative to TMS. However, these values change as magnetic field strength is altered—an absorbance at 2000 Hz on a 400 MHz NMR would absorb at 1000 Hz on a 200 MHz NMR. To normalize these values, we instead report signals in terms of parts per million (ppm), which is defined as:

$$ppm = \frac{v}{R} = \frac{Hz}{MHz}$$

where v is the signal frequency (in Hz) relative to TMS and R is the base resonance frequency of TMS (in MHz). Thus, on a 400 MHz instrument a signal at 2,000 Hz would be reported as 5 ppm (2,000 Hz / 400 MHz). This allows us to establish a universal scale for proton NMR ranging from 0 to about 10 ppm—although it is not terribly uncommon to find protons that absorb outside that range.

Working within this framework, it is important to understand certain features and terminology related to position in the NMR spectrum. First, the ppm scale obscures the fact that frequency increases to the left, so this must be borne in mind. Thus, as protons are deshielded, they are shifted to the left—spectroscopists have dubbed this a "downfield" shift. Similarly, migrating to the right of the spectrum is said to be moving upfield. Phenomenologically, a downfield shift is evidence of deshielding, and this understanding will help us interpret NMR data.

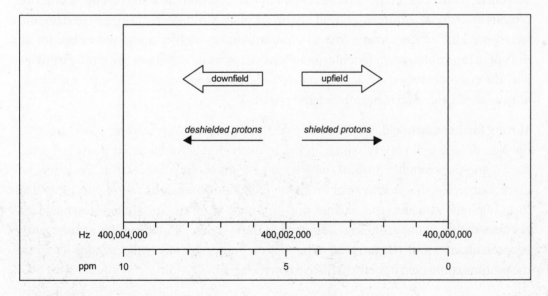

FIGURE 11.47: Important architectural features of the ^{1}H NMR spectrum

Using this idea, we can establish general regions in the NMR spectrum where various proton types tend to congregate (Figure 11.48). For example, most purely aliphatic compounds (hexane, etc.) absorb far upfield in the vicinity of 1 ppm. The attachment of electron-withdrawing groups (e.g., carbonyls) tends to pull resonances downfield.

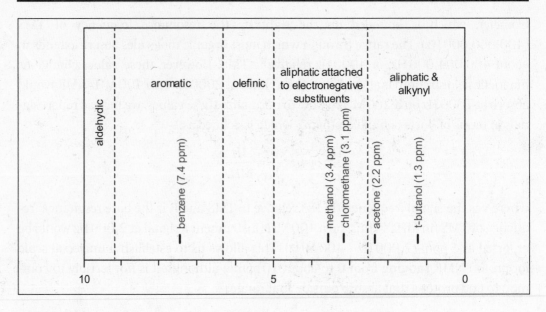

FIGURE 11.48: General regions of the ^{1}H NMR spectrum, with benchmarks

Thus, the protons on acetone show up at around 2.2 ppm. In general, the region between 0 and 2.5 ppm can be thought of as home to protons attached to carbons attached to carbon (H-C-C). This is also where terminal alkyne protons absorb.

As electronegative elements are attached, however, resonances are shifted even farther downfield. Thus, the methyl protons on methanol resonate at about 3.4 ppm, and the protons on chloromethane appear at about 3.1 ppm. Multiple electronegative elements have an additive effect: compared to chloromethane, dichloromethane resonates at 5.35 ppm, and chloroform (trichloromethane) absorbs at 7.25 ppm. As a rough guideline, the region between 2.5 and 5 ppm belongs to protons attached to carbons which are attached to an electronegative element (H-C-X).

Moving farther downfield, we encounter protons attached to sp^{2} carbons, starting with the olefinic (alkenyl) variety, which absorb in the region between about 5 and 6.5 ppm. Next come the aromatic protons, which range from about 6.5 to 9 ppm. As a benchmark, benzene—the prototypical aromatic compound—absorbs at 7.4 ppm. Just like their aliphatic cousins, the olefinic and aromatic protons are shifted downfield as electron-withdrawing groups are attached to the systems. Finally, signals in the region between about 9 and 10 ppm tend to be very diagnostic for aldehydic protons—that is, the protons connected directly to the carbonyl carbon.

Additional information can be derived from a phenomenon known as scalar (or spin-spin) coupling, through which a proton is influenced by its nearest neighbors. For example, consider a proton (H_x) which is vicinal to a pair of protons (H_a and H_b). The latter two protons are either spin up or spin down, and in fact we can imagine four permutations (2^2) of two nuclei with two states to choose from. If both H_a and H_b are aligned with the external magnetic field, they will serve to enhance H_{eff}, thereby increasing the energy gap between the H_x α and β states, which in turn leads to a higher frequency absorbance (a downfield shift). Conversely, the situation in which both H_a and H_b oppose the external magnetic field diminishes the H_{eff}, leading to an upfield shift. The two remaining permutations have one spin up and the other spin down, thereby cancelling each other out. The result is a pattern known as a triplet, in which the three prongs of the signal are present in a 1:2:1 ratio. In other words, the pattern exhibited (or "multiplicity") has one more prong than the number of neighboring protons. Patterns of this type are said to obey the "n+1 rule," where n = the number of neighboring protons, and n + 1 = the multiplicity of the signal. The most common splitting patterns and their abbreviations are summarized in Table 11.10.

Table 11.10. Some common splitting patterns	
Abbr.	**Pattern**
s	singlet
d	doublet
t	triplet
q	quartet
quint	quintet
m	multiplet

So the chemical shift tells us about a proton's electronic environment, and splitting patterns tell us about the number of neighboring protons—but still the spectrum has further information to yield. It turns out that the area under each signal is proportional to the number of protons giving rise to that signal. Therefore, integrating the area under the curves allows us to establish a ratio for all chemically distinct protons in the NMR. As an illustration, Figure 11.49 presents a portion of the NMR spectrum of ethylbenzene corresponding to the ethyl moiety. There are two signals (at 1.15 ppm and 2.58 ppm), corresponding to the two sets of chemically distinct protons on the ethyl substituent (a methyl and methylene group, respectively). The downfield shift of the methylene group is an indication of its being closer to the slightly electron-withdrawing benzene ring. The splitting patterns tell us that the protons resonating at 1.15 (the triplet) are next to two other protons, and the protons at 2.58 (the quartet) are adjacent to three other protons. Furthermore, the integral traces reveal that the two sets of protons are present in a 3:2 ratio.

Generally speaking, protons connected to the same carbon (geminal protons) do not split each other—with one significant exception. Figure 11.50 shows three types of geminal protons: homotopic, enantiotopic, and diastereotopic. To better understand the terminology, consider the imaginary products formed by replacing each of the two geminal protons with another atom, say a chlorine substituent. In the homotopic example, the two "products" are identical (2-chloropropane); for the enantiotopic protons, two enantiomeric "products" are formed (*R*- and *S*-(1-chloroethyl)benzene); and replacing H_a with H_b in the cyclopropane derivative gives diastereomers (*cis*-dichloro vs. *trans*-dichloro).

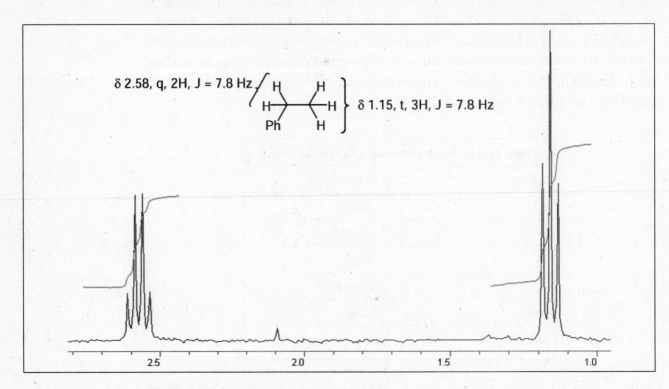

FIGURE 11.49: The ethyl moiety of ethyl benzene

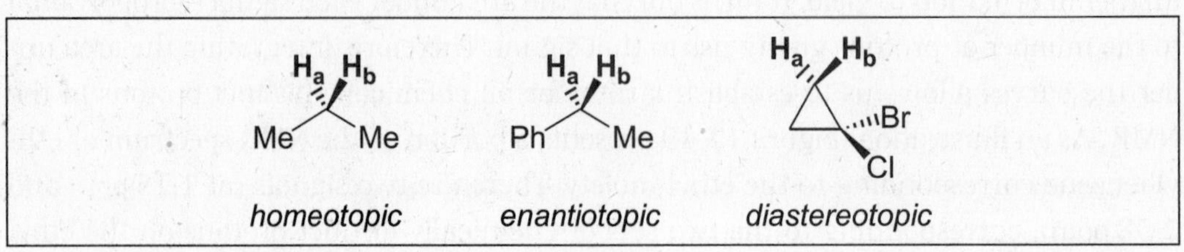

FIGURE 11.50: Three types of geminal protons

Homotopic and enantiotopic geminal protons do not split each other, because they are chemically equivalent. In other words, they are identical through a plane of symmetry (the plane of this page). However, diastereotopic protons are not chemically equivalent—in the example above, H_a is in proximity to the chloro substituent, whereas H_b is close to the bromine. In short, they are in different worlds and therefore behave as individuals. Therefore, in these special cases, geminal protons do split each other, and the magnitude of the *J*-value is relatively large. Figure 11.51 lists this value, along with other representative coupling constants. This summary will be useful for the interpretation of spectra.

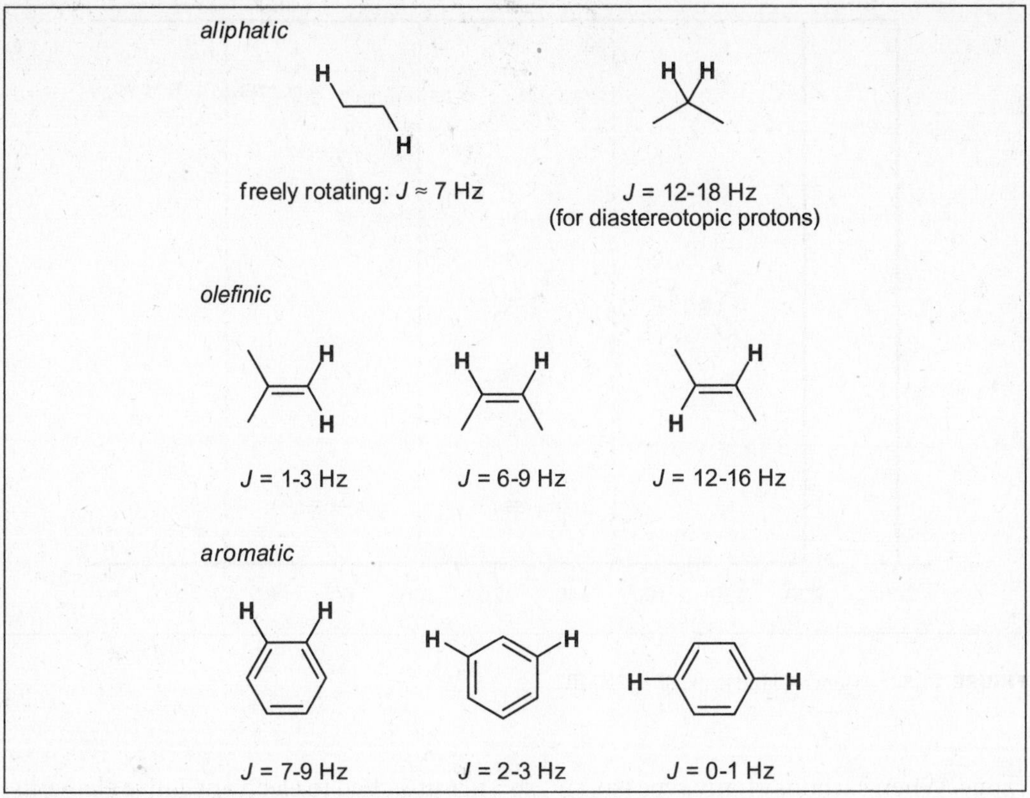

FIGURE 11.51: Some representative coupling constants

CARBON NMR SPECTROSCOPY

The principle of ^{13}C NMR is identical to that of ^{1}H NMR; however, there are a few practical differences that deserve mention. First, while the natural abundance of ^{1}H is almost 100%, the ^{13}C isotope makes up only slightly over 1% of carbon found in nature. This means that the NMR-active carbon nucleus is quite dilute in the typical molecule. As a result, signal-to-noise ratios tend to be lower and data collection times are usually longer. Moreover, although scalar coupling can exist (in principle) between two ^{13}C nuclei, the statistical likelihood that a pair of this species will be situated adjacent to each other is vanishingly small. Carbon can also couple to ^{1}H nuclei, which are plentiful, but most experimental methods wipe out this interaction with a technique known as off-resonance decoupling in order to simplify the spectrum.

Figure 11.52 provides a broad overview of ^{13}C resonances. In the 0-50 ppm range are mostly aliphatic carbons attached to nothing in particular. When π systems are introduced, a dramatic downfield shift occurs through an effect known as anisotropy—areas above and below the π bonds tend to be shielded, while the middle areas tend to be strongly deshielded. Thus, alkenes and aromatic carbons show up in the general region of 100–150 ppm. In alkynes an opposite anisotropic effect occurs: the barrel-like π structure of the alkyne sets up an electronic current whose field lines actually shield at the ends of the triple bond. Therefore, acetylenic carbons resonate in the 50–100

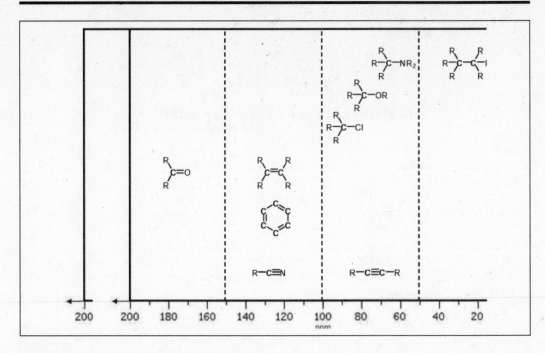

FIGURE 11.52: General landscape of ^{13}C NMR

range. When carbons of any type (sp, sp^2, sp^3) are attached to electronegative elements, a downfield shift occurs. Thus, aliphatics are moved into the 50–100 ppm region, acetylenics (nitriles) are moved into the 100–150 range, and olefinics (carbonyls) migrate to the 150–200 ppm region.

The combination of this wide landscape with the sharp singlet signals means that every unique carbon in a molecule usually can be resolved in a ^{13}C spectrum. This is useful because it can reveal important information about symmetry within a molecule. For example, 2-nitroaniline and 3-nitroaniline (Figure 11.53) exhibit 6 carbon peaks, as we would expect. However, 4-nitroaniline only has 4 carbon signals because of its inherent symmetry.

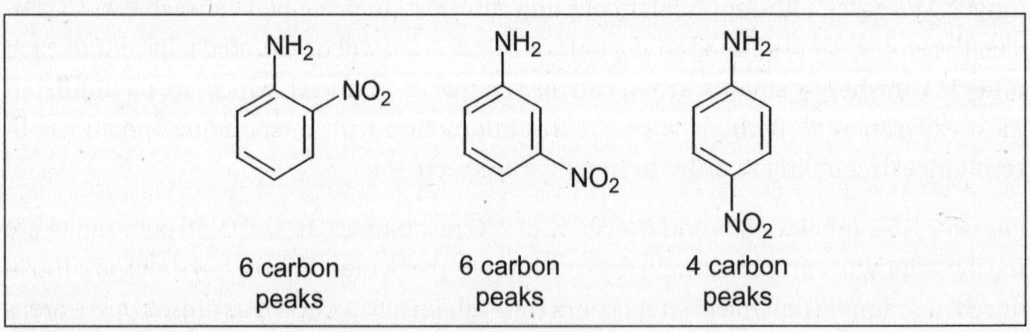

6 carbon
peaks

6 carbon
peaks

4 carbon
peaks

FIGURE 11.53: Impact of symmetry on ^{13}C NMR spectrum

Organic Chemistry

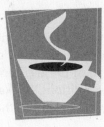

1. Bonding.   The most common bonds found in organic chemistry are:
- ➤ **Covalent bonds** between atoms of very similar electronegativity
- ➤ **Polar covalent bonds** between atoms of moderately differing electronegativity
- ➤ **Ionic bonds** between atoms of vastly differing electronegativity in their ionic form

The connectivity of bonds in molecules can be shown by **Lewis structures,** which sometimes are depicted using multiple **resonance forms**. These forms are evaluated using the following criteria:
- ➤ Each atom should have an octet of electrons (although fewer are possible).
- ➤ No row 2 atom can have more than an octet.
- ➤ Structures should minimize charge separation.
- ➤ Charge separation should follow electronegativity.

2. Molecular Shape.   The shape of a molecule is ultimately driven by the **central atom geometry** at each atomic center, which in turn is determined by **atomic orbital hybridization**. For carbon, these are:
- ➤ **sp hybridization**, which results in linear geometry and 180° bond angles
- ➤ **sp^2 hybridization**, which results in trigonal planar geometry and 120° bond angles
- ➤ **sp^3 hybridization**, which results in tetrahedral geometry and 109.4° bond angles

When a tetrahedral center is surrounded by four unique groups, the center is said to be an **asymmetric center** (or stereocenter). Compounds with asymmetric centers are almost always **chiral** (or handed), and they exist as two **enantiomers** (or nonsuperimposable mirror images).

Molecules can adopt many **conformations** (relative arrangements of atoms or groups), which are usually rapidly interconverting. For open-chain compounds (such as butane), the most important conformations are **staggered** (most stable) and **eclipsed** (least stable). In staggered conformations, substituents on adjacent atoms that are farthest from each other are said to be **antiperiplanar**; those that are next to each other are **gauche**. In eclipsed conformations, all substituents are **eclipsed**.

3. Electronic Structure.   Atomic orbitals are combined by the method of linear combination of atomic orbitals (LCAO) to form new **molecular orbitals** (MOs). The number of molecular orbitals obtained is equal to the number of atomic orbitals used to make them. Usually, there are an equal number of **bonding orbitals** (of lower energy than disconnected atoms) and **antibonding orbitals** (of higher energy than disconnected atoms).

When π bonds are next to each other in a 1,3-relationship, they form **extended π systems**, in which the π bonds are said to be **conjugated**. These conjugated systems form molecular orbitals that are easily predictable from the combination of adjacent p orbitals. In general, conjugated π bonds are more stable than nonconjugated ones. The MO description of conjugated systems offers a fuller understanding of Lewis resonance forms.

Certain cyclic conjugated π bonds can form **aromatic systems**. To be aromatic, a molecule must have a cyclic, contiguous, and coplanar array of p orbitals. Systems that do not fulfill all of these criteria are considered **nonaromatic**. For those that do satisfy all three conditions, **Hückel's Rule** states that aromatic systems must contain $(4n+2)\pi$ electrons, whereas those that contain $4n\pi$ electrons are considered **antiaromatic**.

Aromatic and conjugated systems can be affected by attached substituents. Generally speaking, substituents are classified as either **electron-donating groups** (EDG), such as amino and methoxy, or **electron-withdrawing groups** (EWG), such as nitro and cyano. The impact can be broken down into **inductive effects**, which arise from electronegativity differences and are communicated through σ bonds, and **resonance effects**, in which electron density is moved across extended π systems.

4. Nomenclature. The **IUPAC nomenclature** of organic compounds is driven by consideration of the carbon backbone and functional groups. The process starts by determining the identity of the **parent compound**, which is defined as the longest possible carbon chain bearing the highest order functional group. Once the parent compound is defined, all other groups become **substituents**. Substituents can be **simple** (methyl, ethyl, etc.) or **compound** (such as 2,2-dimethylpropyl). When numbering a compound substituent, the point of attachment is always considered carbon 1. The conversion of alkane chains into substituents is simple: methane becomes methyl. However, functional groups are more subtle: an alkanol becomes a hydroxalkyl substituent, and an alkanone becomes an oxoalkyl substituent. Chiral centers are named using the **Cahn-Ingold-Prelog** (CIP) rules of priority:

➤ prioritize atoms around an asymmetric center according to atomic number
➤ orient the center so that the lowest-priority atom is farthest away
➤ if the priority of the remaining atoms proceeds clockwise from highest to lowest, then it is an **R center**
➤ if the priority of the remaining atoms proceeds counterclockwise from highest to lowest, then it is an **S center.**

The CIP rules are also used to specify the geometry around double bonds. Here the methodology is as follows:

➤ orient the double bond so that it is horizontal
➤ on each side, label the two substituents according to their CIP priority
➤ if the two top-priority substituents are pointing in the same direction, it is a **Z alkene**
➤ if the two top-priority substituents are oriented opposite each other, it is an **E alkene.**

5. Reaction mechanisms. Reactions generally fall into the following classifications:

➤ **radical** reactions, characterized by unpaired electrons
➤ **polar** chemistry, in which charged species are involved, and
➤ **pericyclic** chemistry, which involves concerted electron motion without development of charge separation.

These reactions can be used for **synthetic methodology**, which involves the two major techniques of **carbon-carbon bond formation** and **functional group transformation**. Methods can be organized by the **preparation of** and **reactions of** various functional groups.

6. Isolation and characterization.   Once compounds have been made, they must be purified and identified. The major separation techniques used in the organic laboratory are:
- ➤ **Extraction**, including aqueous workup, which is based on differential solubility
- ➤ **Chromatography**, which depends upon differential affinity to mobile and stationary phases
- ➤ **Distillation** and **sublimation**, in which separation occurs based on differential volatility
- ➤ **Recrystallization**, which relies on differential solubility

Separation techniques can be used both for **preparative purification** and **analysis**. Methods for identifying compounds include:
- ➤ **Combustion analysis**, which can be used to obtain an empirical formula
- ➤ **UV-Vis spectroscopy**, which reveals the nature of extended π systems through electronic transitions
- ➤ **Mass spectrometry**, which can provide information about molecular weight through charge to mass ratios
- ➤ **Infrared spectroscopy**, which indicates the presence or absence of functional groups through molecular vibrations
- ➤ **Nuclear magnetic resonance**, which provides data about the topography of molecules through spin flips of protons and carbons

7. Proton NMR.   Nuclear magnetic resonance (NMR) arises from the absorption of energy in a nuclear **spin flip**, a transition that is extremely sensitive to the electronic density around it. The position of an NMR signal relative to the internal standard TMS is called the **chemical shift**, and these data reveal the nature of a proton's chemical environment. Protons that resonate at much higher frequency than TMS are said to be **downfield**, and those that appear close to the standard are said to be **upfield**. A downfield shift is indicative of an electron-deficient (or **deshielded**) environment, usually caused by the proximity of an electron-withdrawing group (EWG). The **integration** of NMR signals is used to calculate the ratio of the respective protons. The typical range for a proton NMR spectrum is 0–10 ppm, and this can be divided into the following general categories:
- ➤ 0 to ca. 2.5 ppm: aliphatic and and alkynyl C-H protons
- ➤ ca. 2.5 to ca. 5 ppm: aliphatic C-H protons where carbon is attached to an electronegative element
- ➤ ca. 5 to ca. 6.5 ppm: alkenyl (sp^2) C-H protons
- ➤ ca. 6.5 to ca. 9 ppm: aromatic (sp^2) C-H protons
- ➤ ca. 10 ppm: aldehydic C-H protons

In addition, signals often exhibit **splitting patterns**, many of which can be interpreted using the **n + 1 rule**, which states that the **multiplicity** corresponds to the total number of adjacent protons plus one. Thus, a proton with only one next-door proton would give rise to a doublet, and so on. This phenomenon of **scalar splitting** is a **through-bond** effect communicated by the σ backbone. The magnitude of the splitting (otherwise known as the **coupling constant** or **J-value**) is also diagnostic. Freely rotating systems usually exhibit a *J*-value of about 7 Hz; however, this value can be different in constrained systems such as cycloalkanes.

8. Carbon NMR.   Carbon NMR is based on the same principle as proton NMR. However, carbon signals are spread across a wider span than proton absorbances (ca. 200 ppm vs.

10 ppm). Furthermore, since only carbon-13 is observed by NMR, and its natural abundance is about 1%, practically no carbon-carbon splitting is observed. Carbon does couple with hydrogen, but this coupling is artificially suppressed by **off-resonance decoupling**. Consequently, each carbon signal shows up as a singlet, and each unique carbon can usually be resolved.

For this reason, carbon NMR is very useful in identifying **symmetry** within a molecule. In other words, if the molecular formula indicates the presence of ten carbon atoms, but the NMR only reveals nine signals, this is strong evidence that a pair of carbon atoms are related by symmetry.

Like proton NMR, chemical shift can also provide important information. In very general terms, the carbon NMR spectrum can be divided into four regions:
> 0 to ca. 50 ppm: aliphatic (sp^3) carbons
> ca. 50 to ca. 100 ppm: sp^3 carbons attached to heteroatoms; alkynyl (sp) carbons
> ca. 100 to ca. 150 ppm: aromatic and olefinic (sp^2) carbons; nitrile (sp) carbons
> ca. 150 to ca. 200 ppm: carbonyl carbons

PART VI

REVIEWING PCAT MATH SKILLS

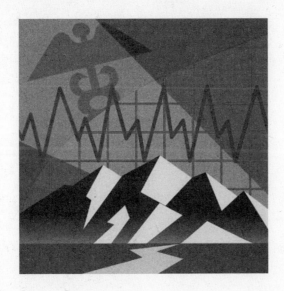

CHAPTER 12

Basic Math

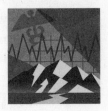

Read This Chapter to Learn About:

➤ Numbers, Number Types, and Number Operations

➤ Fractions, Decimals, and Percents

➤ Averages

NUMBERS

A **number line** is a horizontal line that extends without limit in both directions to represent the entire set of real numbers, as shown below.

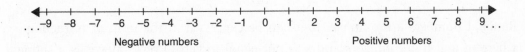

The midpoint of the number line represents zero (0), which is neither a positive nor a negative number. Equally spaced points are used to represent positive and negative numbers, progressively getting larger in the positive *x* (right) direction and progressively getting smaller in the negative *x* (left) direction. Any number positioned to the *left* of a number on the number line is *less* than that number; any number position to the *right* of a number on the number line is *greater* than that number. A number line is used to display the arrangement of all real numbers as well as to conceptualize all arithmetic operations involving real numbers visually.

NUMBER TYPES

Real Numbers

The largest, most inclusive category of numbers (excluding complex numbers, which will not be covered in this review) is real numbers. The real numbers include whole numbers, natural numbers, integers, and rational and irrational numbers. A description and examples of each of these types of numbers are given below.

Natural Numbers

Natural numbers, also referred to as counting numbers, include the entire set of numbers that are used in counting. Natural numbers include the unending set of numbers listed below:

Natural Numbers $\{1, 2, 3, 4, 5, 6, 7, 8 \ldots\}$

Natural numbers are positive, although the numbers above are written without the positive or + sign preceding the number.

Integers

Integers include the set of natural numbers but may be negative as well as positive. Integers also include the number 0. Thus, integers include the unending set of numbers listed below:

Integers $\{\ldots -7, -6, -5, -4, -3, -2, -1, 0, 1, 2, 3, 4, 5, 6, 7 \ldots\}$

Rational Numbers

Rational numbers are numbers that can be expressed in the form of a fraction $\dfrac{m}{n}$ where m and n are integers and n is not equal to zero. Every integer is a rational number because it can be expressed in terms of a fraction, i.e., $-7 = \dfrac{-7}{1}$ and $5 = \dfrac{5}{1}$. The set of rational numbers includes all integers and common fractions, as shown below.

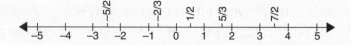

Irrational Numbers

Irrational numbers are real numbers that cannot be expressed as fractions; they are nonterminating, nonrepeating numbers such as

$$\pi = 3.14159\ldots \qquad \sqrt{2} = 1.41421\ldots \qquad e = 2.71828\ldots$$

NUMBER OPERATIONS

Addition

Two numbers (integers) with like signs can be added by adding their numerical values with their common sign as its prefix.

EXAMPLES: $2+4=6; -7+(-8)=-7-8=-15$

Two numbers (integers) with unlike signs can be added by subtracting the smaller numerical value from the larger. The sum is then given the sign of the number having the larger numerical value.

EXAMPLES: $12+(-4)=12-4=8; -17+12=-5$

The sum of two rational numbers expressed with the same denominator is a rational number whose denominator is the common denominator and whose numerator is the sum of the numerators.

EXAMPLES: $\dfrac{1}{4}+\dfrac{3}{8}=\dfrac{2+3}{8}=\dfrac{5}{8}; \dfrac{3}{5}+\dfrac{2}{9}=\dfrac{27+10}{45}=\dfrac{37}{45}$

Subtraction

Any number (integer) can be subtracted from another by changing the sign of the number being subtracted and then adding this number to the other number.

EXAMPLES: $7-3=7+(-3)=4; 23-4=23+(-4)=19$

The difference of two rational numbers expressed with the same denominator is a rational number whose denominator is the common denominator and whose numerator is the difference of the numerators.

EXAMPLES: $\dfrac{3}{4}-\dfrac{3}{8}=\dfrac{6-3}{8}=\dfrac{3}{8}; \dfrac{6}{7}-\dfrac{1}{5}=\dfrac{30-7}{35}=\dfrac{23}{35}$

Multiplication

Multiplication of two numbers (integers) can be done by simply multiplying the numbers together and assigning a positive "+" sign if the two numbers have like signs and a negative "−" sign if the two numbers have unlike signs.

EXAMPLES: $9\times6=54; -4\times-6=24; -3\times7=-21$

Multiplication of two or more rational numbers yields a rational number whose numerator is the product of the numerators and whose denominator is the product of the denominators.

EXAMPLES: $\dfrac{2}{3}\times\dfrac{5}{7}=\dfrac{2\times5}{3\times7}=\dfrac{10}{21}; \dfrac{1}{4}\times-\dfrac{6}{8}=\dfrac{1\times(-6)}{4\times8}=\dfrac{-6}{32}=-\dfrac{6}{32}$

Division

Division of two numbers (integers) can be done by simply dividing the two numbers (making sure that the denominator is not zero), assigning a positive "+" sign if the two numbers have like signs and a negative "−" sign if the two numbers have unlike signs.

EXAMPLES: $4 \div 5 = \dfrac{4}{5}$; $-3 \div -8 = \dfrac{-3}{-8} = \dfrac{3}{8}$; $-7 \div 11 = \dfrac{-7}{11} = -\dfrac{7}{11}$

One rational number can be divided by another rational number by multiplying the first rational number by the reciprocal or inverse of the second rational number. For example, $\dfrac{a}{b}$ divided by $\dfrac{c}{d}$ can be determined by $\dfrac{a}{b} \times \dfrac{d}{c} = \dfrac{a \times d}{b \times c}$.

EXAMPLES: $\dfrac{3}{5} \div \dfrac{7}{9} = \dfrac{\frac{3}{5}}{\frac{7}{9}} = \dfrac{3}{5} \times \dfrac{9}{7} = \dfrac{27}{35}$; $\dfrac{2}{3} \div \dfrac{-5}{6} = \dfrac{\frac{2}{3}}{\frac{-5}{6}} = \dfrac{2}{3} \times \dfrac{6}{-5} = \dfrac{12}{-15} = -\dfrac{12}{15}$

Order of Number Operations

In many cases, such as those illustrated in the properties and laws noted below, calculations can involve a series of operations. The order that operations are made in can make a significant difference in the answer and must be done in the following order according to the acronym PEMDAS (**P**lease **E**xcuse **M**y **D**ear **A**unt **S**ally).

➤ **Rule 1: Parentheses:** Perform any calculations inside parentheses.
➤ **Rule 2: Exponents:** Simplify any exponents, working from left to right.
➤ **Rule 3: Multiplication/Division:** Perform all multiplication and division operations, working from left to right.
➤ **Rule 4: Addition/Subtraction:** Perform all addition and subtraction operations, working from left to right.

EXAMPLES:

a) $531 - (6 \times 3)^2$

$531 - (18)^2$ **Rule 1:** Perform calculations inside parentheses.

$531 - 324$ **Rule 2:** Simplify any exponents.

207 Answer

b) $6 + (4 \times 7) \times 3^4 \div 9$

$6 + (28) \times 3^4 \div 9$ **Rule 1:** Perform calculations inside parentheses.

$6 + (28) \times 81 \div 9$ **Rule 2:** Simplify any exponents.

$6 + 2268 \div 9$ **Rule 3:** Perform multiplication calculations, working from left to right.

6+252

258

Rule 4: Perform division calculations, working from left to right.

Answer

Identity Property of Addition

The addition of zero to any number does not change the number. In other words, if a is any number, then

$$a+0=a \qquad\qquad 0+a=a$$

Note that although $0+a=a$, the same order of operation does not hold true for subtraction, i.e., $0-a=-a \neq a$.

EXAMPLES: $\qquad 16+0=16 \qquad 0+230=230 \qquad 145-0=145$

Identity Property of Multiplication

The multiplication of any number by 1 does not change the number. In other words, if a is any number, then

$$a \times 1=a \qquad\qquad 1 \times a=a$$

Note that although $1 \times a=a$, the same order of operation does not hold true for division, i.e., $1 \div a=\dfrac{1}{a} \neq a$.

EXAMPLES: $\qquad 43 \times 1=43 \qquad\qquad 1 \times 357=357$

The multiplication of any number by -1 does not change the identity of the number, but it does change the sign of the number. In other words, if a is any number, then

$$a \times -1=-a \qquad\qquad -1 \times a=-a$$

EXAMPLES: $\qquad 37 \times -1=-37 \qquad -1 \times 68=-68 \qquad 147 \div -1=\dfrac{147}{-1}=-147$

Commutative Laws of Addition and Multiplication

Addition and multiplication are commutative operations. By commutative, we mean that addition and multiplication can be performed regardless of the order of the numbers without changing the result. In other words, if a and b are numbers, then

Commutative Law of Addition $\quad a+b=b+a$

Commutative Law of Multiplication $\quad a \times b=b \times a$

EXAMPLES: $\qquad 25+8=8+25=33 \qquad 5 \times 3=3 \times 5=15$

The same cannot be said for subtraction and division. Subtraction and division are not commutative operations.

Associative Laws of Addition and Multiplication

Addition and multiplication are associative operations. By associative, we mean that addition and multiplication can be performed regardless of the order of the numbers without changing the result. In other words, if a, b and c are numbers, then

$$\textbf{Associative Law of Addition} \quad (a+b)+c=a+(b+c)$$

$$\textbf{Associative Law of Multiplication} \quad (a\times b)\times c=a\times(b\times c)$$

EXAMPLES:

$$(12+4)+8=12+(4+8) \qquad (3\times10)\times4=3\times(10\times4)$$

$$16+8=12+12 \qquad\qquad 30\times4=3\times40$$

$$24=24 \qquad\qquad\qquad 120=120$$

The same cannot be said for subtraction and division. Subtraction and division are not associative operations.

Distributive Law of Multiplication

Multiplication is a distributive operation. A number multiplied by a group of numbers that are either added or subtracted can be distributed by being multiplied by each number being added or subtracted. In other words, $a\times(b+c)=a\times b+a\times c$ or $a\times(b-c)=a\times b-a\times c$.

EXAMPLES:

$$5\times(8+12)=5\times8+5\times12 \qquad 7\times(15-8)=7\times15-7\times8$$

$$5\times20=40+60 \qquad\qquad 7\times7=105-56$$

$$100=100 \qquad\qquad\qquad 49=49$$

FRACTIONS

Fractions represent a part or portion of a whole and consist of two numbers with one written on top of the other. If a and b are numbers, then a fraction can be written as: $\dfrac{a}{b}$ with $b\neq0$. The top number, a, is known as the *numerator* and the bottom number, b, is known as the *denominator*.

All of the major arithmetic operations (addition, subtraction, multiplication, and division) can be applied to fractions.

Addition with Fractions

Two or more fractions can be added only if they have a common denominator. To find a common denominator, the two denominators are multiplied. Then, each fraction must be converted into a new fraction with the same value yet having a denominator different from its original denominator. Once the fractions have a common denominator, the numerators of each of the fractions are added and written over the common denominator. If a, b, c, d are numbers and b, $d \neq 0$, then $\dfrac{a}{b} + \dfrac{c}{d} = \dfrac{ad + bc}{bd}$ where the product bd is the common denominator.

EXAMPLES: $\dfrac{1}{3} + \dfrac{2}{5} = \dfrac{5+6}{15} = \dfrac{11}{15}$; $\dfrac{3}{8} + \dfrac{2}{11} = \dfrac{33+16}{88} = \dfrac{49}{88}$

Subtraction with Fractions

Just as is the case with addition, fractions can be subtracted only if they have a common denominator. Once the fractions have a common denominator, the numerators of each of the fractions are subtracted and written over the common denominator. If a, b, c, d are numbers and b, $d \neq 0$, then $\dfrac{a}{b} - \dfrac{c}{d} = \dfrac{ad - bc}{bd}$.

EXAMPLES: $\dfrac{4}{5} - \dfrac{2}{9} = \dfrac{36-10}{45} = \dfrac{26}{45}$; $\dfrac{9}{10} - \dfrac{1}{7} = \dfrac{63-10}{70} = \dfrac{53}{70}$

Multiplication with Fractions

Two fractions can be multiplied by multiplying the numerators and denominators. In other words, if a, b, c, and d are numbers (b, $d \neq 0$), then $\dfrac{a}{b} \times \dfrac{c}{d} = \dfrac{a \times c}{b \times d}$.

EXAMPLES: $\dfrac{5}{7} \times \dfrac{1}{8} = \dfrac{5 \times 1}{7 \times 8} = \dfrac{5}{56}$; $\dfrac{11}{13} \times \dfrac{2}{3} = \dfrac{11 \times 2}{13 \times 3} = \dfrac{22}{39}$

Division with Fractions

Given two fractions $\dfrac{a}{b}$ and $\dfrac{c}{d}$, the fraction $\dfrac{a}{b}$ in the numerator can be divided by another fraction $\dfrac{c}{d}$ in the denominator by first taking the reciprocal or flipping the fraction in the denominator and multiplying that fraction by the fraction in the numerator or: $\dfrac{\frac{a}{b}}{\frac{c}{d}} = \dfrac{a \times d}{b \times c} = \dfrac{ad}{bc}$.

EXAMPLES: $\dfrac{3}{7} \div \dfrac{4}{5} = \dfrac{\frac{3}{7}}{\frac{4}{5}} = \dfrac{3}{7} \times \dfrac{5}{4} = \dfrac{15}{28}$; $\dfrac{8}{11} \div \dfrac{7}{9} = \dfrac{\frac{8}{11}}{\frac{7}{9}} = \dfrac{8}{11} \times \dfrac{9}{7} = \dfrac{72}{77}$

Reduction of Fractions

Fractions reveal a specific amount referring to a portion or part of a whole. The fraction $\frac{5}{6}$ means 5 parts out of a whole of six equal parts. However, in some cases, it is possible to express a fraction in a multitude of ways, all having the same numerical value. For example, consider the fractions $\frac{1}{2}$, $\frac{2}{4}$, $\frac{25}{50}$, and $\frac{50}{100}$. All of these fractions are different in expression yet have the same meaning. In problems involving fractions, the goal is to have the basic expression of the fraction, in this case, $\frac{1}{2}$. To achieve such a goal, you will have to reduce fractions. To reduce fractions, you divide the numerator and denominator by a factor common to both numbers. For example, the common factor in the fraction $\frac{2}{4}$ is 2. By dividing the numerator and denominator by 2, you obtain $\frac{1}{2}$. For the fraction $\frac{50}{100}$, the common factor is 50 which, when divided into the numerator and denominator, results in a fraction of $\frac{1}{2}$.

> **EXAMPLE:** Reduce the fraction $\frac{10}{12}$.

The factor common to both the numerator and denominator is 2. Thus, you divide both the numerator and denominator by 2, resulting in the fraction $\frac{5}{6}$.

> **EXAMPLE:** Reduce the fraction $\frac{96}{60}$.

The largest common factor between the numerator and denominator is 12. Dividing both the numerator and denominator by 12 yields the fraction $\frac{8}{5}$.

Mixed Numbers and Fractions

Although fractions are generally presented as $\frac{a}{b}$ or $\frac{1}{3}$, they can also be written in combination with an integer such as $2\frac{1}{3}$ or $6\frac{7}{8}$. These are referred to as *mixed numbers*. Mixed numbers occur when the numerator is greater than the denominator. Consider, for example, the mixed number $2\frac{1}{3}$. This means that the denominator, 3, divided into the numerator two complete times with a remainder of 1. This means that the numerator must have been 7 and the original fraction was $\frac{7}{3}$. Three divides into 7 two times with a remainder of 1 that remains over the denominator of 3. Thus, $2\frac{1}{3} = \frac{7}{3}$. This yields the value that should be placed over the denominator. Referring to the example of $2\frac{1}{3}$ above, the fraction can be determined by multiplying the denominator 3

by the integer 2 and then adding 1, which results in $\frac{7}{3}$.

An easy way to convert between mixed numbers and fractions when given a mixed number is to multiply the denominator by the integer and add the numerator:

$$\text{fraction} = \frac{\left[(\text{denominator}) \times (\text{integer})\right] + \text{numerator}}{\text{denominator}}$$

EXAMPLE: Convert $\frac{34}{5}$ to a mixed number.

Dividing the denominator into the numerator yields 6 with a remainder of 4. The mixed number is therefore $6\frac{4}{5}$.

EXAMPLE: Convert $4\frac{7}{8}$ to a fraction.

The fraction can be found by multiplying the denominator and the integer and then adding the numerator or

$$\text{fraction} = \frac{\left[(\text{denominator}) \times (\text{integer})\right] + \text{numerator}}{\text{denominator}} = \frac{[8 \times 4] + 7}{8} = \frac{39}{8}$$

Ratios and Proportions

A *ratio* is a fraction $\frac{a}{b}$ written as $a{:}b$ where a and b are numbers and $b \neq 0$. If $a = b \neq 0$,

the ratio is 1:1 or $\frac{1}{1}$. The ratio of 6 to 8 is written as $6{:}8 = \frac{6}{8}$. Because the numerator

and denominator are both divisible by two, the fraction $\frac{6}{8}$ can be reduced to $\frac{3}{4}$, which is the ratio.

EXAMPLES: Determine the ratio of $\frac{1}{3}$ to $\frac{5}{6}$.

The ratio of $\frac{1}{3}$ to $\frac{5}{6}$, $\frac{1}{3}{:}\frac{5}{6}$, is $\dfrac{\frac{1}{3}}{\frac{5}{6}} = \frac{1}{3} \times \frac{6}{5} = \frac{6}{15}$, which can be reduced to $\frac{2}{5}$.

Determine the ratio of $6x$ to $\frac{2}{3}y$.

The ratio of $6x$ to $\frac{2}{3}y$ is $6x{:}\frac{2}{3}y = \dfrac{6x}{\frac{2}{3}y} = 6x \times \frac{3}{2y} = \frac{18x}{2y} = \frac{9x}{y}$.

A *proportion* is an equation that relates two ratios $a{:}b = c{:}d$ or $\dfrac{a}{b} = \dfrac{c}{d}$. From this equation, you can derive the following equations known as the *laws of proportion*:

(a) $ad = bc$
(b) $\dfrac{b}{a} = \dfrac{d}{c}$
(c) $\dfrac{a}{c} = \dfrac{b}{d}$
(d) $\dfrac{a+b}{b} = \dfrac{c+d}{d}$

(e) $\dfrac{a-b}{b} = \dfrac{c-d}{d}$
(f) $\dfrac{a+b}{a-b} = \dfrac{c+d}{c-d}$

EXAMPLE: The ratio of boys to girls in a science class is 5:3. If there are 32 students in the class, how many girls are in the science class?

To find the total number of girls in the science class, you must first find the fraction of students in the class who are girls. For every set of 8 students, 3 students are girls, yielding a fraction of $\dfrac{3}{8}$. Thus, the total number of girls in the class is $\dfrac{3}{8} \times 32 = 12$.

DECIMALS

A *decimal* is a means of expressing the numerical value of a fraction. Decimals occur as a result of any fraction but become particularly important when dealing with money ($5.25) and scientific measurements (4.30 mL). An example of a decimal number is 32.1524. The position of a digit in a decimal number bears significance as to its value. A decimal number consists of two parts: a whole part (the numerical value to the left of the decimal point) and a fraction part (the numerical value to the right of the decimal point). From the decimal point, positions to the left begin with ones and increase by a factor of 10 for each additional position to the left of the decimal point. Subsequently, positions to the right begin with tenths and decrease by a factor of 10 for each additional position to the right. Consider, for example, the decimal number noted above 32.1524.

Position	Value of Position		Value of Decimal Number	
3**2**.1524	Tens	10	30	30
3**2**.1524	Ones	1	2	2
32.**1**524	Tenths	0.1	$\dfrac{1}{10}$	0.1
32.1**5**24	Hundredths	0.01	$\dfrac{5}{100}$	0.05
32.15**2**4	Thousandths	0.001	$\dfrac{2}{1000}$	0.002
32.152**4**	Ten Thousandths	0.0001	$\dfrac{4}{10000}$	0.0004

The expanded form of the decimal number 32.1524, which holds for every decimal number, is the sum of each digit value by virtue of its position:

$$32.1524 \rightarrow 30 + 2 + 0.1 + 0.05 + 0.002 + 0.0004$$

Converting Fractions to Decimals

Fractions can be converted to decimals by simply dividing the denominator of the fraction into the numerator. The number of positions in the decimal number depends on the numerator and denominator. For example, $\dfrac{1}{10} = 0.1$, $\dfrac{3}{4} = 0.75$, and $\dfrac{7}{8} = 0.875$.

But what about the fractions $\dfrac{1}{3} = 0.3333333$ and $\dfrac{5}{6} = 0.83333333$? There are many instances in which fractions, when divided, yield a quotient with an unending number of positions in the decimal number. In these cases, the resulting values are often written as $\dfrac{1}{3} = 0.3\overline{3}$ where the bar over the 3 implies that it is a repeating term or $\dfrac{5}{6} = 0.83\overline{3}$.

Converting Decimals to Fractions

Converting a decimal number to a fraction can be done by first noting the number of positions to the right of the decimal point. This is the part of the decimal number that is the fraction. For each position to the right of the decimal, the number decreases by a factor of $\dfrac{1}{10}$. This is illustrated by the chart below.

Decimal Number Without Whole Part		Decimal Number With Whole Part	
Decimal Number	Fraction	Decimal Number	Fraction
0.2	$\dfrac{2}{10}$	4.2	$4\dfrac{2}{10}$
0.02	$\dfrac{2}{100}$	4.02	$4\dfrac{2}{100}$
0.002	$\dfrac{2}{1000}$	4.002	$4\dfrac{2}{1000}$
0.0002	$\dfrac{2}{10000}$	4.0002	$4\dfrac{2}{10000}$

Adding Decimal Numbers

Addition of decimal numbers is done in the same way as addition of ordinary numbers. However, in this case, each number should be written such that all of the decimal points are lined up vertically. For example, the numbers 23.467 and 2.589 are added by:

$$
\begin{array}{r}
23.467 \\
\times\ \ 2.589 \\
\hline
26.056
\end{array}
$$

with the decimal point holding the same position in the sum of the two numbers.

Subtracting Decimal Numbers

Subtraction of decimal numbers is done in a manner similar to addition in that the numbers are positioned with the decimal point lined up. Also, as in the subtraction of ordinary numbers, the smaller decimal number must be subtracted from the larger decimal number. For example, subtracting the number 6.821 from 37.49 can be done as below:

$$
\begin{array}{r}
37.490 \\
-\ \ 6.821 \\
\hline
30.669
\end{array}
$$

Note that the zero added at the end of 37.940 does not alter the value of the number and just serves as a placeholder in the subtraction operation.

Multiplying Decimal Numbers

You multiply two decimal numbers just as you would multiply two ordinary numbers. In this case, however, the decimal points do not have to be lined up. Knowing where to put the decimal point is important, but you can deal with it after you finish multiplying the two numbers. For example, when the two decimal numbers 7.4 and 3.6 are multiplied, the two numbers are multiplied without regard to the decimal point, yielding a result of:

$$
\begin{array}{r}
7.4 \\
\times\ \ 3.6 \\
\hline
2664
\end{array}
$$

To determine the placement of the decimal point in the product, you must first determine the position of the decimal point in each of the two numbers being multiplied. For the first decimal number, because there is only one number following the decimal point, its fraction part is $\dfrac{1}{10}$. The same can be said for the second number; its fraction part is also

$\frac{1}{10}$. The combined fraction part of the product of these two numbers is $\frac{1}{10} \times \frac{1}{10} = \frac{1}{100}$, which is then multiplied by the result of the multiplication to yield the correct answer:

$$2664 \times \frac{1}{100} = 26.64$$

Yet another way of approaching this is to look at each decimal number and count the number of positions it takes to move from the decimal point to the end of the value. For 7.4, it takes one position to move from the decimal point to the end of the number. Similarly, for 3.6, it takes one position to move from the point to the end of the number. For both numbers being multiplied, it takes a combined two positions moved from their decimal point. Once the product is obtained, begin at the end of the number and move to the left the number of combined positions determined for each of the numbers being multiplied. So, once the product of 2664 is obtained, you start to the right of "4" and move to the left two positions. This is where the decimal point should be placed.

EXAMPLE: Find the product of 27.8 and 6.13.

The product of these two decimal numbers can be found by first multiplying the two numbers and ignoring the decimal point:

$$
\begin{array}{r}
20.2 \\
\times\ \ 3.14 \\
\hline
63428
\end{array}
$$

Second, for each number being multiplied, the number of positions that you move from the decimal point to the end of the number must be determined. For 20.2, one position is needed to move from the decimal point to the end. For 3.14, two positions are needed. Adding the number of positions results in a combined number of 3. Finally, returning to the product, you begin at the end of the number and move to the left three positions, or

$$
\begin{array}{r}
20.2 \\
\times\ \ 3.14 \\
\hline
63.428
\end{array}
$$

Dividing Decimal Numbers

Decimal numbers can be divided in the same way as ordinary numbers. The position of the decimal point in the quotient can be determined when division is expressed in long division form. Consider the following division problem: $483.84 \div 38.4$ or $38.4\overline{)483.84}$, where 483.84 is the dividend and 38.4 is the divisor. If there were no decimal point in the divisor, then the decimal point in the quotient would be placed exactly above the dividend. However, because there is a decimal point in the divisor, it is best to move it to the end of the number by multiplying the divisor by an appropriate factor. The factor in this case is 10 because the single digit following the decimal point to the right represents the tenths position. The divisor, when multiplied 10, is equal to 384. In order to multiply the divisor by 10, you must also multiply the dividend by 10, resulting in 4838.4. Now, the division problem becomes 4838.4 ÷ 384 or

$$384 \overline{)4838.4}^{\,12.6}$$

Rounding Decimals

To round decimal numbers to the nearest place, follow these steps:

Consider the decimal number, 3.4925.

Step I: Identify the digit in the decimal number to be rounded.
➤ If asked to round to the nearest tenth, the digit is 4.
➤ If asked to round to the nearest hundredth, the digit is 9.
➤ If asked to round to the nearest thousandth, the digit is 2.

Step II: Then identify the digit immediately to the right of the number that is being rounded.
➤ The digit immediately to the right of the tenth position is 9.
➤ The digit immediately to the right of the hundredth position is 2.
➤ The digit immediately to the right of the thousandth position is 5.

Step III: Depending on the result of Step II, there are two possibilities.
➤ If the digit identified in Step II is 0 – 4 (0, 1, 2, 3, 4), then the digit being rounded remains the same.
➤ If the digit identified in Step II is 5 – 9 (5, 6, 7, 8, 9), then the digit being rounded increases by 1.

Step IV: Apply the result of Step III as follows.
➤ If asked to round 3.4925 to the nearest tenth, then the result is 3.5.
➤ If asked to round 3.4925 to the nearest hundredth, then the result is 3.49.
➤ If asked to round 3.4925 to the nearest thousandth, then the result is 3.493.

Scientific Notation

Scientific notation is a means of expressing numbers, regardless of their size, in powers of ten. Any nonzero number can be expressed in scientific notation when written in the form $a \times 10^b$ where a is a real number such that $1 \le a < 10$ (or $-10 < a \le -1$) [referred to as the *coefficient*] and b is an integer that describes the power of the *exponent*.

To convert a number into scientific notation, follow the steps below. The number 397 serves as an example.

Step I: Express the number in terms of a real number such that $1 \leq a < 10$.

$$397 \Rightarrow 3.97.$$

Step II: Determine the value of b the integer that is the power of the exponent. In order to perform Step I, you divided 397 by 100. Thus, in order to retain our original number, you also need to multiply by 100 which, in terms of exponents, is 10^2. The integer b in this case is 2.

$$397 = 3.97 \times 100 = 3.97 \times 10^2$$

MULTIPLICATION OF NUMBERS EXPRESSED IN SCIENTIFIC NOTATION

To multiply numbers expressed in scientific notation, you multiply the coefficients to reveal the new coefficient and multiply the exponents to reveal the new exponent. However, when exponents are multiplied, the powers add. For example, suppose you want to multiply the numbers 1.36×10^2 and 4.6×10^4.

$$\left(1.36 \times 10^2\right) \times \left(4.6 \times 10^4\right) = \left[1.36 \times 4.6\right] \times \left[10^2 \times 10^4\right]$$
$$= \left[6.256\right] \times \left[10^{2+4}\right] = 6.256 \times 10^6$$

DIVISION OF NUMBERS EXPRESSED IN SCIENTIFIC NOTATION

To divide numbers expressed in scientific notation, you divide the coefficients to reveal the new coefficient and divide the exponents to reveal the new exponent. However, when exponents are divided, the powers subtract. For example, suppose you want to divide 6.75×10^7 and 2.5×10^3.

$$\left(6.75 \times 10^7\right) \div \left(2.5 \times 10^3\right) = \left[6.75 \div 2.5\right] \times \left[10^7 \div 10^3\right] = \left[2.5\right] \times \left[10^{7-3}\right] = 2.5 \times 10^4$$

PERCENTS

Percents, a word meaning "of one hundred," are ratios with a denominator equal to 100. They are represented by the symbol %. Because a percent is a ratio, it can easily be converted into a fraction and decimal number. Percents can be converted to fractions by removing the % symbol and dividing by 100.

$$4\% = \frac{4}{100}, \ 52\% = \frac{52}{100}, \ 84\% = \frac{84}{100}$$

Fractions can be converted to decimals by multiplying the fraction by 100%.

$$\frac{1}{2} = \frac{1}{2} \times 100\% = 50\%; \frac{3}{4} = \frac{3}{4} \times 100\% = 75\%; \frac{7}{9} = \frac{7}{9} \times 100\% = 77.8\%$$

Percents can be converted to decimals by removing the % symbol and placing the decimal point two positions to the left.

$$4\% = 0.04, \ 52\% = 0.52, \ 84\% = 0.84$$

Decimals can be converted to percents by multiplying the fraction by 100%.

$$0.13 = 0.13 \times 100\% = 13\%$$
$$0.47 = 0.47 \times 100\% = 47\%$$
$$0.78 = 0.78 \times 100\% = 78\%$$

AVERAGES

Given a set of numbers, the average can be determined by adding the terms and then dividing by the number of terms in the set. A general formula for calculating the average of a set of numbers is:

$$\text{Average} = \frac{\text{Sum of terms}}{\text{Number of terms}}.$$

To find the average of the set of numbers, 9, 10, 25, 4, 7, 8, 14 you must:

Step I: Add the terms in the set.

$$9 + 10 + 25 + 4 + 7 + 8 + 14 = 77.$$

Step II: Divide the sum by the number of terms in the set. There are seven terms in the set. Thus, the average is:

$$\text{Average} = \frac{\text{Sum of terms}}{\text{Number of terms}} = \frac{77}{7} = 11.$$

ON YOUR OWN

Problems

1. $\dfrac{6}{8} - \dfrac{3}{5} =$

    A. $\dfrac{3}{40}$ **B.** $\dfrac{6}{40}$ **C.** $\dfrac{12}{40}$ **D.** $\dfrac{30}{40}$

2. $\dfrac{2}{3} \div \dfrac{7}{10} =$

    A. $\dfrac{3}{30}$ **B.** $\dfrac{14}{30}$ **C.** $\dfrac{14}{21}$ **D.** $\dfrac{20}{21}$

3. What is the average of the numbers 8, 6, 0, 15, 4, and 9?

   A. 3   **B.** 6   **C.** 7   **D.** 15

4. Converting the mixed number $4\frac{5}{7}$ into a fraction yields

   A. $\frac{5}{7}$ **B.** $\frac{20}{7}$ **C.** $\frac{33}{7}$ **D.** $\frac{45}{7}$

5. A student on average spends 12% of a typical 24-hour day watching TV. Approximately how many hours does this correspond to?

   A. 2.9 hrs   **B.** 5.8 hrs   **C.** 8.6 hrs   **D.** 12.1 hrs

6. Express -532 in scientific notation.

   A. -5.32×10^1 **B.** -5.32×10^2 **C.** -5.32×10^{-1} **D.** -5.32×10^{-1}

7. The mathematical statement $6 \times (4 \times 3) = (6 \times 4) \times 3$ is an example of

   A. associative property of multiplication   **B.** commutative property of multiplication

   C. multiplicative identity property   **D.** multiplicative inverse property

8. Round 8.7356 to the nearest hundredth.

   A. 8.8   **B.** 8.74   **C.** 8.736   **D.** 8.7356

9. $(3.75 \times 10^5) \div (-2.5 \times 10^3) =$

   A. 1.5×10^1 **B.** 1.5×10^2 **C.** -1.5×10^1 **D.** -1.5×10^2

10. $24.11 \times 4.3 =$

   A. 1.03673   **B.** 10.3673   **C.** 103.673   **D.** 1036.73

Solutions

1. Answer: B

In order to subtract two fractions, you must first find a common denominator, which can be found by multiplying the denominator of the two fractions, i.e., 8 and 5. This yields a common denominator of 40. Each fraction must be converted to the new denominator as shown following:

$$\frac{6}{8} = \frac{30}{40} \qquad \text{and} \qquad \frac{3}{5} = \frac{24}{40}$$

Thus, $\frac{6}{8} - \frac{3}{5} = \frac{30-24}{40} = \frac{6}{40}$.

2. Answer: D

To divide the two fractions, you multiply the first fraction $\left(\dfrac{2}{3}\right)$ by the reciprocal of the second fraction $\left(\dfrac{10}{7}\right)$. Thus, the solution can be found by: $\dfrac{2}{3} \div \dfrac{7}{10} = \dfrac{2}{3} \times \dfrac{10}{7} = \dfrac{20}{21}$.

3. Answer: C

To determine the average of a set of numbers, you must first calculate the sum of the terms and then divide by the number of terms in the set:

$$\text{Average} = \frac{\text{Sum of terms}}{\text{Number of terms}}$$
$$= \frac{8+6+0+15+4+9}{6}$$
$$= \frac{42}{6} = 7.$$

4. Answer: C

To convert a mixed number $\left(4\dfrac{5}{7}\right)$ into a fraction, you use the following expression:

$$\text{fraction} = \frac{\left[(\text{denominator}) \times (\text{integer})\right] + \text{numerator}}{\text{denominator}} = \frac{\left[7 \times 4\right] + 5}{7} = \frac{33}{7}.$$

5. Answer: A

The student spends 12% of a 24-hour day watching TV. Expressing the value of 12% as a fraction, it now becomes $12\% = \dfrac{12}{100}$. You must now use a proportional relationship, equating the fraction in terms of percentage to the fraction in terms of the hours in a day. Thus, $\dfrac{12}{100} = \dfrac{x \text{ hrs}}{24 \text{ hrs}}$. Solving this proportion for x yields the desired result:

$$x \text{ hrs} = \frac{12}{100} \times 24 \text{ hrs} = 2.88 \text{ hrs} \approx 2.9 \text{ hrs}.$$

6. Answer: B

The number -532 is expressed in scientific notation by first expressing the value in terms of a real number a such that $1 \leq a < 10$. In this case, the number becomes -5.32. In order to retain the original number, the number must be multiplied by 100 which, in terms of exponents, is 10^2. Thus, in scientific notation,

$$-532 = -5.32 \times 100 = -5.32 \times 10^2.$$

7. Answer: A

The mathematical statement $6 \times (4 \times 3) = (6 \times 4) \times 3$ is an example of the associative property of multiplication. The correct answer is choice A. An example of the commutative property of multiplication is $(21) \times 3 = 3 \times (21)$. An example of the multiplicative identity property is $4321 \times 1 = 4321$. An example of the multiplicative inverse property is $14 \times \left(\dfrac{1}{14}\right) = 1$.

8. **Answer: B**

To round a decimal number, you first identify the digit in the decimal number to be rounded. Since it is to be rounded to the nearest hundredth, the digit is 3. Then, you identify the digit immediately to the right of the number that is being rounded which, in this case, is 5. Because this digit is in the interval 5 – 9, then the digit being rounded increases by 1. Thus, the correct answer is 8.74.

9. **Answer: D**

To divide the two numbers in scientific notation, you have:

$$3.75 \times 10^5 \div -2.5 \times 10^3 = \frac{3.75 \times 10^5}{-2.5 \times 10^3} = \frac{3.75}{-2.5} \times \frac{10^5}{10^3} = -1.5 \times 10^{5-3} = -1.5 \times 10^2.$$

10. **Answer: C**

When multiplying two decimal numbers, the numbers are multiplied as usual, noting the number of positions established by the decimal point for each number. The decimal point in 24.11 is two positions from the end of the number and in 4.3, it is one position from the end of the number. Because each position represents a unit of 10, the combined value that the product must be divided by is 1000. In other words, the decimal point from the end of the number in the product is moved to the left by three positions.

$$
\begin{array}{r}
24.11 \\
\times \quad 4.3 \\
\hline
103.673
\end{array}
$$

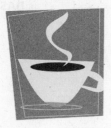

CRAM SESSION

Basic Math

Number Types

Real Numbers   Real numbers include whole numbers, natural numbers, integers, and rational and irrational numbers.

Natural Numbers   Natural numbers, also referred to as counting numbers, include the entire set of numbers that are used in counting.

Natural Numbers   {1, 2, 3, 4, 5, 6, 7, 8 . . . }

Integers   Integers include the set of natural numbers but may be negative as well as positive and include the number 0 (zero).

Integers   { . . . –7, –6, –5, –4, –3, –2, –1, 0, 1, 2, 3, 4, 5, 6, 7 . . . }

Rational Numbers   Rational numbers are numbers that can be expressed in the form of a fraction $\frac{m}{n}$ where *m* and *n* are integers and *n* is not equal to zero.

Irrational Numbers   Irrational numbers are real numbers that cannot be expressed as fractions and are non-terminating, non-repeating numbers such as

$$\pi = 3.14159 \ldots \qquad \sqrt{2} = 1.41.421 \ldots \qquad e = 2.71828 \ldots$$

Number Operations

Addition
➤ Two numbers (integers) with like signs can be added by adding their numerical values with their common sign as its prefix.
➤ Two numbers (integers) with unlike signs can be added by subtracting the smaller numerical value from the larger. The sum is then given the sign of the number having the larger numerical value.
➤ The sum of two rational numbers expressed with the same denominator is a rational number whose denominator is the common denominator and whose numerator is the sum of the numerators.

Subtraction
➤ Any number (integer) can be subtracted from another by changing the sign of the number being subtracted and then adding this number to the other number.
➤ The difference of two rational numbers expressed with the same denominator is a rational number whose denominator is the common denominator and whose numerator is the difference of the numerators.

Multiplication
➤ Multiplication of two numbers (integers) can be done by simply multiplying the numbers together and assigning a positive "+" sign if the two numbers have like signs and a negative "−" sign if the two numbers have unlike signs.
➤ Multiplication of two or more rational numbers yields a rational number whose numerator is the product of the numerators and the denominator is the product of the denominators.

Division
➤ Division of two numbers (integers) can be done by simply dividing the two numbers (making sure that the denominator is not zero) and assigning a positive "+" sign if the two numbers have like signs and a negative "−" sign if the two numbers have unlike signs.
➤ One rational number can be divided by another rational number by multiplying the first rational number by the reciprocal or inverse of the second rational number. For example, $\dfrac{a}{b}$ divided by $\dfrac{c}{d}$ can be determined by $\dfrac{a}{b} \times \dfrac{d}{c} = \dfrac{a \times d}{b \times c}$.

Order of Number Operations

PEMDAS (**P**lease **E**xcuse **M**y **D**ear **A**unt **S**ally)

Rule 1: Parentheses	Perform any calculations inside parentheses.
Rule 2: Exponents	Simplify any exponents, working from left to right.
Rule 3: Multiplication/Division	Perform all multiplication and division operations, working from left to right.
Rule 4: Addition/Subtraction	Perform all addition and subtraction operations, working from left to right.

Identity Property of Addition (and Subtraction)
➤ The addition of zero to any number or the subtraction of zero from any number does not change the identity of the number.

Identity Property of Multiplication (and Division)
➤ The multiplication of any number by 1 or the division of any number by 1 does not change the identity of the number.
➤ The multiplication of any number by −1 or the division of any number by −1 does not change the identity of the number but it does change the sign of the number.

Commutative Law of Addition	$a + b = b + a$
Commutative Law of Multiplication	$a \times b = b \times a$

Subtraction and division are not commutative operations.

Associative Law of Addition	$(a + b) + c = a + (b + c)$
Associative Law of Multiplication	$(a \times b) \times c = a \times (b \times c)$

Subtraction and division are not associative operations.

Distributive Law of Multiplication $a \times (b+c) = a \times b + a \times c$

$a \times (b-c) = a \times b - a \times c$

Fractions

If *a* and *b* are numbers, then a fraction can be written as: $\dfrac{a}{b}$ with $b \neq 0$.

The top number, *a*, is known as the *numerator* and the bottom number, *b*, is known as the *denominator*. In all operations below, *a*, *b*, *c*, *d* are numbers and *b*, *d* $\neq 0$.

Addition with Fractions $\dfrac{a}{b} + \dfrac{c}{d} = \dfrac{ad + bc}{bd}$

Subtraction with Fractions $\dfrac{a}{b} - \dfrac{c}{d} = \dfrac{ad - bc}{bd}$

Multiplication with Fractions $\dfrac{a}{b} \times \dfrac{c}{d} = \dfrac{a \times c}{b \times d}$

Division with Fractions $\dfrac{\frac{a}{b}}{\frac{c}{d}} = \dfrac{a \times d}{b \times c} = \dfrac{ad}{bc}$

Mixed Numbers and Fractions

To convert between mixed numbers and fractions, multiply the denominator of the fraction by the integer and add the numerator.

A *ratio* is a fraction $\dfrac{a}{b}$ but written as *a:b* where *a* and *b* are numbers and $b \neq 0$.

A *proportion* is an equation that relates two ratios *a:b=c:d* or $\dfrac{a}{b} = \dfrac{c}{d}$.

Decimals

A decimal is a means of expressing the numerical value of a fraction. Consider, for example, the decimal number 32.1524.

Position	Value of Position		Value of Decimal Number	
32.1524	Tens	10	30	30
32.1524	Ones	1	2	2
32.1524	Tenths	0.1	$\dfrac{1}{10}$	0.1
32.1524	Hundredths	0.01	$\dfrac{5}{100}$	0.05
32.1524	Thousandths	0.001	$\dfrac{2}{1000}$	0.002
32.1524	Ten Thousandths	0.0001	$\dfrac{4}{10000}$	0.0004

Adding Decimal Numbers: Decimal numbers are added in the same way as ordinary numbers, with all of the decimal points lined up vertically. When the numbers are added, the decimal point holds the same position in the sum of the two numbers.

Subtracting Decimal Numbers: Decimal numbers are subtracted in the same way as ordinary numbers, with all of the decimal points lined up vertically. When the numbers are subtracted, the decimal point holds the same position in the difference of the two numbers.

Multiplying Decimal Numbers: Decimal numbers are multiplied in the same way as ordinary numbers. The position of the decimal point in the product is determined by the sum of the positions of the decimal point in each of the numbers being multiplied.

Dividing Decimal Numbers: Decimal numbers are divided in the same way as ordinary numbers. The position of the decimal point in the quotient can be determined when division is expressed in long division form.

Rounding Decimals
➤ **Step I:** Identify the digit in the decimal number to be rounded.
➤ **Step II:** Identify the digit immediately to the right of the number that is being rounded.
➤ **Step III:** If the digit identified in Step II is 0–4 (0, 1, 2, 3, 4), then the digit being rounded remains the same. If the digit identified in Step II is 5–9 (5, 6, 7, 8, 9), then the digit being rounded increases by 1.

Scientific Notation

Any nonzero number can be expressed in scientific notation when written in the form $a \times 10^b$ where a is a real number such that $1 \le a < 10$ (or $-10 < a \le -1$), (referred to as the *coefficient*), and b is an integer that describes the power of the *exponent*. To convert a number into scientific notation:
➤ **Step I:** Express the number in terms of a real number such that $1 < a < 10$.
➤ **Step II:** Determine the value of b the integer that is the power of the exponent.

To multiply numbers expressed in scientific notation, multiply the coefficients to reveal the new coefficient and multiply the exponents to reveal the new exponent.

To divide numbers expressed in scientific notation, divide the coefficients to reveal the new coefficient and divide the exponents to reveal the new exponent.

Percents

Percents are ratios with a denominator equal to 100 and represented by the symbol %.
➤ Percents can be converted to fractions by removing the % symbol and dividing by 100.
➤ Fractions can be converted to decimals by multiplying the fraction by 100%.
➤ Percents can be converted to decimals by removing the % symbol and placing the decimal point two positions to the left.
➤ Decimals can be converted to percents by multiplying the fraction by 100%.

Averages

$$\text{Average} = \frac{\text{Sum of terms}}{\text{Number of terms}}$$

CHAPTER 13

Algebra

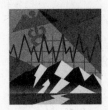

Read This Chapter to Learn About:

➤ **Algebraic Expressions**

➤ **Operations Involving Polynomials**

➤ **Factoring**

➤ **Solving Equations for Unknowns**

➤ **Quadratic Equations**

➤ **Solving Simultaneous Equations**

➤ **Absolute Value Equations and Inequalities**

➤ **Exponents and Logarithms**

ALGEBRAIC EXPRESSIONS

An a*lgebraic expression* is a collection of ordinary numbers, letters, and operational signs. Examples of algebraic expressions include $3t^2$, $4x^2 + 2y$, $6a^4 - 8b^3 - 10c^2$, and $7(4t - s)$. Each individual collection of numbers and letters that are separated by + or − signs is referred to as a *term*. Considering the algebraic expression $4x^2 + 2y$ listed above, $4x^2$ and $2y$ are both terms.

> **EXAMPLE:** Identify the terms in the algebraic expressions $6a^4 - 8b^3 - 10c^2$ and $7(4t - s)$.
>
> $6a^4 - 8b^3 - 10c^2$ 3 terms: ($6a^4$, $8b^3$, and $10c^2$)
> $7(4t - s) = 28t - 7s$ 2 terms: ($28t$ and $7s$)

If an algebraic expression has one term, it is known as a *monomial*. Examples of monomials are: $4rs^2t^3$, $7a$, and $\dfrac{5x^4}{y^2}$. If an algebraic expression has more than one term, it is referred to as a *polynomial*. Examples of polynomials are: $3a + 4b$, $x^2 - 4y^5 - 8z^9$, and $9(4m - n) = 36m - 9n$. A polynomial with two terms is called a *binomial* and a polynomial with three terms is called a *trinomial*.

OPERATIONS INVOLVING POLYNOMIALS

Polynomials can be added, subtracted, multiplied, and divided.

Addition of Polynomials

Two or more polynomials can be added by combining like terms. The process can be simplified by arranging the polynomials with like terms aligned in the same column. The sum can be found by adding each column.

EXAMPLES:

(1) Add the following polynomials: $3x - 2xy + 4y^2$, $5xy + y^2 - 2x$, and $-3y^2 + 7x + 10xy$.

SOLUTION: Arrange the three polynomials for addition such that like terms are in the same column.

$$
\begin{array}{rrr}
3x & -2xy & 4y^2 \\
-2x & 5xy & y^2 \\
+\ \ 7x & 10xy & -3y^2 \\
\hline
8x & 13xy & 2y^2
\end{array}
$$

The result is $8x + 13xy + 2y^2$.

(2) Add the following polynomials: $5x^2 + 3x^2y + 8y^2$ and $-4xy^2 + 6y^2 + 2x^2$.

SOLUTION: Arrange the two polynomials for addition such that like terms are in the same column. If there is one term in one polynomial that is not in the other, create a column for the term and place a "zero" in the column for the polynomial that does not have the term.

$$
\begin{array}{rrrr}
5x^2 & 3x^2y & 0xy^2 & 8y^2 \\
+\ \ 2x^2 & 0x^2y & -4xy^2 & 6y^2 \\
\hline
7x^2 & 3x^2y & -4xy^2 & 14y^2
\end{array}
$$

The result is $7x^2 + 3x^2y - 4xy^2 + 14y^2$.

Subtraction of Polynomials

Two or more polynomials can be subtracted by first changing the sign of every term in the polynomial being subtracted. Like terms between the polynomials undergoing subtraction are then added to provide the difference.

EXAMPLE: Subtract $3a^2 - 2ab - 4b^2$ from $9a^2 - 5ab + 6b^2$.

SOLUTION: First, change the sign of each term in the polynomial being subtracted which, in this problem, is $3a^2 - 2ab - 4b^2$.

$$3a^2 - 2ab - 4b^2 \Rightarrow -3a^2 + 2ab + 4b^2$$

Then, arrange the two polynomials for addition such that like terms are in the same column.

$$
\begin{array}{rrr}
9a^2 & -5ab & 6b^2 \\
+ \ -3a^2 & 2ab & 4b^2 \\
\hline
6a^2 & -3ab & 10b^2
\end{array}
$$

The result is $6a^2 - 3ab + 10b^2$.

Multiplication of Polynomials

Algebraic expressions can be multiplied by multiplying the terms in each expression using the laws of exponents (covered later in the chapter), the rules of signs, and the commutative and associative properties of multiplication. Let us consider some special cases of multiplication of algebraic expressions.

MULTIPLY A MONOMIAL BY ANOTHER MONOMIAL

EXAMPLE: Multiply $4a^2b^4c$ by $-7a^5b^3$.

SOLUTION:

Step 1: Write the product of the two monomials as:

$$\left(4a^2b^4c\right)\left(-7a^5b^3\right).$$

Step 2: Arrange the terms according to the commutative and associative properties:

$$\{(4)(-7)\}\{(a^2)(a^5)\}\{(b^4)(b^3)\}\{(c)\}.$$

Step 3: Use the rules of signs and laws of exponents to obtain the product of the two monomials:

$$-28a^7b^7c.$$

MULTIPLY A POLYNOMIAL BY A MONOMIAL

EXAMPLE: Multiply $5x^2 - 2xy + 7xy^2 + 8y^2$ by $4x^3y^5$.

SOLUTION:

Step 1: Write the product of the polynomial and monomial as:

$$(4x^3y^5)(5x^2 - 2xy + 7xy^2 + 8y^2).$$

Step 2: Multiply each term of the polynomial by the monomial:

$$(4x^3y^5)(5x^2) - (4x^3y^5)(2xy) + (4x^3y^5)(7xy^2) + (4x^3y^5)(8y^2).$$

Step 3: Use the rules of signs and laws of exponents to obtain the product of each term:

$$(20x^5y^5) - (8x^4y^6) + (28x^4y^7) + (32x^3y^7).$$

The product is $20x^5y^5 - 8x^4y^6 + 28x^4y^7 + 32x^3y^7$.

MULTIPLY A POLYNOMIAL BY ANOTHER POLYNOMIAL

EXAMPLE: Multiply $4x - 7x^2 + 8$ by $x + 3$.

SOLUTION:

Step 1: Arrange in descending powers of x and write the product of the two polynomials as:

$$
\begin{array}{r}
-7x^2 \quad +4x \quad +8 \\
\times \underline{\qquad\qquad x \quad +3}\,.
\end{array}
$$

Step 2: Perform the multiplication process:

Multiply $-7x^2 + 4x + 8$ by x which results in $-7x^3 + 4x^2 + 8x$;

Multiply $-7x^2 + 4x + 8$ by 3 which results in $-21x^2 + 12x + 24$.

Step 3: Add the results, making sure to align similar terms in the same column:

$$
\begin{array}{r}
-7x^3 \quad +4x^2 \quad +8x \\
+ \underline{\qquad -21x^2 \quad +12x \quad +24} \\
-7x^3 \quad -17x^2 \quad +20x \quad +24.
\end{array}
$$

Thus, the final solution is $-7x^3 - 17x^2 + 20x + 24$.

Special Products

The following special products of multiplying algebraic expressions occur frequently.

MULTIPLY A MONOMIAL BY A BINOMIAL

$$a(c + d) = ac + ad$$

EXAMPLE: Multiply $2x$ by $5x + y$.

SOLUTION: Using the symbolic expression given above, where $a = 2x$, $c = 5x$ and $d = y$, substitution yields $2x(5x + y) = 2x \cdot 5x + 2x \cdot y = 10x^2 + 2xy$.

MULTIPLY THE SUM AND DIFFERENCE OF TWO TERMS

$$(a + b)(a - b) = a^2 - b^2$$

EXAMPLE: Multiply $4x + 2y$ by $4x - 2y$.

SOLUTION: Using the symbolic expression given above, where $a = 4x$ and $b = 2y$, substitution yields $(4x + 2y)(4x - 2y) = (4x)^2 - (2y)^2 = 16x^2 - 4y^2$.

SQUARE OF A BINOMIAL

$$(a + b)^2 = a^2 + 2ab + b^2$$
$$(a - b)^2 = a^2 - 2ab + b^2$$

EXAMPLE: Determine the product $(2x - 3y)^2$.

SOLUTION: One can first simplify the expression by writing out the product as shown below and then multiply the terms from each expression:

$$(2x - 3y)^2 = (2x - 3y) \cdot (2x - 3y)$$

$$
\begin{array}{r}
2x - 3y \\
\times \quad 2x - 3y \\
\hline
-6xy + 9y^2 \\
+ \quad 4x^2 - 6xy + 0 \\
\hline
4x^2 + 12xy + 9y^2
\end{array}
$$

Division of Polynomials

Algebraic expressions can also be divided. Let us consider some special cases of division.

DIVIDE A MONOMIAL BY ANOTHER MONOMIAL

To divide a monomial by another monomial, first write the two expressions with the first monomial in the numerator and the second monomial in the denominator. Then calculate the quotient of the numerical coefficients, followed by the quotient of the variables. The solution can then be found by multiplying these quotients.

EXAMPLE: Divide $36x^5y^3z^2$ by $-9x^4yz^4$.

SOLUTION:

Step 1: Write the two monomials with the first monomial in the numerator and the second monomial in the denominator:

$$\frac{36x^5y^3z^2}{-9x^4yz^4}.$$

Step 2: Arrange the expressions so that you can calculate the quotients of the coefficients and of the variables:

$$\frac{36x^5y^3z^2}{-9x^4yz^4} = \left(\frac{36}{-9}\right)\left(\frac{x^5}{x^4}\right)\left(\frac{y^3}{y}\right)\left(\frac{z^2}{z^4}\right).$$

Step 3: Calculate the individual quotients:

$$\left(\frac{36}{-9}\right)\left(\frac{x^5}{x^4}\right)\left(\frac{y^3}{y}\right)\left(\frac{z^2}{z^4}\right) = (-4)(x^{5-4})(y^{3-1})(z^{2-4}) = (-4)(x)(y^2)(z^{-2}).$$

Step 4: Report the answer:

$$-4xy^2z^{-2} = -\frac{4xy^2}{z^2}.$$

DIVIDE A POLYNOMIAL BY ANOTHER POLYNOMIAL

To divide a polynomial by a polynomial, one should follow the steps below:

(1) Arrange the terms of both polynomials in descending powers of one of the variables common to both polynomials.
(2) Divide the first term in the dividend by the first term in the divisor. This yields the first term of the quotient.
(3) Multiply the first term of the quotient by the divisor and subtract from the dividend, thus obtaining a new dividend.
(4) Use the dividend obtained in (3) to repeat steps (2) and (3) until a remainder is obtained which is either of degree lower than the degree of the divisor or zero.
(5) The result is written:

$$\frac{\text{dividend}}{\text{divisor}} = \text{quotient} + \frac{\text{remainder}}{\text{divisor}}.$$

EXAMPLE: Divide $x^2 + 2x^4 - 3x^3 + x - 2$ by $x^2 - 3x + 2$.

SOLUTION: Arrange the polynomials in descending powers of x and divide as follows:

$$
\require{enclose}
\begin{array}{r}
2x^2 + 3x + 6 \phantom{{}-2} \\
x^2 - 3x + 2 \enclose{longdiv}{2x^4 - 3x^3 + x^2 + x - 2} \\
\underline{2x^4 - 6x^3 + 4x^2} \\
3x^3 - 3x^2 + x - 2 \\
\underline{3x^3 - 9x^2 + 6x} \\
6x^2 - 5x - 2
\end{array}
$$

FACTORING

Factoring is the mathematical process of simplifying an algebraic expression in terms of two or more algebraic expressions which, when multiplied together, produce the original expression. Examples of polynomials include:

$$x^2 + 2x + 1 = (x+1)(x+1) = (x+1)^2$$
$$4x^2 + 12x = 4x(x+3)$$
$$6x^2 - 7x - 5 = (3x-5)(2x+1)$$
$$x^2 + 2xy - 8y^2 = (x+4y)(x-2y).$$

The following procedures in factoring are very common and useful.

COMMON MONOMIAL FACTOR

$$ac + ad = a(c + d)$$

EXAMPLE: Factor $10x^2y + 2x^3$.

SOLUTION: First, determine any part of a term that is common to both terms in the polynomial. In this problem, the common part of a term is $2x^2$ which becomes **a** in the above expression. Thus, the factored polynomial becomes

$$10x^2y + 2x^3 = 2x^2(5y + x).$$

DIFFERENCE OF TWO SQUARES

$$a^2 - b^2 = (a+b)(a-b)$$

EXAMPLE: Factor $x^2 - 36$.

SOLUTION: $x^2 - 36 = x^2 - 6^2 = (x+6)(x-6).$

PERFECT SQUARE TRINOMIALS

$$a^2 + 2ab + b^2 = (a+b)^2$$
$$a^2 - 2ab + b^2 = (a-b)^2$$

EXAMPLE: Factor $x^2 + 8x + 16$.

SOLUTION: $x^2 + 8x + 16 = (x+4)(x+4) = (x+4)^2.$

GROUPING OF TERMS

$$ac + bc + ad + bd = c(a+b) + d(a+b) = (a+b)(c+d)$$

EXAMPLE: Factor $2ax - 4bx + ay - 2by$.

SOLUTION: $2ax - 4bx + ay - 2by = 2x(a-2b) + y(a-2b) = (a-2b)(2x+y).$

SOLVING EQUATIONS FOR UNKNOWNS

In a typical problem, you are given information in terms of variables with given numerical values and an equation or means of relating these pieces of information. The numerical values are then plugged into the equation with one unknown variable—the answer. Plugging the information into the equation is the easy part. Solving for the unknown variable can be challenging, depending upon its position or location in the equation. Techniques for obtaining the unknown can be found by first understanding that anything can be done to an equation as long as it is done to both sides of the equation. Then application of any mathematical principle and/or operation will yield the solution.

EXAMPLES: Solve for the unknown variable in each of the equations below:

(a) $x+4=10$ (b) $x^2-25=0$ (c) $\dfrac{1}{x+3}=-\dfrac{5}{x}$

(d) $\sqrt{5x+12}=8$ (e) $\ln(e^{3x+1})=13$

SOLUTIONS:

(a) In this problem, the objective is to move all terms with the unknown involved (in this case, x) to one side of the equation and everything else over to the other side. You may leave x on the left side of the equation, but now need to move 4 over to the other side. To eliminate 4 from the left-hand side, you can subtract 4, but if you subtract 4 from the left side of the equation, you must also subtract 4 from the right side of the equation. Thus,

$$x+4-4=10-4$$

and the answer is $x=6$.

(b) In this problem, you need to isolate the unknown variable. That can be done by eliminating 25 from the left-hand side. To do so, you add 25 to the left side of the equation, but then that must also be done to the right side.

$$x^2-25+25=0+25$$
$$x^2=25$$

The answer you are looking for is not x^2 but x. To obtain x, we take the square root of both sides which does yield x, our desired result.

$$\sqrt{x^2}=\sqrt{25}$$

or

$$x=\pm 5$$

The answer is $x=5$ or $x=-5$.

(c) In this problem, it is helpful to remove the unknown variable from the denominator on both sides of the equation. To accomplish this, you should first multiply both sides of the equation by $(x+3)$ followed by multiplication of both sides of the equation by x or:

Multiply both sides by $(x+3)$: $\qquad (x+3)\dfrac{1}{x+3} = -\dfrac{5}{x}(x+3)$

$$1 = -\dfrac{5(x+3)}{x}$$

Multiply both sides by x: $\qquad (x)1 = -\dfrac{5(x+3)}{x}(x)$

$$x = -5(x+3) = -5x - 15$$

Isolate the unknown variable on the left-hand side of the equation by adding $5x$ to both sides of the equation. This yields:

$$x + 5x = -5x - 15 + 5x$$
$$x + 5x = -15$$
$$6x = -15$$

The unknown variable can be determined by dividing both sides of the equation by 6:

$$\dfrac{6x}{6} = -\dfrac{15}{6}$$
$$x = -\dfrac{15}{6}$$

(d) The unknown variable is under a square root. To solve the expression for the unknown variable, x must be brought out from under the square root by squaring both sides of the equation:

$$\left(\sqrt{5x+12}\right)^2 = 8^2$$
$$5x + 12 = 64$$

To solve for x, first subtract 12 from both sides of the equation and then divide both sides of the equation by 5:

$$5x + 12 - 12 = 64 - 12$$
$$5x = 52$$
$$\dfrac{5x}{5} = \dfrac{52}{5}$$
$$x = \dfrac{52}{5} = 10\dfrac{2}{5}$$

(e) In this problem, it is important to note that the natural logarithm is the inverse operation of the exponential function or $\ln(e^x) = x$. Thus, the left-hand side of the equation is simply $3x+1$ or

$$\ln(e^{3x+1}) = 13$$
$$3x + 1 = 13$$

To solve for the unknown x, subtract 1 from both sides of the equation and then divide both sides of the equation by 3:

$$3x + 1 - 1 = 13 - 1$$
$$3x = 12$$
$$x = 4$$

Note: If you are unsure which technique to employ given a particular problem or do not seem to be getting the correct response, remember that the equation sign means that the left side is equal to the right side—they are both identical. Thus, you can always consider substituting each of the four possible options for the multiple-choice question into one side of the equation and, after calculating, see if your answer equals the other side of the equation.

QUADRATIC EQUATIONS

A quadratic equation is an equation of the form $ax^2 + bx + c = 0$. You may be given an equation which is exactly in this form, such as $2x^2 + 5x - 3 = 0$, or you may be given an equation such as $x^2 + 3x = -4$ which can easily be arranged to follow the form of the quadratic equation: $x^2 + 3x + 4 = 0$. In either case, you must solve the quadratic equation for the unknown variable, x.

One way to solve quadratic equations is the factor method. In this method, the equation is factored with each factor separately set to zero, yielding the two solutions of the quadratic equation. Consider, for example, the equation $x^2 + 3x - 10 = 0$. The left-hand side of the equation can be factored as:

$$x^2 + 3x - 10 = 0$$
$$(x - 2)(x + 5) = 0$$

The solution can be found by setting each of the factors equal to 0 and solving for x:

$$(x - 2) = 0 \Rightarrow x = 2 \qquad (x + 5) = 0 \Rightarrow x = -5$$

So the solution to the quadratic equation $x^2 + 3x - 10 = 0$ is $x = 2$ or $x = -5$.

Yet another way to solve quadratic equations is to use the quadratic formula. If the quadratic equation is given in the form $ax^2 + bx + c = 0$, then the quadratic formula can be applied in every instance by plugging the coefficients into:

$$x = \frac{-b \pm \sqrt{b^2 - 4ac}}{2a}$$

Let us solve the same example as above, $x^2 + 3x - 10 = 0$, using the quadratic formula. You should obtain the same results. In this case, $a = 1$, $b = 3$, and $c = -10$. Substituting these values into the quadratic formula yields:

$$x = \frac{-3 \pm \sqrt{3^2 - 4(1)(-10)}}{2(1)} = \frac{-3 \pm \sqrt{9 + 40}}{2} = \frac{-3 \pm \sqrt{49}}{2} = \frac{-3 \pm 7}{2}$$

The two solutions are

$$x = \frac{-3+7}{2} = \frac{4}{2} = 2 \quad \text{and} \quad x = \frac{-3-7}{2} = \frac{-10}{2} = -5.$$

These are the same solutions or roots you achieved using the factoring method.

The nature of the roots of the quadratic equation is determined by the value of the term under the radical, $b^2 - 4ac$. Assuming a, b, and c are real numbers, then

if $b^2 - 4ac > 0$, the roots are *real* and *unequal*.
if $b^2 - 4ac = 0$, the roots are *real* and *equal*.
if $b^2 - 4ac < 0$, the roots are *imaginary*.

SOLVING SIMULTANEOUS EQUATIONS

Most problems encountered in science will involve a scenario in which the student will be asked to solve for an unknown quantity using an equation relating the information given in the problem to the unknown quantity. Simple substitution of numerical values and possible elementary algebra operations will yield the desired answer. In some instances, a problem might involve a scenario with two unknown quantities. Solving a problem with two unknown quantities will require the student to use two equations that each describe the same system but in terms of more than one variable. The desired answers can be obtained by solving the system of equations simultaneously. The best way to explain the simultaneous solution of a system of equations is through an example.

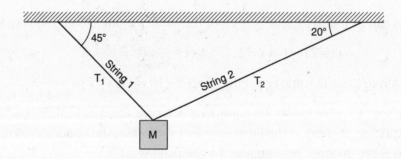

EXAMPLE: Consider an object of mass, M = 25 kg, suspended by two strings of different lengths oriented at different angles, as shown in the figure above.

String 1 is of length L = 0.5 m, oriented at an angle of 45° with respect to the horizontal, and is exerting a force on the object equal to T_1. String 2 is of length, L = 0.8 m, oriented at an angle of 20° with respect to the horizontal, and is exerting a force on the object equal to T_2. One is asked to find the magnitude of the tension forces, T_1 and T_2.

To solve the problem, begin by noting all given information:

Object	String 1	String 2
M = 25 kg	$L_1 = 0.5$ m	$L_2 = 0.8$ m
	$\theta_1 = 45°$	$\theta_2 = 20°$
$W = (25 \text{ kg})\left(9.8\dfrac{m}{s^2}\right) = 245$ N	$T_1 = ?$	$T_2 = ?$

Newton's Second Law of motion, namely $\Sigma F = ma$, applies to this problem. In words, Newton's Second Law says:

The sum of the forces (ΣF) acting on an object is equal to the mass (m) of the object times its acceleration (a).

Applying Newton's Second Law to the sum of the forces in the x direction and the y direction yields the two equations from which the two unknowns can be determined:

$\Sigma F_x = ma_x$ and $\Sigma F_y = ma_y$. Because the object is not accelerating in either direction, both a_x and $a_y = 0$. Identifying all of the forces acting only in the x direction yields:

$$\Sigma F_x = ma_x$$
$$-T_1 \cos\theta_1 + T_2 \cos\theta_2 = 0$$
$$-T_1 \cos(45°) + T_2 \cos(20°) = 0$$
$$-T_1(0.707) + T_2(0.940) = 0 \qquad \text{Equation A}$$

Similarly, identifying the forces acting only in the y direction yields:

$$\Sigma F_y = ma_y$$
$$T_1 \sin\theta_1 + T_2 \sin\theta_2 - W = 0$$
$$T_1 \sin(45°) + T_2 \sin(20°) - 245\,N = 0$$
$$T_1(0.707) + T_2(0.342) - 245N = 0 \qquad \text{Equation B}$$

You now have two equations (Equation A and Equation B) to solve for the two unknowns, T_1 and T_2. From Equation A, you can solve for T_1 in terms of T_2:

$$T_1 = \frac{T_2(0.940)}{(0.707)} = 1.3T_2 \qquad \text{Equation C}$$

You can then substitute Equation C into Equation B and solve for T_2:

$$1.3T_2(0.707) + T_2(0.342) - 245\,N = 0$$
$$1.26T_2 = 245\,N$$
$$T_2 = \frac{245N}{1.26} = 194N$$

This value is now substituted into Equation A to determine the second unknown, T_1:

$$-T_1(0.707) + (194\,N)(0.940) = 0$$
$$T_1 = \frac{182.17}{0.707} = 258N$$

ABSOLUTE VALUE EQUATIONS AND INEQUALITIES

Let us begin by defining the absolute value of a quantity. The absolute value of a real number, written as $|x|$, is defined as the distance between that number and zero on the number line. That distance can be in the positive direction, that is, $+x$ or in the negative direction, that is, $-x$. The formal definition of an absolute value of a real number is:

$$|x| = \begin{cases} -x \text{ if } x < 0 \\ +x \text{ if } x \geq 0 \end{cases}.$$

When an absolute value is present in an equation, it becomes helpful to consider the single equation as two equations. For example, the equation

$$|x + 10| = 5$$

can be rewritten as

$$x + 10 = +5 \quad \text{and} \quad x + 10 = -5.$$

Thus, the solutions of the equation $|x + 10| = 5$ are $x = +5$ and -5.

Next, let us discuss inequalities. An inequality is a mathematical equation in which the two sides are unequal—one side of the equation is either greater than or less than the other side of the equation. Inequalities are represented with the following symbols:

$a > b$ means that a is greater than b (or b is less than a)

$a \geq b$ means that a is greater than or equal to b (or b is less than or equal to a)

$a < b$ means that a is less than b (or b is greater than a)

$a \leq b$ means that a is less than or equal to b (or b is greater than or equal to a)

> **EXAMPLES:** (a) $0 < x < 4$ means that x is greater than 0 but less than 4
> (b) $-5 \leq x < 8$ means that x is greater than or equal to -5 but less than 8

In a problem involving absolute value inequalities, the goal is to solve the inequality for the unknown variable.

> **EXAMPLE:** Solve the inequality $|x + 4| < 7$ for x.

> **SOLUTION:** The inequality can be rewritten as $-7 < x + 4 < +7$. To isolate x, you must eliminate 4, which means you will have to subtract 4 from all terms of the inequality. The solution becomes $-7 - 4 < x + 4 - 4 < +7 - 4$ or $-11 < x < 3$. The solution interval is written as $(-11, 3)$.

EXPONENTS

Consider a number x that is multiplied by itself n times. Its product is $x \cdot x \cdot x \cdots x = x^n$ where x^n is referred to as "the nth power of x" or "x to the nth power". The number x is called the *base* and the positive integer n is the *exponent*. The term is referred to as an *exponential function*.

The following are the laws of exponents (m and n are positive integers):

(1) $x^m \cdot x^n = x^m$

EXAMPLE: $3^2 \cdot 3^3 = 3^{2+3} = 3^5 = 243$

(2) $\dfrac{x^m}{x^n} = x^{m-n} = \dfrac{1}{x^{n-m}}$ if $x \neq 0$

EXAMPLE: $\dfrac{5^5}{5^2} = 5^{5-2} = 5^3 = 125$

(3) $(x^m)^n = x^{mn}$

EXAMPLE: $(2^2)^4 = 2^{2 \cdot 4} = 2^8 = 256$

(4) $(xy)^m = x^m y^m, \left(\dfrac{x}{y}\right)^m = \dfrac{x^m}{y^m}$

EXAMPLE: $\left(\dfrac{5}{3}\right)^2 = \dfrac{5^2}{3^2} = \dfrac{25}{9}$

(5) $x^{-m} = \dfrac{1}{x^m}$

EXAMPLE: $6^{-2} = \dfrac{1}{6^2} = \dfrac{1}{36}$

LOGARITHMS

Logarithms are mathematical functions that are related to exponents—they are inverses of one another. Consider the exponential function $y = x^n$. Then the logarithmic counterpart can be written as $n = \log_x y$ for $y > 0$, $x > 0$, $x \neq 1$ where x is the base of the logarithm. The value of the logarithm, n, is the exponent to which the base x must be raised to obtain the value y. The following are the laws of logarithms:

(1) $\log_x mn = \log_x m + \log_x n$ such that $m, n > 0$

EXAMPLE: $\log_2(5 \cdot 6) = \log_2 5 + \log_2 6$

(2) $\log_x\left(\dfrac{m}{n}\right) = \log_x m - \log_x n$ such that $n \neq 0, \dfrac{m}{n} > 0$

EXAMPLE: $\log_{10}\left(\dfrac{36}{42}\right) = \log_{10} 36 - \log_{10} 42$

(3) $\log_x m^p = p \log_x m$ such that $m > 0$

EXAMPLE: $\log_7 8^4 = 4\log_7 8$

ON YOUR OWN

Problems

1. Solve for x: $2x - 3 > 3 - 4x$.

  A. $x > 1$ **B.** $x < 1$ **C.** $x > 2$ **D.** $x < 2$

2. Solve for x: $\dfrac{24}{3x + 42} = \dfrac{2}{9}$.

  A. 10   **B.** 22   **C.** 31   **D.** 42

3. What are the roots of the quadratic equation $x^2 - 3x + 1 = 0$?

  A. $x = 1, 3$ **C.** $x = \dfrac{3 + \sqrt{5}}{2}, \dfrac{3 - \sqrt{5}}{2}$

  B. $x = \dfrac{\sqrt{5}}{2}, -\dfrac{\sqrt{5}}{2}$ **D.** $x = \dfrac{3 + 3\sqrt{5}}{2}, \dfrac{3 - 3\sqrt{5}}{2}$

4. Solve the system of equations $x - 3y = -7$ and $4x + 3y = 2$.

  A. $x = 1, y = 2$ **B.** $x = -1, y = 2$ **C.** $x = -1, y = -2$ **D.** $x = 1, y = -2$

5. If $\dfrac{x}{y} = 5$ and $x = 25$, then what is the sum $x + y$?

  A. 5   **B.** 15   **C.** 20   **D.** 30

6. $(6x^3y^4z^2) \div (2xy^3z^5) =$

  A. $\dfrac{3x^2y}{z^3}$ **B.** $\dfrac{x^2y}{3z^3}$ **C.** $\dfrac{z^3}{3x^2y}$ **D.** $3x^2yz^3$

7. Solve for x: $\dfrac{x^2 - 4x - 21}{x + 3} = 1$.

  A. 1   **B.** 2   **C.** 8   **D.** 16

8. What are the roots of the equation $2x^2 - 6x - 20 = 0$?

  A. $2, -5$ **B.** $-2, 5$ **C.** $2, 5$ **D.** $-2, -5$

9. What is the solution set for the absolute value equation $|2x - 4| = 20$?

  A. $\{8, -12\}$ **B.** $\{8, 12\}$ **C.** $\{-8, 12\}$ **D.** $\{-8, -12\}$

10. Solve for x: $\sqrt[3]{\dfrac{27}{x - 4}} = 3$.

  A. 5   **B.** 4   **C.** 3   **D.** 1

Solutions

1. Answer: A

To solve the inequality $2x - 3 > 3 - 4x$, you need to collect like terms of x on one side of the inequality and all other values to the other side. First add 3 to both sides of the inequality:

$$2x - 3 + 3 > 3 - 4x + 3$$
$$2x > 6 - 4x$$

Then add $4x$ to both sides of the inequality:

$$2x + 4x > 6 - 4x + 4x$$
$$6x > 6$$

Dividing both sides by 6 yields $x > 1$.

2. Answer: B

To solve for the unknown in the equation $\dfrac{24}{3x + 42} = \dfrac{2}{9}$, the goal is to isolate the unknown variable x on one side of the equation with all other terms on the other side. Begin by multiplying both sides of the equation by $3x + 42$:

$$\left(3x + 42\right) \cdot \frac{24}{3x + 42} = \frac{2}{9} \cdot \left(3x + 42\right)$$
$$24 = \frac{2}{9} \cdot \left(3x + 42\right)$$

Then divide both sides by $\dfrac{2}{9}$ which, in essence, means multiply both sides of the equation by its reciprocal $\dfrac{9}{2}$:

$$\frac{9}{2} \cdot 24 = \frac{2}{9} \cdot \left(3x + 42\right) \cdot \frac{9}{2}$$
$$\frac{216}{2} = \left(3x + 42\right)$$

Then subtract 42 from both sides and divide both sides by 3, giving the desired result.

$$108 - 42 = 3x$$
$$\frac{108 - 42}{3} = x$$
$$x = 22$$

3. Answer: C

The equation is in the form of a quadratic equation $ax^2 + bx + c = 0$, where $a = 1$, $b = -3$, and $c = 1$. To solve this problem, you use the quadratic formula or

$$x = \frac{-b \pm \sqrt{b^2 - 4ac}}{2a} = \frac{-(-3) \pm \sqrt{(-3)^2 - 4(1)(1)}}{2(1)} = \frac{3 \pm \sqrt{9 - 4}}{2} = \frac{3 \pm \sqrt{5}}{2}.$$

The roots of the quadratic equation are:

$$x = \frac{3+\sqrt{5}}{2}, \frac{3-\sqrt{5}}{2}.$$

4. Answer: B

Write the equations as

$$(1) \quad x - 3y = -7$$

$$(2) \quad 4x + 3y = 2$$

Solve Equation (1) for x in terms of y or

$$(3) \quad x = 3y - 7$$

Substitute Equation (3) into Equation (2) to yield:

$$4(3y - 7) + 3y = 2$$

$$12y - 28 + 3y = 2$$

$$15y = 30$$

$$y = \frac{30}{15} = 2.$$

Substituting this value for y into Equation (1) yields the value for x:

$$x - 3(2) = -7$$

$$x = -7 + 6 = -1$$

So the solution for the system of equations is $x = -1, y = 2$.

5. Answer: D

From the first equation, multiply both sides by y resulting in

$$x = 5y$$

Because $x = 25$, you can write

$$25 = 5y$$

$$\text{or} \quad y = \frac{25}{5} = 5.$$

Substituting the given information regarding x and y into its sum yields:

$$x + y = 25 + 5 = 30$$

6. Answer: A

To determine the quotient of $6x^3 y^4 z^2$ divided by $2xy^3 z^5$, write the two monomials as a division problem with one expression on top of another:

$$\frac{6x^3 y^4 z^2}{2xy^3 z^5}.$$

The expressions are then arranged and presented such that you can calculate the quotients of the coefficients and of the variables:

$$\frac{6x^3y^4z^2}{2xy^3z^5} = \left(\frac{6}{2}\right)\left(\frac{x^3}{x}\right)\left(\frac{y^4}{y^3}\right)\left(\frac{z^2}{z^5}\right) = 3 \cdot x^2 \cdot y \cdot z^{-3} = \frac{3x^2y}{z^3}$$

7. Answer: C

Given the equation $\dfrac{x^2 - 4x - 21}{x + 3} = 1$, you must first try to simplify the numerator by

expressing the polynomial in terms of its factors or

$$\frac{x^2 - 4x - 21}{x + 3} = \frac{(x - 7)(x + 3)}{(x + 3)} = 1$$

The term $(x + 3)$ can be eliminated from the numerator and denominator because any term divided by itself is 1. Thus, the equation above can be simplified as:

$$(x - 7) = 1$$
$$\text{or } x = 8$$

8. Answer: B

To determine the roots of a quadratic equation, you can first try to see if the equation can be factored. In this case, the equation $2x^2 - 6x - 20 = 0$ can be factored as:

$$2x^2 - 6x - 20 = (2x + 4)(x - 5) = 0.$$

Thus, the roots can be found by the two equations:

$$2x + 4 = 0 \quad \text{which yields the root } x = -2$$

$$x - 5 = 0 \quad \text{which yields the root } x = 5.$$

9. Answer: C

When asked to solve an absolute value equation, it is helpful to write the equation in its two forms:

$$(1) \quad 2x - 4 = 20$$

$$(2) \quad 2x - 4 = -20$$

Solving for x in equation (1) yields $x = 12$ and in equation (2) yields $x = -8$.

10. Answer: A

In order to determine the value of x from the expression, you must perform mathematical operations to isolate x. The first step is to undo the cube root by raising each side of the equation by an exponent equal to 3 or

$$\left(\sqrt[3]{\frac{27}{x - 4}}\right)^3 = (3)^3$$

$$\frac{27}{x - 4} = 27$$

$$27 = 27 \cdot (x - 4)$$
$$27 = 27x - 108$$
$$27 + 108 = 27x$$
$$x = 5.$$

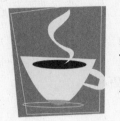

CRAM SESSION

Algebra

➤ An *algebraic expression* is a collection of ordinary numbers, letters, and operational signs. Examples include $3t^2$, $4x^2+2y$, $6a^4-8b^3-10c^2$, and $7(4t-s)$. Each individual collection of numbers and letters is referred to as a *term*.
➤ An algebraic expression with one term is called a *monomial*.
➤ An algebraic expression with more than one term is called a *polynomial*.
➤ A polynomial with two terms is a *binomial*. A polynomial with three terms is a *trinomial*.

OPERATIONS INVOLVING POLYNOMIALS

Addition of Polynomials

EXAMPLE: Add the following polynomials: $3x-2xy+4y^2$, $5xy+y^2-2x$, and $-3y^2+7x+10xy$.

SOLUTION: Arrange the three polynomials for addition such that like terms are in the same column.

$$
\begin{array}{rrr}
3x & -2xy & 4y^2 \\
-2x & 5xy & y^2 \\
+\ 7x & 10xy & -3y^2 \\
\hline
8x & 13xy & 2y^2
\end{array}
$$

Thus, the sum of the three polynomials is $8x+13xy+2y^2$.

Subtraction of Polynomials

EXAMPLE: Subtract $3a^2-2ab-4b^2$ from $9a^2-5ab+6b^2$.

SOLUTION: First, change the sign of each term in the polynomial being subtracted:

$$3a^2-2ab-4b^2 \Rightarrow -3a^2+2ab+4b^2.$$

Arrange the two polynomials for addition such that like terms are in the same column.

$$
\begin{array}{rrr}
9a^2 & -5ab & 6b^2 \\
-3a^2 & 2ab & 4b^2 \\
\hline
6a^2 & -3ab & 10b^2
\end{array}
$$

Thus, the difference of the two polynomials is $6a^2-3ab+10b^2$.

Multiplication of a Monomial by Another Monomial

EXAMPLE: Multiply $4a^2b^4c$ by $-7a^5b^3$.

SOLUTION:

Step 1: Write the product of the two monomials as:

$$(4a^2b^4c)(-7a^5b^3).$$

Step 2: Arrange the terms according to the commutative and associative properties:

$$\{(4)(-7)\}\{(a^2)(a^5)\}\{(b^4)(b^3)\}\{(c)\}.$$

Step 3: Use the rules of signs and laws of exponents to obtain the product of the two monomials:

$$-28a^7b^7c.$$

Multiplication of a Polynomial by a Monomial

EXAMPLE: Multiply $5x^2 - 2xy + 7xy^2 + 8y^2$ by $4x^3y^5$.

SOLUTION:

Step 1: Write the product of the polynomial and monomial as:

$$(4x^3y^5)(5x^2 - 2xy + 7xy^2 + 8y^2).$$

Step 2: Multiply each term of the polynomial by the monomial:

$$(4x^3y^5)(5x^2) - (4x^3y^5)(2xy) + (4x^3y^5)(7xy^2) + (4x^3y^5)(8y^2).$$

Step 3: Use the rules of signs and laws of exponents to obtain the product of each term:

$$(20x^5y^5) - (8x^4y^6) + (28x^4y^7) + (32x^3y^7).$$

Multiplication of a Polynomial by Another Polynomial

EXAMPLE: Multiply $4x - 7x^2 + 8$ by $x + 3$.

SOLUTION:

Step 1: Arrange in descending powers of x and write the product of the two polynomials as:

$$-7x^2 \qquad +4x \qquad +8$$
$$\underline{\times \qquad\qquad\quad x \qquad +3}$$

Step 2: Perform the multiplication process:

(1) Multiply $-7x^2+4x+8$ by x which results in $-7x^3+4x^2+8x$

(2) Multiply $-7x^2+4x+8$ by 3 which results in $-21x^2+12x+24$.

Step 3: Add the results making sure to align similar terms in the same column:

$$
\begin{array}{r}
-7x^3 \quad\; +4x^2 \quad\; +8x \\
+ \quad\quad\quad -21x^2 \quad +12x \quad +24 \\
\hline
-7x^3 \quad -17x^2 \quad +20x \quad +24.
\end{array}
$$

Thus, the product of the two polynomials is $-7x^3-17x^2+20x+24$.

Division of a Monomial by Another Monomial

EXAMPLE: Divide $36x^5y^3z^2$ by $-9x^4yz^4$.

SOLUTION:

Step 1: Write the two monomials with the first monomial in the numerator and the second monomial in the denominator.

$$\frac{36x^5y^3z^2}{-9x^4yz^4}.$$

Step 2: Arrange the expressions so that you can calculate the quotients of the coefficients and of the variables.

$$\frac{36x^5y^3z^2}{-9x^4yz^4} = \left(\frac{36}{-9}\right)\left(\frac{x^5}{x^4}\right)\left(\frac{y^3}{y}\right)\left(\frac{z^2}{z^4}\right).$$

Step 3: Calculate the individual quotients:

$$\left(\frac{36}{-9}\right)\left(\frac{x^5}{x^4}\right)\left(\frac{y^3}{y}\right)\left(\frac{z^2}{z^4}\right) = (-4)\left(x^{5-4}\right)\left(y^{3-1}\right)\left(z^{2-4}\right) = (-4)(x)\left(y^2\right)\left(z^{-2}\right).$$

Step 4: Report the answer:

$$-4xy^2z^{-2} = -\frac{4xy^2}{z^2}.$$

Division of a Polynomial by Another Polynomial

EXAMPLE: Divide $x^2+2x^4-3x^3+x-2$ by x^2-3x+2.

SOLUTION: Arrange polynomials in descending powers of x and divide:

$$
\begin{array}{r}
2x^2+3x+6 \\
x^2-3x+2{\overline{\smash{\big)}\,2x^4-3x^3+x^2+x-2}} \\
\underline{2x^4-6x^3+4x^2} \\
3x^3-3x^2+x-2 \\
\underline{3x^3-9x^2+6x} \\
6x^2-5x-2
\end{array}
$$

Factoring is the mathematical process of simplifying an algebraic expression in terms of two or more algebraic expressions which, when multiplied together, produce the original expression.

A. **Common monomial factor** $ac + ad = a(c + d)$

B. **Difference of two squares** $a^2 - b^2 = (a + b)(a - b)$

C. **Perfect square trinomials** $a^2 + 2ab + b^2 = (a + b)^2$

   $a^2 - 2ab + b^2 = (a - b)^2$

D. **Grouping of terms** $ac + bc + ad + bd = c(a + b) + d(a + b)$

   $= (a + b)(c + d)$

Solving Equations for Unknowns involves the use of mathematical relationships and operations applied to both sides of an equation to isolate and then solve for the unknown variable.

QUADRATIC EQUATIONS

A quadratic equation is an equation of the form $ax^2 + bx + c = 0$. You may be given an equation that is in exactly this form, such as $2x^2 + 5x - 3 = 0$, or you may be given an equation such as $x^2 + 3x = -4$ that can easily be arranged to follow the form of a quadratic equation—in this case, $x^2 + 3x + 4 = 0$. In either case, you must solve for the unknown variable, x.

To solve quadratic equations by the factor method, set each factor separately to zero, yielding the two solutions of the quadratic equation.

You can also solve quadratic equations by using the quadratic formula. If the quadratic equation is given in the form $ax^2 + bx + c = 0$, then the quadratic formula can be applied in every instance by plugging the coefficients into:

$$
x = \frac{-b \pm \sqrt{b^2 - 4ac}}{2a}
$$

The nature of the roots of the quadratic equation is determined by the value of the term under the radical, $b^2 - 4ac$. Assuming a, b, and c are real numbers, then

➤ If $b^2 - 4ac > 0$, the roots are *real* and *unequal*.

➤ If $b^2 - 4ac = 0$, the roots are *real* and *equal*.

➤ If $b^2 - 4ac < 0$, the roots are *imaginary*.

ABSOLUTE VALUE

The absolute value of a real number, written as $|x|$, is defined as the distance between that number and zero on the number line.

$$|x| = \begin{cases} -x \text{ if } x < 0 \\ +x \text{ if } x \geq 0 \end{cases}$$

INEQUALITIES

An inequality is a mathematical equation in which the two sides are unequal; one side of the equation is either greater than or less than the other side. Inequalities are represented as follows:

$a > b$ a is greater than b (or b is less than a)

$a \geq b$ a is greater than or equal to b (or b is less than or equal to a)

$a < b$ a is less than b (or b is greater than a)

$a \leq b$ a is less than or equal to b (or b is greater than or equal to a)

EXPONENTS

An exponential function is given by x^n or "the nth power of x" or "x to the nth power." The number x is called the *base* and the positive integer n is the *exponent*.

These are the laws of exponents (m and n are positive integers):

(1) $x^m \cdot x^n = x^{m+n}$

(2) $\dfrac{x^m}{x^n} = x^{m-n} = \dfrac{1}{x^{n-m}}$ if $x \neq 0$

(3) $(x^m)^n = x^{mn}$

(4) $(xy)^m = x^m y^m$, $\left(\dfrac{x}{y}\right)^m = \dfrac{x^m}{y^m}$

(5) $x^{-m} = \dfrac{1}{x^m}$

LOGARITHMS

Logarithms are inversely related to exponents. If you consider the exponential function $y = x^n$, then the logarithmic counterpart can be written as $n = \log_x y$ for $y > 0$, $x > 0$, $x \neq 1$ where x is the base of the logarithm. The value of the logarithm, n, is the exponent to which the base x must be raised to obtain the value y.

These are the laws of logarithms:

(1) $\log_x mn = \log_x m + \log_x n$ such that $m, n > 0$

(2) $\log_x \left(\dfrac{m}{n} \right) = \log_x m - \log_x n$ such that $n \neq 0, \dfrac{m}{n} > 0$

(3) $\log_x m^p = p \log_x m$ such that $m > 0$

CHAPTER 14

Probability and Statistics

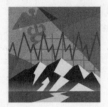

Read This Chapter to Learn About:

➤ **Probability**

➤ **Single-Event Probability**

➤ **Multiple-Event Probability**

➤ **Statistics**

➤ **Mean, Median, Mode, and Range**

PROBABILITY

A flip of the coin, a roll of the dice, or a card picked from a deck are just three examples of *probability*. The probability of an event is a numerical measure of the likelihood that the given event will occur. The calculations involving probability depend on how many and in what order are the successful outcomes and the total number of desired outcomes. If you assume that there are n different but equally possible outcomes of an event, with a number s of these outcomes considered successes and a number $f = n - s$, considered failures, then the probability of success for a given event, p, is $p = \dfrac{s}{n}$ and the probability of failure for a given event, q, is $q = \dfrac{f}{n}$.

SINGLE-EVENT PROBABILITY

Single-event probability is the probability of a single event occurring within a given set of possible outcomes. If you were to apply this to the probability of obtaining heads in a coin flip, there is one successful outcome (heads) and two possible outcomes (heads or tails). So the probability of obtaining heads in a coin flip is:

$$p = \frac{s}{n} = \frac{1}{2}.$$

Since the probability is a fraction, it can be expressed as a percentage, with the probability of obtaining heads in a coin flip being 50 percent. Single-event probability can also be applied to a single playing card drawn from a standard deck of 52 cards. To determine the probability that a selected card is of a black suit, you first note that a card can be selected from a deck in $n = 52$ different ways. Since there are two black suits (clubs and spades) with 13 cards per suit, a card of a black suit can be drawn from the deck in $s = 26$ different ways. Thus, the probability that the selected card is a card of a black suit is:

$$p = \frac{s}{n} = \frac{26}{52} = \frac{1}{2}.$$

EXAMPLE: What is the probability of not selecting the king of hearts from a deck of cards?

SOLUTION: To determine the probability of *not* selecting the king of hearts, let's determine the probability of selecting the king of hearts. Since the king of hearts is but one of 52 cards, the probability of selecting the king of hearts is $p = \frac{s}{n} = \frac{1}{52}$. Thus, the probability, q, of not selecting the king of hearts is $q = 1 - p = \frac{52}{52} - \frac{1}{52} = \frac{51}{52}$.

MULTIPLE-EVENT PROBABILITY

In single-event probability, you seek to determine the probability or likelihood of a single successful outcome out of a set of possible outcomes. In multiple-event probability, you seek to determine the probability or likelihood of two or more successful outcomes occurring, but not at the same time (referred to as mutually exclusive events) or the probability of one outcome occurring and another outcome not occurring (referred to as independent events).

Probability Involving Mutually Exclusive Events

Let us say that the probability of one successful event is P(A), the probability of another is P(B), and the two events have no common outcomes. Then the probability that either of these events occurring P(A or B) is the sum of their individual probabilities, P(A) + P(B) or P(A or B) = P(A) + P(B).

EXAMPLE: Upon rolling a pair of dice, what is the probability that the sum of the two numbers on the dice is either 6 or 12?

SOLUTION: The number of total possible outcomes from the roll of two dice is 36. In other words, there are 36 different pairs of numbers that can be obtained. You first need to determine the number of possible outcomes yielding a sum of 6 and 12 from the two dice. The number of possible outcomes yielding a sum of 6 is 5 or

$$\{(1, 5), (2, 4), (3, 3), (4, 2), (5, 1)\}.$$

The probability of yielding a sum of 6 between the two dice is

$$P(A) = P(6) = \frac{5}{36}.$$

The number of possible outcomes yielding a sum of 12 is 1 or

$$\{(6, 6)\}.$$

The probability of yielding a sum of 12 between the two dice is

$$P(B) = P(12) = \frac{1}{36}$$

Upon the roll of two dice, you cannot obtain a sum of 6 and a sum of 12 at the same time; the two successful outcomes thus are mutually exclusive. The probability that the sum of the two dice is either 6 or 12 is:

$$P(A \text{ or } B) = P(A) + P(B) = P(6) + P(12) = \frac{5}{36} + \frac{1}{36} = \frac{6}{36} = \frac{1}{6}.$$

Probability Involving Independent Events

In this case, you are being asked to determine the probability of two events that are independent and that occur in sequence. Two events are independent if the success of one event does not influence the success of the second event. The probability of two independent events, $P(A \text{ and } B)$, can be determined by first calculating the probability of each event occurring separately, $P(A)$ and $P(B)$, then multiplying these probabilities, $P(A) \cdot P(B)$, or

$$P(A \text{ and } B) = P(A) \cdot P(B).$$

EXAMPLE: What is the probability that two cards drawn from a deck of cards are face cards (king, queen, or jack) if the first card drawn is replaced before the second card is drawn?

SOLUTION: Because the two drawings are made from a full deck of cards, the two events are independent of one another. You first need to determine the probability of drawing a face card from a deck of cards. Out of a total of 52 cards, there are 3 face cards in each of the four suits, resulting in 12 face cards in a deck. The probability of drawing a face card, $P(A)$, is $\frac{12}{52}$. Because the first card is replaced before the second drawing, the probability of drawing a face card, P(B), is also $\frac{12}{52}$. Thus, the probability of drawing two face cards is

$$P(A \text{ and } B) = P(A) \cdot P(B) = \frac{12}{52} \cdot \frac{12}{52} = \frac{144}{2704}.$$

Because both the numerator and denominator are divisible by 16, the probability fraction can be simplified to $P(A \text{ and } B) = \frac{9}{169}$.

STATISTICS

Statistics is a branch of mathematics that reveals important information about variables and their relationships from groups or sets of data. Several statistical terms that are used in describing an individual variable from a data set include *mean*, *median*, *mode*, and *range*. As these terms are explained and discussed, consider the example of a student who has received the eleven following classroom grades for a certain grading period:

$$\{72, 86, 97, 95, 81, 79, 81, 67, 70, 65, 83\}.$$

Mean, Median, Mode, and Range

The *mean* is the average value of the data set. To determine the mean, the terms in the data set are added and then divided by the number of terms in the set. In other words, the mean can be determined by:

$$\text{Mean} = \frac{\text{Sum of all terms in data set}}{\text{Number of values in data set}}.$$

Applying this calculation to the set of classroom grades shown above,

$$\text{Mean} = \frac{72+86+97+95+81+79+81+67+70+65+83}{11} = \frac{876}{11} = 79.6 \approx 80.$$

The *median* is the middle term in a data set. In order to identify the median, it is helpful to arrange the terms of the data set in ascending order. If there is an odd number of terms in the data set, the single term in the middle is the median. However, if there is an even number of terms in the data set, the median is the average of the two terms that are in the middle of the data set. The median of the data set given above can be found by first arranging the terms of the data set in ascending order:

$$\{65, 67, 70, 72, 79, 81, 81, 83, 86, 95, 97\}.$$

The middle term of the data set, the median, is 81.

The *mode* is the term that occurs most frequently in the data set. Referring to the afore-mentioned data set, the term 81 occurs twice and is therefore the mode of the data set. The *range* is the difference between the largest and smallest terms in the data set. The largest term of the data set is 97 and the smallest term is 65. Thus, the range of the data set is:

$$\text{Range} = 97 - 65 = 32.$$

ON YOUR OWN
Problems

1. What is the probability of getting tails on a single coin toss?

   A. $\dfrac{1}{2}$ B. $\dfrac{1}{3}$ C. $\dfrac{2}{3}$ D. $\dfrac{3}{4}$

2. On a single roll of a die, what is the probability of not getting a 5?

   A. $\dfrac{1}{6}$ B. $\dfrac{3}{6}$ C. $\dfrac{4}{6}$ D. $\dfrac{5}{6}$

3. What is the probability of selecting an ace from a standard deck of cards?

   A. $\dfrac{1}{52}$ B. $\dfrac{4}{52}$ C. $\dfrac{48}{52}$ D. $\dfrac{51}{52}$

4. What is the probability of selecting a card of a spade suit from two standard decks of cards?

   A. $\dfrac{1}{104}$ B. $\dfrac{13}{104}$ C. $\dfrac{26}{104}$ D. $\dfrac{52}{104}$

5. When rolling a pair of dice, what is the probability that the sum of the two numbers on the dice is either 3 or 7?

   A. $\dfrac{1}{36}$ B. $\dfrac{3}{36}$ C. $\dfrac{5}{36}$ D. $\dfrac{8}{36}$

6. What is the probability that two cards drawn from a deck of cards are of the same suit (hearts, diamonds, clubs, or spades) if the first card drawn is replaced before the second card is drawn?

   A. $\dfrac{169}{2704}$ B. $\dfrac{26}{2704}$ C. $\dfrac{26}{52}$ D. $\dfrac{1}{52}$

Questions 7–10

A group of students working on a measurement lab were asked to measure the mass of seven objects found around the classroom and they obtained the following set of measurements:

$$\{2.0\,\text{g}, 3.5\,\text{g}, 2.0\,\text{g}, 5.5\,\text{g}, 8.4\,\text{g}, 9.1\,\text{g}, 12.3\,\text{g}\}.$$

7. What is the mean of the data set?

    A. 6.1 g   **B.** 5.5 g   **C.** 10.3 g   **D.** 2.0 g

8. What is the median of the data set?

    A. 6.1 g   **B.** 5.5 g   **C.** 10.3 g   **D.** 2.0 g

9. What is the mode of the data set?

    A. 6.1 g   **B.** 5.5 g   **C.** 10.3 g   **D.** 2.0 g

10. What is the range of the data set?

    A. 6.1 g   **B.** 5.5 g   **C.** 10.3 g   **D.** 2.0 g

Solutions

1. **Answer: A**

Obtaining tails in a coin flip requires one successful outcome (tails) out of two possible outcomes (heads or tails). So the probability of obtaining tails in a coin flip is: $p = \dfrac{s}{n} = \dfrac{1}{2}$.

2. **Answer: D**

The probability of not getting a 5 on the roll of the dice can be found using the equation $q = \dfrac{f}{n} = \dfrac{n-s}{n}$ where n is the total number of possible outcomes ($n=6$) and s is the number of outcomes considered a success ($s=1$). So $q = \dfrac{n-s}{n} = \dfrac{6-1}{6} = \dfrac{5}{6}$. Another way of looking at this problem would be that the probability of *not* rolling a 5 is equal to the probability of rolling a 1, 2, 3, 4, and 6 which is five out of a possible six outcomes.

3. **Answer: B**

To determine the probability that a selected card is an ace, you should first note that a card can be selected from a deck in $n=52$ different ways. Since there are four aces, one ace for each of the four suits, an ace can be drawn from the deck in $s=4$ different ways. Thus, the probability that the selected card is an ace is: $p = \dfrac{s}{n} = \dfrac{4}{52}$.

4. **Answer: C**

You are asked to determine the probability of selecting a spade from two standard decks of cards. Because there are two decks of cards, a single card can be selected from two decks in $n=104$ different ways. Since there are 13 spades in one deck of cards, a spade can be drawn from the two decks in $s=26$ different ways. Thus, the probability that the selected card is a spade is: $p = \dfrac{s}{n} = \dfrac{26}{104}$.

5. Answer: D

The number of total possible outcomes from the roll of two dice is 36. In other words, there are 36 different pairs of numbers that can be obtained. You first need to determine the number of possible outcomes yielding a sum of 3 and 7 from the two dice. The number of possible outcomes yielding a sum of 3 is 2 or

$$\{(1, 2), (2, 1)\}.$$

The probability of yielding a sum of 3 between the two dice is

$$P(A) = P(3) = \frac{2}{36}.$$

The number of possible outcomes yielding a sum of 7 is 6 or

$$\{(1, 6), (2, 5), (3, 4), (4, 3), (5, 2), (6, 1)\}.$$

The probability of yielding a sum of 7 between the two dice is

$$P(B) = P(7) = \frac{6}{36}.$$

Upon the roll of two dice, you cannot obtain a sum of 3 and a sum of 7 at the same time; the successful outcomes thus are mutually exclusive. The probability that the sum of the two dice is either 3 or 7 is:

$$P(A \text{ or } B) = P(A) + P(B) = P(3) + P(7) = \frac{2}{36} + \frac{6}{36} = \frac{8}{36}.$$

6. Answer: A

Because the two drawings are made from a full deck of cards, the two events are independent of one another. You first need to determine the probability of drawing a card of any suit from a deck of cards. Out of a total of 52 cards, there are 13 cards of any suit. The probability of drawing a card of any suit, $P(A)$, is $\frac{13}{52}$. Because the first card is replaced before the second drawing, the probability of drawing a card of the same suit, $P(B)$, is also $\frac{13}{52}$. Thus, the probability of drawing two cards of the same suit is

$$P(A \text{ and } B) = P(A) \cdot P(B) = \frac{13}{52} \cdot \frac{13}{52} = \frac{169}{2704}.$$

7. Answer: A

The mean of a data set is the arithmetic average of the terms of the data set or

$$\frac{2.0g + 3.5g + 2.0g + 5.5g + 8.4g + 9.1g + 12.3g}{7} = \frac{42.8g}{7} = 6.1g.$$

8. Answer: B

The median is the middle or center term of the data set when the data are in ascending numerical order, or 5.5 g.

9. **Answer: D**

The mode is the measurement that is the most frequent or common term in the data set. In this example, the mode is 2.0 g, because it occurs twice, more than any of the other measurements that occur only once.

10. **Answer: C**

The range or difference between the largest and smallest terms in this data set is 12.3 g −2.0 g = 10.3 g.

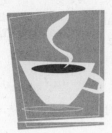

CRAM SESSION

Probability and Statistics

Probability   The probability of an event is a numerical measure of the likelihood that the given event will occur. If you assume that there are n different but equally possible outcomes to an event, with a number s of these outcomes considered successes and a number, $f = n - s$, considered failures, then the probability of

$$\text{success for a given event, } p, \text{ is } p = \frac{s}{n};$$

$$\text{failure for a given event, } q, \text{ is } q = \frac{f}{n}$$

Single-Event Probability   This is the probability of a single event occurring within a given set of possible outcomes. If you were to apply this to the probability of obtaining heads in a coin flip, there is one successful outcome (heads) and two possible outcomes (heads or tails). So the probability of obtaining heads in a coin flip is:

$$p = \frac{s}{n} = \frac{1}{2}.$$

Since the probability is a fraction, it can be expressed as a percentage, with the probability of obtaining heads in a coin flip being 50 percent.

Multiple-Event Probability   In multiple-event probability, you seek to determine the probability or likelihood of two or more successful outcomes occurring, but not at the same time (referred to as mutually exclusive events) or the probability of one outcome occurring and another outcome not occurring (referred to as independent events).

Probability Involving Mutually Exclusive Events   Suppose that the probability of one successful event is P(A) and the probability of a second event that does not depend on the success of the first event is P(B). Then the probability that either of these events occur, P(A or B), is the sum of their individual probabilities, P(A)+P(B), or

$$P(A \text{ or } B) = P(A) + P(B).$$

Probability Involving Independent Events   Two events are independent if the success of one event does not influence the success of the second event. The probability of two independent events, P(A and B), can be determined by first calculating the probability of each event occurring separately, P(A) and P(B), then multiplying each of these probabilities, P(A)·P(B), or

$$P(A \text{ and } B) = P(A) \cdot P(B).$$

Statistics   Statistics is a branch of mathematics that reveals important information about variables and their relationships from groups or sets of data. Statistical terms that are used to describe an individual variable from a data set include *mean*, *median*, *mode*, and *range*.

Mean: the average term of the data set. To determine the mean, the terms in the data set are added and then divided by the number of terms in the set. In other words, the mean can be determined by:

$$\text{Mean} = \frac{\text{Sum of all terms in data set}}{\text{Number of terms in data set}}.$$

Median: the middle term in a data set. In order to identify the median, arrange the terms of the data set in ascending order.

➤ If there is an odd number of terms in the data set, the single term in the middle is the median.

➤ If there is an even number of terms in the data set, the median is the average of the two terms that are in the middle of the data set.

Mode: the term that occurs most frequently in the data set.

Range: the difference between the largest and smallest terms in the data set.

Precalculus

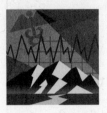

FUNCTIONS

A *function* is defined as a mathematical relationship between elements of a given set $X = \{x\}$, referred to as the *domain*, and another set $Y = \{y\}$, referred to as the *range*. A function represents a mathematical relationship between a dependent variable y and an independent variable x, which can represent any number within a specified range or interval. A function, denoted typically as $y = f(x)$, allows one to mathematically characterize a physical system in terms of variables that directly influence the system's behavior and stability. Two types of functions that will be discussed in this review are *polynomial functions* and *power functions*.

Polynomial Functions

Polynomial functions are presented in the form

$$y = f(x) = a_0 + a_1 x + a_2 x^2 + a_3 x^3 + \ldots + a_n x^n,$$

where a_0, a_1, a_2, a_3, a_n are coefficients (constants) and n is a whole number that describes the degree or order of the polynomial. Special cases of the polynomial function include the first-order polynomial function (linear function) given by

$$y = f(x) = a_0 + a_1 x \qquad a_1 \neq 0.$$

Another special case of the polynomial function is the second-order polynomial function (quadratic equation) given by

$$y = f(x) = a_0 + a_1 x + a_2 x^2 \qquad a_1, a_2 \neq 0.$$

Consider the quadratic equation expressed in the form $ax^2 + bx + c$ and equal to zero or

$$ax^2 + bx + c = 0.$$

The solution x can be determined for the quadratic equation from the following formula:

$$x = \frac{-b \pm \sqrt{b^2 - 4ac}}{2a}$$

Two items of note:

1. It is possible that the solution from the above formula may result in complex roots, that is, the square root of a negative quantity.
2. The calculation from the formula will reveal two possible solutions. When applied to a science problem, it becomes readily clear by either the sign or the magnitude of the values that one solution is not physically realistic or possible, with the other solution being the correct solution.

Graphs of polynomial functions are shown below.

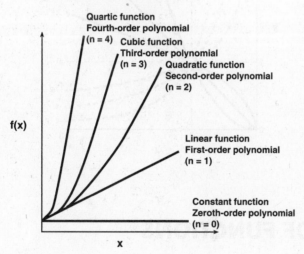

Polynomial Functions

Power Functions

Power functions are defined by

$$y = ax^n,$$

where a is a constant and n is a real number, representing the mathematical power of the function. Mathematical rules involving powers are summarized below. If p and q are any numbers and $a > 0$ but $a \neq 1$:

$$a^p a^q = a^{p+q} \qquad a^p + a^q \neq a^{p+q} \qquad \frac{a^p}{a^q} = a^{p-q} \qquad \left(a^p\right)^q = a^{pq}$$

$$a^{m/n} = \sqrt[n]{a^m} \qquad a^{-n} = \frac{1}{a^n} \qquad a^{1/n} = \sqrt[n]{a} \qquad a^0 = 1$$

Several forms of the power function include:

$$n = -2: y = x^{-2} = \frac{1}{x^2} \qquad n = -1: y = x^{-1} = \frac{1}{x} \qquad n = -\frac{1}{2}: y = x^{-1/2} = \frac{1}{\sqrt{x}}$$

$$n = 0: y = x^0 = 1 \qquad n = \frac{1}{2}: y = x^{1/2} = \sqrt{x} \qquad n = 1: y = x^1 = x$$

$$n = 2: y = x^2 = x^2$$

Graphs of power functions are shown below.

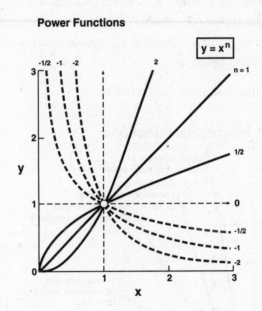

Power Functions

GRAPHS OF FUNCTIONS

An important aspect of science is the ability to evaluate and interpret data presented in graphs. Graphs represent an important means for illustrating information obtained from a scientific experiment or observations. Graphs can reveal relationships and trends between the graphed variables and allow the scientist to draw relevant conclusions about the experimental variables and the underlying principles involved in the scientific question being answered. When you are asked to evaluate and interpret graphs, consider the following points:

1. All graphs should have a short title that will describe the experiment that was conducted. What does the title tell you about the experiment in general and the variables being investigated?

2. The variable represented on each axis should be clearly labeled on its relevant axis with appropriate units noted. The *independent variable* (the variable that is free to move) is displayed on the horizontal *x*-axis while the *dependent variable* (the variable that depends upon the value of the independent variable) is displayed on the vertical *y*-axis.

3. The scale and range for each axis should be evident from the graph. On the grid on which the data are presented, a legend should be noted, for example, that 1 square = 1 meter or 5 squares = 10 meters per second.

4. Given the features involved in the presentation of the graph, you should then look at the data points themselves. Questions that a scientist might pose include:

    ➤ Is there a general trend exhibited by the data and, if so, is the relationship between the two variables linear, inverse, quadratic or something else?

    ➤ If the trend is linear, is the relationship between the two variables constant (represented by a straight horizontal line), increasing (represented by an upward slanted line), or decreasing (represented by a downward slanted line)?

    ➤ If the relationship between the two variables is constant, what is the numerical value of the dependent variable that holds throughout the entire experiment?

    ➤ If the relationship between the two variables is increasing or decreasing, by how much is the trend increasing or decreasing (that is, what is the slope of the curve?) and where do these functions begin on the *y*-axis (that is, what is the *y*-intercept of the curve?). This information can be quantified for a linear function by calculating its slope and y-intercept.

Calculating the Slope and *y*-Intercept

Consider the function describing a line:

$$y = mx + b.$$

Two important features of a function presented by the above equation are the *slope*, *m*, and the *y-intercept*, *b*, of the function. These features are illustrated in the figure below.

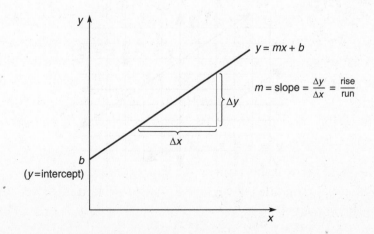

Some relationships between variables may originate at the origin (0,0) of the coordinate system while others may originate from or pass through a point along the y-axis other than the origin. This value, the point at which the line intercepts or passes through the y-axis, is known as the y-intercept.

The *slope* defines the rate of change of the line in the y-axis with respect to the corresponding change in the x axis (also known as the rise over the run) and is given mathematically as

$$\text{Slope} = m = \frac{\Delta y}{\Delta x} = \frac{y_2 - y_1}{x_2 - x_1}.$$

Important features to note about the slope are:

➤ If the slope is positive, y increases as x increases.
➤ If the slope is negative, y decreases as x increases.
➤ A horizontal line (that is, $y = c$ where c is a constant) has zero slope.
➤ A vertical line (that is, $x = c$ where c is a constant) has an undefined slope.

PROPERTIES OF FUNCTIONS
Parallel Lines

Two lines are parallel if they do not intersect, have the same slope, and have different y-intercepts.

EXAMPLE: Determine whether the lines $y = -\frac{3}{4}x + 2$ and $y = -\frac{3}{4}x - 3$ are parallel.

SOLUTION: By plotting the graphs of the lines $y = -\frac{3}{4}x + 2$ and $y = -\frac{3}{4}x - 3$ shown below, you can see that the lines are parallel. This is the case because their slopes are equal.

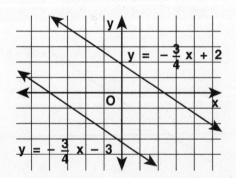

Perpendicular Lines

Two nonvertical lines are perpendicular if the product of their slopes is -1. The two intersecting lines form right angles.

> **EXAMPLE:** Determine whether the lines $y = -\frac{3}{5}x + 6$ and $y = \frac{5}{3}x + 2$ are perpendicular.
>
> **SOLUTION:** By plotting the graphs of the lines $y = -\frac{3}{5}x + 6$ and $y = \frac{5}{3}x + 2$ shown below, you can see that the lines are perpendicular. The slope of the line $y = -\frac{3}{5}x + 6$ is $m = -\frac{3}{5}$ and the slope of the line $y = \frac{5}{3}x + 2$ is $m = \frac{5}{3}$. The lines are perpendicular if the product of their slopes is -1 or $\left(-\frac{3}{5}\right)\left(\frac{5}{3}\right) = -1$.

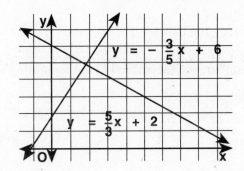

ON YOUR OWN

Problems

1. Solving the equation $9x^2 - 81x = 0$ for x yields the roots

   A. $12, 9$ **B.** $6, 9$ **C.** $3, 9$ **D.** $0, 9$

2. Solve for x: $6x^4 - 96 = 0$

   A. ± 2 **B.** ± 4 **C.** ± 16 **D.** ± 32

3. Solve for x: $(3x + 3)^3 = 729$

   A. -2 **B.** -3 **C.** 2 **D.** 3

4. What is the equation of a line that passes through the point $(2, -5)$ and has a slope of 4?

   A. $y = 4x + 13$ **B.** $y = 4x$ **C.** $y = 4x - 13$ **D.** $y = 4x + 26$

5. What is the slope of a line that passes through the points (3, 3) and (6, 8)?

A. $\dfrac{5}{3}$ **B.** $-\dfrac{5}{3}$ **C.** $\dfrac{3}{5}$ **D.** $-\dfrac{3}{5}$

Questions 6, 7, and 8

The following position (meters) versus time (seconds) data were collected for a remote-controlled car as it moved along a straight track.

Time (seconds)	0	15	30	45	60	75
Position (meters)	0	5	10	15	20	25

6. What is the velocity of the car as it moves along the track?

A. $-\dfrac{1}{3}\dfrac{m}{s}$ **B.** $\dfrac{1}{3}\dfrac{m}{s}$ **C.** $3\dfrac{m}{s}$ **D.** $-3\dfrac{m}{s}$

7. The position, P, of the car at any time, t, would best be described by which of the following equations?

A. $P=\left(-3\dfrac{m}{s}\right)t$ **B.** $P=\left(-\dfrac{1}{3}\dfrac{m}{s}\right)t$ **C.** $P=\left(3\dfrac{m}{s}\right)t$ **D.** $P=\left(\dfrac{1}{3}\dfrac{m}{s}\right)t$

8. Which of the following lines is not parallel to the remaining three lines?

A. $y=-\dfrac{3}{5}x+3$ **B.** $y=-\dfrac{3}{5}x$ **C.** $y=-\dfrac{3}{5}x-5$ **D.** $y=-\dfrac{5}{3}x-\dfrac{3}{5}$

Questions 9 and 10

Consider two lines, $3x-y=1$ and $x+3y=5$, that are perpendicular to one another.

9. These two lines are perpendicular to one another because the product of their slopes equals -1.

What are the slope values for the two lines, respectively?

A. $3,-\dfrac{1}{3}$ **B.** $3,\dfrac{1}{3}$ **C.** $5,-\dfrac{1}{5}$ **D.** $3,-3$

10. What are the x and y-coordinates of the point where the two perpendicular lines intersect?

A. $\left(\dfrac{4}{5},\dfrac{5}{7}\right)$ **B.** $\left(\dfrac{5}{4},\dfrac{7}{5}\right)$ **C.** $\left(\dfrac{4}{5},\dfrac{7}{5}\right)$ **D.** $\left(\dfrac{7}{5},\dfrac{4}{5}\right)$

Solutions

1. Answer: D

The first thing to do in solving the equation $9x^2-81x=0$ for x is to factor out common terms, which leads to

$$9x(x-9)=0.$$

The roots of x can now be determined by solving for x from the two equations

$$9x = 0 \text{ or } x = 0,$$

$$(x - 9) = 0 \text{ or } x = 9.$$

The roots for the equation are 0, 9.

2. **Answer: A**

In order to solve the equation $6x^4 - 96 = 0$ for x, you need to isolate x:

$$6x^4 = 96;$$

$$x^4 = \frac{96}{6} = 16.$$

Taking the fourth root of each side of the equation yields $x = \pm 2$.

3. **Answer: C**

This equation can be solved by first taking the cube root of both sides of the equation $(3x + 3)^3 = 729$ or $3x + 3 = 9$. Solving for x yields $x = 2$.

4. **Answer: C**

You can use the information provided by the specific point and the value of the slope to derive the equation for the line:

$$m = \frac{y_2 - y_1}{x_2 - x_1}$$

$$4 = \frac{y_2 - (-5)}{x_2 - 2} = \frac{y_2 + 5}{x_2 - 2}$$

$$y_2 + 5 = 4 \cdot (x_2 - 2)$$

$$y_2 + 5 = 4x_2 - 8$$

$$y_2 = 4x_2 - 8 - 5$$

$$y_2 = 4x_2 - 13$$

$$y = 4x - 13.$$

5. **Answer: A**

The slope is defined as: $m = \frac{y_2 - y_1}{x_2 - x_1}$. If the first point $(3, 3) = (x_1, y_1)$ and the second point $(6, 8) = (x_2, y_2)$, then substituting these coordinate values into the definition for the slope yields

$$m = \frac{8 - 3}{6 - 3} = \frac{5}{3}.$$

6. **Answer: B**

When given data, you should create a graph to determine the relationship between the y-variable (position) and the x-variable (time). By creating such a graph, as shown below, you can see a linear relationship. The slope of the line, the change in position over the change in time, reveals the velocity. Because it is a line, any two points will reveal the slope, so we will select the first and last data points.

$$m = \frac{25m - 0m}{75s - 0s} = \frac{25}{75}\frac{m}{s} = \frac{1}{3}\frac{m}{s}.$$

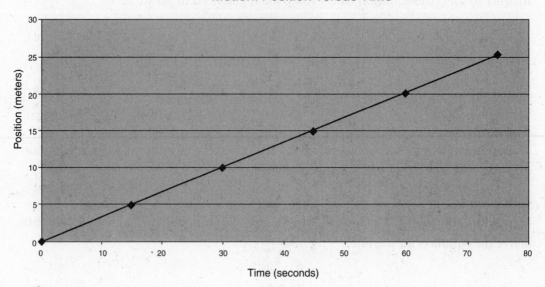

Motion: Position versus Time

7. Answer: D

From the previous problem, the velocity or slope of the data was found to be $m = \frac{1}{3}\frac{m}{s}$. Using the definition of the equation of a line or $y = mx + b$, you get $P = \left(\frac{1}{3}\frac{m}{s}\right)t$ where $y = P$, $x = t$, and $b = y\text{-intercept} = 0$.

8. Answer: D

Lines are parallel if they have the same slope. The lines in answer choices A, B, and C, all have the same slope, $-\frac{3}{5}$. Choice D has a different slope, $-\frac{5}{3}$, and is thus not parallel to the remaining three lines.

9. Answer: A

To find the slope of each line, you must rearrange the equation to conform to the definition of a line or $y = mx + b$.

Equation 1: $3x - y = 1$ Equation 2: $x + 3y = 5$

$y = 3x - 1$ $3y = -x + 5$ or $y = -\left(\frac{1}{3}\right)x + \frac{5}{3}$

$m = 3.$ $m = -\frac{1}{3}.$

10. **Answer: C**

The coordinates of the point where the two perpendicular lines intersect can be found by simultaneously solving the two equations $3x - y = 1$ and $x + 3y = 5$ for x and y.

Starting with the first equation and solving for y:

$$y = 3x - 1.$$

Substituting into the second equation yields

$$x + 3(3x - 1) = 5$$

$$x + 9x - 3 = 5$$

$$10x = 8$$

$$x = \frac{8}{10} = \frac{4}{5}.$$

Substituting this value for x into the first equation yields:

$$y = 3\left(\frac{4}{5}\right) - 1 = \frac{12}{5} - 1 = \frac{12}{5} - \frac{5}{5} = \frac{7}{5}.$$

The coordinates of the point of intersection are $\left(\frac{4}{5}, \frac{7}{5}\right)$.

CRAM SESSION

Basic Math

Function   A *function* is a mathematical relationship between elements of a given set $X=\{x\}$, referred to as the *domain*, and another set $Y=\{y\}$, referred to as the *range*. A function describes a mathematical relationship between a dependent variable y and an independent variable x, which can represent any number within a specified interval.

Polynomial functions are represented by the form

$$y=f(x)=a_0+a_1x+a_2x^2+a_3x^3+\ldots+a_nx^n,$$

where a_0, a_1, a_2, a_3, a_n are coefficients (constants) and n is a positive integer or zero that describes the degree or order of the polynomial.

Special cases

➤ A first-order polynomial function (linear function) is given by

$$y=f(x)=a_0+a_1x \qquad\qquad a_1\neq0.$$

➤ A second-order polynomial function (quadratic equation) is given by

$$y=f(x)=a_0+a_1x+a_2x^2 \qquad\qquad a_1,a_2\neq0.$$

➤ If the quadratic equation is written in the form

$$ax^2+bx+c=0,$$

then the solution x can be determined from the following formula:

$$x=\frac{-b\pm\sqrt{b^2-4ac}}{2a}.$$

Power Functions

Power functions are defined by

$$y=ax^n,$$

where a is a constant and n is a real number, representing the mathematical power of the function. If p and q are any numbers and $a>0$ but $a\neq1$:

$$a^pa^q=a^{p+q} \qquad a^p+a^q\neq a^{p+q} \qquad \frac{a^p}{a^q}=a^{p-q} \qquad \left(a^p\right)^q=a^{pq}$$

$$a^{m/n} = \sqrt[n]{a^m} \qquad a^{-n} = \frac{1}{a^n} \qquad a^{1/n} = \sqrt[n]{a} \qquad a^0 = 1$$

Graphs of Functions

Graphs, a means for illustrating information from scientific observations, can reveal relationships and trends between the graphed variables and can allow the scientist to draw relevant conclusions about the variables and the underlying principles involved in the scientific question being answered.

Important Features of a Graph

1. All graphs should have a title that describes the experiment and variables being investigated.
2. The *independent variable* (the variable that is free to move) is displayed on the horizontal x-axis, while the *dependent variable* (the variable that depends upon the value of the independent variable) is displayed on the vertical y-axis.
3. The scale and range for each variable should be noted in a legend on the graph.
4. Looking at the data points in the graph, you should note:
   ➤ Is there a general trend exhibited by the data and, if so, is the relationship between the two variables linear, inverse, quadratic or something else?
   ➤ If the trend is linear, is the relationship between the two variables constant (represented by a straight horizontal line), increasing (represented by an upward slanted line), or decreasing (represented by a downward slanted line)?
   ➤ If the relationship between the two variables is constant, what is the numerical value of the dependent variable that holds throughout the entire experiment?
   ➤ If the relationship between the two variables is increasing or decreasing, by how much is the trend increasing or decreasing (i.e., what is the slope of the curve?) and where does the function begin on the y-axis (i.e., what is the y-intercept of the curve?).

Calculating the Slope and y-Intercept

For the function describing a line, $y = mx + b$, m is the slope and b is the y-intercept of the function. The *y-intercept* is the point at which the line intercepts or passes through the y-axis. The *slope* defines the rate of change of the line in the y-axis with respect to the corresponding change in the x axis (also known as the rise over the run) and is given as

$$\text{Slope} = m = \frac{\Delta y}{\Delta x} = \frac{y_2 - y_1}{x_2 - x_1}.$$

Important features to note about the slope are:

➤ If the slope is positive, y increases as x increases.

➤ If the slope is negative, y decreases as x increases.

➤ A horizontal line (that is, $y = c$ where c is a constant) has zero slope.

➤ A vertical line (that is, $x = c$ where c is a constant) has an undefined slope.

Properties of Functions

➤ Two lines are *parallel* if they do not intersect, have the same slope and have different *y*-intercepts.

➤ Two lines are *perpendicular* if the product of their slopes is –1. The two intersecting lines form right angles.

Calculus

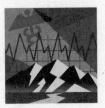

DIFFERENTIATION

The basis for differential calculus is the derivative, a mathematical operation very similar to the calculation of the slope of a function. Given any two coordinate points (x_1, y_1) and (x_2, y_2) along the line, the slope of a straight line can be calculated from the formula

$$\text{Slope} = m = \frac{\Delta y}{\Delta x} = \frac{y_2 - y_1}{x_2 - x_1}.$$

How would you calculate the slope of a function if it were not a straight line? If it were a polynomial function? If it were a power function? In fact, the majority of functions that occur in nature are not linear. Given the importance of the slope to the behavior of a function, could a slope be calculated for such a function and, if so, how? The answer is yes, using differential calculus and the derivative.

THE DERIVATIVE

When dealing with a curved function, you cannot simply pick two coordinate points and calculate the change of these points along both the x and y axes. If you did, you would get different values for the slope depending on which two coordinate points you chose. If a range of x was chosen that was so small that you were essentially looking at a point, then the slope for the function could be determined from a line that is tangent to the point.

The derivative of a function, described symbolically as $\frac{df(x)}{dx} = \frac{dy}{dx}$ or $f'(x)$, describes the rate of increase (or decrease) along the y-axis with respect to the x-axis at a point on the curve, as shown in the figure below.

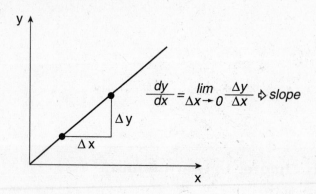

From the expression above, dx and dy are termed differentials. The differentials dx and dy are the same as Δx and Δy in meaning but represent infinitesimal or very small changes along their respective axes. The derivative $\frac{dy}{dx}$ can be equated with the slope $\frac{\Delta y}{\Delta x}$ only in the limit as Δx becomes very small and approaches 0. This is expressed mathematically

$$\frac{dy}{dx} = \lim_{\Delta x \to 0} \frac{\Delta y}{\Delta x} \Rightarrow \text{slope}.$$

Differentiation can be applied to the entire spectrum of functions by using specific differentiation formulas. For the purpose of this review, differentiation will be limited to differentiation of polynomial functions as well as a constant. The formulas are listed below:

$\frac{d}{dx}(c) = 0$ where c is a constant. The constant can be any real number or variable

other than the differentiating variable, x.

$\frac{d}{dx}(cx^n) = ncx^{n-1}$ where c is a constant and n is a real number that is not equal to

zero.

EXAMPLE: Calculate the first and second derivative of $f(x) = x^4 - 5x^3 + 7x - 2$.

SOLUTION: Since you are asked to determine the derivative of a polynomial function,

$$f'(x) = \frac{d}{dx}(x^4 - 5x^3 + 7x - 2)$$

$$= \frac{d}{dx}(x^4) - \frac{d}{dx}(5x^3) + \frac{d}{dx}(7x) - \frac{d}{dx}(2) = 4x^3 - 15x^2 + 7 - 0$$

$$f'(x) = 4x^3 - 15x^2 + 7.$$

To calculate the second derivative of the function, you calculate the derivative of the differentiated function, $f'(x)$ or

$$f''(x) = \frac{d}{dx}\left(f'(x)\right) = \frac{d}{dx}\left(4x^3 - 15x^2 + 7\right)$$

$$= \frac{d}{dx}\left(4x^3\right) - \frac{d}{dx}\left(15x^2\right) + \frac{d}{dx}\left(7\right) = 12x^2 - 30x + 0$$

$$f''(x) = 12x^3 - 30x.$$

APPLICATIONS OF THE DERIVATIVE

One important application of the derivative is motion. Let us consider the position of a particle, $\Delta x(t)$ (measured in units of centimeters, cm), that moves over a time t (measured in units of seconds, s) according to the function

$$\Delta x(t) = 4t^3 - 10t^2 + 6.$$

You can determine the velocity and acceleration of the particle through differentiation.

Velocity

The velocity can be determined by calculating the derivative of the position of the particle. Because the motion of the particle is described by a polynomial function, the velocity, v (in units of cm/s), can be determined by:

$$v(t) = \frac{d}{dt}\left(4t^3 - 10t^2 + 6\right) = \frac{d}{dt}\left(4t^3\right) - \frac{d}{dt}\left(10t^2\right) + \frac{d}{dt}\left(6\right)$$

$$= 12t^2 - 20t + 0$$

$$= 12t^2 - 20t$$

The velocity of the particle for any time t is $v(t) = 12t^2 - 20t$. To find the velocity of the particle at a particular time, say three seconds, substitute the value given for time for each mention of t or

$$v(t = 3s) = 12(3s)^2 - 20(3s) = 108\frac{cm}{s} - 60\frac{cm}{s} = 48\frac{cm}{s}.$$

Acceleration

From the velocity of the particle, you can now determine the acceleration or rate of change of velocity of the particle by once again taking the derivative—of the velocity function, not the position function. The acceleration, a, can be found by:

$$a(t) = \frac{d}{dt}\left(v(t)\right) = \frac{d}{dt}\left(12t^2 - 20t\right) = \frac{d}{dt}\left(12t^2\right) - \frac{d}{dt}\left(20t\right) = 24t - 20.$$

So the acceleration of the particle at any time, t is

$$a(t) = 24t - 20.$$

INTEGRATION

The integral is to integral calculus as the derivative is to differential calculus. Differentiation is used to determine the slope or the rate of change of a function—regardless of whether the function is linear or nonlinear. Integration is used to determine the area under the curve. If the curve is linear, you can subdivide the area into rectangular strips. But using a true rectangular strip oversteps the line of the graph and thus overestimates the area calculated by summing the area of the rectangular strips. One way to address this problem is to make the rectangular strips very small—infinitesimally small such that each strip is not Δx in width but dx, which makes the length of each strip dy. Each of these infinitesimally small rectangular strips is summed through the use of an integral.

THE INTEGRAL

Integration of a given function, $f(x)$, is the inverse of differentiation and is performed using an integral defined mathematically as

$$\int f(x)dx,$$

where dx is the differential along the x-axis. The integral, referred to as an indefinite integral, represents the area under the curve $y = f(x)$. The area under the curve is subdivided into equal regions of size dx, as shown in the figure below. By integrating the function, you are, in effect, summing all of the dx regions bounded by the function curve.

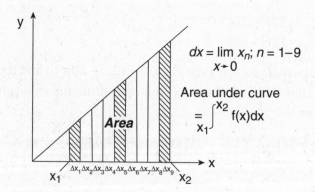

Although integration formulas exist for all types of functions, the formulas that will be covered in this review are:

$$\int k\,dx = kx + C \qquad\qquad \text{where } C \text{ is an integration constant;}$$

$$\int x^n dx = \frac{1}{n+1}x^{n+1} + C.$$

If you are concerned about the area under the curve bounded by limits of x_1 and x_2 along the x-axis and predefined limits along the y-axis, then you can apply the definite integral or

$$\int_{x_1}^{x_2} f(x)dx = F(x)\Big|_{x_1}^{x_2} = F(x_2) - F(x_1),$$

where $F(x)$ is the integrated result of the original function.

EXAMPLE: Evaluate the indefinite integral $\int 3x^4 dx$.

SOLUTION: The integral is evaluated by:

$$\int 3x^4 dx = 3 \cdot \frac{1}{4+1} x^{4+1} = \frac{3}{5} x^5 + C.$$

EXAMPLE: Evaluate the definite integral $\int_2^5 9dy$.

SOLUTION: The integral is evaluated by:

$$\int_2^5 9dy = 9y\Big|_2^5 = 9(5) - 9(2) = 45 - 18 = 27.$$

APPLICATIONS OF THE INTEGRAL

To show the relationship between the integral and the derivative, consider the same example of motion that was introduced in a previous section of this chapter. Now, however, let us start with the acceleration of the particle.

Velocity

To determine the velocity of the particle, the acceleration of the particle is integrated with respect to time. The acceleration of the particle in the prior example was determined to be $a(t) = 24t - 20$. Using the integral formula $\int x^n dx = \frac{1}{n+1} x^{n+1} + C$, then

$$v(t) = \int adt = \int (24t - 20)dt = \int 24tdt - \int 20dt = 12t^2 - 20t + C.$$

Position

From the velocity of the particle, you can now determine the position of the particle by once again performing integration on the velocity function. The position, Δx, can be found by:

$$\Delta x(t) = \int vdt = \int (12t^2 - 20t)dt = \int 12t^2 dt - \int 20tdt = 4t^3 - 10t^2 + C.$$

If you compare the expression for position just obtained to the one with which you originally started out, there is a slight difference. By comparing the two expressions for position, the difference is that the term "6" is missing, which can actually be shown to equal the integration constant, C.

ON YOUR OWN

Problems

1. Evaluate the following derivative: $\dfrac{d}{dx}(5)$.

   A. 0   **B.** 5   **C.** $5x$ **D.** $5x^2$

2. Evaluate the following derivative: $\dfrac{d}{dx}\left(x^4\right)$.

   A. $3x^3$ **B.** $4x^3$ **C.** $3x^4$ **D.** $4x^4$

3. Evaluate the following derivative: $\dfrac{d}{dx}\left(\dfrac{3}{x^5}\right)$.

   A. $-\dfrac{15}{x^5}$ **B.** $\dfrac{15}{x^5}$ **C.** $\dfrac{15}{x^6}$ **D.** $-\dfrac{15}{x^6}$

4. Evaluate the following derivative: $\dfrac{d}{dx}\left(2x^3 - 4x^2\right)$.

   A. $2x^2 - 4x$ **B.** $6x^3 - 8x^2$ **C.** $6x^2 - 8x$ **D.** $6x^2 + 8x$

5. Evaluate the following derivative: $\dfrac{d}{dx}\left(7x^8 + 9x^4 + 3x - 15\right)$ at $x = 1$.

   A. 68   **B.** 82   **C.** 95   **D.** 104

6. Evaluate the following indefinite integral: $\int t^2 (4 - t^2)\,dt$.

   A. $\dfrac{4}{3}t^3 + \dfrac{1}{5}t^5 + C$ **B.** $\dfrac{4}{3}t^3 - \dfrac{1}{5}t^5 + C$ **C.** $-\dfrac{4}{3}t^3 - \dfrac{1}{5}t^5 + C$ **D.** $-\dfrac{4}{3}t^3 + \dfrac{1}{5}t^5 + C$

7. Evaluate the following indefinite integral: $\int (3 - t^2)\,dt$.

   A. $3 - t^2 + C$ **B.** $3 - \dfrac{t^2}{2} + C$ **C.** $3t - \dfrac{t^3}{3} + C$ **D.** $3t - t^3 + C$

8. Evaluate the following definite integral: $\displaystyle\int_{1}^{7} r^2\,dr$.

   A. 114   **B.** 256   **C.** 342   **D.** 512

9. Evaluate the following definite integral: $\displaystyle\int_{1}^{4} \left(x^3 - 6x^2 + 9x + 1\right)dx$.

   A. 4.90   **B.** 8.25   **C.** 10.64   **D.** 12.50

10. Evaluate the following definite integral: $\displaystyle\int_{2}^{10} \dfrac{2}{x^3}\,dx$.

    A. $\dfrac{6}{25}$ **B.** $\dfrac{13}{50}$ **C.** $\dfrac{24}{25}$ **D.** $\dfrac{51}{100}$

Solutions

1. **Answer: A**

In evaluating the derivative, you should note that the function is a number or a constant because it has no dependence on the variable, x. Thus, the derivative of a constant can be determined by:

$$\frac{d}{dx}(5) = 0.$$

2. **Answer: B**

The derivative of a power function can be found according to the general equation

$$\frac{d}{dx}(x^n) = nx^{n-1}.$$

In the problem, $n = 4$ and therefore the derivative can now be calculated as:

$$\frac{d}{dx}(x^4) = 4x^{4-1} = 4x^3.$$

3. **Answer: D**

The derivative of this function can be performed by arranging it in the form of a power function by:

$$\frac{3}{x^5} = 3x^{-5}$$

$$\frac{d}{dx}(3x^{-5}) = -15x^{-5-1} = -15x^{-6} = -\frac{15}{x^6}.$$

4. **Answer: C**

The derivative of a polynomial is the sum of the derivatives of the terms of the polynomial or:

$$\frac{d}{dx}(2x^3 - 4x^2) = \frac{d}{dx}(2x^3) + \frac{d}{dx}(-4x^2)$$

$$= \frac{d}{dx}(2x^3) - \frac{d}{dx}(4x^2)$$

$$= 6x^2 - 8x.$$

5. **Answer: C**

You first must calculate the derivative before you can evaluate the derivative at a given point.

$$\frac{d}{dx}(7x^8 + 9x^4 + 3x - 15) = \frac{d}{dx}(7x^8) + \frac{d}{dx}(9x^4) + \frac{d}{dx}(3x) + \frac{d}{dx}(-15)$$

$$= 56x^7 + 36x^3 + 3.$$

The derivative can now be evaluated at $x = 1$ by plugging in the value of 1 for x in the derivative or

$$\frac{d}{dx}(7x^8 + 9x^4 + 3x - 15)\bigg|_{x=1} = 56(1)^7 + 36(1)^3 + 3 = 56 + 36 + 3 = 95.$$

6. Answer: B

Evaluating this integral becomes an easier task if the function is distributed as:

$$\int t^2 \left(4 - t^2 \right) dt = \int \left(4t^2 - t^4 \right) dt = \int \left(4t^2 \right) dt - \int t^4 dt = \frac{4}{3} t^3 - \frac{1}{5} t^5 + C.$$

7. Answer: C

Evaluation of this integral proceeds by:

$$\int \left(3 - t^2 \right) dt = \int 3 dt - \int t^2 dt = 3t - \frac{t^3}{3} + C.$$

8. Answer: A

You begin by solving the integral and then evaluating the result between the limits of 1 and 7.

$$\int_1^7 r^2 dr = \frac{r^3}{3} \bigg|_1^7 = \frac{(7)^3}{3} - \frac{(1)^3}{3} = \frac{343}{3} - \frac{1}{3} = \frac{342}{3} = 114.$$

9. Answer: B

You begin by solving the integral and then evaluating the result between the limits of 1 and 4.

$$\int_1^4 \left(x^3 - 6x^2 + 9x + 1 \right) dx = \left(\frac{x^4}{4} - \frac{6x^3}{3} + \frac{9x^2}{2} + x \right) \bigg|_1^4$$

$$= \left(\frac{(4)^4}{4} - \frac{6(4)^3}{3} + \frac{9(4)^2}{2} + (4) \right) - \left(\frac{(1)^4}{4} - \frac{6(1)^3}{3} + \frac{9(1)^2}{2} + (1) \right)$$

$$= \left(\frac{256}{4} - \frac{384}{3} + \frac{144}{2} + 4 \right) - \left(\frac{1}{4} - \frac{6}{3} + \frac{9}{2} + 1 \right)$$

$$= \frac{144}{12} - \frac{45}{12} = \frac{99}{12} = 8.25.$$

10. Answer: A

You begin by solving the integral and then evaluating the result between the limits of 2 and 10.

$$\int_2^{10} \frac{2}{x^3} dx = \int 2 \left(x^{-3} \right) dx = \frac{2 \left(x^{-2} \right)}{-2} = -\frac{1}{x^2} \bigg|_2^{10} = \left(-\frac{1}{10^2} \right) - \left(-\frac{1}{2^2} \right) = \left(-\frac{1}{100} \right) + \left(\frac{1}{4} \right)$$

$$= \frac{24}{100} = \frac{6}{25}.$$

Calculus

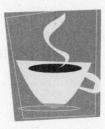

➤ **Differentiation:** the basis for differential calculus is the derivative, a mathematical operation very similar to the calculation of the slope of a function.

➤ The **derivative** of a function, described symbolically as $\dfrac{df(x)}{dx} = \dfrac{dy}{dx}$ or $f'(x)$, describes the rate of increase (or decrease) along the y-axis with respect to the x-axis at a point on the curve.

➤ The derivative $\dfrac{dy}{dx}$ can be equated with the slope $\dfrac{\Delta y}{\Delta x}$ only in the limit as Δx becomes very small and approaches 0. This is expressed mathematically as:

$$\frac{dy}{dx} = \lim_{\Delta x \to 0} \frac{\Delta y}{\Delta x}.$$

➤ Differentiation can be applied to the entire spectrum of functions by using specific differentiation formulas such as:

$\dfrac{d}{dx}(c) = 0$ where c is a constant. The constant can be any real number or variable other than the differentiating variable, x.

$\dfrac{d}{dx}(cx^n) = ncx^{n-1}$ where c is a constant and n is a real number not equal to zero.

➤ **Integration** is used to determine the area under the curve. The integral is to integral calculus as the derivative is to differential calculus.

➤ Integration of a given function, $f(x)$, is the inverse of differentiation and is performed using an **integral** defined mathematically as

$$\int f(x)dx,$$

where dx is the differential along the x-axis. The integral, referred to as an indefinite integral, represents the area under the curve $y = f(x)$. The area under the curve is subdivided into equal regions of size dx. By integrating the function, one is summing all of the dx regions bounded by the function curve.

➤ Integration formulas covered in this review are:

$\int k\,dx = kx + C$ where C is an integration constant;

$$\int x^n dx = \frac{1}{n+1} x^{n+1} + C.$$

➤ The area under the curve bounded by limits of x_1 and x_2 along the x-axis and predefined limits along the y-axis can be found through the definite integral or

$$\int_{x_1}^{x_2} f(x)dx = F(x)\Big|_{x_1}^{x_2} = F(x_2) - F(x_1),$$

where $F(x)$ is the integrated result of the original function.

REVIEWING PCAT WRITING

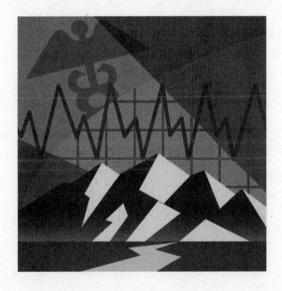

REVIEWING PCAT WRITING

Conventions of Language

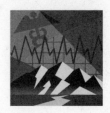

WHY YOU NEED THIS CHAPTER

You will write two essays for the PCAT, one at the beginning of the first session, and one at the beginning of the second session. Your essays will be graded for content, but they will also be graded for Conventions of Language—how well you follow the rules of English grammar, usage, mechanics (punctuation and capitalization), and spelling.

The Handbooks here do not present an exhaustive study of English. They focus on the basic skills many students at your level tend to forget when faced with a standardized test. For a more comprehensive review of grammar, usage, mechanics, and spelling, visit the library or your local bookstore and find a book dedicated to those skills.

GRAMMAR HANDBOOK

Fragments	To avoid fragments, make sure each sentence has a subject and a verb. **CORRECT:** The sun rises in the east. **INCORRECT:** Rising in the east.
Run-ons	When you are writing quickly, it is easy to connect too many thoughts in a river of language. As you revise, cut down run-on sentences to a more reasonable length.

CORRECT:	I enjoyed the concert. The orchestra was outstanding.
INCORRECT:	I enjoyed the concert the orchestra was outstanding.

Verb agreement Use singular verb forms with singular subjects or with compound singular subjects joined with *or* or *nor*.

> **EXAMPLES:** Dr. Ming examines me.
> Neither Dr. Ming nor his nurse examines me.

Use plural verb forms with plural subjects or with compound subjects joined with *and*.

> **EXAMPLES:** The doctors examine me.
> Dr. Ming and his nurse examine me.

Use singular verb forms with the pronouns *anybody, anyone, each, either, everybody, everyone, nobody, no one, somebody,* and *someone.*

> **EXAMPLES:** Each examines me.
> Nobody examines me.

Use plural verb forms with the pronouns *both, few, several,* and *many.*

> **EXAMPLES:** Both examine me.
> Few examine me.

The pronouns *all, any, most, none,* and *some* may take singular or plural verbs depending on their antecedents.

Verb tense Maintain consistency of tenses. When in doubt, read your writing "aloud" in your head to check whether your tenses work.

> **CORRECT:** Our visit to Montreal was exciting. We visited the Old City.

> **INCORRECT:** Our visit to Montreal was exciting. We visit the Old City.

USAGE HANDBOOK

Abbreviations Avoid abbreviations in formal writing.

> **CORRECT:** The embassy is on K Street.
> **INCORRECT:** The embassy is on K St.

Exception: Use abbreviations of personal titles.

> **EXAMPLE:** We shook hands with Mr. Alvarez.

Adjectives/ Adverbs

Use *good* as an adjective; use *well* as an adverb.

> **EXAMPLES:** He is a good teacher.
> He teaches well.

Exception: Use *well* to describe a state of being.

> **EXAMPLE:** I don't feel well.

Affect/Effect

Affect is a verb meaning "to influence" or "to have an effect on." *Effect* is a noun meaning "the result of a cause." It can also be a verb meaning "to bring about."

> **EXAMPLES:** How does hot weather affect you?
> What is the effect of radiation?
> How can we best effect change in a democracy?

Antecedents

Make sure that your pronouns match their preceding nouns.

> **CORRECT:** The horse tossed its mane.
> **INCORRECT:** The horses tossed its mane.

Between/Among

Use *between* to refer to two things. Use *among* to refer to three or more.

> **EXAMPLES:** The argument is between Jo and me.
> Split the cake among the four cousins.

Dangling participle

Keep modifiers close to the words they modify.

> **CORRECT:** Nailed to the wall, a special bulletin caught my eye.
> **CORRECT:** I noticed a special bulletin nailed to the wall.
> **INCORRECT:** Nailed to the wall, I noticed a special bulletin.

Fewer/Less

Use *fewer* with plural words. Use *less* with singular words.

> **EXAMPLES:** He has fewer coins than I have.
> He has less money than I have.

Its/It's

Its is a possessive pronoun. *It's* means "it is."

	EXAMPLES:	The car lost its muffler. It's the third muffler I've replaced.

Lay/Lie

You can lie down, or you can lay something down. You cannot lay down in the present tense or lie something down. *Lie* never takes an object. *Lay* may be used as the past tense of *lie*.

CORRECT:	I will lie down on the bed.
INCORRECT:	I will lay down on the bed.
CORRECT:	I lay the plates on the table.
INCORRECT:	I lie the plates on the table.
CORRECT:	Last night I lay down to sleep.

Misplaced modifier

Keep modifiers close to the words they modify.

CORRECT:	My mother taught me to read when I was three years of age.
INCORRECT:	At three years of age, my mother taught me to read.

Negatives

Use only one negative per sentence.

CORRECT:	He does not own any pets.
INCORRECT:	He does not own no pets.

Exception: neither/nor.

EXAMPLE:	Neither fog nor rain stopped the game.

Passive voice

Eschew the passive voice. Write actively.

CORRECT:	Use active verbs to write your essay.
INCORRECT:	Your essay should be written using active verbs.

Principal/ Principle

A *principal* heads a school. Something that is *principal* is critically important. A *principle* is a law or code of conduct.

EXAMPLES:	The principal hired those teachers. That principal beam holds up the barn. Courtesy is a principle by which we should live.

Slang

Slang is never appropriate in formal writing.

Who/Whom

Who is used as a subject or predicate nominative. *Whom* is used as a direct or indirect object. In other words, if you would use *he*, use *who*. If you would use *him*, use *whom*.

EXAMPLES: Who told her the secret?
That is who heard the secret.
To whom did he tell the secret?

MECHANICS HANDBOOK

Apostrophes   Use an apostrophe and *s* to show possession in a singular noun.

>**EXAMPLE:**   Is that your brother's car?

Use an apostrophe alone to show possession in a plural noun.

>**EXAMPLE:**   Are those your brothers' cars?

Exceptions are *children's, men's, women's.*

>**EXAMPLE:**   Are those the children's toys?

Capital letters   Use capital letters for proper nouns and adjectives.

>**EXAMPLE:**   Is it best to study French in France?

Capitalize the first, last, and all important words in a title or multiple-word proper noun.

>**EXAMPLE:**   I recently read *A Year in Provence.*

Do not capitalize the names of seasons.

>**EXAMPLE:**   I spent one summer in the French
countryside.

Commas   Use a comma between two independent clauses in a compound sentence.

>**EXAMPLE:**   We could fly, but I prefer driving.

Use a comma to separate all parts of a series.

>**EXAMPLE:**   She bought soda, lemonade, and milk.

Use a comma after a long introductory prepositional phrase or after a pair of short introductory prepositional phrases.

>**EXAMPLE:**   During the first part of the season,
they fished for small-mouth bass.

Use a comma to separate city and state and after the state in a sentence.

>**EXAMPLE:**   He likes Missoula, Montana, better
than Naples, Florida.

Use a comma to set off an appositive.

> **EXAMPLE:** My father, a brilliant scientist, won a prize.

Use a comma to set off nonessential phrases and clauses.

> **EXAMPLE:** Her eyes, which were an unusual shade of aqua, held Joe's attention.

Italics

In a handwritten paper, use underlining to represent the italicizing of book or other titles.

> **EXAMPLE:** I recently read <u>A Year in Provence</u>.

Paragraph

Make sure a reader can tell where your new paragraphs begin. Do not write a one-page response in a single block paragraph.

Quotation marks

Use quotation marks around direct quotations or around titles of stories or poems.

> **EXAMPLES:** Juan asked, "What should we read?"
> The class enjoyed "Annabel Lee."

Keep commas and periods inside quotation marks; keep colons and semicolons outside.

> **EXAMPLES:** I replied, "Nothing is certain."
> He whispered, "Come closer"; no one responded.

If question marks and exclamation points are part of the quotation itself, they go inside. If not, they go outside.

> **EXAMPLES:** "What a great poem!" cried Lisa.
> Who wrote "The Raven"?

Semicolons

Use a semicolon to separate two independent clauses.

> **EXAMPLE:** My pet frog is lost; I expect to find him in the bathtub any day now.

Use a semicolon before *for example* followed by a list.

> **EXAMPLE:** Cecile participates in many sports; for example, she plays soccer, basketball, and softball.

Use a semicolon between items in a series when the items themselves include commas.

> **EXAMPLE:** Jon carried the blanket; the picnic basket; and the red, white, and blue bunting.

SPELLING HANDBOOK

Ei/Ie

Use pronunciation to guide you. If the sound is long /ē/, write *ie*.

EXAMPLES: belief, chief, piece

If the sound is long /ā/, write *ei*.

EXAMPLES: eight, neighbor, rein

If the sound is a short vowel, there is no rule.

EXAMPLES: foreign, forfeit, friend, mischief

Exceptions: If the long /ē/ follows the letter *c*, write *ei*.

EXAMPLES: ceiling, deceive, receipt

And some words break the rules entirely.

EXAMPLES: neither, seize, weird

Inflected endings

If the base word ends in a single consonant preceded by a vowel, double the consonant before adding *ed* or *ing* or a suffix.

EXAMPLES: bat/batted
shop/shopping

Plural nouns

Add *s* to most singular nouns.

EXAMPLE: bear/bears

Add *es* to nouns ending in *s*, *x*, *sh*, *ch*, or *z*.

EXAMPLE: fox/foxes

Change *y* to *i* and add *es* to nouns ending in a consonant and *y*.

EXAMPLE: bunny/bunnies

Add *es* to nouns that end in a consonant and *o*.

EXAMPLE: hero/heroes

Exceptions: If a noun ending in *o* relates to music, form the plural by adding *s*.

EXAMPLES: soprano/sopranos
virtuoso/virtuosos

If a vowel precedes the *o*, just add *s*.

EXAMPLE: radio/radios

For some words ending in *f* or *fe*, change *f* to *v* and add *es* or *s*.

> **EXAMPLES:** leaf/leaves
> knife/knives

Exceptions: Some nouns that end in *f* or *fe* do not follow the rule above.

> **EXAMPLES:** fife/fifes
> roof/roofs

Prefixes

Adding a prefix does not change the spelling of a base word.

> **EXAMPLES:** logical/illogical
> regular/irregular

Suffixes

If the base word ends with silent *e*, and the suffix begins with a consonant, keep the *e*.

> **EXAMPLES:** nice/nicely
> pride/prideful

Exception: Some words that end with a soft *g* sound drop the *e*.

> **EXAMPLES:** acknowledge/acknowledgment
> judge/judgment

Another exception: If the base word ends with two vowels, drop the *e*.

> **EXAMPLES:** due/duly
> true/truly

If the base word ends with silent *e*, and the suffix begins with a vowel, drop the *e*.

> **EXAMPLES:** create/creative
> move/movable

Exception: Some words that end with a soft *g* sound keep the *e*.

> **EXAMPLES:** change/changeable
> knowledge/knowledgeable

If the base word ends in *y* preceded by a consonant, change the *y* to *i* before adding the suffix.

> **EXAMPLES:** hasty/hastily
> mercy/merciless

180 Frequently Misspelled Words

aberrant
abhor
absence
absorption
abstention
accelerate
accompanist
accordion
acknowledge
acquaint
affidavit
albeit
allegiance
ascend
average
bankruptcy
belligerent
buoyant
censor
chancellor
circuit
clientele
college
committee
congratulate
conscience
curiosity
debt
defendant
dependence
desperate
diphtheria
disciple
doubt
eczema
egregious
eligible
embarrass
endeavor
environment
exaggerate
exercise

exorbitant
extraordinary
facsimile
fascist
fluorescent
foreign
forfeit
fraudulent
fruit
gauge
gauze
gesture
gonorrhea
grievance
gymnasium
harass
heifer
hiatus
hypocrite
illusory
inauguration
independent
indict
intermittent
irrelevant
italicize
itinerary
jaguar
jealous
jeopardy
judgment
juvenile
kiosk
knowledge
laity
lawyer
legislature
liquor
luscious
maelstrom
maintenance
mandatory

mediocre
milieu
miscellaneous
mischievous
muscle
nadir
nauseous
necessary
nonchalant
obscene
occupant
occurrence
omniscient
onomatopoeia
ophthalmology
opossum
oscillate
overture
pageant
paradigm
parallel
pedestrian
penicillin
personnel
pharmaceutical
physician
playwright
precinct
privilege
professor
pronunciation
psyche
quandary
questionnaire
rarity
rebellion
recruit
reference
renown
repertoire
rescind
reservoir

restaurant	soliloquy	unctuous
resuscitate	souvenir	unnecessary
risqué	spatial	vaccinate
rural	species	vacuum
sabotage	stomach	vague
saccharine	strategy	vehement
sanctuary	subpoena	victual
savage	success	vigilant
scalpel	succumb	volatile
scenario	supersede	voyeur
schedule	surgeon	weird
schizophrenia	surveillance	wholly
scholar	synthesize	withhold
segregate	tacit	women
separate	tenor	yacht
severance	tetanus	yearn
signature	thorough	zealous
solemn	unanimous	zoological

ON YOUR OWN

Directions: Each sentence below violates two of the rules of Standard English. Circle the errors. Then rewrite the sentence correctly.

1. Two pharmacutical salesmen presents a pitch for a new diabetes drug.

   _____

2. One asks the clinician whom is in charge, "How many patients do you see"?

   _____

3. She replies, Between all of us, we may see one hundred patients per day."

   _____

4. The salesmen seem to be earnest well-spoken, and knowledgable.

   _____

5. Both the clinician and her aide has questions about the occurence of side effects.

   _____

6. According to the salesmen, most drs. find that patients tolerate the drug good.

   _____

7. Some test subjects felt dizzy although most had no such ill affects.

8. After feeling dizzy, the drug was replaced with a lower dosage.

9. Was the original testing done in mexico, or did they take place in Canada?

10. The companys initial expenditure on research did not result in no firm data.

Answers and Explanations

1. Two pharmaceutical salesmen present a pitch for a new diabetes drug.
   Error 1: The word *pharmaceutical* is frequently misspelled.
   Error 2: The verb *presents* does not fit the plural subject *salesmen*.

2. One asks the clinician who is in charge, "How many patients do you see?"
   Error 1: The correct pronoun is *who*, not the object pronoun *whom*.
   Error 2: The question mark is part of the quotation and should therefore go within the quotation marks.

3. She replies, "Among all of us, we may see one hundred patients per day."
   Error 1: Quotation marks must come before and after the direct quotation.
   Error 2: Because the clinician is referring to more than two people, the correct word is *among*, not *between*.

4. The salesmen seem to be earnest, well-spoken, and knowledgeable.
   Error 1: A series of adjectives requires commas to separate each.
   Error 2: *Knowledgeable* has a soft *g* sound and therefore requires an *e* before the suffix.

5. Both the clinician and her aide have questions about the occurrence of side effects.
   Error 1: The subject is plural (Both the clinician and her aide) and requires a plural verb.
   Error 2: *Occur* ends with a vowel and *r*, so you double the *r* before adding the suffix.

6. According to the salesmen, most doctors find that patients tolerate the drug well.
   Error 1: Do not abbreviate *doctors* in formal writing unless it is used as a title.
   Error 2: *Good* is an adjective. The adverb *well* modifies the verb *tolerate*.

7. Some test subjects felt dizzy, although most had no such ill effects.
   Error 1: Omitting the comma between independent clauses leads to a run-on sentence.
   Error 2: *Affects* is a verb; the word required is the noun that means "results of a cause."

8. After patients felt dizzy, doctors replaced the drug with a lower dosage.
   Error 1: The drug did not feel dizzy. The original sentence had a misplaced modifier. Rewording may vary.
   Error 2: Adding the subject *doctors* keeps this from being in the passive voice. Again, rewording may vary.

9. Was the original testing done in Mexico, or did it take place in Canada?
   Error 1: Mexico is a proper noun and must be capitalized.
   Error 2: The pronoun in the second clause must agree with the singular noun *testing* in the first clause.

10. The company's initial expenditure on research did not result in any firm data.
   Error 1: *Company's* is a possessive noun and requires an apostrophe.
   Error 2: Replace the double negative with *not . . . any* or "resulted in no firm data."

Conventions of Language

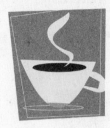

The essay portion of the test measures your ability to respond to a prompt, to present ideas in a logical way, and to write using the rules of Standard English. Conventions of Language include rules of English grammar, usage, mechanics, and spelling.

➤ **GRAMMAR:** As you write, be sure to use complete sentences, not fragments or run-ons. Make sure that your subjects and verbs agree. Use consistent tenses.

➤ **USAGE:** Choose the correct word in confusing pairs such as *lay/lie*, *between/among*, and *its/it's*. Avoid dangling participles, misplaced modifiers, the passive voice, abbreviations, and slang. Make sure that your pronouns match their antecedents

➤ **MECHANICS:** Use paragraphing to separate sections of your essay. Capitalize proper nouns and adjectives and the first, last, and all important words in the title of a written work. Review the Mechanics Handbook for some critical rules involving punctuation.

➤ **SPELLING:** Remember that a prefix does not change the spelling of a base word, but a suffix often does. Follow spelling rules as specified in the Spelling Handbook. Where there are exceptions to the rules, you may need to memorize examples.

CHAPTER 18

Problem Solving Essays

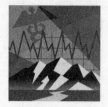

> ### Read This Chapter to Learn About:
> ➤ Problem Solving Essays and What They Test
> ➤ How Your Essays Are Scored
> ➤ How to Use the Writing Process to Create a First-Rate Essay

WHAT PROBLEM SOLVING ESSAYS TEST

The PCAT recently added a second essay to the test, reducing the number of multiple-choice items in favor of requiring additional writing. Both essays require you to suggest a solution to a problem that is given in a prompt like this one:

Discuss a solution to the problem of voter apathy, especially among young people.

Topics vary among health-related, science-related, or social/cultural/political subject areas. Although you will write two essays, only one will be formally scored. The other is considered experimental, and your results on that essay will not be sent to schools.

The PCAT Problem Solving Essays do not test specific knowledge of a topic. They test your ability to express a logical solution to a given problem in organized Standard English. You are not graded on whether your solution is correct, simply on whether it is presented clearly.

HOW THE ESSAYS ARE SCORED

Three or more separate readers may read your essays. One reader addresses the Conventions of Language (see Chapter 17)—your grammar, usage, mechanics, and spelling. That reader assigns a score from 1.0 to 5.0, using a rubric like this one:

CONVENTIONS OF LANGUAGE SCORING RUBRIC	
0	Paper blank, illegible, or not in English.
1.0	Multiple errors in capitalization, punctuation, grammar, and/or usage, seriously affecting flow and meaning.
2.0	Multiple errors in capitalization, punctuation, grammar, and/or usage, affecting both flow and meaning.
3.0	Several errors in capitalization, punctuation, grammar, and/or usage. Errors may affect flow, but they do not affect meaning.
4.0	Some errors in capitalization, punctuation, grammar, and/or usage, but errors do not affect meaning or flow.
5.0	Few errors in capitalization, punctuation, grammar, and/or usage.

Next, a pair of readers evaluates your essay for its achievement of the essay's purpose: solving a problem. Each reader assigns a score, based on a rubric like this one:

PROBLEM SOLVING SCORING RUBRIC	
0	Paper blank, illegible, on a topic other than that assigned, or not in English.
1.0	Lack of understanding evident. Organization nonexistent or unclear. Ideas undeveloped.
2.0	Organization unclear or scattershot. Ideas underdeveloped and unsupported.
3.0	Organization fairly coherent. Ideas developed and supported with relevant details that lack complexity.
4.0	Organization coherent and focused. Ideas complex, well developed, and clearly supported.
5.0	Organization coherent and focused. Ideas complex, sophisticated, and substantially developed, with logical, convincing support.

If the scores given by the pair of readers differs by more than one point, a third reader may be assigned to read your test. If the pair of readers assigns you, say, a 3.0 and a 4.0, your final problem solving score will be 3.5. The Conventions of Language and the Problem Solving scores will appear as two separate numbers on your test score report. You will also see your two scores compared to the mean for everyone who took the PCAT that same day, so that you can get some sense of where you stand in relation to other test takers.

PREPARING FOR THE ESSAYS

You probably know by now whether you are a good writer, a competent writer, or a person who cannot communicate using the written word. The PCAT Problem Solving Essay requires a very specific type of writing. By reviewing this section and practicing with some prompts, you can improve your ability to submit the kind of writing the PCAT scorers expect.

Write

Practice on letters to the editor, which are a form of writing that is often quite similar to the one required on the PCAT. You do not have to submit your letters, just write them. Think of a problem that is facing your community. Then write a letter that suggests a solution and gives solid reasons and examples to support your ideas.

Pace Yourself

It is not easy to write under time pressure. The essays begin each session of the test, which means that you will be writing each one while relatively refreshed. However, you will have only 30 minutes per essay. You should spend part of that time preparing to write and part of that time reviewing your writing (see Using the Writing Process later in this chapter). As you complete sample essays in this book, time yourself. Think about breaking each half hour as shown here:

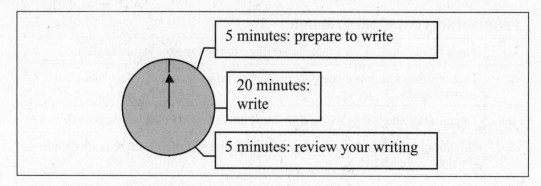

FIGURE 18.1: Budgeting time for PCAT Writing.

Spending a little time organizing your thoughts and a little time cleaning up your mechanics will pay off in your score. Remember, you are judged on your organization and on your proper use of Standard English. The more you write and time yourself, the better you will be at judging when your 20-minute writing period is up.

Preview

The PCAT Problem Solving Essay is a very specific piece of writing on a very specific kind of prompt. Knowing what a typical prompt looks like will help you understand how to address the two prompts you will see later on the PCAT.

THE PCAT PROMPT

Discuss a solution to the problem of voter apathy, especially among young people.

The PCAT Prompt begins with the words "discuss a solution." This is your task. The type of writing is defined for you: You will write a solution to a problem.

The opening words are followed by the problem, which is circled above. This is usually quite a broad topic, and it does not require specific background knowledge. Often, it will be something you have thought about or talked over with friends. Occasionally, it will be a topic that is new to you.

Your response will incorporate these steps:

1. **Explanation of the problem.** You will tell the reader what the problem is and why it is a problem. For example, why should we be concerned about voter apathy among young people? Why do we care?

2. **Description of your solution(s).** Although the prompt asks for a single solution, the highest-scored essays will always offer multiple solutions. Here you will detail your solution(s) and provide in-depth support for your ideas. You will tell why your solutions will work and how they will solve the problem.

3. **Summary of the main ideas.** Do not simply end with step 2. Try to wrap up your essay with a concluding paragraph that sums up your key points.

This is a lot to do in 30 minutes, which is why your initial preparation is so important. The PCAT scorers are looking for an integrated response that progresses logically and addresses the prompt precisely.

USING THE WRITING PROCESS

You may have used the writing process in school, in which case you have a leg up on your competition. Here is a quick review of that process, which you can and should apply to the PCAT Problem Solving Essay.

1. **Prewrite (5 minutes).** Prewriting consists of everything you do up to the moment of creating your draft. In timed writing such as that on the PCAT, prewriting is a brief but critical step in the writing process.
   - ➤ **READ** the prompt. Restate it in your mind.
   - ➤ **PLAN** your response.

Think about why the problem is a problem. Brainstorm two or three solutions that might solve the problem.

Problem because young people who don't vote 1) aren't represented, 2) aren't expressing themselves at the ballot box
1) Have young candidates reach out
2) Link voter registration to driver's license
3) More Rock the vote-type events

2. **Draft (20 minutes).** Drafting is getting your ideas on paper. Use your prewriting notes to assist you with organization. Separate ideas into paragraphs. Focus on answering the prompt, not on introducing new concepts, expressing personal asides, or using big vocabulary words.

Notice how this writer fused her Prewriting ideas into her Draft. By doing that, she made sure to address the prompt in her essay.

Because young people are, as a rule, apathetic toward elections, they miss out on allowing their voice to be heard. A quick look at the average age of senators proves that they are underrepresented. Improving the voting record of young people should be a goal of all Americans especially those my age.

How can we energize young voters. First, let's make voter registration easier. Linking it to getting a driver's license is easy to do, and it would ensure that whenever a new driver received a license, he or she would automatically be registered to vote.

Second, events such as "Rock the vote" have helped to remind young people of upcoming elections. Certain celebrities have worked hard to point out the relevance of voting to young people's lives. I think that more of this kind of event, even at the local level, can improve turnout for young people at the polls.

Finally, there are young candidates out there who might benefit from reaching out to a younger crowd while helping the young crowd learn about issues. Campaigning on college campuses, going-door-to-door in college towns, or even speaking at high schools can all be ways to improve connections between politics and youth.

Young people need to see that voting has meaning for people their age. By improving access, exciting interest, and explaining issues, we can help eliminate voter apathy among American youth.

3. **Revise and Edit (5 minutes).** In timed writing like that on the PCAT, no one expects a perfectly clean draft. You do not have time to rewrite your draft neatly, but you do have time to check it for errors. As you have seen, grammar, usage, mechanics, and spelling errors count against you. So do errors involving faulty organization and inadequate support. It is better to insert and cross out than to leave a deficient but neat draft intact.

This writer corrected some minor errors—an unclear antecedent, an incorrect punctuation mark, and a misspelling—and added a clarifying line to the introduction.

Because young people are, as a rule, apathetic toward elections, they miss out on allowing their voice to be heard. A quick look at the average age of senators proves that
young people
~~they~~ are underrepresented. *Improving the voting record of young people should be a goal of all Americans especially those my age. We can do that by improving access to voting, exciting interest, and explaining the issues in a clear and meaningful way.*

?
How can we energize young voters. First, let's make voter registration easier. Linking it to getting a driver's license is easy to do, and it would ensure that whenever a new driver received a license, he or she would automatically be registered to vote.

Second, events such as "Rock the vote" have helped to remind young people of
celebrities
upcoming elections. Certain ~~celebraties~~ *have worked hard to point out the relevance of voting to young people's lives. I think that more of this kind of event, even at the local level, can improve turnout for young people at the polls.*

Finally, there are young candidates out there who might benefit from reaching out to a younger crowd while helping the young crowd learn about issues. Campaigning on college campuses, going door-to-door in college towns, or even speaking at high schools can all be ways to improve connections between politics and youth.

Young people need to see that voting has meaning for people their age. By improving access, exciting interest, and explaining issues, we can help eliminate voter apathy among American youth.

ON YOUR OWN

Try your hand at the following Sample Essay prompts. Use the steps in the Writing Process. Afterward, compare your response to the rated responses that follow to see how your writing measures up. The final two prompts allow you to grade another test taker's response to see whether you are able to read and respond the way PCAT graders might. As you respond to these prompts, time yourself to make sure you can complete an essay within the 30-minute period required for the PCAT.

Sample Essay 1

Discuss a solution to the problem of increased obesity in elementary-school-age children.

_____

_____

_____

_____

_____

_____

_____

_____

_____

_____

_____

_____

_____

_____

_____

_____

_____

_____

_____

_____

_____

_____

_____

_____

Essay 1A

The era of the Couch Potato kid bodes ill for the health of the adults those kids will become. Childhood obesity may not be the epidemic some have titled it, but it is certainly a problem Americans need to address. Obesity in childhood leads directly to diabetes, hypertension, and high cholesterol. These problems that were once "adults only" are increasingly rated "G."

Just as for adults, the solution to obesity in children lies with the dual factors of diet and exercise. With adults, however, we expect self-control and personal goal-setting. When it comes to children, we may need an approach that is more external.

Children spend much of their waking-life in school. Although it is problematic to place additional burdens on schools, they simply must be on the frontlines of the struggle against childhood obesity. Schools can begin by offering better choices on the lunch line. Many schools are moving from high-fat offerings to lower-fat foods, and this must continue. In addition, schools must restock soda machines with water and replace high-calorie snacks in vending machines with more healthful options.

When it comes to exercise, too many schools have removed play time from the curriculum. Students of all ages need regular P.E. sessions and a period after lunch for movement and play.

Besides the schools, parents are the number one influence in their children's healthy lives. Parents must not use food as a punishment or a reward. They should replace packaged foods with healthful snacks. They should encourage family mealtime, making it a leisurely, fun experience. The meals they serve should be colorful, implying that they are including a variety of healthful foods.

When it comes to exercise, parents must be the ones to get kids off the couch and into physical activity. This does not have to mean organized sports going on a family walk after dinner can be a good way to share exercise painlessly. Above all, parents need to provide a model for their children, a living good example of how to eat and be active.

Hitting kids where they live is the way to combat childhood obesity. By making minor changes at school and at home, we can control the health of America's children.

Conventions of Language Score: 5.0

The writer shows a strong command of the English language and makes almost no mistakes, despite using a variety of sentence types and advanced punctuation.

Problem Solving Score: 5.0

This essay responds clearly and coherently to the prompt. In paragraph 1, the writer restates and explains the problem, using colorful language that is stylish and precise, and offering specific examples to support opinions. In paragraph 2, the writer presents the outline of the solution: diet and exercise. In paragraphs 3 and 4, the writer applies those two solutions to schools. In paragraphs 5 and 6, the writer applies the solutions to the home. Whether or not one agrees with the writer's premise, the writing itself is strong, reasoned, and easy to follow.

The essay is organized in a pattern that could be easily outlined as follows:

I. Introduction
II. Solution: Diet and Exercise
III. Diet in School
IV. Exercise in School
V. Diet at Home
VI. Exercise at Home
VII. Conclusion

Clearly, the writer used the Prewriting period to good effect, or the finished essay would not break down as neatly and logically.

Essay 1B

Children in America are increasingly obese. This is a problem because of the health issues it raises. Fat children become fat adults. This cannot go on.

My solution is to educate parents. For example, at the birth of a child, parents ought to receive pamphlets on proper nutrition at age 1, age 3, elementary school age, and so on. That education could continue as the children go to school, bringing articles on proper nutrition home to parents in their backpacks, and so on. Especially when children are involved in sports teams, their parents could learn from coaches how to feed the little athletes so that they get the most from their nutrition. It might even be possible to have a parent-child cooking club at the middle school level which would enable parents to learn along with their children the rules of good nutrition.

Unless we get the parents involved we will see no change in the level of obesity in children. Only parents can control what their children eat, limiting sugary snacks, and sodas, and providing well rounded meals three times a day. But unless we educate the parents so that they know how nutrition impacts their children's health we will see no change.

Conventions of Language Score: 3.0

The writer is fairly comfortable making points in English. Although there are missing punctuation marks and occasional awkward phrasings, they do not detract from the essay's essential meaning.

Problem Solving Score: 3.0

This essay addresses the prompt, but the smoothness and sophistication of Essay 1A are missing here. In paragraph 1, the writer explains the problem. In paragraph 2, the writer proposes a solution: to educate parents. The rest of that paragraph gives examples that explain how that might happen. The final paragraph provides a conclusion that stresses the writer's key points.

Support for the writer's ideas is limited; the writer mentions "health issues" without naming them, and only gives a reason for the "parent-child club," not for any of the other ideas for educating parents. This writer seems to have written paragraph 2 off the top of his or her head rather than taking a few minutes to outline ideas. A clue to this stream-of-consciousness composition is the repeated use of "and so on."

Essay 1C

Obesity is one of the main problems of children in America, they are increasingly obese from not getting enough excersize eating too much Macdonnalds as well as not excercizing or actively. For one thing, they watch too much tv. also play computer games wich do not be active for moving musels or brething correctly. So this lead to obesity for children or adults.

Sometime obesity run in familys, this is very common, for example, if a mother gain a lot of weit in pregnantcy then her babies fat and feeding her babies too much at one sitting can make this worst. Especialy if both parents have a weit problem it will be much more likely to be the childs problem as well. This can lead to many problems at school like teesing or they cant do the excercises in P.E. classes. How would a child get thin if everone at home is fat, it is nearly imposible to see how. Especialy if every meal is full of calores which is usully true in familes like that.

It is important not to be obese or have obese children which requires a lot of self control, if you see yourselve eating too much in front of your child make sure to stop or eat carrots insted to give your child a good roll model which could make children want to act more like a good eater not an obese person. Being thin could make your child want more like you.

Conventions of Language Score: 1.0

The essay is riddled with errors in grammar, usage, mechanics, and spelling. The errors combine to make the essay extremely difficult to understand.

Problem Solving Score: 1.0

Although it is possible to distill meaning from this essay, it is difficult to do so because of the writer's misspellings, awkward phrasing, and illogical flow of ideas. The writer has restated the problem without really explaining why it is a problem. Paragraph 2 is really a continuation of a discussion of the problem, not a solution for it. It is possible that the writer means the end of paragraph 3 (the discussion of being a role model) to be a solution for childhood obesity, but that connection is never clear. There is no conclusion at all.

Most of the response seems to be the ramblings of someone who has not formulated a cogent argument. Although the response is actually longer than that in Essay 1B, much of its verbiage is incoherence that neither supports a main idea nor offers a logical response to the prompt.

Sample Essay 2

Discuss a solution to the problem of encouraging middle-class Americans to conserve energy.

Grade It Yourself

Read the following essay. Use the scoring rubric found earlier in the chapter to give it two number scores. Then turn the page to compare your scores with the ones given by a reader.

ESSAY 2

If we are ever going to be free from dependence on foreign oil, we need to convince middle-class Americans that conservation must be a way of life. Too many of us think it's enough to recycle every other week. Sadly, that is not enough to make the kind of difference we need to make.

I believe that this kind of change needs to come from the top down. To solve the problem, I would have the federal government provide incentives for conservation. People who buy hybrid vehicles ought to get a tax break. People who install wind or solar instruments need to be able to sell excess energy back to the electric company. Companies that use less energy should be on special lists that encourage consumer support.

It might seem as though I'm bribing citizens to do something they should be doing anyway. That's true, but sometimes people need to be jumpstarted to do the right thing. I think that if our government truly wants us to change, government incentives are a sensible way to inspire us to do so. Within a generation or so, conservation could become a common way of life, and incentives would no longer be needed.

MY SCORE

Conventions of Language: _____

Problem Solving: _____

READER'S SCORE

Conventions of Language: 5.0

The essay contains no serious errors in grammar, usage, mechanics, or spelling.

Problem Solving: 4.0

This response is well written and thoughtful. It provides a clear response to the prompt, with the writer's solution being to provide government incentives to stimulate a variety of citizen responses. Paragraph 2 contains a series of examples to support the writer's ideas, and paragraph 3 gives a summary as well as a response to an anticipated argument. Only an occasional vagueness ("Sadly, that is not enough to make the kind of difference we need to make") keeps this response from achieving a higher score.

Sample Essay 3

Discuss a solution to the problem of educating children to compete in a global economy.

Grade It Yourself

Read the following essay. Use the scoring rubric found earlier in the chapter to give it two number scores. Then turn the page to compare your scores with the ones given by a reader.

ESSAY 3

There's been a lot of talk about how American students don't do as well on tests as students in other developed countries, so they can't compete in a global market. To do so, we need to make sure students are learning the skills they need for that competing.

For example, it's not enough to teach reading, writing, and arithmetic, we need to be teaching computer skills and forein languages at a more important rate. We need to be looking ahead, like: "What are the skills that will be important in 2010? 2015? 2020?" Then, with that knowledge in hand, we can go ahead and tell the schools what they should be teaching.

One thing every student should have is computer skills. Without understanding of that, it is hard to see how anyone can succeed in today's global economy. So the first thing is to make sure these are being taught in our schools. In the past we didn't need this so much. Most students took typing for secretarial jobs, but it was not required. Today it is absolutely essential for getting ahead with any sort of success.

So I would be teaching forein languages and computer skills in every school in America, which would allow our students to compete in a global market.

MY SCORE

Conventions of Language: _____

Problem Solving: _____

READER'S SCORE

Conventions of Language: 3.0

Although they do not necessarily inhibit meaning, the essay contains several mistakes in grammar, usage, mechanics, and spelling.

Problem Solving: 2.0

This response attempts to maintain an introduction-body-conclusion structure, but the fuzzy thinking exhibited by the writer drags the essay down. The writer begins by mentioning American students' scores on tests, but neither of the writer's solutions (computer skills, foreign language instruction) really addresses this problem. The fuzziness continues in the language used, which is vague and sometimes meaningless ("at a more important rate," "We need to be looking ahead, like. . ."). Even the use of "we" is confusing; how are "we" going to tell the schools what to teach? The writer goes off on a tangent about typing and secretarial skills that adds nothing to the main idea. If not for a haphazard attempt to follow the rules of organization, this essay might rate a 1.0.

Problem Solving Essays

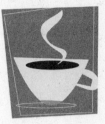

The PCAT Problem Solving Essays consist of two 30-minute essays in response to two given prompts. The essay portion of the test measures your ability to respond to a prompt, present ideas in a logical way, and write using the conventions of Standard English.

You cannot **study** for the Problem Solving Essays, but you can **prepare**. Here are some ideas you can use to prepare:

➤ **Write**, practicing especially your persuasive writing.

➤ **Pace Yourself** by dividing your 30-minute writing period into sections.

➤ **Preview** the test.

Each writing prompt asks you to provide a logical solution to a familiar problem. You must explain what the problem is and why it is a problem and then present some well-thought-out solutions to the problem. You should end with a conclusion that summarizes your key points.

Use the Writing Process as you complete your response.

➤ **Prewrite** for 5 minutes, reading the prompt and planning your response.

➤ **Draft** for 20 minutes, using your prewriting notes to organize your ideas.

➤ **Revise** for 5 minutes, checking for grammar, usage, mechanics, and spelling errors as well as errors of organization and support.

PART VIII

PCAT PRACTICE TEST

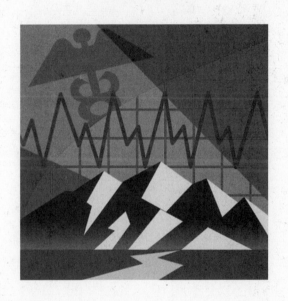

PCAT Practice Test

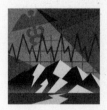

In This Section You Will Find

➤ A full-length PCAT Practice Test covering all subjects tested

➤ Hundreds of sample questions like the ones on the real exam

➤ Answer explanations for every question

This chapter contains a complete, full-length PCAT Practice Test. It is designed to help you test your knowledge of each subject area and sharpen your test-taking skills. The questions are modeled on the questions in the real exam. They cover the same topics and are designed to be at the same level of difficulty. Answer explanations are given at the end of the test.

The test begins with an Answer Sheet that you may want to remove from the book. Use this sheet to mark your answers. When you are finished with the test, carefully read the answer explanations, especially for any questions that you answered incorrectly. Identify any weak areas by determining the subjects in which you made the most errors. Then go back and review the corresponding chapters in this book. If time permits, you may also want to review your stronger areas.

This practice test will help you gauge your test readiness if you treat it as an actual examination. Here are some hints on how to take the test under conditions similar to those of the actual exam.

➤ Find a time when you will not be interrupted.

➤ Complete the test in a single session, following the suggested time limits.

➤ If you run out of time on any section, take note of where you ended when time ran out. This will help you determine if you need to speed up your pacing.

PCAT Practice Test Answer Sheet

SECTION 2. VERBAL ABILITY

1 Ⓐ Ⓑ Ⓒ Ⓓ	17 Ⓐ Ⓑ Ⓒ Ⓓ	33 Ⓐ Ⓑ Ⓒ Ⓓ
2 Ⓐ Ⓑ Ⓒ Ⓓ	18 Ⓐ Ⓑ Ⓒ Ⓓ	34 Ⓐ Ⓑ Ⓒ Ⓓ
3 Ⓐ Ⓑ Ⓒ Ⓓ	19 Ⓐ Ⓑ Ⓒ Ⓓ	35 Ⓐ Ⓑ Ⓒ Ⓓ
4 Ⓐ Ⓑ Ⓒ Ⓓ	20 Ⓐ Ⓑ Ⓒ Ⓓ	36 Ⓐ Ⓑ Ⓒ Ⓓ
5 Ⓐ Ⓑ Ⓒ Ⓓ	21 Ⓐ Ⓑ Ⓒ Ⓓ	37 Ⓐ Ⓑ Ⓒ Ⓓ
6 Ⓐ Ⓑ Ⓒ Ⓓ	22 Ⓐ Ⓑ Ⓒ Ⓓ	38 Ⓐ Ⓑ Ⓒ Ⓓ
7 Ⓐ Ⓑ Ⓒ Ⓓ	23 Ⓐ Ⓑ Ⓒ Ⓓ	39 Ⓐ Ⓑ Ⓒ Ⓓ
8 Ⓐ Ⓑ Ⓒ Ⓓ	24 Ⓐ Ⓑ Ⓒ Ⓓ	40 Ⓐ Ⓑ Ⓒ Ⓓ
9 Ⓐ Ⓑ Ⓒ Ⓓ	25 Ⓐ Ⓑ Ⓒ Ⓓ	41 Ⓐ Ⓑ Ⓒ Ⓓ
10 Ⓐ Ⓑ Ⓒ Ⓓ	26 Ⓐ Ⓑ Ⓒ Ⓓ	42 Ⓐ Ⓑ Ⓒ Ⓓ
11 Ⓐ Ⓑ Ⓒ Ⓓ	27 Ⓐ Ⓑ Ⓒ Ⓓ	43 Ⓐ Ⓑ Ⓒ Ⓓ
12 Ⓐ Ⓑ Ⓒ Ⓓ	28 Ⓐ Ⓑ Ⓒ Ⓓ	44 Ⓐ Ⓑ Ⓒ Ⓓ
13 Ⓐ Ⓑ Ⓒ Ⓓ	29 Ⓐ Ⓑ Ⓒ Ⓓ	45 Ⓐ Ⓑ Ⓒ Ⓓ
14 Ⓐ Ⓑ Ⓒ Ⓓ	30 Ⓐ Ⓑ Ⓒ Ⓓ	46 Ⓐ Ⓑ Ⓒ Ⓓ
15 Ⓐ Ⓑ Ⓒ Ⓓ	31 Ⓐ Ⓑ Ⓒ Ⓓ	47 Ⓐ Ⓑ Ⓒ Ⓓ
16 Ⓐ Ⓑ Ⓒ Ⓓ	32 Ⓐ Ⓑ Ⓒ Ⓓ	48 Ⓐ Ⓑ Ⓒ Ⓓ

SECTION 3. BIOLOGY

1 Ⓐ Ⓑ Ⓒ Ⓓ	17 Ⓐ Ⓑ Ⓒ Ⓓ	33 Ⓐ Ⓑ Ⓒ Ⓓ
2 Ⓐ Ⓑ Ⓒ Ⓓ	18 Ⓐ Ⓑ Ⓒ Ⓓ	34 Ⓐ Ⓑ Ⓒ Ⓓ
3 Ⓐ Ⓑ Ⓒ Ⓓ	19 Ⓐ Ⓑ Ⓒ Ⓓ	35 Ⓐ Ⓑ Ⓒ Ⓓ
4 Ⓐ Ⓑ Ⓒ Ⓓ	20 Ⓐ Ⓑ Ⓒ Ⓓ	36 Ⓐ Ⓑ Ⓒ Ⓓ
5 Ⓐ Ⓑ Ⓒ Ⓓ	21 Ⓐ Ⓑ Ⓒ Ⓓ	37 Ⓐ Ⓑ Ⓒ Ⓓ
6 Ⓐ Ⓑ Ⓒ Ⓓ	22 Ⓐ Ⓑ Ⓒ Ⓓ	38 Ⓐ Ⓑ Ⓒ Ⓓ
7 Ⓐ Ⓑ Ⓒ Ⓓ	23 Ⓐ Ⓑ Ⓒ Ⓓ	39 Ⓐ Ⓑ Ⓒ Ⓓ
8 Ⓐ Ⓑ Ⓒ Ⓓ	24 Ⓐ Ⓑ Ⓒ Ⓓ	40 Ⓐ Ⓑ Ⓒ Ⓓ
9 Ⓐ Ⓑ Ⓒ Ⓓ	25 Ⓐ Ⓑ Ⓒ Ⓓ	41 Ⓐ Ⓑ Ⓒ Ⓓ
10 Ⓐ Ⓑ Ⓒ Ⓓ	26 Ⓐ Ⓑ Ⓒ Ⓓ	42 Ⓐ Ⓑ Ⓒ Ⓓ
11 Ⓐ Ⓑ Ⓒ Ⓓ	27 Ⓐ Ⓑ Ⓒ Ⓓ	43 Ⓐ Ⓑ Ⓒ Ⓓ
12 Ⓐ Ⓑ Ⓒ Ⓓ	28 Ⓐ Ⓑ Ⓒ Ⓓ	44 Ⓐ Ⓑ Ⓒ Ⓓ
13 Ⓐ Ⓑ Ⓒ Ⓓ	29 Ⓐ Ⓑ Ⓒ Ⓓ	45 Ⓐ Ⓑ Ⓒ Ⓓ
14 Ⓐ Ⓑ Ⓒ Ⓓ	30 Ⓐ Ⓑ Ⓒ Ⓓ	46 Ⓐ Ⓑ Ⓒ Ⓓ
15 Ⓐ Ⓑ Ⓒ Ⓓ	31 Ⓐ Ⓑ Ⓒ Ⓓ	47 Ⓐ Ⓑ Ⓒ Ⓓ
16 Ⓐ Ⓑ Ⓒ Ⓓ	32 Ⓐ Ⓑ Ⓒ Ⓓ	48 Ⓐ Ⓑ Ⓒ Ⓓ

SECTION 4. CHEMISTRY

1 (A) (B) (C) (D)   17 (A) (B) (C) (D)   33 (A) (B) (C) (D)
2 (A) (B) (C) (D)   18 (A) (B) (C) (D)   34 (A) (B) (C) (D)
3 (A) (B) (C) (D)   19 (A) (B) (C) (D)   35 (A) (B) (C) (D)
4 (A) (B) (C) (D)   20 (A) (B) (C) (D)   36 (A) (B) (C) (D)
5 (A) (B) (C) (D)   21 (A) (B) (C) (D)   37 (A) (B) (C) (D)
6 (A) (B) (C) (D)   22 (A) (B) (C) (D)   38 (A) (B) (C) (D)
7 (A) (B) (C) (D)   23 (A) (B) (C) (D)   39 (A) (B) (C) (D)
8 (A) (B) (C) (D)   24 (A) (B) (C) (D)   40 (A) (B) (C) (D)
9 (A) (B) (C) (D)   25 (A) (B) (C) (D)   41 (A) (B) (C) (D)
10 (A) (B) (C) (D)   26 (A) (B) (C) (D)   42 (A) (B) (C) (D)
11 (A) (B) (C) (D)   27 (A) (B) (C) (D)   43 (A) (B) (C) (D)
12 (A) (B) (C) (D)   28 (A) (B) (C) (D)   44 (A) (B) (C) (D)
13 (A) (B) (C) (D)   29 (A) (B) (C) (D)   45 (A) (B) (C) (D)
14 (A) (B) (C) (D)   30 (A) (B) (C) (D)   46 (A) (B) (C) (D)
15 (A) (B) (C) (D)   31 (A) (B) (C) (D)   47 (A) (B) (C) (D)
16 (A) (B) (C) (D)   32 (A) (B) (C) (D)   48 (A) (B) (C) (D)

SECTION 6. READING COMPREHENSION

1 (A) (B) (C) (D)   17 (A) (B) (C) (D)   33 (A) (B) (C) (D)
2 (A) (B) (C) (D)   18 (A) (B) (C) (D)   34 (A) (B) (C) (D)
3 (A) (B) (C) (D)   19 (A) (B) (C) (D)   35 (A) (B) (C) (D)
4 (A) (B) (C) (D)   20 (A) (B) (C) (D)   36 (A) (B) (C) (D)
5 (A) (B) (C) (D)   21 (A) (B) (C) (D)   37 (A) (B) (C) (D)
6 (A) (B) (C) (D)   22 (A) (B) (C) (D)   38 (A) (B) (C) (D)
7 (A) (B) (C) (D)   23 (A) (B) (C) (D)   39 (A) (B) (C) (D)
8 (A) (B) (C) (D)   24 (A) (B) (C) (D)   40 (A) (B) (C) (D)
9 (A) (B) (C) (D)   25 (A) (B) (C) (D)   41 (A) (B) (C) (D)
10 (A) (B) (C) (D)   26 (A) (B) (C) (D)   42 (A) (B) (C) (D)
11 (A) (B) (C) (D)   27 (A) (B) (C) (D)   43 (A) (B) (C) (D)
12 (A) (B) (C) (D)   28 (A) (B) (C) (D)   44 (A) (B) (C) (D)
13 (A) (B) (C) (D)   29 (A) (B) (C) (D)   45 (A) (B) (C) (D)
14 (A) (B) (C) (D)   30 (A) (B) (C) (D)   46 (A) (B) (C) (D)
15 (A) (B) (C) (D)   31 (A) (B) (C) (D)   47 (A) (B) (C) (D)
16 (A) (B) (C) (D)   32 (A) (B) (C) (D)   48 (A) (B) (C) (D)

SECTION 7. QUANTITATIVE ABILITY

1 Ⓐ Ⓑ Ⓒ Ⓓ	17 Ⓐ Ⓑ Ⓒ Ⓓ	33 Ⓐ Ⓑ Ⓒ Ⓓ
2 Ⓐ Ⓑ Ⓒ Ⓓ	18 Ⓐ Ⓑ Ⓒ Ⓓ	34 Ⓐ Ⓑ Ⓒ Ⓓ
3 Ⓐ Ⓑ Ⓒ Ⓓ	19 Ⓐ Ⓑ Ⓒ Ⓓ	35 Ⓐ Ⓑ Ⓒ Ⓓ
4 Ⓐ Ⓑ Ⓒ Ⓓ	20 Ⓐ Ⓑ Ⓒ Ⓓ	36 Ⓐ Ⓑ Ⓒ Ⓓ
5 Ⓐ Ⓑ Ⓒ Ⓓ	21 Ⓐ Ⓑ Ⓒ Ⓓ	37 Ⓐ Ⓑ Ⓒ Ⓓ
6 Ⓐ Ⓑ Ⓒ Ⓓ	22 Ⓐ Ⓑ Ⓒ Ⓓ	38 Ⓐ Ⓑ Ⓒ Ⓓ
7 Ⓐ Ⓑ Ⓒ Ⓓ	23 Ⓐ Ⓑ Ⓒ Ⓓ	39 Ⓐ Ⓑ Ⓒ Ⓓ
8 Ⓐ Ⓑ Ⓒ Ⓓ	24 Ⓐ Ⓑ Ⓒ Ⓓ	40 Ⓐ Ⓑ Ⓒ Ⓓ
9 Ⓐ Ⓑ Ⓒ Ⓓ	25 Ⓐ Ⓑ Ⓒ Ⓓ	41 Ⓐ Ⓑ Ⓒ Ⓓ
10 Ⓐ Ⓑ Ⓒ Ⓓ	26 Ⓐ Ⓑ Ⓒ Ⓓ	42 Ⓐ Ⓑ Ⓒ Ⓓ
11 Ⓐ Ⓑ Ⓒ Ⓓ	27 Ⓐ Ⓑ Ⓒ Ⓓ	43 Ⓐ Ⓑ Ⓒ Ⓓ
12 Ⓐ Ⓑ Ⓒ Ⓓ	28 Ⓐ Ⓑ Ⓒ Ⓓ	44 Ⓐ Ⓑ Ⓒ Ⓓ
13 Ⓐ Ⓑ Ⓒ Ⓓ	29 Ⓐ Ⓑ Ⓒ Ⓓ	45 Ⓐ Ⓑ Ⓒ Ⓓ
14 Ⓐ Ⓑ Ⓒ Ⓓ	30 Ⓐ Ⓑ Ⓒ Ⓓ	46 Ⓐ Ⓑ Ⓒ Ⓓ
15 Ⓐ Ⓑ Ⓒ Ⓓ	31 Ⓐ Ⓑ Ⓒ Ⓓ	47 Ⓐ Ⓑ Ⓒ Ⓓ
16 Ⓐ Ⓑ Ⓒ Ⓓ	32 Ⓐ Ⓑ Ⓒ Ⓓ	48 Ⓐ Ⓑ Ⓒ Ⓓ

SECTION 1. WRITING

1 Question　　　**Time: 30 minutes**

Discuss a solution to the problem of parental concern about childhood vaccinations.

_____
_____
_____
_____
_____
_____
_____
_____
_____
_____
_____
_____
_____
_____
_____
_____
_____
_____
_____
_____
_____
_____
_____
_____
_____
_____
_____
_____
_____
_____

SECTION 2. VERBAL ABILITY

48 Questions   Time: 30 minutes

Directions: Questions 1–19 consist of sentences with one or two blanks where words or phrases have been left out. Choose the word or set of words that **best** completes each sentence from the choices given.

1. In sickle-cell anemia, the red blood cells are misshapen, _____ crescents rather than round discs.
   A. inferring
   B. resulting
   C. manufacturing
   D. resembling

2. Population density is a comparison of the _____ of organisms in a population to the size of the area in which they live.
   A. population
   B. number
   C. size
   D. concentration

3. Chemical reactions in mitochondria produce ATP, which is the _____ of energy for the cell.
   A. limit
   B. fault
   C. source
   D. name

4. Inexpensive and _____ available, aspirin has been used for decades to _____ fever and inflammation and to reduce pain.
   A. readily . . . treat
   B. currently . . . barricade
   C. easily . . . enhance
   D. modestly . . . inhibit

5. Because twins are so _____ physically, they will usually _____ similarly to the same diet.
   A. alike . . . endure
   B. familiar . . . act
   C. similar . . . respond
   D. close . . . consume

6. Unlike the less complex roundworms or flatworms, annelids have a circulatory system and _____ nervous and digestive systems.
   A. simpler
   B. representative
   C. nonessential
   D. well-developed

7. Sometimes there is more than one bond between the same two atoms; for example, ethylene has a _____ bond between its two carbon atoms.
   A. single
   B. strong
   C. dual
   D. chemical

8. A grasshopper's exoskeleton performs two key functions: to protect the insect and to _____ it from drying out.
   A. maintain
   B. cover
   C. secure
   D. prevent

9. Although no one understands _____ how some animals sense that an earth-quake is imminent, it is clear that they _____ stimuli that humans cannot detect.
   A. exactly . . . create
   B. directly . . . hear
   C. precisely . . . sense
   D. thoroughly . . . know

10. As the earth formed, enormous quantities of hydrogen and oxygen were trapped beneath the crust, and these elements _____ to form water.
   A. aspired
   B. evolved
   C. required
   D. combined

11. It may seem that the only _____ in a predator-prey relationship is the predator, but in fact, the prey benefits from having its population _____.
   A. recipient . . . eradicated
   B. beneficiary . . . controlled
   C. winner . . . underestimated
   D. consumer . . . eaten

12. If one species reproduces more rapidly than its competitors, it may _____ others out of the immediate area.
   A. crowd
   B. inhibit
   C. expend
   D. deduce

13. Smoking crack causes a lung _____ known as "cracklung," which does not re-spond to antibiotics or other _____ pneumonia treatments but must instead be treated with corticosteroids.
   A. irritation . . . shielding
   B. disorder . . . traditional
   C. addiction . . . standard
   D. disease . . . harmonizing

14. Drug testing on humans _____ consists of three phases, with Phase I being a test for negative reactions and _____.
   A. generally . . . toxicity
   B. typically . . . volunteers
   C. eventually . . . disease
   D. potentially . . . dosages

15. Although we tend to _____ the plague with medieval times, several cases a year _____ occur in the American Southwest.
   A. remember . . . residually
   B. identify . . . rarely
   C. equate . . . sporadically
   D. associate . . . still

16. People with panic disorder have a high _____ for suicide, usually brought on by _____ depression.
   A. likelihood . . . normative
   B. propensity . . . secondary
   C. frequency . . . severe
   D. tolerance . . . illogical

17. The rediscovery of the *Titanic* was made during sea trials of a remote-controlled sled, the *Argo*, _____ descending to depths of 20,000 feet (6,100 meters).
   A. having often
   B. capable of
   C. which could
   D. in the process

18. A stroke does not affect all areas of the brain the same way, nor are all aspects of intellectual functioning affected _____.

A. as well

B. in fact

C. also

D. equally

19. Since obesity is the single most common nongenetic factor in the _____ of diabetes, weight control is absolutely essential.

A. carrier

B. practice

C. development

D. heredity

Directions: For questions 20–48, choose the word that best completes the analogy so that the third and fourth terms have a relationship parallel to that of the first and second terms.

20. GLUCOSE : SUGAR :: ETHANOL :

A. Oil

B. Gas

C. Salt

D. Alcohol

21. COLD : VIRUS :: HEADACHE :

A. Pain

B. Stress

C. Bacterium

D. Heat

22. PUMP : HEART :: FILTER :

A. Kidney

B. Bladder

C. Lung

D. Aorta

23. FOND : INDIFFERENT :: JOCULAR :

A. Morose

B. Uncaring

C. Jolly

D. Laugh

24. PYRAMID : TRIANGLE :: CUBE :

A. Prism

B. Square

C. Cone

D. Rectangle

25. POUCH : MARSUPIAL :: HOOF :

A. Elephant

B. Antler

C. Mammal

D. Ungulate

26. SCURVY : VITAMIN C :: GOITER :

A. Vitamin D

B. Beriberi

C. Iodine

D. Iron

27. FRANTIC : CALM :: COMPLAINING :

A. Carping

B. Belligerent

C. Frenetic

D. Stoic

28. PETAL : ATTRACT :: PISTIL :

A. Repel

B. Manufacture

C. Consume

D. Reproduce

29. CRANIOTOMY : SKULL :: PHLEBOTOMY :
  A. Brain
  B. Limb
  C. Vein
  D. Sensory organ

30. EVEREST : K2 :: NILE :
  A. Mississippi
  B. Amazon
  C. Yangtze
  D. Niger

31. HERPETOLOGIST : PYTHON :: ICHTHYOLOGIST :
  A. Atlantic
  B. Cod
  C. Cobra
  D. Macaw

32. DIET : WEIGHT :: FOG :
  A. Translucency
  B. Droplets
  C. Visibility
  D. Pollutant

33. MELANCHOLY : HILARITY :: MALICE :
  A. Fecundity
  B. Mirth
  C. Spite
  D. Benevolence

34. NAVIGATOR : COURSE :: REFEREE :
  A. Game
  B. Ruling
  C. Competition
  D. Amendment

35. GROUNDHOG : WOODCHUCK :: POLECAT :
  A. Bobcat
  B. Raccoon
  C. Skunk
  D. Cougar

36. OXYGEN : ELEMENT :: WATER :
  A. Property
  B. Atom
  C. Ion
  D. Molecule

37. PROVISIONAL : PERPETUAL :: VOLUNTARY :
  A. Charitable
  B. Compulsory
  C. Optional
  D. Regular

38. WORD PROCESSOR : TYPEWRITER :: CALCULATOR :
  A. Abacus
  B. Arithmetic
  C. Numerals
  D. Computer

39. ARTERY : ARTERIOLE :: VEIN :
  A. Varicose
  B. Heart valve
  C. Venule
  D. Vena cava

40. STRIDENT : SHRILL :: SONOROUS :
  A. Clamorous
  B. Resonant
  C. Agreeable
  D. Reedy

41. FURRIER : HIDE :: FARRIER :
    - **A.** Iron
    - **B.** Shoe
    - **C.** Beat
    - **D.** Horse

42. INGENIOUS: CLEVER :: INFURIATING :
    - **A.** Brainy
    - **B.** Irksome
    - **C.** Terrible
    - **D.** Furious

43. PROD : STAB :: DISOBEY :
    - **A.** Wound
    - **B.** Punish
    - **C.** Flout
    - **D.** Conform

44. AREA : HECTARE :: DEPTH :
    - **A.** Liter
    - **B.** Furlong
    - **C.** Fathom
    - **D.** Angstrom

45. FOX : SLYNESS :: OWL :
    - **A.** Night vision
    - **B.** Wisdom
    - **C.** Predation
    - **D.** Craftiness

46. NICKEL : QUARTER :: DIME :
    - **A.** Nickel
    - **B.** Penny
    - **C.** Half-dollar
    - **D.** Dollar

47. ELEVATOR : SKYSCRAPER :: FUNICULAR :
    - **A.** Cathedral
    - **B.** Edifice
    - **C.** Road
    - **D.** Mountain

48. IMPROVE : DETERIORATE :: IMPRESS :
    - **A.** Decline
    - **B.** Disappoint
    - **C.** Electrify
    - **D.** Bolster

**STOP. IF YOU HAVE TIME LEFT OVER,
CHECK YOUR WORK ON THIS SECTION ONLY.**

SECTION 3. BIOLOGY

48 Questions   **30 Minutes**

1. The number of mitochondria in a particular cell type probably relate to
   A. the size of the cell and the amount of space available
   B. the number of proteins the cell needs to produce
   C. the amount of materials in the cell that need to be degraded and removed
   D. the amount of ATP the cell needs to produce

2. Oncogenic viruses are associated with cancer and are known to become latent as they enter into the host cell's chromosomes. Many of these oncogenic viruses are retroviruses. In order for a retrovirus to insert into the host cell's chromosomes, it must first
   A. convert its RNA to DNA   C. initiate transcription
   B. translate its RNA   D. recombine with the host cell's chromosomes

3. Endosymbiotic theory explains why mitochondria have their own DNA. This theory essentially states that at one point, free living prokaryotic cells were engulfed by another cell, eventually becoming mitochondria. The best support for this theory is that
   A. mitochondria are membrane-bound organelles
   B. mitochondrial DNA resembles that of prokaryotic DNA
   C. mitochondria have more than one copy of their DNA
   D. mitochondria are found in multiple copies in each cell

4. The hormones FSH and LH are involved in oogenesis in women. When LH surges in the ovarian cycle, what event will result?
   A. endometrium proliferation
   B. ovulation
   C. menstruation
   D. corpus luteum degradation

5. Mitochondrial DNA within the cells of a given individual is present in a single copy because it is derived from a single source (the individual's mother). Which of the following processes should not occur within mtDNA?
   A. transcription   C. crossing over and recombination
   B. translation   D. spontaneous mutation

6. Conjugation is one method bacteria use to pass their antibiotic resistance genes to other bacteria. During conjugation, the genes transferred are typically located on the (a)
   A. bacterial chromosome   C. mRNA
   B. ribosome   D. plasmid

7. The repeated use of antibiotics puts selective pressure on bacteria so that the population quickly becomes antibiotic resistant. What type of selection is going to occur with this type of selective pressure?
   - A. artificial selection
   - B. stabilizing selection
   - C. directional selection
   - D. disruptive selection

8. If a patient has a condition called pulmonary arterial hypertension (PAH), the heart can become overly stressed. PAH can ultimately lead to heart failure. Which area of the heart is most likely to be initially affected by increased blood pressure in the pulmonary arteries?
   - A. the right and left atria
   - B. the right and left ventricles
   - C. the right ventricle
   - D. the left ventricle

9. When changes occur to DNA, they are often corrected by a proofreading mechanism. If the change is not corrected, a permanent mutation is the result. This must be the result of which enzyme not functioning properly?
   - A. helicase
   - B. ligase
   - C. DNA polymerase
   - D. RNA polymerase

10. The strains of the bacterium *Staphylococcus aureus* associated with osteomyelitis (a bone infection) have a variety of cell adhesion molecules called adhesins that help them to attach to and be internalized by osteoblasts. These molecules are likely found in which of the following bacterial structures?
    - A. the nucleoid
    - B. the ribosomes
    - C. the capsule
    - D. spores

11. Cells that perform apoptosis are ultimately able to activate enzymes within the cell that damage and destroy cellular contents. Which of the following organelles is most likely to become involved with apoptosis?
    - A. the endoplasmic reticulum
    - B. the Golgi complex
    - C. lysosomes
    - D. mitochondria

12. Procaine (also known as novocaine) and lidocaine are both drugs used for local anesthesia, and they have similar mechanisms of action. The drugs affect neurons in the local areas to which they are applied by preventing the opening of Na^+ gated channels in the neurons. How would blocking gated Na^+ channels prevent the transmission of messages in nerves?
    - A. If gated Na^+ channels are blocked, Na^+ concentrations remain higher inside the neuron than outside of the neuron.
    - B. If gated Na^+ channels are blocked, the neuronal membrane cannot depolarize.
    - C. Blocking Na^+ channels would prevent the Na^+/K^+ pumps from properly functioning.
    - D. Blocking Na^+ channels would prevent neurotransmitters from binding to receptors at the synapse.

13. Drugs such as AZT and ddI are nucleoside analogs used in HIV-infected patients. Both are chemically modified versions of the nucleotides that make up DNA and RNA. These modified nucleotides interfere with normal replication and transcription. The most important goal of these drugs would be

   A. to prevent the replication of host cell DNA so that the host cell cannot function

   B. to prevent the transcription of host cell RNA so that no proteins can be expressed

   C. to prevent the viral nucleic acid from entering the host cells

   D. to prevent replication of the viral genome

14. When a certain bacterium encounters the antibiotic tetracycline, the antibiotic molecule enters the cell and attaches to a repressor protein. This keeps the repressor from binding to the bacterial DNA that allows certain genes to be transcribed. These genes code for enzymes that break down tetracycline. This set of genes is best described as

   A. an operator   **C.** a repressible operon

   B. an inducible operon   **D.** a regulator

15. In Mendel's experiments with the pea plant, the gene for height exists in two allelic forms designated *T* for tall stature and *t* for short stature. In the second generation of a cross between a homozygous tall parent (*TT*) and a homozygous short parent (*tt*), the phenotypic ratio of dominant to recessive pea plants is

   A. 1:1   **C.** 3:1

   B. 2:1   **D.** 4:1

16. The regulation of water and sodium levels in the nephrons is adjusted in two regions of the kidneys where water and sodium can be reabsorbed from the nephron and returned to circulation. Those regions are the

   A. proximal convoluted tubule and distal convoluted tubule

   B. the loop of Henle and the distal convoluted tubule

   C. the distal convoluted tubule and the collecting duct

   D. the proximal convoluted tubule and the loop of Henle

17. Suppose plasma levels of carbon dioxide are elevated. On a cellular level, where does this carbon dioxide come from?

   A. It is produced during protein synthesis.

   B. It is a by-product of nucleic acid metabolism.

   C. It is a by-product of glucose metabolism.

   D. It is produced as a direct conversion from oxygen gas in the cells.

18. The genes for antibiotic resistance are often carried on bacterial plasmids. These plasmids can be transferred from one bacterium to another. The most likely method for plasmid transfer would be

   A. transduction   **C.** conjugation

   B. transformation   **D.** binary fission

19. Many dialysis patients do not produce any urine, so dialysis must be used to manage their fluid levels. In order to remove excess fluids from the blood during dialysis, the patient's blood must be

A. isotonic as compared to the dialysis solution

B. hypertonic as compared to the dialysis solution

C. hypotonic as compared to the dialysis solution

D. the same pH as the dialysis solution

20. The cystic fibrosis transmembrane regulator (CTFR protein) is 1480 amino acids in length. How many codons must have been present in the mRNA used to make the protein?

A. 493   C. 1481

B. 1480   D. 4440

21. An unknown cell type has been isolated. It is suspected that this cell is prokaryotic; tests are performed in order to confirm this suspicion. The presence of which of these cell structures would confirm that the cells are prokaryotic?

A. cytoplasm   C. a peptidoglycan cell wall

B. a flagellum   D. spores

22. If two parents do not have cystic fibrosis but are carriers for the disease, what are their odds of having a child with cystic fibrosis?

A. 0%   C. 50%

B. 25%   D. 75%

23. Which of the following statements is true about peptide hormones?

A. They cross the cell membrane.

B. They use second messengers like cAMP.

C. They activate the expression of certain genes.

D. They are lipid-soluble.

24. Vegetables that have been left in a dish of fresh water will tend to swell up and become stiff while vegetables soaked in salt water tend to shrivel and become limp. The best explanation is that fresh water is _____ to the cells and salt water is _____ to the cells.

A. hypertonic; hypotonic   C. hypotonic; hypertonic

B. hypertonic; isotonic   D. isotonic; hypertonic

25. Fungi are typically characterized based on reproductive methods and structures. A fungus that always reproduces asexually is most likely classified as

A. Zygomycetes   C. Deuteromycetes

B. Ascomycetes   D. Basidomycetes

26. A cell is exposed to a substance that prevents it from dividing. The cell becomes larger and larger. This situation
    A. should present no problem to the cell since it can continue to perform all other necessary functions
    B. should present no problem to the cell since the surface area of the cell will increase as the volume of the cell increases
    C. will eventually be problematic to the cell since the surface-area-to-volume ratio is decreasing
    D. will eventually be problematic to the cell since the nutritional requirements will increase

27. You touch a hot stove and your hand jerks back. Which of the following describes the pathway of nerve impulses responsible for this reflex?
    A. motor neuron → sensory neuron → interneuron
    B. sensory neuron → interneuron → motor neuron
    C. interneuron → sensory neuron → motor neuron
    D. motor neuron → interneuron → sensory neuron

28. A living plant is exposed to H_2O labeled with ^{18}O and exposed to sunlight. The ^{18}O will end up in which of the following molecules at the end of photosynthesis?
    A. glucose
    B. CO_2
    C. H_2O
    D. O_2

29. A bacteriophage that is in the lysogenic cycle will do all of the following except
    A. lyse the host
    B. be passed on as the bacterial host cell divides
    C. eventually enter the lytic cycle
    D. insert into the host's DNA

30. The drug DNP destroys the H^+ gradient that forms in the electron transport chain. The most likely consequence would be
    A. the cells will be forced to perform fermentation
    B. ATP production will increase
    C. glycolysis will stop
    D. oxygen consumption will increase

31. Guillain-Barré Syndrome affects the myelin of the peripheral nervous system. Which neurons in the body should not be affected by GBS?
    A. those in the arms and legs
    B. those in the abdominal cavity
    C. those that innervate the heart
    D. those in the spinal cord

32. A child is born with an unusual condition in which mitochondria are missing from his skeletal muscles (the mitochondria are present in all other body cells). Physicians find that this child's muscle can function. They also find that

    A. the muscles contain large quantities of lactic acid even after very mild activity

    B. the muscles require extremely large amounts of oxygen to function

    C. the muscle cells cannot convert glucose to pyruvate

    D. the muscle cells require large amounts of CO_2 to function

33. Which of the following characteristics distinguishes retroviruses from all other types of viruses?

    A. They are viruses that use RNA as their genetic material.

    B. They must interact with a receptor on the host to infect it.

    C. They enter latent phases.

    D. They utilize the enzyme reverse transcriptase.

34. A lab technician allows a cell to perform semiconservative replication in the presence of radioactive nucleotides. Which of the following would occur?

    A. The DNA in one of the double helices would be radioactive but not in the other double helix.

    B. The DNA in each of the double helices would be radioactive.

    C. The DNA would not be radioactive in either of the double helices.

    D. The mRNA made from this DNA would be radioactive.

35. A person is on medication to increase the pH of the stomach. A side effect is that the increased pH causes the normal stomach enzymes to be unable to function. Which component of this person's diet may not be completely digested?

    A. proteins   **C.** fats

    B. carbohydrates   **D.** nucleic acids

36. A diploid human cell that is dividing will contain _____ chromosomes. These chromosomes will each consist of _____ chromatid(s).

    A. 46 . . . 1   **C.** 46 . . . 2

    B. 23 . . . 1   **D.** 23 . . . 2

37. Host cells are often killed by a virus as the direct result of

    A. integrating into the host cell chromosomes

    B. lysis of the host to release new viruses

    C. replication of the viral genetic material within the host

    D. toxic enzymes that damage the host cell that are coded for in the viral genome

38. RNA
   A. is usually found as a double helix
   B. is made during translation
   C. is distinguished from DNA by the use of ribose sugar in the nucleotides
   D. is produced in the cytoplasm

39. Which of the following choices indicates the correct pathway of CO_2 leaving the body?
   A. alveoli, bronchioles, bronchi, trachea, larynx, pharynx
   B. pharynx, larynx, trachea, bronchi, bronchioles, alveoli
   C. alveoli, bronchi, bronchioles, larynx, trachea, pharynx
   D. alveoli, bronchioles, bronchi, trachea, pharynx, larynx

40. Why are mutations that cause changes to amino acid sequences not more common?
   A. because the DNA polymerase enzyme proofreads and usually corrects its mistakes
   B. because tRNAs can correct mistakes and bring the proper amino acid to the ribosome
   C. because RNA polymerase can correct DNA mistakes during transcription
   D. Any of the above are acceptable explanations.

41. An allele known as BRCA1 is often found in women with breast and ovarian cancer. However, some women develop these cancers and do not have the BRCA1 allele. In addition, some women who have BRCA1 never develop breast or ovarian cancer. How can this be explained?
   A. This must be an example of pleiotropy.
   B. These types of cancers are in no way associated with specific alleles.
   C. Something other than the gene must factor into whether cancer develops or not.
   D. The BRCA1 gene must be dominant inheritance.

42. A person has been lost in the desert for two days with no water or fluids to drink. Concerning the excretory system you would expect all of the following except a(n)
   A. decrease in urine volume
   B. increase in antidiuretic hormone secretion
   C. increase in aldosterone secretion
   D. increase in blood volume

43. Phenylketonuria is caused by an autosomal recessive allele. A man is the carrier of the disorder; his wife does not have PKU and is not a carrier of the disorder. What is the probability that some of their offspring will have the disorder and others will be carriers?

   A. 0% of the offspring will have the disorder; 0% of the males will be carriers; 100% of the females will be carriers.

   B. 0% of the offspring will have the disorder; 50% will be carriers.

   C. 50% of the offspring will have the disorder; 50% will be carriers.

   D. 25% of the offspring will have the disorder; 75% will be carriers.

44. Duchene muscular dystrophy is caused by a sex-linked allele. Its victims are almost always boys who die before the age of 20. Why is this disorder rarely seen in girls?

   A. The allele is carried on the Y chromosome.

   B. Girls must receive the allele from both their mother and their father to have the disease.

   C. Males carrying the allele do not usually live long enough to reproduce.

   D. Sex-linked traits are never seen in girls.

45. Which of the following is not part of the Calvin cycle?

   A. ATP production   **C.** fixation of carbon dioxide

   B. regeneration of RuBP   **D.** oxidation of NADPH

46. If a sperm cell contains 12 chromosomes, it must have come from an original parent cell that contained _____ chromosomes.

   A. 4   **C.** 12

   B. 6   **D.** 24

47. Darwin's theory of natural selection is often referred to as "survival of the fittest." The "fittest" organisms in a population are those which

   A. are the biggest and strongest   **C.** live the longest

   B. mutate the fastest   **D.** reproduce the most

48. In a certain population, 81% of individuals have a homozygous recessive genotype. Using the Hardy-Weinberg equations, what percentage of individuals in the next generation will be heterozygous?

   A. 10%   **C.** 18%

   B. 19%   **D.** 9%

STOP. IF YOU HAVE TIME LEFT OVER,
CHECK YOUR WORK ON THIS SECTION ONLY.

SECTION 4. CHEMISTRY

48 Questions   30 Minutes

1. How many neutrons are there in an atom of ^{31}P?
   (The atomic number of P is 15.)
   A. 15   C. 47
   B. 31   D. 16

2. What is the mass percent of oxygen in Na_2CO_3?
   (atomic masses $Na = 23$ $^g/_{mol}$, $C = 12$ $^g/_{mol}$, and $O = 16$ $^g/_{mol}$)
   A. 16.9 %   C. 31.3 %
   B. 57.8 %   D. 45.3 %

3. How many hydrogen atoms are there in 48 g of methane, CH_4?
   (Avogadro's number $= 6 \times 10^{23}$, atomic masses $C = 12$ $^g/_{mol}$, and $H = 1$ $^g/_{mol}$)
   A. 7.2×10^{24} C. 6.4×10^{24}
   B. 2.9×10^{25} D. 1.8×10^{24}

4. What is the maximum amount of ammonia that can be formed by reaction
   of 70 g of nitrogen and 12 g of hydrogen?
   (atomic masses $N = 14$ $^g/_{mol}$, and $H = 1$ $^g/_{mol}$)

   $$N_2(g) + 3H_2(g) \rightarrow 2NH_3(g)$$

   A. 85 g   C. 45
   B. 170 g   D. 68 g

5. A reaction is carried out with 372 g of P_4 and excess Cl_2, and 1000 g of PCl_3 is
   isolated. What is the percent yield of the reaction?
   (atomic masses $P = 31$ $^g/_{mol}$, and $Cl = 35.5$ $^g/_{mol}$)

   $$P_4(s) + 6Cl_2(g) \rightarrow 4PCl_3(l)$$

   A. 37.2 %   C. 60.6 %
   B. 15.2 %   D. 46.7 %

6. A graduated cylinder is filled with water to the 10.0 mL mark. A metal cylinder
   of mass 10.3 g is immersed in the water, and the water level rises to 13.8 mL.
   What is the density of the metal?
   A. 0.75 $^g/_{mL}$ C. 2.7 $^g/_{mL}$
   B. 39 $^g/_{mL}$ D. 0.37 $^g/_{mL}$

7. A compound that contains only sulfur, oxygen, and bromine is analyzed and found
   to contain 9.6 g sulfur, 4.8 g oxygen, and 48 g bromine. What is the empirical
   formula of the compound?
   (atomic masses $S = 32$ $^g/_{mol}$, $O = 16$ $^g/_{mol}$, and $Br = 80$ $^g/_{mol}$)

A. S_2OBr_5

B. $SOBr_2$

C. S_2OBr_4

D. SO_2Br_2

8. A solution is made by adding 10.5 g of NaF (molar mass = 42 $^g/_{mol}$) to make a solution with a total volume of 750 mL. A sample of 100 mL of this solution is added to 200 mL of water to make a second solution. What is the molarity of the second solution?

   A. 1.00 M

   B. 0.33 M

   C. 0.22 M

   D. 0.11 M

9. A 20.0 mL solution of oxalic acid ($H_2C_2O_4$) of unknown concentration required 24.0 mL of 0.250 M potassium permanganate to reach the end point. What is the molarity of the oxalic acid solution?

$$2\,MnO_4^-\,(aq) + 5\,H_2C_2O_4\,(aq) + 6\,H^+(aq) \rightarrow 2\,Mn^{2+}(aq) + 10\,CO_2\,(g) + 8\,H_2O(l)$$

   A. 0.75 M

   B. 0.30 M

   C. 1.30 M

   D. 0.12 M

10. At a fixed temperature and number of moles of gas, the pressure of a gas increases if the volume is decreased. According to the kinetic molecular theory, which of the following is the explanation for this effect?

   A. Decreasing the volume increases the energy of the molecules so they hit the walls of the container more frequently.

   B. At a reduced volume the gas molecules collide with the walls of the container more frequently, increasing the pressure.

   C. Decreasing the volume crowds the molecules together, thus increasing the pressure.

   D. The molecules react to the reduced volume by expanding in size and the larger molecules create more pressure.

11. A 2.46 g sample of $KClO_3$ (molar mass = 123 $^g/_{mol}$) is completely decomposed and the oxygen generated is collected in a 0.82 L container at 27°C. What is the pressure of the oxygen?

$$2KClO_3(s) \rightarrow 2KCl(s) + 3O_2(g)\ (R = 0.82^{L\cdot atm}/_{mol\cdot K})$$

   A. 0.60 atm

   B. 0.75 atm

   C. 0.035 atm

   D. 0.90 atm

12. Calculate the standard enthalpy of formation of PbO from the following data:

   $PbO(s) + C(graphite) \rightarrow Pb(s) + CO(g)$ $\qquad \Delta H° = 107\,kJ$

   $2C(graphite) + O_2(g) \rightarrow 2CO(g)$ $\qquad \Delta H° = -221\,kJ$

   A. −328 kJ

   B. −114 kJ

   C. +217.5 kJ

   D. −217.5 kJ

13. The light emitted from an atom has a wavelength of 9.0×10^{-8} m. What is the energy of the photon associated with this light?
($c = 3.0 \times 10^8$ m/s and $h = 6.6 \times 10^{-34}$ J·s)

A. 1.8×10^{-32} J
B. $4.5 \times 10^{+17}$ J
C. 2.2×10^{-18} J
D. 5.0×10^{-18} J

The portion of the periodic table shown below is to be used for questions 14–18.

1	2	3	4	5	6	7	8	9	10	11	12	13	14	15	16	17	18
H																	He
Li	Be											B	C	N	O	F	Ne
Na	Mg											Al	Si	P	S	Cl	Ar
K	Ca	Sc	Ti	V	Cr	Mn	Fe	Co	Ni	Cu	Zn	Ga	Ge	As	Se	Br	Kr

14. Arrange the atoms or ions O, F, F^+, and S in order by ionization energy, from smallest to largest.

A. $S < O < F^+ < F$
B. $S < O < F < F^+$
C. $F^+ < F < O < S$
D. $O < F < F^+ < S$

15. Which of the following is a possible excited state for a Cl atom?

A. $1s^2 2s^2 2p^6 3s^2 3p^4 3d^1$
B. $1s^2 2s^2 2p^6 3s^2 3p^5$
C. $1s^2 2s^2 2p^6 3s^2 3p^6$
D. $1s^2 2s^2 2p^6 3s^2 3p^5 3d^1$

16. Which is the most polar bond?

A. O-O
B. C-N
C. Si-O
D. N-O

17. What is the formal charge on each atom in the OCN^- ion for the resonance structure with a single bond between O and C and a triple bond between C and N?

A. $O = +1, C = 0, N = -2$
B. $O = -1, C = 0, N = 0$
C. $O = 0, C = 0, N = -1$
D. $O = 0, C = -1, N = 0$

18. What is the geometry of the ion ClO_3^-?

A. trigonal pyramidal
B. tetragonal
C. trigonal planar
D. trigonal bipyramidal

19. The vapor pressure of an unknown liquid is measured at 25°C. The vapor pressure is twice the vapor pressure of water at this temperature. Which of the following statements is true about the unknown liquid?

A. The unknown liquid has a larger enthalpy of vaporization than water.
B. The intermolecular forces in the unknown liquid are weaker than the intermolecular forces in water.
C. The unknown liquid has a higher boiling point than water.
D. The average energies of the molecules in the vapor phase of the unknown liquid are greater than the energies of the water molecules in the vapor phase.

20. A 24.0 gram sample of urea (structure below, a nonelectrolyte) is dissolved in 250 g of benzene. What is the boiling point of the solution? The normal boiling point of benzene is 80.10°C and $K_b = 2.53 \,°C \cdot kg/mol$. (atomic masses C = 12 $^g/_{mol}$, O = 16 $^g/_{mol}$, H = 1 $^g/_{mol}$ and N = 14 $^g/_{mol}$)

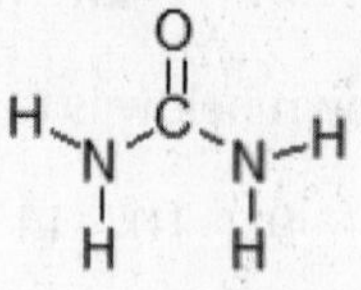

$$
\begin{array}{c}
\text{O} \\
\| \\
H_2N - C - NH_2
\end{array}
$$

A. 4.05°C
C. 84.15°C
B. 76.05°C
D. −4.05°C

21. A chemical reaction has a first order rate constant of 6.93×10^{-2} ($^1/_{min}$). How long will it take for the concentration of the reactant to decay to 10 % of its initial value?

A. 90 min
C. 1.4 min
B. 14 min
D. 33 min

22. A catalyst is added to a reaction. Which if the following is true about the catalyzed reaction?

A. The equilibrium constant increases, shifting the reaction to the products.
B. The activation energy is lowered, which speeds up the reaction.
C. The activation energy is raised, which speeds up the reaction.
D. The energy of the products is lowered, stabilizing the reaction and thus increasing the rate of the reaction.

23. The formation of HI at some temperature has an equilibrium constant, K = 64. At equilibrium, $[H_2] = 1.0$ M and $[I_2] = 0.25$ M. What is the concentration of [HI] at equilibrium at this temperature?

$$H_2(g) + I_2(g) \rightleftharpoons 2HI(g)$$

A. 16 M
C. 0.25 M
B. 4.0 M
D. 0.063 M

24. What is the pH of a solution that is 1.0 M in benzoic acid, C_6H_5COOH? ($K_a = 6.3 \times 10^{-5}$)

A. 2.10
C. 8.20
B. 4.20
D. 7.00

25. Which of the following will dissolve to produce a basic solution? (CH_3COOH, $K_a = 1.8 \times 10^{-5}$; NH_3, $K_b = 1.8 \times 10^{-5}$)

A. $NaCH_3COO$
C. NH_4Cl
B. CH_3COOH
D. $Mg(NO_3)_2$

26. A buffer is made by mixing solutions such that $[HF] = 3.0\,M$ and $[F^-] = 0.30\,M$. What is the pH of this buffer? (HF, $K_a = 7.2 \times 10^{-4}$, $pK_a = 3.14$)
    A. 1.14
    B. 3.14
    C. 4.14
    D. 2.14

27. The K_{sp} for copper(I) thiocyanate, CuSCN, is 1.6×10^{-11}. What is the molar solubility of CuSCN in a saturated solution?
    A. $8.0 \times 10^{-12}\,M$
    B. $4.0 \times 10^{-6}\,M$
    C. $2.5 \times 10^{-4}\,M$
    D. $4.0 \times 10^{-5}\,M$

28. For the following reaction at 25°C, $\Delta H° = -20.6\,^{kJ}/_{mol}$ and $\Delta S° = +43.3\,^{J}/_{mol \cdot K}$. At 25°C, which is true about the spontaneity of this reaction?

    $$S(s) + H_2(g) \rightleftharpoons H_2S(g)$$

    A. It is spontaneous (product favored).
    B. It is nonspontaneous (reactant favored).
    C. It is at equilibrium.
    D. It cannot be determined.

29. In the following overall reaction, what is the half reaction for the reactant that is reduced?

    $$Ca(s) + Sn^{2+}(aq) \rightarrow Ca^{2+}(aq) + Sn(s)$$

    A. $Ca^{2+}(aq) + 2\,e^- \rightarrow Ca(s)$
    B. $Ca(s) \rightarrow Ca^{2+}(aq) + 2\,e^-$
    C. $Sn^{2+}(aq) + 2\,e^- \rightarrow Sn(s)$
    D. $Sn(s) \rightarrow Sn^{2+}(aq) + 2\,e^-$

30. Which of the following is a valid propagation step for the chlorination of methane?
    A. $Cl \cdot + \cdot CH_3 \rightarrow Cl\text{-}CH_3$
    B. $H_3C\text{-}H \rightarrow H_3C \cdot + H \cdot$
    C. $Cl \cdot + H_3C\text{-}H \rightarrow H\text{-}Cl + H_3C \cdot$
    D. $H_3C \cdot + H\text{-}Cl \rightarrow H_3C\text{-}Cl + H \cdot$

31. The most likely major product from the radical bromination of 2,2,4-trimethylpentane is:

    A.

    C.

    B.

    D.

32. Consider the termination step shown below.

    $$H_3C \cdot + H_3C \cdot \rightarrow H_3C\text{-}CH_3$$

Which of the following is the most accurate description of this reaction's thermodynamic properties?

A. ΔH is positive; ΔS is positive.   C. ΔH is negative; ΔS is positive.

B. ΔH is positive; ΔS is negative.   D. ΔH is negative; ΔS is negative.

33. What is the most likely product of the Bayer-Villiger reaction shown below?

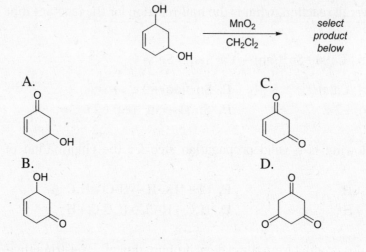

34. What is the most likely product of the oxidation shown below?

35. Which is the best leaving group?

A. chloride   C. iodide

B. fluoride   D. hydroxide

36. Which is the best nucleophile?

A. chloride   C. iodide

B. fluoride   D. hydroxide

37. Consider the chemical transformation shown below.

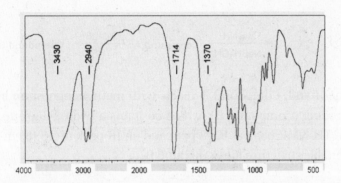

Which of the following are the most suitable conditions to provide the indicated product?

A. 1. MeLi, Et$_2$O; 2. EtBr

B. 1. Me$_2$CuLi, Et$_2$O; 2. EtBr

C. 1. EtLi, Et$_2$O; 2. MeBr

D. 1. Et$_2$CuLi, Et$_2$O; 2. MeBr

38. Consider the following infrared spectrum for an oxygen-containing compound.

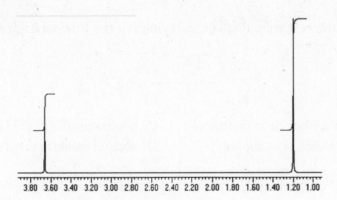

The compound most likely to have generated this spectrum is

A. 5-oxopentanal

B. 5-hydroxypentan-2-one

C. 4-penten-2-ol

D. 4-penten-2-one

39. The 1H NMR spectrum below was taken from a compound with molecular formula C$_6$H$_{12}$O$_2$.

The compound most consistent with these NMR data is

A. 2-methylpropanoic acid, ethyl ester

B. propanoic acid, 1-methylethyl ester

C. 2,2-dimethylpropanoic acid, methyl ester

D. ethanoic acid, 1,1-dimethylethyl ester

40. For the structure

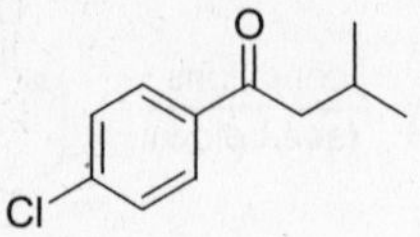

how many signals would be present in the 13C NMR spectrum?

A. 8   **C.** 10

B. 9   **D.** 11

41. Treatment of Compound A with dimethylamine in the presence of sodium cyanoborohydride results in the formation of N,N,2,2-tetramethylpropan-1-amine (shown below).

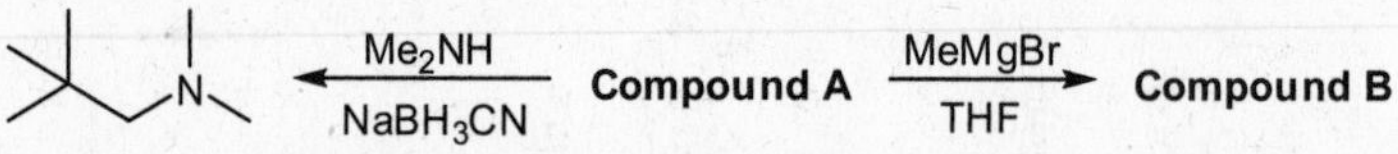

Compound A

Compound B

On the other hand, Compound A reacts with methylmagnesium bromide to give another product (Compound B), which contains a hydroxyl group. Compound A exhibits an 1H-NMR peak at 9.48 ppm and an IR peak at 2698 cm-1. What is the most reasonable structure for Compound B?

A.

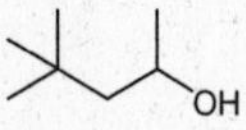

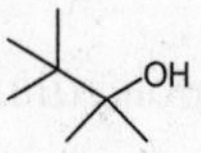

C.

B.

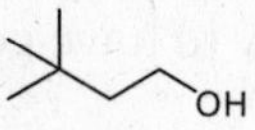

D.

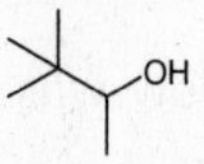

42. What are the best conditions for carrying out the transformation shown below?

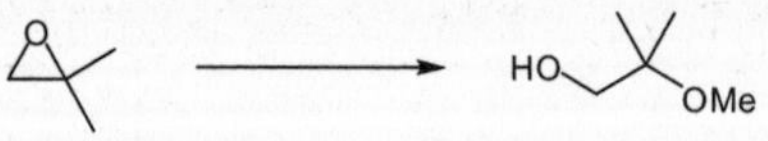

A. sodium methoxide in methanol   **C.** p-toluenesulfonic acid in methanol

B. methyl iodide in methanol   **D.** sodium iodide in methanol

43. The orbital containing the lone pair of the methyl anion is best described as a(n)

A. p orbital   **C.** sp_2 orbital

B. sp orbital   **D.** sp_3 orbital

44. What is the most reasonable starting material for the ozonolysis shown below?

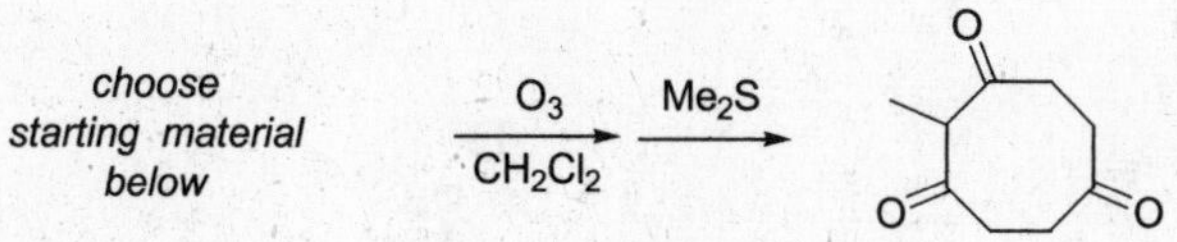

A.

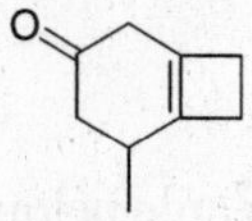

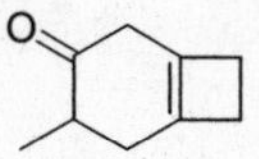

B.

C.

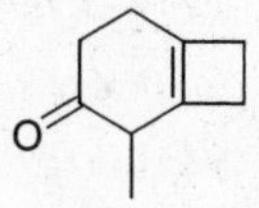

D.

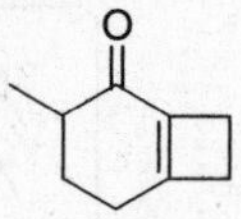

45. What is the best set of conditions for the following transformation?

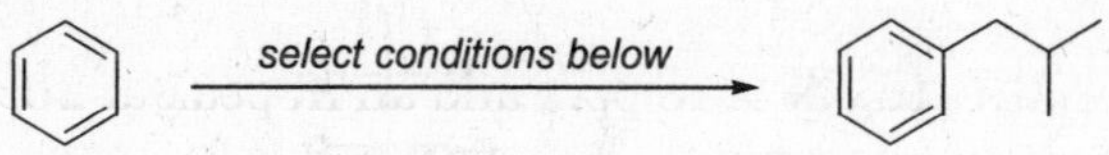

A. 1. $(CH_3)_2CHCOCl$, $AlCl_3$; 2. $Zn(Hg)/HCl$
B. $(CH_3)_2CHCH_2Cl$, $AlCl_3$
C. 1. $HCOCl$, $AlCl_3$; 2. $(CH_3)_2CHMgBr$
D. $(CH_3)_2CHCH_2OH$, BF_3OEt_2

46. What is the most reasonable major product of the reaction sequence below?

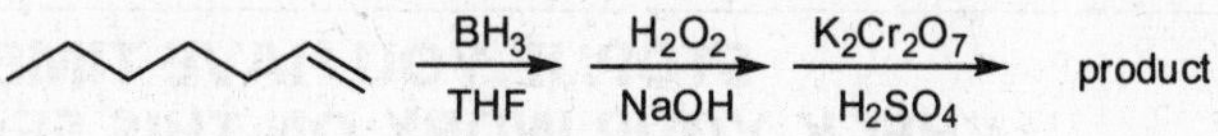

A.

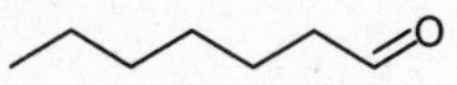

C.

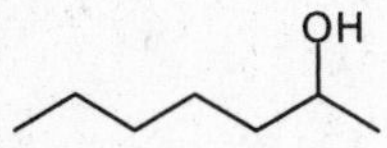

B.

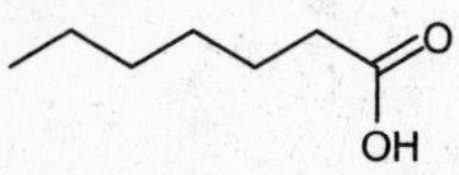

D.

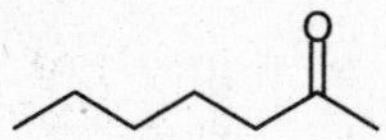

47. What is the best starting material to give the indicated stereochemistry?

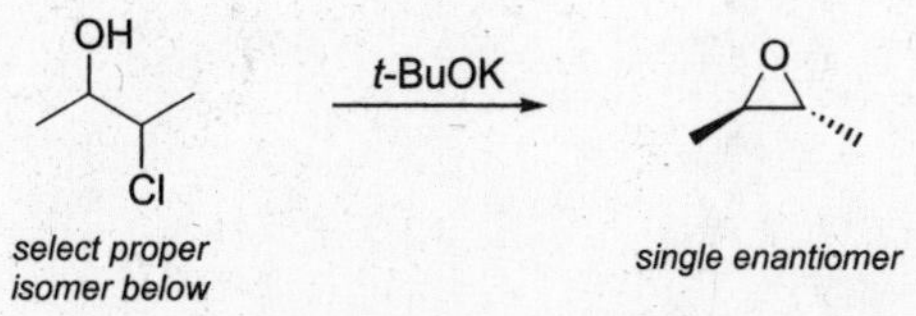

select proper
isomer below

single enantiomer

A.

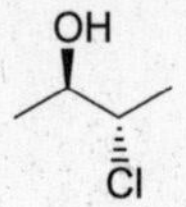

OH

Cl

C.

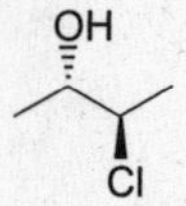

OH

Cl

B.

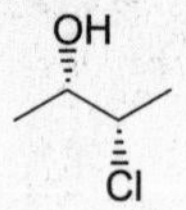

OH

Cl

D.

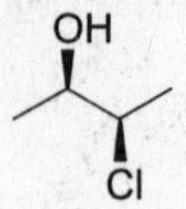

OH

Cl

48. Which Fischer projection most accurately describes the boxed molecule below?

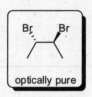

Br   Br

optically pure

A.

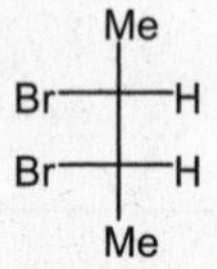

```
      Me
Br ——|—— H
Br ——|—— H
      Me
```

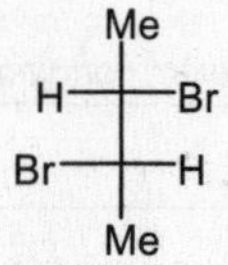

B.

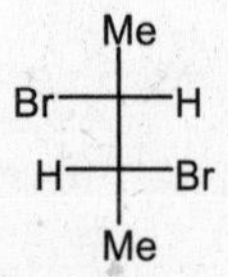

```
      Me
Br ——|—— H
 H ——|—— Br
      Me
```

C.

```
      Me
 H ——|—— Br
Br ——|—— H
      Me
```

D.

```
      Me
 H ——|—— Br
 H ——|—— Br
      Me
```

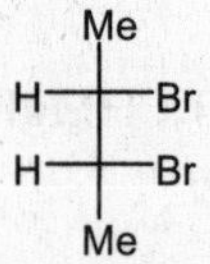

STOP. IF YOU HAVE TIME LEFT OVER,
CHECK YOUR WORK ON THIS SECTION ONLY.

SECTION 5. WRITING

1 Question   **Time: 30 minutes**

Discuss a solution to the problem of protecting endangered species in populated areas.

_____
_____
_____
_____
_____
_____
_____
_____
_____
_____
_____
_____
_____
_____
_____
_____
_____
_____
_____
_____
_____
_____
_____
_____
_____
_____
_____
_____
_____

SECTION 6. READING COMPREHENSION

Questions: 48   **Time: 50 minutes**

Directions: Read each passage. Answer the questions that follow by choosing the best answer from the choices given.

PASSAGE 1

1   According to Professor John MacKinnon, certain places are more likely than others to house new or rediscovered species. First, scientists should look in areas that are geologically <u>stable.</u> Areas with regular earthquakes or volcanic eruptions are less likely to contain species that go back thousands of years, because frequent upheavals are not conducive to steady growth or a comfortable way of life. Second, scientists are most likely to find undiscovered or rediscovered species in remote, isolated areas. Often, cultivation eliminates the trees or shrubs that house and protect animal life. A stable climate is a third thing to look for. Stability of climate ensures that the animals that live in the region have had no reason to leave for warmer or wetter environments.

2   A fourth key thing scientists should look for, according to MacKinnon, is an area with a variety of unusual species that are specific to that area. Of course, this requirement refers back to requirement number two, isolation. An area that is very isolated or difficult to access will naturally have species that cannot be found anywhere else.

3   In 1994 American biologist Peter Zahler took his second trip to the isolated valleys of the Diamer region in northern Pakistan. He was searching for the woolly flying squirrel, a dog-sized squirrel last seen in 1924. Working with a guide, Zahler moved from valley to valley. He quizzed the local residents about the squirrel. Many recalled hearing tales about the strange animal, but all insisted that it was extinct.

4   One day, two men entered Zahler's camp. After some small talk, one asked whether he would be willing to pay for a live squirrel. Zahler agreed to pay top dollar, never envisioning that two hours later, he would be presented with a woolly flying squirrel in a bag. Following that surprise, Zahler located evidence of live squirrels throughout the region. The squirrel certainly obeyed all of MacKinnon's regulations. Despite frequent avalanches, the Himalayas are a geologically stable area with a harsh but stable climate and a number of rare species. Not only were the squirrels' caves remote and isolated, it was often necessary to rappel down or climb up sheer cliffs to reach them.

1. According to the passage, all of these statements are true **except**
    A. "Woolly flying squirrels are larger than most squirrels."
    B. "The Himalayas contain a variety of unique species."
    C. "Animals in a drought may leave for a wetter habitat."
    D. "The woolly flying squirrel was extinct for many years."

2. In the context of the first paragraph, the word *stable* is used to mean
   A. a place to house animals
   B. fixed and secure
   C. group or gang
   D. unwavering or committed

3. Which of these would be the **best** title for the passage?
   A. "A Subtropical Find"
   B. "Rediscovering Our Planet"
   C. "A Squirrel Supports a Theory"
   D. "The Animals of Pakistan"

4. The author includes the story of the woolly flying squirrel to
   A. provide an example that supports McKinnon's premise
   B. demonstrate that new species are not always new
   C. refute McKinnon's notion that climate matters to rediscovery
   D. contrast one recent rediscovery with another

5. According to the article, one reason new or long-lost species may be found in areas with stable climates is that
   A. stable climates are often found in areas that are difficult to access
   B. an unstable climate can decimate an animal population
   C. without a stable climate, animals may need to migrate or leave
   D. stable climates appear in regions with geological stability

6. How is the information in the third paragraph organized?
   A. by reasons and examples
   B. using comparisons and contrasts
   C. in time order
   D. using cause-and-effect relationships

7. Information in the passage suggests that the jungles of Borneo would be more likely than the edge of the Sahara Desert to house a new species of animal because
   A. Borneo is not as isolated as the Sahara.
   B. The Sahara does not have a stable climate.
   C. Volcanic eruptions in Borneo lend it stability.
   D. The Sahara Desert is largely cultivated.

8. Which of the following statements from the passage provides the **least** support for the author's claim that Zahler's rediscovery obeyed McKinnon's regulations?
   A. "Despite frequent avalanches, the Himalayas are a geologically stable area with a harsh but stable climate and a number of rare species."
   B. "In 1994 American biologist Peter Zahler took his second trip to the isolated valleys of the Diamer region in northern Pakistan."
   C. "Not only were the squirrels' caves remote and isolated, it was often necessary to rappel down or climb up sheer cliffs to reach them."
   D. "Zahler agreed to pay top dollar, never envisioning that two hours later, he would be presented with a woolly flying squirrel in a bag."

PASSAGE 2

1   Aluminum is the most abundant metallic element in the earth's crust, but it is never found naturally as an element. Instead, it always appears naturally in its oxidized form as a hydroxide we call bauxite.

2   The extraction of aluminum from bauxite requires three stages. First, the ore is mined. Then it is <u>refined</u> to recover alumina. Finally, the alumina is smelted to produce aluminum.

3   The mining is done via the open-cut method. Bulldozers remove the topsoil, and excavators or other types of power machinery are used to remove the underlying layer of bauxite. The bauxite may be washed to remove clay and other detritus.

4   Refining is done via the Bayer refining process, named after its inventor, Karl Bayer. Ground bauxite is fed into a digester, where it is mixed with a caustic soda. The aluminum oxide reacts with the soda to form a solution of sodium aluminate and a precipitate of sodium aluminium silicate. The solution is separated from the silicate through washing and pumping, and the alumina is precipitated from the solution, where it appears as crystals of alumina hydrate. The crystals are washed again to remove any remaining solution. Then they are heated to remove water, leaving the gritty alumina.

5   Smelting is done via the Hall-Heroult smelting process. An electric current is passed through a molten solution of alumina and cryolite, which is in a cell lined at the bottom and top with carbon. This forces the oxygen to combine with the carbon at the top of the cell, making carbon dioxide, while the molten metallic aluminum collects at the bottom of the cell, where it is siphoned off, cleaned up, and cast into bars, sheets, or whatever form is needed.

6   As with all mining of metals, bauxite mining presents certain hazards. Along with the usual mining issues of degraded soil and polluted runoff, chief among them is the omnipresent bauxite dust, which clogs machinery and lungs, sometimes for miles around the mining site. Jamaica and Brazil have seen widespread protests recently against the major bauxite mining companies, which continue to insist that no link between bauxite dust and pervasive lung problems has been proved.

9. In the context of the second paragraph, the word *refined* means
    A. superio   C. processed
    B. polished   D. restricted

10. Based on the information in the third paragraph, you can conclude that bauxite is located
    A. within the topsoil   C. below the topsoil
    B. wherever clay is found   D. below the earth's crust

11. All of these are produced by the Bayer process **except**
    A. sodium aluminum silicate   C. aluminum manganese
    B. sodium aluminate   D. alumina hydrate

12. The ideas in the third, fourth, and fifth paragraphs are related because they are
  A. steps in a process
  B. examples of a mineral
  C. reasons for mining
  D. comparisons among theories

13. When the author says in the last paragraph that bauxite dust is *omnipresent*, she means that it is
  A. hazardous
  B. pervasive
  C. despoiled
  D. impenetrable

14. The process by which aluminum is extracted from bauxite is most similar to
  A. the building of steel bridges
  B. the making of copper tubing
  C. the manufacturing of glass
  D. the mixing of cement

15. The author includes the discussion of protests primarily to show that
  A. Bauxite mining takes place in the Third World.
  B. Workers are starting to fight back against the dangers of mining.
  C. Mining companies have misled people for decades.
  D. The government of Brazil works with the mining companies.

16. The **tone** of the passage suggests that the author would most likely believe that
  A. Bauxite mining poses health problems.
  B. The U.S. should use less aluminum.
  C. Australian bauxite is the best quality.
  D. Karl Bayer was something of a genius.

PASSAGE 3

1   A land bridge is land exposed when the sea recedes, connecting one expanse of land to another. One of the most famous land bridges was the Bering Land Bridge, often known as Beringia, which connected Alaska to Siberia across what is now the Bering Strait.

2   The Bering Land Bridge was not terribly long. If it still existed today, you could drive it in your car in about an hour. It appeared during the Ice Age, when enormous sheets of ice covered much of Europe and America. The ice sheets contained huge amounts of water north of the Equator, and because of this, the sea level dropped precipitously, perhaps as much as 400 feet, revealing landmasses such as the Bering Land Bridge.

3   At this time, the ecology of the northern hemisphere was that of the Mammoth Steppe. It was a dry, frigid land filled with grasses, sedges, and tundra vegetation. It supported many large grazing animals including reindeer, bison, and musk oxen, as well as the lions that fed upon them. It also contained large camels, giant short-faced bears, and woolly mammoths. Many of the animals of the Mammoth Steppe used the bridge

to cross from east to west and back again. Eventually, their human hunters tracked them from Asia to North America.

4 Ethnologists and geologists generally believe that humans used the Bering Land Bridge to populate the Americas, which up until about 24,000 years ago had no sign of human life. Ethnologists use evidence such as shared religions, similar houses and tools, and unique methods of cleaning and preserving food to show the link between the people of coastal Siberia and the people of coastal Alaska.

5 There are those among the Native American population who dispute the land bridge theory. For one thing, it contradicts most native teachings on the origins of the people. For another, it seems to undermine the notion that they are truly "native" to the North American continent.

17. According to this passage, the first people in North America lived
    A. in what is now Central America
    B. west of the Bering Strait
    C. below sea level
    D. in what is now Alaska

18. Based on information in the passage, about how long was the Bering Land Bridge?
    A. between 50 and 75 miles long
    B. between 90 and 120 miles long
    C. around 150 miles long
    D. around 200 miles long

19. According to the passage, which of these would be considered a land bridge?
    A. the isthmus of Panama
    B. the Chesapeake Bay
    C. the Strait of Hormuz
    D. the Khyber Pass

20. In the third paragraph, the author includes information about large mammals in order to
    A. explain patterns of growth among animals of the Mammoth Steppe
    B. indicate how tough animals needed to be to survive the Ice Age
    C. contrast the climate of North America with the climate of Asia
    D. suggest a reason for human migration from Asia to North America

21. The author's purpose in the fourth paragraph is to
    A. introduce a theory and show some support for it
    B. compare some processes used by geologists and ethnologists
    C. list some possible reasons for the migrations of early humans
    D. contradict a theory about an early use of the land bridge

22. The author suggests that some contemporary Native Americans object to the land bridge theory because
    A. It equates them with Pleistocene man.
    B. It challenges their history and status.
    C. It relies on disputed science.
    D. It belies the importance of southern tribes.

23. Which of the following findings **best** supports the author's contention that Siberia was once connected to North America?

    A. Native American legends from the American Northwest feature enormous whales and large fish.

    B. People of coastal Siberia have features that distinguish them from people in the rest of Russia.

    C. Hunters in both Siberia and coastal Alaska continue to hunt seals, walrus, and sea lions.

    D. Large animal fossils found in both places prove that identical species once populated both regions.

24. Which new information, if true, would most **challenge** the claim that humans first moved to North America across the Bering Land Bridge?

    A. a new translation of an Inuit legend about Raven and a giant flood

    B. new fossil records that place the Ice Age 1,000 years earlier than believed

    C. the discovery of human fossils in Kansas that predate the Ice Age

    D. DNA proof that the musk ox of Siberia differed from the musk ox of Alaska

PASSAGE 4

1   Ballast waifs are seeds that arrive on one shore from another in the soil placed in a ship's hold as ballast. One remarkably lovely and dreadfully damaging ballast waif is *Lythrum salicaria*, the bright purple, spiky flower known commonly as purple loosestrife. Purple loosestrife is not a newcomer to U.S. shores; it arrived from Eurasia, almost certainly via ship, some 200 years ago.

2   For all its beauty, purple loosestrife is a menace. The same long growing season that makes it so beloved by gardeners makes it a seed-making machine. A mature plant may produce two or three million seeds a year. It also propagates underground, sending out shoots and stems in all directions.

3   Scientists took little notice of purple loosestrife until sometime in the 1930s, when a particular strain began colonizing along the St. Lawrence River, an area rife with the sort of wetlands purple loosestrife likes best. Purple loosestrife does not just propagate wildly; it also adapts easily to changes in environment. As it starts up in a new area, it quickly outcompetes native grasses, sedges, and other flowering plants, forming <u>dense</u> stands of purple loosestrife where once heterogeneous wetland meadows existed. This not only eradicates the native plants, but also it removes food sources for migratory birds and other animals.

4   In recent years, purple loosestrife has had a devastating impact on native cattails and wild rice. It has invaded and destroyed spawning areas for fish. In rural areas, it is beginning to move away from wetlands and adapt to drier areas, encroaching on agricultural lands. In urban areas, it is blocking pipes and drainage canals. It has moved steadily westward and is now found in all states but Florida.

5   Attempts to control purple loosestrife have been only partially successful. It has proved resistant to many herbicides, and it is impervious to burning, as its rootstock lies beneath the surface and can reproduce from there. It can be mowed down and plowed under, and then replaced with a less invasive plant. This is very labor-intensive in marshy areas that are substantially overgrown, but it may be the only way of eliminating the pest.

25. According to the passage, all of these are true **except**
    A. Purple loosestrife propagates through an underground system.
    B. Purple loosestrife is found in urban and rural settings.
    C. Purple loosestrife is best eradicated through controlled burning.
    D. Purple loosestrife is not native to North and South America.

26. Which of these would be the **best** title for the passage?
    A. "A Floral Invasion"   **C.** "Migrating Plants"
    B. "A Gardener's Worst Nightmare"   **D.** "Controlling Pesky Plants"

27. The author's mention of the St. Lawrence River shows primarily that
    A. Ballast waifs prefer to travel on freshwater conveyances.
    B. Purple loosestrife does well in marshy areas along rivers.
    C. Most ballast waifs survive best in northern regions.
    D. Purple loosestrife can be replaced by less damaging plants.

28. Which fact about purple loosestrife adds to its power of endurance?
    A. easy adaptability   **C.** introduction as a ballast waif
    B. spiky stems and flowers   **D.** preference for wetlands

29. The author suggests that people enjoy growing purple loosestrife because it
    A. keeps out other weeds   **C.** has a long growing season
    B. makes millions of seeds   **D.** reduces weevils and insects

30. In the context of the third paragraph, the word *dense* is used to mean
    A. intense   **C.** complicated
    B. opaque   **D.** concentrated

31. According to the passage, where would purple loosestrife **least** easily thrive?
    A. among swampy areas of northern New Jersey
    B. in the wetland meadows of eastern Michigan
    C. along the inland waterways of North Carolina
    D. above the treeline in the mountains of Utah

32. According to the author, purple loosestrife can be eradicated by being mowed down, plowed under, and planted with other species. Which of the following information, if true, would provide the **least** support for this argument?

A. *Lythrum salicaria* has been removed from some gardens through the careful use of an Australian slug.

B. Replanted meadows where purple loosestrife once grew are slowly being taken over by a new, hardier strain of *Lythrum salicaria.*

C. Cattails are coming back to some New York swampland once devastated by the incursion of *Lythrum salicaria.*

D. Chopping up the rootstock of *Lythrum salicaria* with a plow adds an unexpected bonus in the form of nitrogen-rich fertilizer.

PASSAGE 5

1   Elk were once found in the East, from Georgia north to New York and Connecticut. By the time of the Civil War, hunting and habitat destruction had caused their extinction in most eastern states. All of the eastern subspecies are now extinct. Elk County, Pennsylvania, was without elk for over a century.

2   At the beginning of the twentieth century, herds of elk in the Rocky Mountains faced death by starvation as encroaching farms depleted their winter feeding grounds, and finally the government decided to intercede. They gathered up elk from Yellowstone National Park and shipped 50 of them to Pennsylvania.

3   At that early date, 1913, there was little understanding of the kind of acclimatization required when moving large animals from one habitat to another. The elk were released from cattle cars and chased into the wild to fend for themselves. Two years later, 95 more elk were moved from Yellowstone to Pennsylvania.

4   The elk tended to move toward farming areas because that was where the food was. Although they were protected, their destruction of farmland caused farmers to poach them illegally. In a 1971 survey, researchers found about 65 animals. Intensive work by the Bureau of Forestry to improve elk habitat, especially through reclamation of old strip mines, brought those numbers up to 135 by the early 1980s. By the year 2000, there were over 500 elk in Pennsylvania, including many in Elk County.

5   In 1984, hunters established the Rocky Mountain Elk Foundation, whose mission is to reintroduce elk in the states where they once roamed. At present, new herds are established in Arkansas, Kentucky, Michigan, and Wisconsin, in addition to Pennsylvania. There is talk of moving herds to Tennessee and to the Adirondack range in New York. It seems fairly clear that improving habitat for elk reintroduction improves conditions for other wildlife—wild turkey, whitetail deer, and black bear, among others.

5   Unlike in the 1910s, today reintroduction is vastly improved—far more closely monitored and controlled. Animals are checked for disease. Land trusts are used to preserve habitat and to keep the elk from moving too close to cropland.

33. According to this passage, a major early threat to elk populations was

A. wolves and cougars

B. vehicular traffic

C. disease

D. hunting

34. Based on information in the passage, about how many elk were moved from Yellowstone to Pennsylvania in the mid-1910s?

A. 65

B. 95

C. 135

D. 145

35. According to the passage, where might you see elk today?

A. The Tennessee Valley

B. Georgia

C. The Adirondacks

D. Arkansas

36. According to the passage, what is true of the elk in Pennsylvania today?

A. They are the same as the elk who lived there 200 years ago.

B. They are a different subspecies from the old Pennsylvania elk.

C. They are a different subspecies from the elk found in the Rockies.

D. They are only distantly related to the elk found in Yellowstone.

37. The passage implies that

A. Reclamation of land is a bad idea.

B. Hunters have ulterior motives for reintroducing elk.

C. Species reintroduction has improved over time.

D. Elk reintroduction may be doomed to failure.

38. Which of the following findings **best** supports the author's contention that elk repopulation is carefully monitored?

A. Farming to raise deer, elk, and reindeer is increasingly popular.

B. Before 1997, there had not been a wild elk in Kentucky in 150 years.

C. Rocky Mountain elk were among the original animals at the Hearst Zoo.

D. Jackson County is testing potential elk herds for chronic wasting disease.

39. Which new information, if true, would provide the **least** support for the claim that elk reintroduction benefits other species as well?

A. Record sightings of wild turkey, pheasant, and grouse on reclaimed land in Pennsylvania

B. Surprising numbers of multiple births in moose from central and western Maine and New Hampshire

C. A census showing that whitetail deer were migrating northward from Pennsylvania into New York

D. An increase in temperature of one or two degrees in the headwaters of the Yellowstone River

40. Which of these statements from the passage expresses a personal **opinion**?

A. "Elk County, Pennsylvania, was without elk for over a century." (Paragraph one)

B. "Although they were protected, their destruction of farmland caused farmers to poach them illegally." (Paragraph four)

C. "By the year 2000, there were over 500 elk in Pennsylvania, including many in Elk County." (Paragraph four)

D. "Unlike in the 1910s, today reintroduction is vastly improved—far more closely monitored and controlled." (Paragraph five)

PASSAGE 6

1   The discovery of electrons came about in a roundabout way. In the latter part of the nineteenth century, a popular demonstration by lecturers involved the cathode ray. They would <u>evacuate</u> air from the tube, pass high voltage through it, and show audiences the patterns of light that appeared. Were these really waves traveling through "ether"? Heinrich Hertz and Phillip Lenard conducted experiments that made this seem possible. On the other hand, English physicists had long posited that there must be a fundamental unit of electricity, a particle that connected matter and electricity. The Irish physicist George Johnstone Stoney had even gone so far as to calculate its size and to name it *electron*.

2   French physicist Jean Perrin determined that the cathode rays had negative charges. But it was not until English physicist J.J. Thomson designed an elegant set of experiments that the electron's existence was proved.

3   The first experiment determined that the negative charge of cathode rays could not be separated from the rays themselves using magnetism. The second found that the rays could bend when influenced by an electric field. The third measured the ratio of charge to mass of the rays by comparing the energy they carried and the amount of deflection possible when an electric field was introduced. Thomson discovered that the ratio was enormous, meaning that the rays were tiny or very highly charged or both.

4   His conclusions, published in 1897, were of the existence of a subatomic particle with a negative charge. It was not until Thomson's son George proved that electrons, although particles, had many of the properties of a wave, that the mysteries of the cathode ray were truly solved.

5   George Thomson's concept of wave-particle duality, the notion that matter and light have properties of both waves and particles, was critical to the development of quantum mechanics. It was not a particularly new concept, having roots as far back as Isaac Newton's insistence that light was composed of particles, which he called *corpuscles*, the very word J.J. Thomson used to describe the particles of atoms he found in cathode rays.

41. In the context of the passage, the word *evacuate* refers to

A. abandoning a location

B. removing a substance

C. sending someone away

D. relinquishing control

42. Which of the following examples is presented as evidence that J.J. Thomson's theory about subatomic particles was not new?

    A. the work of George Johnstone Stoney   **C.** the work of Heinrich Hertz

    B. the work of George Thomson   **D.** the work of Phillip Lenard

43. Thomson's first experiment indicated that

    A. Unlike most rays, cathode rays were negatively charged.

    B. Cathode rays could be diverted using electromagnetism.

    C. The ray's negative charge was embedded within particles.

    D. Most subatomic particles are tiny and highly charged.

44. The discussion of corpuscles in the fifth paragraph shows primarily that

    A. People in the 1600s understood the parts of an atom.

    B. Thomson borrowed a term from a much older theory.

    C. Atoms and blood cells are linked by similar structures.

    D. Isaac Newton was trained as a medical doctor.

45. The statement in the first paragraph that "the discovery of electrons came about in a roundabout way" indicates that the author believes that

    A. There is more to discover about electrons.

    B. The discovery of electrons did not proceed step-by-step.

    C. Electrons could never have been discovered by a single scientist.

    D. Scientists ended up at the beginning when they searched for an answer.

46. The **tone** of this passage suggests that the author

    A. considers J.J. Thomson a splendid scientist

    B. prefers Isaac Newton to more recent scientists

    C. would like to know more about George Thomson

    D. believes that English scientists surpass the French

47. The author's claim that George Thomson's work was critical to quantum mechanics could **best** be supported by the inclusion of

    A. the theories of light proposed by Isaac Newton and Christiaan Huygens

    B. experiments showing the results of gravity on light and sound waves

    C. de Broglie's equation relating wavelength to momentum

    D. a definition of quantum mechanics that mentions wave-particle duality

48. Which of these inventions **most** relies on wave-particle duality in its everyday workings?

    A. a vacuum cleaner   **C.** an electron microscope

    B. a high-voltage electric line   **D.** a short-wave radio

---

STOP. IF YOU HAVE TIME LEFT OVER,
CHECK YOUR WORK ON THIS SECTION ONLY.

SECTION 7. QUANTITATIVE ABILITY

48 Questions   40 Minutes

1. The mixed number $4\frac{5}{7}$ expressed as a fraction is

   A. $\frac{5}{7}$ B. $\frac{20}{7}$ C. $\frac{33}{7}$ D. $\frac{45}{7}$

2. $4\frac{5}{6} - 2\frac{3}{4} =$

   A. $\frac{12}{25}$ B. $\frac{25}{12}$ C. $\frac{29}{6}$ D. $\frac{11}{12}$

3. A student obtained an average of 86 for a series of seven assignments. Six of the grades were 85, 78, 83, 91, 89, and 86. The grade of the seventh assignment is

   A. 74   B. 86   C. 90   D. 98

4. A full-time employee works 40 hours during a five-day week. The percentage of a five-day week that the employee is at work is

   A. 20%   B. 33%   C. 40%   D. 50%

5. $(2.4 \times 10^6) \div (1.2 \times 10^3) =$

   A. -2.0×10^3 B. -2.0×10^4 C. 2.0×10^3 D. 2.0×10^6

6. $35.2 \times 4.16 =$

   A. 13.213   B. 13.312   C. 13.320   D. 13.023

7. Express in scientific notation: 13.9

   A. 1.39×10^{-1} B. 1.39×10^1 C. 13.9×10^{-1} D. 13.9×10^1

8. The ratio of boys to girls in the graduating class of a school is 3:2. If there are a total of 430 students in the class, how many girls are in the graduating class?

   A. 74   B. 86   C. 172   D. 215

9. $(6x^2y^5z^3) \div (3x^2y^3z^6) =$

   A. $\frac{z^2}{2y^3}$ B. $\frac{y^2}{2z^3}$ C. $\frac{2y^2}{z^3}$ D. $\frac{2z^2}{y^3}$

10. Solve for x: $\dfrac{x^2 + x - 42}{x + 7} = 1$

    A. -7 B. 2   C. 6   D. 7

11. What are the roots of the equation $x^2 - 7x - 18 = 0$?

    A. $4.5, -1$ B. $-2, 4.5$ C. $3.5, 8$ D. $-1, -4.5$

12. $(4a^2b^4c) \times (-7a^5b^3) =$
    A. $-11a^7b^7c$ B. $-28a^7b^7c$ C. $28a^7b^7c$ D. a^7b^7c

13. What is the sum of the following polynomials? $5x + 3xy - 6y^2$, $9xy + 7y^2 - 4x$ and $-8y^2 + 7x + 12xy$
    A. $12x + 15xy - 14y^2$ C. $8x + 24xy - 7y^2$
    B. $x + 9xy - 6y^2$ D. $5x + 12xy + 7y^2$

14. $3^3 \cdot 3^2 \cdot 3^1 =$
    A. 81   B. 243   C. 729   D. 2187

15. What are the roots of the quadratic equation $3x^2 - x - 10 = 0$?
    A. $x = \sqrt{2}, \ -\dfrac{5}{3}$ B. $x = 2, \ -\sqrt{\dfrac{5}{3}}$ C. $x = -2, \ \sqrt{\dfrac{5}{3}}$ D. $x = 2, \ -\dfrac{5}{3}$

16. What is the solution of the following system of equations? $x + y = 4$ and $2x - 6y = 3$
    A. $x = -\dfrac{27}{8}, y = \dfrac{5}{8}$ B. $x = \dfrac{27}{8}, y = -\dfrac{5}{8}$ C. $x = \dfrac{27}{8}, y = \dfrac{5}{8}$ D. $x = \dfrac{8}{27}, y = \dfrac{8}{5}$

17. If $\sqrt[3]{x} = y^4$, then what is x in terms of y?
    A. $x = y^{12}$ B. $x = y^7$ C. $x = y^4$ D. $x = y$

18. A bag of Skittles® contains 10 red, 9 yellow, 8 orange, 6 green, and 4 blue colored candies. What is the probability of randomly choosing an orange-colored candy from the bag?
    A. $\dfrac{8}{37}$ B. $\dfrac{37}{8}$ C. $\dfrac{8}{27}$ D. $\dfrac{3}{4}$

19. What is the probability of selecting an ace of a red suit from a standard deck of cards?
    A. $\dfrac{1}{52}$ B. $\dfrac{2}{52}$ C. $\dfrac{48}{52}$ D. $\dfrac{50}{52}$

20. What is the probability of selecting a face card of a spade suit from two standard decks of cards?
    A. $\dfrac{3}{52}$ B. $\dfrac{6}{52}$ C. $\dfrac{6}{104}$ D. $\dfrac{46}{104}$

21. Upon rolling a pair of dice, what is the probability that the sum of the two numbers on the dice is either 7 or 12?
    A. $\dfrac{1}{6}$ B. $\dfrac{1}{36}$ C. $\dfrac{5}{36}$ D. $\dfrac{7}{36}$

22. What is the probability that two cards drawn from a deck of cards are of a black suit (e.g., either clubs or spades) if the first card drawn is replaced before the second card is drawn?
    A. $\dfrac{1352}{2704}$ B. $\dfrac{676}{2704}$ C. $\dfrac{6}{2704}$ D. $\dfrac{2}{2704}$

Questions 23–26

Chemistry students performed nine volume measurements of a solution during a lab and obtained the following results:

$$\{2.4\,\text{mL}, 3.2\,\text{mL}, 3.7\,\text{mL}, 3.7\,\text{mL}, 4.5\,\text{mL}, 6.8\,\text{mL}, 7.3\,\text{mL}, 8.1\,\text{mL}, 12.2\,\text{mL}\}$$

23. What is the mean of the data set?
   A. 3.7 mL   **B.** 4.5 mL   **C.** 5.8 mL   **D.** 9.8 mL

24. What is the median of the data set?
   A. 3.7 mL   **B.** 4.5 mL   **C.** 5.8 mL   **D.** 9.8 mL

25. What is the mode of the data set?
   A. 3.7 mL   **B.** 4.5 mL   **C.** 5.8 mL   **D.** 9.8 mL

26. What is the range of the data set?
   A. 3.7 mL   **B.** 4.5 mL   **C.** 5.8 mL   **D.** 9.8 mL

27. Solve for x: $x^2 - 12x = -36$
   A. 2   **B.** 3   **C.** 4   **D.** 6

28. Solve for x: $x^3 - 64x = 0$
   A. $x = \pm 8$ **B.** $x = \pm 6$ **C.** $x = \pm 4$ **D.** $x = \pm 2$

29. Solve for x: $(4x - 1)^2 = 121$
   A. −3   **B.** 2   **C.** 3   **D.** 6

30. What is the slope of a line that passes through the points (5, 2) and (1, 3)?
   A. $\dfrac{1}{3}$ **B.** $-\dfrac{1}{3}$ **C.** 3   **D.** 5

31. What is the slope of a line described by $3x + 2y - 12 = 0$?
   A. $\dfrac{3}{2}$ **B.** $-\dfrac{3}{2}$ **C.** $\dfrac{2}{3}$ **D.** $-\dfrac{2}{3}$

32. What is the equation of a line that passes through the point (−3, −1) and has a slope of $-\dfrac{2}{3}$?

   A. $y = -\dfrac{2}{3}x$ **B.** $y = -\dfrac{2}{3}x + 3$ **C.** $y = -\dfrac{2}{3}x - 3$ **D.** $y = \dfrac{2}{3}x - 3$

Questions 33–35

The three most commonly used temperature scales are Fahrenheit (°F), Celsius (°C), and Kelvin (K). They are based on the freezing point and boiling point of water as shown below.

Temperature Scale	Freezing Point of Water	Boiling Point of Water
Fahrenheit (°F)	32	212
Celsius (°C)	0	100
Kelvin (K)	273	373

The formula for temperature conversion between the Fahrenheit and Celsius scales is

$$T_F = \frac{9}{5}T_C + 32$$

33. What is the slope of the conversion formula relating temperature in Fahrenheit to temperature in Celsius?

A. $\dfrac{9}{5}\dfrac{°F}{°C}$ **B.** $\dfrac{5}{9}\dfrac{°F}{°C}$ **C.** $\dfrac{9}{5}\dfrac{°C}{°F}$ **D.** $\dfrac{5}{9}\dfrac{°C}{°F}$

34. What is the linear equation relating temperature in Celsius to temperature in Fahrenheit?

A. $T_c = -\dfrac{5}{9}T_F + 17.8$ **C.** $T_c = \dfrac{5}{9}T_F - 17.8$

B. $T_c = -\dfrac{5}{9}T_F - 17.8$ **D.** $T_c = \dfrac{5}{9}T_F + 17.8$

35. What is the linear equation relating temperature in Fahrenheit to temperature in Kelvin?

A. $T_F = -\dfrac{9}{5}T_K + 459.4$ **C.** $T_F = \dfrac{9}{5}T_K + 459.4$

B. $T_F = \dfrac{9}{5}T_K + 459.4$ **D.** $T_F = \dfrac{9}{5}T_K - 459.4$

36. Which line is perpendicular to the line $y + 3x = 8$?

A. $y + \dfrac{1}{3}x = -5$ **B.** $y - \dfrac{1}{3}x = -5$ **C.** $y + 3x = -5$ **D.** $y - 3x = -5$

37. Which line is parallel to the line $y + 3x = 8$?

A. $y + \dfrac{1}{3}x = -5$ **B.** $y - \dfrac{1}{3}x = -5$ **C.** $y + 3x = -5$ **D.** $y - 3x = -5$

38. Evaluate the following derivative: $\dfrac{d}{dx}(100)$

A. 0   **B.** 10   **C.** $10x$ **D.** 100

39. Evaluate the following derivative: $\dfrac{d}{dx}(5a^4)$

A. 0   **B.** $5a^4$ **C.** $20a^3$ **D.** $5a^3$

40. Evaluate the following derivative: $\dfrac{d}{dx}(5x^4)$

A. 0   **B.** $5x^4$ **C.** $20x^3$ **D.** $5x^3$

41. Evaluate the following derivative: $\dfrac{d}{dx}\left(\dfrac{15}{3x^8}\right)$

   A. $-\dfrac{40}{x^9}$ **B.** $\dfrac{40}{x^9}$ **C.** $-\dfrac{40}{x^{-9}}$ **D.** $\dfrac{40}{x^{-9}}$

42. Evaluate the following derivative: $\dfrac{d}{dx}\left(6x^4 - 4x^3\right)$

   A. $-24x^3 - 12x^2$ **B.** $-24x^3 + 12x^2$ **C.** $24x^3 - 12x^2$ **D.** $24x^3 + 12x^2$

43. Evaluate the following derivative $\dfrac{d}{dx}\left(9x^5 - 3x^4 + 3x^2 - 10\right)$ at $x = 1$.

   A. 24   **B.** 39   **C.** 47   **D.** 58

44. Evaluate the following derivative $\dfrac{d}{dx}\left(24x^3 - 9x^2 + 3x - 11\right)$ at $x = 3$.

   A. 597   **B.** 325   **C.** 154   **D.** 96

45. Evaluate the following indefinite integral: $\int t^2\left(\dfrac{5}{t} - \dfrac{t}{5}\right)dt$

   A. $\dfrac{5t^2}{2} + \dfrac{t^4}{20} + C$ **B.** $\dfrac{5t^2}{2} - \dfrac{t^4}{20} + C$ **C.** $-\dfrac{5t^2}{2} - \dfrac{t^4}{20} + C$ **D.** $-\dfrac{5t^2}{2} + \dfrac{t^4}{20} + C$

46. Evaluate the following indefinite integral: $\int (8 - t^3)dt$

   A. $-8t + \dfrac{t^4}{4} + C$ **B.** $-8t - \dfrac{t^4}{4} + C$ **C.** $8t - \dfrac{t^4}{4} + C$ **D.** $8t + \dfrac{t^4}{4} + C$

47. Evaluate the following definite integral: $\int_{1}^{9} 3t^3 dt$

   A. 4920   **B.** 2560   **C.** 2179   **D.** 1659

48. Evaluate the following definite integral: $\int_{2}^{4}\left(x^5 - 6x^3 + 8x + 2\right)dx$

   A. 110   **B.** 364   **C.** 148   **D.** 250

**STOP. IF YOU HAVE TIME LEFT OVER,
CHECK YOUR WORK ON THIS SECTION ONLY.**

Answer Key

Section 2. Verbal Ability

1. D	17. B	33. D
2. B	18. D	34. B
3. C	19. C	35. C
4. A	20. D	36. D
5. C	21. B	37. B
6. D	22. A	38. A
7. C	23. A	39. A
8. D	24. B	40. B
9. C	25. D	41. A
10. D	26. C	42. B
11. B	27. D	43. C
12. A	28. D	44. C
13. B	29. C	45. B
14. A	30. B	46. C
15. D	31. B	47. D
16. B	32. C	48. B

Section 3. Biology

1. D	17. C	33. D
2. A	18. C	34. B
3. B	19. C	35. A
4. B	20. C	36. C
5. C	21. C	37. B
6. D	22. B	38. C
7. C	23. B	39. A
8. C	24. C	40. A
9. C	25. C	41. C
10. C	26. C	42. D
11. C	27. B	43. C
12. B	28. D	44. B
13. D	29. A	45. A
14. B	30. A	46. D
15. C	31. D	47. D
16. B	32. A	48. C

Section 4. Chemistry

1. D	17. B	33. D
2. D	18. A	34. A
3. A	19. B	35. C
4. D	20. C	36. C
5. C	21. D	37. B
6. C	22. B	38. B
7. B	23. B	39. C
8. D	24. A	30. A
9. A	25. A	41. D
10. B	26. D	42. C
11. D	27. B	43. D
12. D	28. A	44. B
13. C	29. C	45. A
14. B	30. C	46. B
15. A	31. C	47. A
16. C	32. D	48. C

Section 6. Reading Comprehension

1. D	17. D	33. D
2. B	18. A	34. D
3. C	19. A	35. D
4. A	20. D	36. B
5. C	21. A	37. C
6. C	22. B	38. D
7. B	23. D	39. C
8. D	24. C	40. D
9. C	25. C	41. B
10. C	26. A	42. A
11. C	27. B	43. C
12. A	28. C	44. B
13. B	29. C	45. B
14. B	30. D	46. A
15. B	31. D	47. D
16. A	32. B	48. C

Section 7. Quantitative Ability

1. C	17. A	33. A
2. B	18. A	34. C
3. C	19. B	35. D
4. B	20. C	36. B
5. A	21. D	37. C
6. B	22. B	38. A
7. B	23. C	39. A
8. C	24. B	40. C
9. C	25. A	41. A
10. D	26. D	42. C
11. A	27. D	43. B
12. B	28. A	44. A
13. C	29. C	45. B
14. C	30. A	46. C
15. D	31. B	47. A
16. C	32. C	48. B

ANSWER EXPLANATIONS
SECTION 1. WRITING

Ask a teacher or another student to score your essay, or score it yourself using the following scoring rubrics.

CONVENTIONS OF LANGUAGE SCORING RUBRIC	
0	Paper blank, illegible, or not in English.
1.0	Multiple errors in capitalization, punctuation, grammar, and/or usage, seriously affecting flow and meaning.
2.0	Multiple errors in capitalization, punctuation, grammar, and/or usage, affecting both flow and meaning.
3.0	Several errors in capitalization, punctuation, grammar, and/or usage. Errors may affect flow, but they do not affect meaning.
4.0	Some errors in capitalization, punctuation, grammar, and/or usage, but errors do not affect meaning or flow.
5.0	Few errors in capitalization, punctuation, grammar, and/or usage.

PROBLEM SOLVING SCORING RUBRIC	
0	Paper blank, illegible, on a topic other than that assigned, or not in English.
1.0	Lack of understanding evident. Organization nonexistent or unclear. Ideas undeveloped.
2.0	Organization unclear or scattershot. Ideas underdeveloped and unsupported.
3.0	Organization fairly coherent. Ideas developed and supported with relevant details that lack complexity.
4.0	Organization coherent and focused. Ideas complex, well developed, and clearly supported.
5.0	Organization coherent and focused. Ideas complex, sophisticated, and substantially developed, with logical, convincing support.

SECTION 2. VERBAL ABILITY

1. Answer: D
The clues in this sentence include the word *misshapen*. The cells resemble crescents rather than round discs. Choice B might be acceptable if it were "resulting in" rather than "resulting."

2. Answer: B
Whether you know this definition or not, it should be easy enough to infer that density equals the number of organisms compared to the size of their habitat. Choice A is redundant, and choice D is a synonym for *density*.

3. Answer: C
Logical thinking should result in your choosing choice C.

4. Answer: A
Choices A, B, and C would work for the first blank, but only choice A fits the second blank. *Barricade* (choice B) would be an odd choice of verb to describe what aspirin does, and you would not want it to *enhance* pain (choice C).

5. Answer: C
Any of the answer choices might work for the first blank, but only choice C fits the second blank. Neither *endure* (choice A) nor *consume* (choice D) makes sense in context, and *act* (choice B) is ungrammatical.

6. Answer: D
The clue in this sentence is *less complex*. Annelids are more complex than the other worms mentioned; therefore, their systems are not *simpler* (choice A) but rather *well-developed* (choice D). Choice B has little meaning, and choice C would not support the author's point that annelids are more complex.

7. Answer: C

The clue here is *more than one.* If you missed that key point, any of the answer choices might work. Ethylene is presented as an example of something with more than one bond—a dual bond, in fact.

8. Answer: D

The correct answer here is the one that is most idiomatic in English. We would say "prevent X from drying out."

9. Answer: C

Try all the pairs in turn before choosing one. Of the four, only choice C has the precise meaning you want. Animals sense stimuli; they do not create it, as in choice A.

10. Answer: D

The elements did not *aspire* to something (choice A), which would indicate that they had conscious thought. Nor did they *evolve* (choice B), which is an action we ascribe only to living things. Instead, they simply *combined* (choice D) to create water.

11. Answer: B

Prey could not benefit from being *eradicated* (choice A) or win by being *underestimated* (choice C). If the prey benefits, that does not mean that it, too, is a *consumer* (choice D). Only choice B fits both parts of the sentence.

12. Answer: A

To answer this one, you should have a good idea of the meaning of each answer choice. Remember that one species is reproducing fast. What is the likely result? Not that it will *inhibit* (restrain) others (choice B), *expend* (use up) others (choice C), or *deduce* (reason) others, but rather that it will *crowd* them out (choice A).

13. Answer: B

Cracklung might be an *irritation* (choice A), *disorder* (choice B), or *disease* (choice C). It may not respond to *traditional* (choice B) or *standard* (choice C) treatments. Since *disorder* and *traditional* fit, the answer is choice B.

14. Answer: A

Think about the meaning of the whole sentence. Drug testing has three phases. Phase I usually considers negative reactions and something else. That "something else" is most logically *toxicity* (choice A). Since the first word fits, too, choice A is the best answer.

15. Answer: D

We might *identify* the plague with medieval times (choice B) or *associate* it with medieval times (choice D). We would not *equate* it with medieval times (choice C); that implies that the two are equal. If there were *rarely* cases now (choice B), there would be no need to make this statement. The fact that there are *still* cases (choice D) makes the statement interesting.

16. Answer: B

Again, this answer depends on your understanding of idiomatic English. We would never say *likelihood for* (choice A); the term is *likelihood of.* Nor would we say *frequency for* (choice C), and *tolerance for suicide* (choice D) makes no sense. The best answer is choice B—people with panic disorder often have secondary depression, giving them a *propensity for* (tendency toward) suicide.

17. Answer: B
Plug all four answers into the blank to find the best one. Only choice B makes sense grammatically as well as contextually.

18. Answer: D
The structure of this sentence involves two parallel clauses. The stroke does not affect all areas of the brain the same way. It does not affect all aspects of intellectual functioning the same way. "The same way" can be restated as "equally," making choice D the best answer.

19. Answer: C
Think: Obesity is the most common nongenetic factor in the WHAT of diabetes? One can be a *carrier* of diabetes (choice A), but obesity is not a factor in the carrier of diabetes. You would never refer to the *practice* of diabetes (choice B). If the factor is nongenetic, it has nothing to do with the *heredity* of diabetes (choice D). The only answer that makes sense is choice C.

20. Answer: D
Glucose is one form of *sugar*, and *ethanol*, sometimes used as fuel, is one form of *alcohol*.

21. Answer: B
A *virus* is the cause of a *cold*. *Stress* may be the cause of a *headache*.

22. Answer: A
The job of the *heart* is to *pump* blood. The job of the *kidney* is to *filter* waste.

23. Answer: A
Fond is the opposite of *indifferent*. *Jocular* is the opposite of *morose*.

24. Answer: B
This is a Part/Whole analogy. Most or all of a pyramid's faces are *triangles*. A cube's faces are *squares*.

25. Answer: D
A *marsupial* is a mammal that typically uses a pouch rather than a placenta in which to carry its young. An *ungulate* is a hoofed mammal such as a horse, antelope, or bison.

26. Answer: C
Lack of Vitamin C can lead to the deficiency disease called *scurvy*. Lack of iodine can cause the swelling of the thyroid known as a *goiter*.

27. Answer: D
If you are *calm*, you are not *frantic*. If you are *stoic*, you are patient and uncomplaining.

28. Answer: D

The *petal* is a part of a flower whose job is *attraction* (of birds, butterflies, and so on). The *pistil* is a part of a flower whose job is *reproduction*.

29. Answer: C

Craniotomy requires opening of the skull. *Phlebotomy* requires opening of a vein.

30. Answer: B

Mount Everest is the tallest mountain in the world, and K2 is the second-tallest. The Nile is the longest river in the world, and the Amazon is second-longest.

31. Answer: B

A *herpetologist* might study pythons or other species of snake. An *ichthyologist* might study cod or other species of fish.

32. Answer: C

A *diet* reduces *weight*, and *fog* reduces *visibility*.

33. Answer: D

Hilarity is the opposite of *melancholy*, and *benevolence* (kindness) is the opposite of *malice* (meanness).

34. Answer: B

A *navigator* generates a *course*, and a *referee* generates a *ruling*.

35. Answer: C

Groundhog and *woodchuck* are regional names for the same rodent. *Skunk* and *polecat* are regional names for the same mustelid.

36. Answer: D

Oxygen is an *element*, which may be defined as a substance that cannot be broken down into simpler substances. Water is a *molecule*, a group of two or more atoms held together by chemical bonds that is also the smallest part of a compound that retains the properties of that compound. A water molecule contains two elements—two atoms of hydrogen and one of oxygen.

37. Answer: B

Something that is *perpetual*, or ongoing, is not *provisional*, or short-term. Something that is *compulsory*, or required, is not *voluntary*.

38. Answer: A

A *word processor* may be considered a modern version of the *typewriter*. A *calculator* may be considered a modern version of the *abacus*.

39. Answer: A

An *arteriole* is the tiniest of arteries; it connects the artery with capillaries. A *venule* is the tiniest of veins; it connects the vein with capillaries.

40. Answer: B

A sound that is sharp and *strident* is *shrill*. A sound that is deep and *resonant* is *sonorous*.

41. Answer: A

A *furrier* makes or repairs fur (or *hide*) garments. A *farrier* is a blacksmith who works with *iron* and shoes horses.

42. Answer: B

This is a Degree analogy. If you are very *clever*, you are *ingenious*. If you are very *irksome*, you are *infuriating*.

43. Answer: C

To *prod* with vigor is to *stab*. To *disobey* with vigor is to *flout*.

44. Answer: C

The *hectare* is a unit used to measure *area* of land. One hectare equals 10,000 square meters. The *fathom* is a unit used to measure *depth* of water. One fathom equals six feet.

45. Answer: B

In literature, a *fox* is used as a symbol of *slyness*, and an *owl* is used as a symbol of *wisdom*.

46. Answer: C

Five *nickels* equal one *quarter*. Five *dimes* equal one *half dollar*.

47. Answer: D

An *elevator* carries passengers up a *skyscraper*. A *funicular* carries passengers up a *mountain*.

48. Answer: B

To *improve* is the opposite of to *deteriorate*. To *impress* is the opposite of to *disappoint*.

SECTION 3. BIOLOGY

1. Answer: D

This question is simply asking about the function of mitochondria in the cell. Mitochondria are involved in aerobic respiration and are the site of the Krebs cycle and the electron transport chain. Aerobic cellular respiration produces large amounts of ATP. Therefore the more mitochondria a cell has, the more ATP it can produce. Cells with higher ATP demands should have more mitochondria than cells with lower ATP demands.

2. Answer: A

Retroviruses are unique in that they enter their host as RNA but most convert themselves to DNA in order to enter the latent phase and insert into the host's chromosomes, which are also DNA. This is indicated by choice A. This conversion of RNA to DNA is carried out by the enzyme reverse transcriptase.

3. Answer: B

This question relies on some basic knowledge of endosymbiotic theory. Choice A suggests that this theory is supported because mitochondria are membrane bound. Since cells have many other membrane-bound organelles, this would not provide any compelling evidence for mitochondria being unique. Choice C indicates that mitochondria are found in multiple copies within a cell and that this would be evidence to support endosymbiosis. Since other organelles are found in multiple copies, this would not be a plausible explanation. The best choice to support the idea that mitochondria were once free-living prokaryotic cells is that they have their own DNA. Since mitochondria have their own DNA and it resembles that of prokaryotes, choice B would lend the best support to the endosymbiotic theory.

4. **Answer: B**

This question relies on your knowledge of the female reproductive cycle. In women, as FSH levels climb, follicles are stimulated to grow. These follicles produce estrogen that exerts positive feedback on LH, whose levels begin to climb. When LH levels peak on the fourteenth day of the cycle, the follicle ruptures, releasing the egg from the ovary and leaving the corpus luteum behind in the ovary. After ovulation, the corpus luteum secretes both estrogen and progesterone to inhibit GnRH. When GnRH is inhibited, FSH and LH will also be inhibited.

5. **Answer: C**

The question explains that mtDNA comes from a single source, which we know is the mother. In the nucleus of diploid cells, each gene is present in duplicate copies that can recombine during crossing over. Since mtDNA comes from a single source, recombination should not occur. The remaining choices listed, such as transcription and translation, should still be able to happen within the mitochondria. Any DNA is subject to spontaneous mutation, including the mtDNA.

6. **Answer: D**

This question is asking about a basic knowledge of bacterial conjugation. During conjugation, a bacterial cell copies a plasmid and transfers that plasmid to a recipient that is lacking the plasmid. Since the question tells us that the resistance genes are often passed by conjugation and we know conjugation passes plasmids, then we can assume that the resistance genes are located on plasmids.

7. **Answer: C**

The repeated use of antibiotics forces the entire bacterial population to become resistant to the antibiotic. This selective pressure forces the population to drive towards a single phenotype, which is characteristic of directional selection. Stabilizing selection leads to most of the population having an intermediate phenotype while disruptive selections leads to the development of two extreme phenotypes in the population.

8. **Answer: C**

To answer this question, you must be familiar with the anatomy of the heart. The right side of the heart is the pulmonary circuit, while the left side is the systemic circuit. Deoxygenated blood enters the right atrium of the heart via the superior and inferior vena cava. Blood from the right atrium passes through the tricuspid valve to the right ventricle and then leaves the heart through the pulmonary semilunar valve. Blood is carried via the pulmonary arteries to the lungs, where gas exchange occurs. After gas exchange occurs, oxygenated blood returns to the heart via pulmonary veins to enter the left atrium. From there blood passes through the bicuspid valve into the left ventricle. Blood leaves the left side of the heart by passing through the aortic valve into the aorta. If there were a pressure increase in the pulmonary arteries, the right ventricle of the heart would most likely be affected, as it is the last chamber that blood is located in before it moves towards the lungs in the pulmonary arteries.

9. **Answer: C**

The question suggests that errors that occur during DNA replication are caught by a proofreading mechanism. The only enzyme that is responsible for DNA replication is DNA polymerase, which is known to proofread and correct many of its errors. Helicase is an enzyme that unwinds the DNA double helix. Ligase is an enzyme that seals DNA fragments. RNA polymerase is responsible for transcription, the conversion of DNA to RNA.

10. **Answer: C**

This question relies on your knowledge of bacterial cell structures and functions. The nucleoid is the region of the cell where the one circular loop of chromosomal DNA is located. The ribosomes are responsible for protein synthesis. Bacteria can convert themselves to spores when environmental conditions are poor, allowing them to survive for extended periods of time in harsh conditions. The capsule is a sticky layer surrounding the cell that helps in the attachment of the cell to a surface. It is likely that the adhesins are located here.

11. **Answer: C**

A familiarity with eukaryotic cell structures and organelles is needed to answer this question. The organelles that normally contain digestive enzymes are the lysosomes, which makes them the most likely candidate for being involved with apoptosis. Each of the other choices listed does not deal with destruction of cellular components. The endoplasmic reticulum has two sides—rough and smooth. The rough endoplasmic reticulum is involved with protein production and modification, while the smooth endoplasmic reticulum is involved with lipid synthesis. The Golgi complex sorts and routes contents from the endoplasmic reticulum. Mitochondria are involved with aerobic cellular respiration and the production of ATP.

12. **Answer: B**

This question requires an understanding of resting potentials and action potentials in the neurons. Recall that resting potentials (polarization) of neuronal membranes are maintained due to an unequal balance of ions that allows for the inside of the neuron to be more negative than the outside of the neuron. This is primarily due to the action of Na^+/K^+ pumps which utilize large amounts of ATP to maintain an unequal balance of ions such that Na^+ is found in high concentrations outside the neuron and K^+ is found in high concentrations inside the neuron. The neuron also contains a variety of negatively charged molecules. In order for a message to be sent, the membrane needs to depolarize. This is characterized by the opening of Na^+ gated channels, which allow Na^+ to flood the inside of the neuron, temporarily (and locally) making that area of the neuron more positive inside than outside. This action potential will propagate the length of the neuron, where it will ultimately coerce the release of neurotransmitters to the synapse. Blockage of the Na$^+$ channels would essentially keep the neuron in resting potential, where Na$^+$ is restricted outside the neuron. This eliminates choice A. Choice C alleges that blocking Na$^+$ channels would in some way interfere with Na$^+$/K$^+$ pumps which are used for the maintenance of resting potential. Since Na$^+$ channels are only needed to initiate an action potential, this choice can be eliminated. Neurotransmitters are not released until an action potential has made its way down the length of the neurons so choice D can also be eliminated. This leaves us with choice B. Blocking Na$^+$ channels prevents the initiation of the action potential, or depolarization, of the membrane.

13. **Answer: D**

The question explains that AZT and ddI interfere with replication and transcription. During a viral infection, the ideal situation would be to interfere with viral processes while leaving host cell processes unaffected. Choice A suggests that host cell DNA replication should be prevented in order to keep the host cell from functioning and mentions nothing about how this would affect the virus. Choice B is similar in that it does not mention how the virus would be affected. Choice C is not appropriate because it discusses preventing infection. If the patient is already confirmed as infected, then this choice wouldn't make sense. If a person is infected with HIV, then the viral genetic material has already entered the host cells. If replication of the viral genome can be prevented as suggested by choice D, then the progression of the infection can be slowed.

14. **Answer: B**

The question describes a system of gene regulation using repressors. Since the organism described is bacterial, and the question is asking about gene regulation, this should narrow the choices to operons. Since the enzymes produced in this question are only used when the antibiotic tetracycline is present, this would be an example of an inducible operon.

15. **Answer: C**

This problem requires a Punnett square to be performed for each generation. For the first generation, the Punnett square for the genetic cross of $TT \times tt$ should be performed. In the first generation, the T and t gametes unite to produce individuals with a Tt (heterozygous) genotype. In the second generation, the Punnett square is conducted for the genetic cross of $TT \times Tt$ or:

	T	t
T	TT	Tt
t	Tt	tt

The phenotypic results from this cross are that three of the four pea plants will be tall (*TT*, *Tt*, and *Tt*) and one of the four is short (*tt*). Thus, the phenotypic ratio of dominant to recessive pea plants is 3:1.

16. **Answer: B**

In the proximal convoluted tubule the primary events are the reabsorption of nutrients and water. There are two regions in the nephron where large amounts of sodium and water are reabsorbed. In the loop of Henle the countercurrent multiplier system is used which leads to salts (sodium and chloride) and water being reabsorbed. In the distal convoluted tubule, the hormone aldosterone influences the reabsorption of salts and water follows by osmosis.

17. **Answer: C**

This question is simply asking for how carbon dioxide is produced on the cellular level. Choice D can be eliminated because carbon dioxide is not directly produced from oxygen gas in the cells. You should recall your knowledge of the process of cellular respiration. During aerobic respiration, glucose goes through glycolysis, the Krebs cycle, and the electron transport chain. During the Krebs cycle, carbon dioxide is released. Therefore carbon dioxide is formed in the cells as a by-product of glucose metabolism. Protein synthesis and nucleic acid metabolism do not produce carbon dioxide as by-products.

18. **Answer: C**

To answer this question you need to be familiar with methods of bacterial gene transfer. Since the question says that a plasmid is being transferred, this would indicate that conjugation is the most likely method. Transformation involves taking up excess DNA from the environment and transduction involves bacteriophage transfer. Binary fission is normal bacterial cell division.

19. **Answer: C**

This question is about osmotic effects. The process of dialysis needs to remove excess fluids (water) from the blood. In order to do this, the dialysis fluid must have more solutes and less water than the blood. This would mean that the dialysis fluid must be hypertonic compared to the blood. Another way to say this is that the blood must be hypotonic (contain less solutes and more water) compared to the dialysis fluid (choice C). If the patient's blood was isotonic to the dialysis fluid, there would be no net movement of water and if the blood were hypertonic to the dialysis fluid then water would enter the blood. In this example, pH is not a major factor in determining osmotic effects, so choice D can be eliminated.

20. **Answer: C**

A codon is a sequence of three nucleotides found on the mRNA that specifies particular amino acids to be added to a protein. The genetic code lists all possible codons. One codon always specifies one amino acid. If the protein is 1480 amino acids long, we might suspect that the mRNA had 1480 codons. However, there would be an additional codon present that served as the stop codon. The stop codon does not code for an amino acid, but instead signals the end of translation and the release of the protein. Therefore 1481 codons would be present on the mRNA.

21. **Answer: C**

This question is asking you to identify a cell structure that is only found in bacterial cells. Cytoplasm can be eliminated, since it is found in all types of cells. Flagella can be found in many types of cells that need to move. Spores can be found in bacteria but also in fungi. The only choice that is unique to bacteria is a cell wall that contains peptidoglycan.

22. **Answer: B**

Carriers are heterozygotes. In the case of a recessive inheritance, a carrier will not necessarily know that they are carrying a single allele for the disease. When two heterozygotes are crossed in a Punnett square, the result is that 25% will be homozygous dominant (normal), 50% will be heterozygous carriers, and 25% will be homozygous recessive and will have cystic fibrosis.

23. **Answer: B**

This question is asking about the general differences in mechanisms of action between steroid and peptide hormones. Steroid hormones are derived from cholesterol, enter their target cells where they bind to a receptor, and act to influence gene expression. Peptide hormones are not lipid-soluble and do not enter their target cells. They act as first messengers to activate second messengers such as cAMP in their target cells.

24. **Answer: C**

Fresh water will contain more water and less solute relative to the cells of the vegetable. This makes the fresh water hypotonic to the vegetables. Osmosis will then move the water into the cells of the vegetables, causing them to swell. Salt water has a higher solute concentration and less water than the cells of the vegetables. The salt water is a hypertonic solution which causes the movement of water out of the cells due to osmosis.

25. **Answer: C**

Fungi tend to be classified based on their means of reproduction and reproductive structures. Of the groups listed, only Deuteromycetes lacks a sexual reproduction phase and only reproduces asexually. While the other classes of fungi can also reproduce asexually, they have sexual phases of the life cycle as well.

26. **Answer: C**

This question is essentially asking why cells need to be small in size. As a cell gets larger its surface area and volume increase. Cells typically need a large surface area relative to a small volume, or a large surface-area-to-volume ratio. This allows the cell to get the substances it needs into and out of itself quickly. The larger a cell gets, the smaller the surface-area-to-volume ratio becomes.

27. **Answer: B**

Messages are picked up by sensory neurons in the peripheral nervous system and passed to interneurons in the central nervous system; responses are passed on to motor neurons in the peripheral nervous system.

28. **Answer: D**

During the light-dependent reactions, water molecules will be split to release electrons. As a byproduct, O_2 gas will be formed. Carbon dioxide is used in the light-independent reactions to eventually produce glucose.

29. **Answer: A**

During the lysogenic cycle, the virus inserts into the host chromosome and stays latent. Each time the cell divides, the bacteriophage DNA will be passed on to the progeny. Eventually, lysogeny ends and the lytic cycle will begin. During the lysogenic cycle the host cell will not be damaged or lysed.

30. **Answer: A**

If the proton gradient of the electron transport chain were to be destroyed, you would need to look for the choice that relates to how a cell would perform cellular respiration without an electron transport chain. The only option would be to move to anaerobic respiration, which requires fermentation, as indicated by choice A.

31. **Answer: D**

This question is asking for a simple understanding of the structures of the peripheral nervous system as compared to the central nervous system. The central nervous system is composed of the brain and spinal cord, while the peripheral nervous system is composed of nerves outside of the brain and spinal cord. Since GBS only affects the peripheral nervous system, the neurons in the central nervous system should be unaffected. Of the choices listed, the neurons of the arms and legs, abdominal cavity, and heart are all part of the peripheral nervous system and subject to GBS. The neurons of the spinal cord are part of the central nervous system and should be unaffected by GBS.

32. **Answer: A**

Since the Krebs cycle and electron transport chain of aerobic respiration occur in the mitochondria, a situation where mitochondria were absent would prevent aerobic respiration. The only option would be anaerobic respiration. In animals, the form of anaerobic respiration used would be lactate fermentation, which converts pyruvate to lactic acid.

33. **Answer: D**

Each of the choices listed is characteristic of a retrovirus; however, some of these characteristics are common to other viruses. For example, viruses other than retroviruses use RNA as their genetic material. The unique feature of retroviruses is that they code for the enzyme reverse transcriptase. This enzyme allows the RNA virus to convert itself into DNA form.

34. **Answer: B**

During semiconservative replication, the DNA double helix unwinds, unzips, and each strand serves as a template. DNA polymerase copies each strand, producing complementary strands. The resulting double helices contain one original template strand and one newly synthesized strand.

35. **Answer: A**

The question is essentially asking about what substances are normally digested in the stomach. The stomach produces the enzyme pepsin, which is activated by the low pH (high acidity) of the stomach. Pepsin is used to digest proteins. If stomach pH were increased, pepsin would not be activated and protein digestion in the stomach would not happen properly.

36. **Answer: C**

The diploid number for humans is 46 and the haploid number is 23. When cells are dividing, each chromosome is present in duplicate copy. These chromosomes are composed of two chromatids each when they are replicated.

37. **Answer: B**

Host cells tend to be killed as newly formed viruses try to exit the cell. Lysis is one means a virus can use to leave the cell. This ruptures the cell membrane, which ultimately kills the host cell.

38. **Answer: C**

RNA and DNA differ in several ways. RNA exists as a single strand that is copied from DNA in the nucleus during the process of transcription. The nucleotides that are used to make RNA are cytosine, guanine, adenine, and uracil. The sugar that is used in RNA nucleotides is ribose (as compared with deoxyribose in DNA).

39. **Answer: A**

The alveoli are the site of gas exchange, which is where CO_2 will be picked up. Moving up from the alveoli will lead to the bronchioles, the bronchi, the trachea, the pharynx, and the larynx.

40. **Answer: A**

Mutations are changes to the DNA. While it does not catch all mistakes, DNA polymerase does catch many errors and allows for their correction during a proofreading process. RNA polymerase does not have proofreading or correcting abilities; nor do tRNAs correct errors in the process of translation.

41. **Answer: C**

The question indicates that breast cancer can be associated with the BRCA1 allele. However, not all cases of breast cancer are associated with this allele, and some individuals that have the allele do not develop cancer. The only reasonable explanation in this case is that something other than a genetic factor must be involved. Environmental influences, in addition to certain alleles, are known to influence the development of certain phenotypes in some cases.

42. **Answer: D**

If a person has no incoming fluids, we would expect that urine volume would decrease in an attempt to retain the fluids already present in the body. The signal to increase water reabsorption in the nephrons comes from antidiuretic hormone and aldosterone.

Since the body is trying to conserve the fluids it has and there are no incoming fluids, the blood volume should not increase.

43. Answer: C

The parents in this case are a carrier father and a normal (noncarrier) mother. This is not a sex-linked trait, so we can indicate the genotype of the father as Aa and the mother as AA. If you work out the Punnett square, 50% will be carriers (Aa) and 50% will be normal (AA). None of the children will have the disease.

44. Answer: B

The question indicates that Duchene muscular dystrophy is a sex-linked allele that affects males more than females. However, the question indicates that the disorder does occur in females although it is more rare than in males. This indicates that the allele is on the X chromosome. Since a male only has one X chromosome that he inherited from his mother, he will express whatever allele is on that X chromosome. Therefore males only need to inherit the alleles from their mother to be affected. For a female to have this disease, she must receive it on both X chromosomes (from both parents). It would be more likely for a male to inherit this from one parent (his mother) than for a female to inherit the allele from both parents.

45. Answer: A

ATP is produced during the light-dependent reactions of photosynthesis by PSII. During the Calvin cycle carbon dioxide is fixed by combining with RuBP, which is regenerated by the cycle. NADPH donates electrons causing it to be oxidized to $NADP^+$.

46. Answer: D

A sperm cell would be the result of cells that had completed meiosis II. The question indicates that the number of chromosomes in the haploid sperm cell would be 12. The original parent cell that started meiosis would be diploid, or twice that of the haploid number. In this question, the diploid number of the starting cell would be 24.

47. Answer: D

This question relies on an understanding of the fitness concept. Fitness is relative to the specific population. Fit individuals carry alleles that make them more likely to reproduce and pass those alleles to the next generation. Therefore, those that reproduce the most in a certain population would be considered the most fit under the conditions of that population.

48. Answer: C

The two equations of Hardy-Weinberg are $p + q = 1$ and $p2 + 2pq + q2 = 1$ where $p =$ the frequency of the dominant allele and $q =$ the frequency of the recessive allele. The question says that the homozygous recessive genotype is 81% of the population. This means that $q2 = 0.81$. Now solve for q and p. If $q2 = 0.81$ then $q = 0.9$ and $p = 0.1$. The question asks for the frequency of heterozygous individuals, which is $2pq$ or $2(0.9)(0.1) = 0.18$.

SECTION 4. CHEMISTRY

1. Answer: D

The superscript is the mass number, which is the sum of protons and neutrons. The number of neutrons is the mass number minus the atomic number. In this case $31 - 15 = 16$.

2. Answer: D

To calculate the mass percent, you first need the molar mass of Na_2CO_3.

Molar mass $= (2 \times Na) + (1 \times C) + (3 \times O) = (2 \times 23) + (1 \times 12) + (3 \times 16)\ ^g/_{mol} = 106\ ^g/_{mol}$. Of this 106g, 48g is oxygen.

$$\text{Mass \% O} = \frac{48\,g\,O}{106\,g\,\text{total}} \times 100\% = 45.3\,O\,\%$$

3. Answer: A

$$g\,CH_4 \rightarrow mol\,CH_4 \rightarrow \text{molecules}\,CH_4 \rightarrow H\,\text{atoms}$$

The molar mass needed is $CH_4 = 16\ ^g/_{mol}$.

$$48\,g\,\text{of}\,CH_4 \times \frac{1\,mol\,CH_4}{16\,g\,CH_4} = 3.0\,mol\,CH_4$$

$$3.0\,mol\,CH_4 \times \frac{6 \times 10^{23}\,\text{molecules}\,CH_4}{1\,mol\,CH_4} = 1.8 \times 10^{24}\,\text{molecules}\,CH_4$$

$$1.8 \times 10^{24}\,\text{molecules}\,CH_4 \times \frac{4\,H\,\text{atoms}}{1\,\text{molecule}\,CH_4} = 7.2 \times 10^{24}\,\text{atom}\,H$$

A common error is omitting the last step (choice D).

4. Answer: D

This problem is a limiting reactant problem because two reactants are given. You must determine the limiting reactant. One method is to calculate the mass of product that can be formed from each reactant. The one that forms the smaller amount is the limiting reactant. The molar masses needed are $N_2 = 28\ ^g/_{mol}$, $H_2 = 2\ ^g/_{mol}$, and $NH_3 = 17\ ^g/_{mol}$. The two possible reactants are:

$$g\,N_2 \rightarrow mol\,N_2 \rightarrow mol\,NH_3 \rightarrow g\,NH_3$$

$$g\,H_2 \rightarrow mol\,H_2 \rightarrow mol\,NH_3 \rightarrow g\,NH_3$$

For N_2:

$$70\,g\,\text{of}\,N_2 \times \frac{1\,mol\,N_2}{28\,g\,N_2} = 2.50\,mol\,N_2$$

$$2.50\,mol\,N_2 \times \frac{2\,mol\,NH_3}{1\,mol\,N_2} = 5.0\,mol\,NH_3$$

$$5.0\ \text{mol NH}_3 \times \frac{17\ \text{g NH}_3}{1\ \text{mol NH}_3} = 85\ \text{g NH}_3$$

For H_2:

$$12\ \text{g of H}_2 \times \frac{1\ \text{mol H}_2}{2\ \text{g H}_2} = 6.0\ \text{mol H}_2$$

$$6.0\ \text{mol H}_2 \times \frac{2\ \text{mol NH}_3}{3\ \text{mol H}_2} = 4.0\ \text{mol NH}_3$$

$$4.0\ \text{mol NH}_3 \times \frac{17\ \text{g NH}_3}{1\ \text{mol NH}_3} = 68\ \text{g NH}_3$$

Because the amount of NH_3 formed from the H_2 given is less than that formed from the N_2, the H_2 is the limiting reactant, and the maximum amount of NH_3 formed will be 68 g.

5. **Answer: C**

To find percent yield, you must calculate the maximum amount of product that can form, which is the theoretical yield. The percent yield is defined as:

$$\text{Percent yield} = \frac{\text{actual yield}}{\text{theoretical yield}} \times 100\%$$

The necessary molar masses are $P_4 = 124\ ^\text{g}/_\text{mol}$, and $PCl_3 = 137.5\ ^\text{g}/_\text{mol}$. The theoretical yield is calculated by:

$$\text{g P}_4 \rightarrow \text{mol P}_4 \rightarrow \text{mol PCl}_3 \rightarrow \text{g PCl}_3$$

$$372\ \text{g of P}_4 \times \frac{1\ \text{mol P}_4}{124\text{g P}_4} = 3.0\ \text{mol P}_4$$

$$3.0\ \text{mol P}_4 \times \frac{4\ \text{mol PCl}_3}{1\ \text{mol P}_4} = 12.0\ \text{mol PCl}_3$$

$$12.0\ \text{mol PCl}_3 \times \frac{137.5\ \text{g PCl}_3}{1\ \text{mol PCl}_3} = 1650\ \text{g PCl}_3$$

$$\text{Theoretical yield} = \frac{1000\ \text{g}}{1650\ \text{g}} \times 100\% = 60.6\%$$

6. **Answer: C**

The amount of the increase of the water level in the graduated cylinder is equal to the volume of the metal ($13.8 - 10.0\ \text{mL} = 3.8\ \text{mL}$). The density is given by:

$$\text{Density} = \frac{10.3\ \text{g}}{3.8\ \text{mL}} = 2.7\ \text{g / mL}$$

7. **Answer: B**

To determine the empirical formula you must determine the simplest whole number ratio of atoms in the compound. This is related to the ratio of the moles of each element. First calculate the moles of each element.

$$9.6 \text{ g of S } \times \frac{1 \text{ mol S}}{32 \text{ g S}} = 0.30 \text{ mol S}$$

$$4.8 \text{ g of O } \times \frac{1 \text{ mol O}}{16 \text{ g O}} = 0.30 \text{ mol O}$$

$$48 \text{ g of Br} \times \frac{1 \text{ mol Br}}{80 \text{ g Br}} = 0.60 \text{ mol Br}$$

The ratio of moles is clearly S:O:Br = 030:0.30:0.60 = 1:1:2. The empirical formula is $SOBr_2$.

The incorrect answers come from ratio of the masses instead of the moles (choice A) and from using 32 for the mass of oxygen (choice C). Choice D is random.

8. **Answer: D**

This problem prepares two solutions. Solution 1 is prepared from NaF and water. Solution 2 is a dilution of a portion of solution 1. For solution 1, you must find the moles of NaF, and use the definition of molarity. The molar mass of NaF is 42 $^g/_{mol}$. The steps in this problem are:

g NaF → M NaF solution 1 → mol NaF used in solution 2 → M NaF solution 2

$$10.5 \text{ g of NaF } \times \frac{1 \text{ mol NaF}}{42. \text{ g NaF}} = 0.25 \text{ mol NaF}$$

$$\text{Molarity solution 1} = \frac{\text{mol solute}}{\text{L solution}} = \frac{0.25 \text{ mol NaF}}{0.750 \text{ L soln}} = 0.33 \text{ M NaF}$$

A dilution does not change the number of mol of solute. Dilution simply spreads the solute out over a greater volume. The number of moles taken from solution 1 is:

$$0.10 \text{ L of soln } \times \frac{0.33 \text{ mol NaF}}{1 \text{ L soln}} = 0.033 \text{ mol NaF}$$

The total volume of solution 2 is 100 + 200 mL = 300 mL

$$\text{Molarity solution 2} = \frac{0.033 \text{ mol NaF}}{0.300 \text{ L soln}} = 0.11 \text{ M NaF}$$

9. **Answer: A**

This problem is a titration using solution stoichiometry. The steps in the solution are:

$$\text{mL MnO}_4^- \rightarrow \text{mol MnO}_4^- \rightarrow \text{mol H}_2\text{C}_2\text{O}_4 \rightarrow \text{M H}_2\text{C}_2\text{O}_4$$

$$0.024\,\text{L of MnO}_4^- \times \frac{0.250\,\text{mol MnO}_4^-}{1\,\text{L soln}} = 0.0060\,\text{mol MnO}_4^-$$

$$0.0060\,\text{mol MnO}_4^- \times \frac{5\,\text{mol H}_2\text{C}_2\text{O}_4}{2\,\text{mol MnO}_4^-} = 0.015\,\text{mol H}_2\text{C}_2\text{O}_4$$

$$\text{Molarity} = \frac{0.015\,\text{mol H}_2\text{C}_2\text{O}_4}{0.020\,\text{L soln}} = 0.75\,\text{M H}_2\text{C}_2\text{O}_4$$

10. Answer: B

According to kinetic molecular theory, the average energy of the molecules is proportional to the Kelvin temperature. In this example the temperature is fixed, so the average energy is fixed. Choice A is wrong. When the volume is decreased, the distance that the molecules must travel before hitting the walls of the container is shorter. If temperature is fixed, the average energy and thus the average speed is fixed, so the molecules hit the walls of the container more frequently. Choice B is correct. The molecules of a gas are well separated, so only when the volume becomes very small will the molecules "crowd" each other. Choice C is wrong. Molecules do not change shape appreciably with volume changes. Choice D is wrong.

11. Answer: D

This is a gas law stoichiometry problem. The steps are:

$$\text{g KClO}_3 \rightarrow \text{mol KClO}_3 \rightarrow \text{mol O}_2 \rightarrow \text{P O}_2$$

$$2.46\,\text{g of KClO}_3 \times \frac{1\,\text{mol KClO}_3}{123\,\text{g KClO}_3} = 0.020\,\text{mol KClO}_3$$

$$0.020\,\text{mol KClO}_3 \times \frac{3\,\text{mol O}_2}{2\,\text{mol KClO}_3} = 0.030\,\text{mol O}_2$$

For the last step the ideal gas law is used. The temperature must be converted to Kelvin. $(27 + 273 = 300\,\text{K})$.

$$PV = nRT$$

$$P = \frac{(0.030\,\text{mol O}_2)\left(0.082\,\dfrac{\text{L} \cdot \text{atm}}{\text{mol} \cdot \text{K}}\right)(300\,\text{K})}{0.82\,\text{L}} = 0.90\,\text{atm}$$

Common errors are skipping the stoichiometry step (choice A) and not converting the temperature to K (choice C).

12. Answer: D

The standard enthalpy of formation is the enthalpy of the reaction for the formation of one mole of a substance from the elements in their standard states. For PbO this reaction is:

$$\text{Pb(s)} + \tfrac{1}{2}\,\text{O}_2(\text{g}) \rightarrow \text{PbO(s)}$$

You must use the given reactions to add up to this formation reaction. Pb is in the product side of the first reaction, but needs to be on the reactant side in the target reaction. The first reaction must be reversed and the ΔH multiplied by -1. In the second reaction O_2 is on the correct side, but must be multiplied by ½ to get the correct number of O_2 molecules. The value of ΔH must also be multiplied by ½.

$$Pb(s) + CO(g) \rightarrow PbO(s) + C(graphite) \qquad \Delta H° = -1 \times (107.0\,kJ) = -107.0\,kJ$$
$$C(graphite) + \tfrac{1}{2}O_2(g) \rightarrow CO(g) \qquad \Delta H° = \tfrac{1}{2} \times (-221\,kJ) = -110.5\,kJ$$

$$Pb(s) + \tfrac{1}{2}O_2(g) \rightarrow PbO(s) \qquad \Delta H°_{total} = -217.5\,kJ$$

13. Answer: C

This problem is done in two steps:

$$\lambda\,photon \rightarrow \nu\,photon \rightarrow E\,photon$$

The equation for the first step is $\nu\lambda = c$ rearranged to $\nu = c/\lambda$.

$$\nu = \frac{3.0 \times 10^8\,\frac{m}{s}}{9.0 \times 10^{-8}\,m} = 0.33 \times 10^{15}\,\tfrac{1}{s}\ \text{or}\ 3.3 \times 10^{15}\,\tfrac{1}{s}$$

The next step uses Planck's relationship, $E = h\nu$

$$E = (6.6 \times 10^{-34}\,J{\cdot}s) \times (3.3 \times 10^{+15}) = 2.2 \times 10^{-18}\,J$$

14. Answer: B

The general trend in ionization energy for atoms across a period is that the ionization energy increases from left to right. The trend in a column is that the ionization energy increases from the bottom to the top of a column. The trend across a period means that O < F. The trend in the column means that S < O. Putting these two results together gives S < O < F. For cations, the ionization energy is always greater than the atom from which the cation is derived, so F < F⁺ giving a final order of S < O < F < F⁺.

15. Answer: A

Chlorine is element number 17 so its atom must have 17 electrons. This rules out choices C and D, which have 18 electrons. Choice B is the ground state electron configuration of Cl. Choice A has one of the 3p electrons promoted to the higher 3d level. This is the correct answer.

16. Answer: C

The trend in electronegativity in the periodic table is that electronegativity increases across a period from left to right and up a column from bottom to top. The relative order of electronegativity would thus be Si < C < N < O. An O-O bond would be nonpolar. The greatest difference in electronegativity is between Si and O, and that will be the most polar bond.

17. Answer: B
The resonance structure in question is:

$$:\ddot{O}-C\equiv N:$$
$$\ominus$$

The formal charge is calculated by the formula:

Formal charge = valence electrons − [(lone pair electrons + ½ (bond pair electrons)]

Formal charge (O) = $6 - (6 + \frac{1}{2}(2)) = -1$

Formal charge (C) = $4 - (0 + \frac{1}{2}(8)) = 0$

Formal charge (N) = $5 - (2 + \frac{1}{2}(6)) = 0$

18. Answer: A
The ion has $7 + (3 \times 6) + 1 = 26$ electrons. Following the rules for drawing Lewis structures, the correct Lewis structure is shown on the left. The molecule has four effective electron pairs and one lone pair, so its geometry is trigonal pyramidal. The molecular geometry (without lone pairs on oxygen) is shown on the right.

19. Answer: B
At a given temperature, if a substance has a higher vapor pressure than another, this means that there are more molecules in the vapor phase. There are more molecules in the vapor phase because the intermolecular forces are weaker, and it is easier for the molecules to break apart from one another. In the liquid phase, molecules are touching, but in the vapor or gas phase the molecules are well separated. Water has quite strong intermolecular interactions, so it is relatively difficult for the molecules to break free from one another and enter the vapor phase. The unknown will have a lower boiling point than water because the vapor pressure will reach 1 atm before water. Because the intermolecular forces in the unknown are less than water, the enthalpy of vaporization will be smaller than water. The energy of molecules in the gas phase depends on the temperature, so the vapors at the same temperature will have the same average kinetic energies.

20. Answer: C
The formula for the boiling point elevation of a non-electrolyte is $\Delta T_b = K_b m$ where ΔT_b is the change in boiling point, K_b is the boiling point elevation constant, and m is the molality of solute. The molar mass of urea is 60 $^g/_{mol}$. This problem has the steps:

$$g \text{ urea} \rightarrow \text{mol urea} \rightarrow \text{m urea} \rightarrow \Delta T_b \rightarrow \text{boiling point}$$

$$24 \text{g of urea} \times \frac{1 \text{ mol urea}}{60 \text{ g urea}} = 0.40 \text{ mol urea}$$

$$\text{Molality} = \frac{\text{mol solute}}{\text{kg solvent}} = \frac{0.40 \text{ mol urea}}{0.250 \text{ kg}} = 1.6 \text{ }^{mol}/_{kg}$$

$$\Delta T = (2.53 \text{ }^{°C \cdot kg}/_{mol}) (1.6 \text{ }^{mol}/_{kg}) = 4.05 \text{ °C}$$

$$\text{Boiling point of the solution} = 80.10 + 4.05 \text{ °C} = 84.15 \text{ °C}$$

21. **Answer: D**

To get the correct answer, you must use the formula for a first order reaction, but you can also estimate the answer with half lives. The equation for the relationship between concentration and time for a first order reaction is:

$$\ln[A]_t = -kt + \ln[A]_o$$

In this case $[A]_t = 0.1[A]_o$

$$\ln(0.1[A]_o) = -6.93 \times 10^{-2} (^1/_{min}) \times t + \ln[A]_o$$

$$\ln(0.1[A]_o) - \ln[A]_o = -6.93 \times 10^{-2} (^1/_{min}) \times t$$

$$\ln(0.1) = -6.93 \times 10^{-2} (^1/_{min}) \times t$$

$$-2.30 = -6.93 \times 10^{-2} (^1/_{min}) \times t$$

$$33 \text{ min} = t$$

Even without a calculator with logarithms, you can estimate the time using the half lives. The half life of a first order reaction is $\frac{\ln 2}{k}$ or $\frac{0.693}{k}$. For this reaction,

$$t_{1/2} = \frac{0.693}{0.0693 \left(\dfrac{1}{\min} \right)} = 10 \text{ min}$$

For a first order reaction, the half life is constant. So you can tabulate the fraction remaining after each half life has elapsed.

# of half lives	time (min)	% left
0	0	100
1	10	50

# of half lives	time (min)	% left
2	20	25
3	30	12.5
4	40	6.25
5	50	3.125

The time for 10% remaining is between 3 and 4 half lives elapsed. Only choice D falls within this window and agrees with the exact calculation.

22. **Answer: B**

The function of a catalyst is to lower the activation energy of a reaction. With a lower activation energy, a larger fraction of molecules will have sufficient energy to react, which increases the rate of the reaction. The catalyst does not affect the energies of the reactants or products or the value of the equilibrium constant. The catalyst simply allows equilibrium to be reached faster.

23. **Answer: B**

The equilibrium constant expression appropriate for this equation is given below. The only unknown in the equation is [HI]. The equation is solved for [HI].

$$K = \frac{[HI]^2}{[H_2][I_2]} \Rightarrow K[H_2][I_2] = [HI]^2 \Rightarrow \sqrt{K[H_2][I_2]} = [HI]$$

$$\sqrt{64(1.0)(0.25)} = [HI]$$

$$\sqrt{16} = [HI]$$

$$4.0M = [HI]$$

Common errors in these types of problems include forgetting an exponent such as the square on [HI].

24. **Answer: A**

The equilibrium equation, ICE table, and corresponding K_a expression are:

	$C_6H_5COOH(aq) + H_2O(l)$ ⇌	$H_3O^+(aq) +$	$C_6H_5COO^-(aq)$
Initial	1.0	0	0
Change	− x	+x	+x
Equilibrium	1.0 − x	x	x

$$K_a = \frac{[H_3O^+][C_6H_5COO^-]}{[C_6H_5COOH]}$$

Because the equilibrium constant is small, x is expected to be small and you can approximate $1.0 - x \approx 1.0$. Substituting the equilibrium values with the approximation gives:

$$6.3 \times 10^{-5} = \frac{[x][x]}{[1.0]}$$

$$6.3 \times 10^{-5} = x^2$$

$7.9 \times 10^{-3} = x$, which is the concentration of H_3O^+

$$pH = -\log[H_3O^+] = -\log(7.9 \times 10^{-3}) = 2.10$$

Even without a calculator, you can estimate the pH. Starting with $6.3 \times 10^{-5} = x^2$, you can rewrite this in a more convenient form: $63 \times 10^{-6} = x^2$. This is very close to 64×10^{-6}, which has a square root of $8 \times 10^{-3} = x$. You can estimate the pH by using powers of 10. The value of x is between 10^{-3} and 10^{-2}, but closer to 10^{-2}. The pH is between $-\log(10^{-3})$ and $-\log(10^{-2})$ or between 3.0 and 2.0, but closer to 2.0. The only value that meets these criteria is choice A.

25. **Answer: A**

The weak acid CH_3COOH dissolves to produce an acidic solution. NH_4Cl contains NH_4^+, which is the conjugate acid of a weak base and produces an acidic solution. The anion Cl^- is the conjugate base of a strong acid which has no acidic or basic properties. The salt $Mg(NO_3)_2$ will not affect the pH because neither ion is acidic or basic. The salt $NaCH_3COO$ dissolves to form Na^+ ions and CH_3COO^- ions. Sodium ion has no acid or basic properties, but CH_3COO^- is the conjugate base of the weak acid, CH_3COOH. This anion will make the solution basic by removing a proton from water according to the following equilibria:

$$CH_3COO^-(aq) + H_2O(l) \rightleftharpoons CH_3COOH(aq) + OH^-(aq)$$

26. **Answer: D**

The pH of buffers is determined by the Henderson-Hasselbalch equation:

$$pH = pK_a + \log\frac{[A^-]}{[HA]}$$

For this problem:

$$pH = 3.14 + \log\frac{[(0.3)]}{[(3.0)]}$$
$$pH = 3.14 + \log(0.10)$$
$$pH = 3.14 + (-1.0) = 2.14$$

27. **Answer: B**

The solubility equilibrium equation, ICE table, and solubility product constant are:

$CuSCN(s) \rightleftharpoons$	$Cu^+(aq) +$	$SCN^-(aq)$
Initial	0	0
Change	+x	+x
Equilibrium	x	x

$$K_{sp} = [Cu^+][SCN^-] = x^2$$
$$1.6 \times 10^{-11} = x^2$$
$$4.0 \times 10^{-6}\ M = x$$

To work this problem without a calculator with a square root key, rewrite the equation as $16 \times 10^{-12} = x^2$ The left side is now two perfect squares and the solution is easily obtained as 4.0×10^{-6} M $= x$.

28. Answer: A

The spontaneity of a reaction is given by the value of the free energy, $\Delta G°$, which is defined by:

$$\Delta G° = \Delta H° - T\Delta S°$$

If the value of $\Delta G°$ is negative, the reaction is spontaneous (product favored), a positive value means the reverse reaction is spontaneous, and a value of 0 means the system is at equilibrium. For this reaction, the $\Delta H°$ term is negative and the term $-T\Delta S°$ is also negative, because $\Delta S°$ is positive. The two terms make the overall value of $\Delta G°$ negative, which means the reaction is spontaneous as written.

29. Answer: C

The species that is reduced will have a decrease in the oxidation number. The oxidation number of each species is given in the equation below.

$$Ca(s) + Sn^{2+}(aq) \rightarrow Ca^{2+}(aq) + Sn(s)$$
$$0 \qquad +2 \qquad\quad +2 \qquad 0$$

The oxidation number of Ca changes from 0 to +2, which is an oxidation. The Sn changes from +2 to 0, which is a reduction. The Sn^{2+} ion picks up two electrons and is reduced to Sn metal. The correct half reaction for the species that is reduced is: $Sn^{2+}(aq) + 2 e^- \rightarrow Sn(s)$

30. Answer: C

Choice A is a termination step, and choice B is a highly endothermic fragmentation. Choice D resembles a propagation step, but it actually consumes product. Choice C obeys all the guidelines of a propagation step: it provides a continuation of the radical cycle, it consumes stoichiometric reagent, and it provides one of the observed products.

31. Answer: C

Since the first step in bromination is highly endothermic, the transition state energies resemble those of the intermediate carbon radicals. This is why bromination is a selective process. Therefore, the most highly substituted center is most rapidly brominated.

32. Answer: D

This step represents bond formation, which is always exothermic; therefore, ΔH is negative. Since two species are combining to form one, translational degrees of freedom are lost, and ΔS is also negative.

33. Answer: D

The Baeyer-Villiger reaction converts ketones to esters; thus choices C and D are the most valid. These two choices differ with regard to which alkyl group has migrated.

Keep in mind that this is a migration of an electron-deficient center; therefore, the substituent which can best support a positive charge will be the most likely to migrate. Thus, the isopropyl group is attached to the ester oxygen.

34. **Answer: A**

Manganese dioxide is a selective oxidant for allylic and benzylic alcohols. The substrate in this problem has two alcohol moieties, both secondary, but only one with an allylic character—only this will be oxidized.

35. **Answer: C**

Remember that the stronger the conjugate acid, the better the leaving group. Here we compare HCl, HF, HI, and H2O. Since HI is the strongest acid, iodide is the best leaving group.

36. **Answer: C**

Ironically, iodide is also the best nucleophile, by virtue of its great polarizability.

37. **Answer: B**

The first decision to make here is what the nucleophilic moiety should be: methyl or ethyl. Since the methyl is attached to the β-position of the enone, which is electrophilic, it is reasonable to choose a nucleophilic methyl group. This reduces our options to choices A and B. The next decision is between methyllithium and the corresponding cuprate. Here it is necessary to recognize that alkyllithiums tend to add in a 1,2-fashion to enones, while cuprates add 1,4.

38. **Answer: B**

The three functional groups in question are the carbonyl, the hydroxyl, and the alkene. There is no absorption band in the alkene region, but there are strong bands in the carbonyl ($1714\,\mathrm{cm}^{-1}$) and hydroxyl ($3430\,\mathrm{cm}^{-1}$) regions. This molecule is the only choice that exhibits both of these functionalities.

39. **Answer: C**

The only two choices that would give only singlets in the NMR are choices C and D. We can distinguish between these two choices by the chemical shift of the 3-proton singlet—the value of 3.7 tells us that it is connected directly to the oxygen. In choice D, the methyl group is attached to a carbonyl ($\delta = $ca. 2).

40. **Answer: A**

Because of symmetry in the molecule, some carbon atoms are chemically identical—for example, the two methyl carbons of the isopropyl group (triangles), the aromatic carbons ortho to the chloro (circles), and the aromatic carbons meta to the chloro (squares).

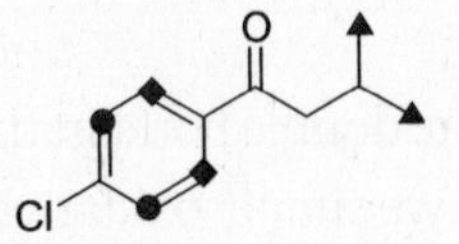

41. **Answer: D**

The conditions leading to the formation of $N,N,2,2$-tetramethylpropan-1-amine represent reductive amination, which occurs between amines and carbonyl compounds in the presence of a reducing agent such as sodium cyanoborohydride. Since the amine component is given as dimethylamine, then consideration of the remaining carbon fragment leads to the conclusion that Compound A is the aldehyde shown below. The conditions leading to Compound B are evocative of the Grignard reaction, which proceeds by nucleophilic addition to a carbonyl.

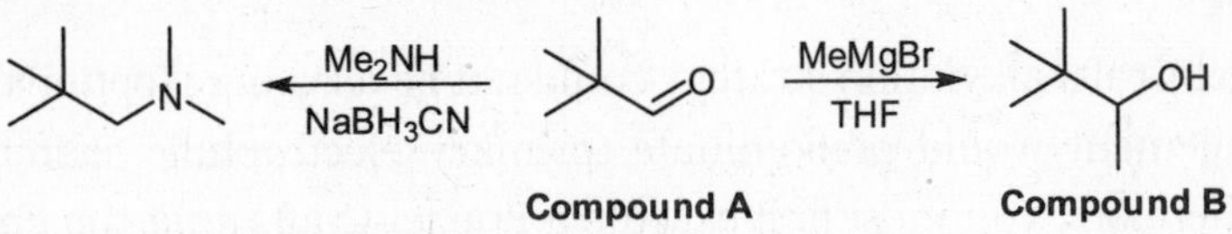

Compound A   **Compound B**

42. **Answer: C**

The product shown is the result of a nucleophilic ring opening of an epoxide. Methyl iodide can be discounted because it does not represent a competent nucleophile. Sodium iodide does provide a good nucleophile (iodide), but it would not provide the product shown. The choice then becomes one of base-catalyzed or acid-catalyzed ring opening in methanol. Here the regiochemistry is the deciding factor. Note that the methoxy group ends up at the more substituted position; yet methoxide (Conditions A) would attack at the least hindered (less substituted) position. However, under acidic conditions, the protonated epoxide already starts to open, elongating the bond between the oxygen and the more substituted carbon (i.e., more able to sustain positive character). The lone pair on the methanol is then attracted to the developing positive charge at that site, leading to the product shown.

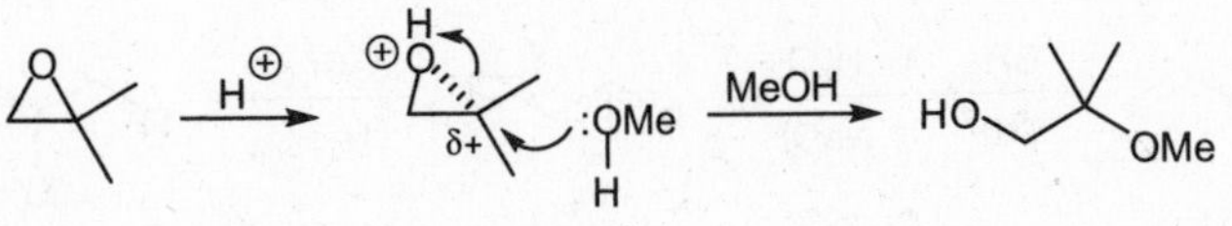

43. **Answer: D**

To make this decision, an electronic picture of the methyl anion must be envisioned. The carbon atom is surrounded by three hydrogen atoms and a lone pair, as shown below:

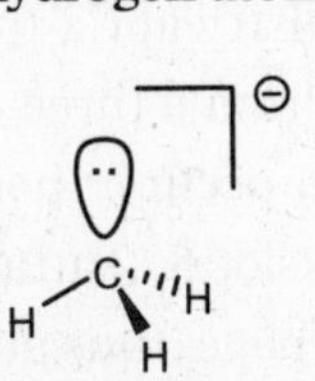

Thus, the methyl anion is isoelectronic with ammonia (:NH$_3$). As with ammonia, since the central atom has four centers of electron density to accommodate, an sp^3 hybridization scheme is the most probable. In the methyl anion, three of these hybrid orbitals are used for bonding, and the one remaining houses the lone pair.

44. **Answer: B**

The key here is to recognize that the double bond in the starting material represents two carbonyl groups in the product. If we simply oxidatively cleave the double bond without moving any bonds (as shown below), it is clear that the chosen starting material will give the desired product—three carbonyl groups separated by one, two, and two carbons, with a methyl group attached to the one-carbon tether.

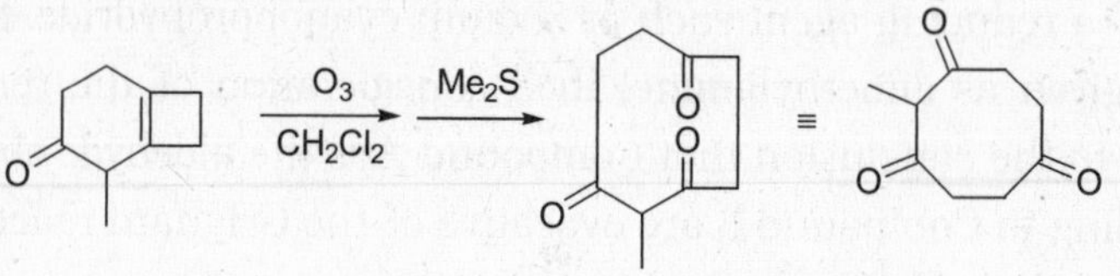

45. **Answer: A**

A simple Friedel-Crafts alkylation strategy could not be used here (options B and D), because rearrangement would predominate (primary electrophilic center adjacent to branching). Therefore, you must first execute a Friedel-Crafts *acylation*, followed by reduction of the carbonyl.

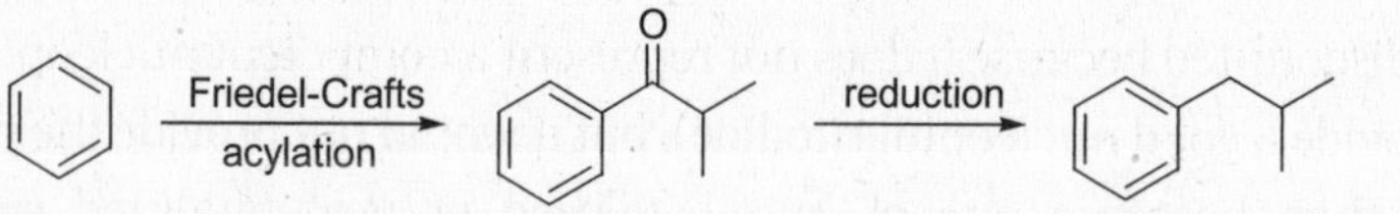

46. **Answer: B**

The reaction conditions represent a multistep synthetic sequence. The first set of conditions corresponds to hydroboration, a method of anti-Markovnikov hydration of alkenes; thus, the hydroxyl group is attached to the less substituted site, providing a primary alcohol. The second step is oxidation under Jones conditions, which converts primary alcohols to the corresponding carboxylic acids.

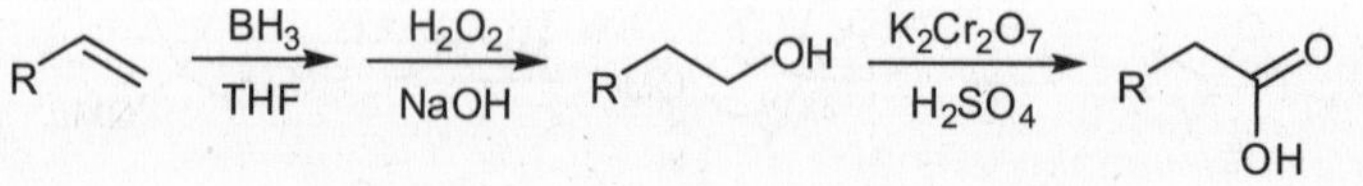

47. **Answer: A**

This represents the chlorohydrin synthesis of epoxides, which is a stereospecific process. In other words, the stereochemistry at C2 (hydroxyl) is retained, while that of C3 (chloro) is inverted. It is easy to see from a three-dimensional mechanistic standpoint, as shown below. First deprotonation occurs; then the nucleophile (alkoxide) must be oriented so that it can engage in backside S$_N$2 attack at C3. Think of this as nudging the alkoxide moiety into the plane of the page (thus pushing the left-hand methyl group out towards us) and pulling the chloro substituent into the plane (thereby rotating the right-hand methyl group away from us). The nucleophilic displacement does not change the dash-wedge relationship of the methyl groups.

48. Answer: C

The molecule in the box is already in an eclipsed conformation required for a Fischer projection. Therefore, since the bromines are on opposite sides in the dash-wedge projection, they must also be on opposite sides in the Fischer, and we can exclude choices A and D. The remaining choices (B and C) are enantiomeric—distinguishing between the two is best carried out by imagining a vantage point from above the dash-wedge representation, as shown:

It is then apparent that the upper bromine would point to the right and the lower bromine would be directed to the left of the observer.

SECTION 5. WRITING

Ask a teacher or another student to score your essay, or score it yourself using the following scoring rubrics.

CONVENTIONS OF LANGUAGE SCORING RUBRIC	
0	Paper blank, illegible, or not in English.
1.0	Multiple errors in capitalization, punctuation, grammar, and/or usage, seriously affecting flow and meaning.
2.0	Multiple errors in capitalization, punctuation, grammar, and/or usage, affecting both flow and meaning.
3.0	Several errors in capitalization, punctuation, grammar, and/or usage. Errors may affect flow, but they do not affect meaning.
4.0	Some errors in capitalization, punctuation, grammar, and/or usage, but errors do not affect meaning or flow.
5.0	Few errors in capitalization, punctuation, grammar, and/or usage.

PROBLEM SOLVING SCORING RUBRIC	
0	Paper blank, illegible, on a topic other than that assigned, or not in English.
1.0	Lack of understanding evident. Organization nonexistent or unclear. Ideas undeveloped.
2.0	Organization unclear or scattershot. Ideas underdeveloped and unsupported.
3.0	Organization fairly coherent. Ideas developed and supported with relevant details that lack complexity.
4.0	Organization coherent and focused. Ideas complex, well developed, and clearly supported.
5.0	Organization coherent and focused. Ideas complex, sophisticated, and substantially developed, with logical, convincing support.

SECTION 6. READING COMPREHENSION

1. Answer: D

The woolly flying squirrel was not extinct or it could not have been found again in 1994. Choices A, B, and C are supported by information in the passage.

2. Answer: B

The word *stable* has multiple meanings, but only one works in context here. The article refers to areas that are "geologically stable," meaning areas that are not altered by earthquakes or volcanoes. Only choice B provides this sense of fixed and secure stability.

3. Answer: C

The Himalayan find was not "subtropical" (choice A). Choice B is too broad to fit the specificity of this passage, as is choice D—the passage speaks only of a single animal of Pakistan. Choice C is best. The passage tells how one rediscovery confirmed McKinnon's theory.

4. Answer: A

The inclusion of the woolly flying squirrel story can have only one purpose: to provide an example that confirms McKinnon's theory. Choice B is incorrect; nowhere in the passage does it suggest that the woolly flying squirrel is a "new" species. Choice C is wrong because the rediscovery does not refute anything McKinnon said; instead, it confirms it. Choice D cannot be correct because only one rediscovery is mentioned.

5. Answer: C

To answer this question, you should look for the part of the passage in which information on stable climates appears; that is, the first paragraph. According to the author, "A stable climate is a third thing to look for. Stability of climate ensures that the animals that live in the region have had no reason to leave for warmer or wetter environments." In other words, a stable climate means that animals need not migrate or leave. There is no support in the passage for any other answer choice.

6. Answer: C

The third paragraph is a narrative that tells the beginning of Zahler's story of rediscovery. As many narratives are, it is told in sequence of time, making choice C the correct answer.

7. Answer: B

This question requires you to make a prediction based on information you are given in the passage. You don't need to know much about Borneo or the Sahara to recognize that if Borneo is more likely to house a new species, that must be because it conforms to McKinnon's four key requirements: stable geology, isolation, stable climate, and abundant species. You can immediately eliminate choice A; if Borneo were less isolated, it would be less likely to house a new species. Choice C makes no sense; volcanic eruptions would not make a place stable. If you know anything about deserts, you know that choice D is unlikely. The best answer is choice B; the climate in the Sahara is unstable, meaning that animals need to move around to seek water and food. According to McKinnon, that makes the Sahara an unlikely site for a rediscovery.

8. Answer: D

Notice that the question asks for the statement that offers the **least** support for the claim that Zahler's rediscovery obeyed McKinnon's regulations. You should read each statement and decide whether it supports the claim. Choice A does, because the rediscovery was made in a geologically stable region. Choices B and C do, because the rediscovery was made in an isolated region. Choice D, on the other hand, has nothing to do with McKinnon's regulations, so that is the correct choice.

9. Answer: C

Refining is one of the three steps in the creation of aluminum. It involves the separation of a solution through distillation and addition of chemicals. Although *refined* is a multiple-meaning word that in context may have any of the four definitions listed, only choice C works in the context of this passage.

10. Answer: C

According to the third paragraph, "Bulldozers remove the topsoil, and excavators or other types of power machinery are used to remove the underlying layer of bauxite." In other words, a layer of bauxite lies underneath the layer of topsoil. Although clay is then often removed from the bauxite, there is no indication that bauxite is found wherever clay is found (choice B), and the first paragraph stated directly that aluminum is *in* the earth's crust, not *below* it (choice D).

11. Answer: C

The fourth paragraph describes the process of refinement and its byproducts. Those that are mentioned in the paragraph include choices A, B, and D. There is no mention of choice C, which is an alloy of aluminum and an element not involved in this refining process.

12. Answer: A

A quick scan of the third, fourth, and fifth paragraphs indicates that the third is about mining, the fourth about refining, and the fifth about smelting. All three are steps in the process of making aluminum, so choice A is correct.

13. Answer: B

Omnipresent means "present everywhere." Although the implication is that the dust is harmful (choice A), the denotative meaning is that it is pervasive (choice B). There is no support for choice C, and choice D is not synonymous with *omnipresent*.

14. Answer: B

The three-step process that produces aluminum is described as involving mining, refining, and smelting. It is typical of the process that results in most metal products that we use, so it is parallel to copper production (choice B). None of the other three products results from the same three-step process.

15. Answer: B

Choice A is true, but it has nothing to do with the protests. There is no evidence to support choice D. Choice C may or may not be true; it is implied, but it is not a major point. The mention of protests mainly indicates choice B, that working people are beginning to question the dangers of mining.

16. Answer: A

There is nothing to support choice B or choice C, and the author is completely objective when it comes to the discussion of Karl Bayer (choice D). In the final paragraph, the author states, "As with all mining of metals, bauxite mining presents certain hazards," indicating that choice A is the best answer.

17. Answer: D

The Bering Land Bridge is described as connecting Siberia to what is now Alaska. If humans walked across from Siberia, the first ones in North America would have emerged into Alaska.

18. Answer: A

According to the passage, you could drive across the bridge, if it still existed, in about an hour. Based on that information, you can infer that the bridge was about as long as a typical mileage per hour, which would put it at choice A, between 50 and 75 miles.

19. Answer: A

A land bridge is a piece of land with water on either side that connects two larger pieces of land. That makes it equivalent to an isthmus (choice A). A bay (choice B) is a body of water, a strait (choice C) is a channel of water connecting two pieces of land, and a pass (choice D) is a narrow piece of land between mountains.

20. Answer: D

The third paragraph begins with a description of the ecology of the Mammoth Steppe and ends by explaining that the movement of large mammals across the Bering Land Bridge led to the movement of human hunters across that same bridge. Since the main topic of the passage is the Bering Land Bridge, the author's reason for including this information is to show how the bridge was used to move animals and then human hunters. There is no information about animal growth (choice A), the author does not emphasize the need for toughness in animals (choice B), and the author does not contrast the two climates (choice C). The only possible answer is choice D.

21. Answer: A

Although the paragraph mentions geologists and ethnologists (choice B), it does not compare their methodology. Nor does it list reasons for migration (choice C) or contradict a theory (choice D). The paragraph primarily puts forth a theory about migration across the land bridge, supporting the theory with discoveries made by ethnologists, from shared religions to similarities in tools and food preservation. The best answer is choice A.

22. Answer: B

According to the passage, some Native Americans object to the theory because "it contradicts most native teachings on the origins of the people," and "it seems to undermine the notion that they are truly 'native' to the North American continent." In other words, it challenges their history and status.

23. Answer: D

Your challenge is to find the response that **best** supports the idea that the continents were once connected. Choice (A) affects only North America. Choice B affects only Siberia. Choice C is possible, but it does not provide the unambiguous evidence that choice D does.

24. Answer: C

Again, you must look for the answer that **best** challenges the idea that humans first moved from Siberia to North America. Neither choice A nor choice B would prove or disprove the notion. Choice D would throw some doubt on the theory that the two continents were connected, but only choice C would indicate that humans were already in North America prior to the forming of the land bridge.

25. Answer : C

Skim to locate mention of three out of four assertions. The underground system (choice A) appears in the second paragraph, rural and urban settings are mentioned in the fourth paragraph, and the fact that purple loosestrife is not native (choice D) appears in the first paragraph. The fifth paragraph says that it is "impervious to burning," making choice C the best answer.

26. Answer: A

Gardeners (choice B) don't really object to purple loosestrife, as the second paragraph makes clear. Although many plants migrate, the passage is concerned only with one, making choice C too broad a title. Only the final paragraph has to do with largely unsuccessful attempts at controlling purple loosestrife, so choice D is not correct, either. The best title is choice A—the entire passage deals with a floral invader.

27. Answer: B

This question indirectly asks you to locate an author's reasons for including a detail. Returning to the passage will help you see that the mention of the St. Lawrence refers to a type of wetland where purple loosestrife does well. The only answer supported by the text is choice B.

28. Answer: C

All four details are facts about purple loosestrife, but only its easy adaptability is a fact that "adds to its power of endurance," so the answer is choice C.

29. Answer: C

The answer appears in the second paragraph: "The same long growing season that makes it so beloved by gardeners makes it a seed-making machine." It is the long growing season (choice C) that gardeners like.

30. Answer: D

The context is this: "*dense* stands of purple loosestrife." Although *dense* has a variety of meanings, here the author is referring to the thickness of the stands, not their opacity (choice B) or complexity (choice C). The weeds are tightly concentrated; the answer is choice D.

31. Answer: D

You must infer the answer based on what you have learned about purple loosestrife from the passage. Because it thrives in wetlands and along rivers, the places it would **most** easily thrive include swamps (choice A), wetland meadows (choice B), and along inland waterways (choice C). By process of elimination, then, choice D is the best answer.

32. Answer: B

Your choice must weaken the argument that purple loosestrife is best eradicated by digging it up, plowing it under, and reseeding. Choice A would suggest another means of eradication, but would not weaken the original argument. Choices C and D do not weaken or strengthen the argument, although both may suggest benefits of the eradication plan. Only choice B throws a monkey wrench in the works: If a new strain of purple loosestrife is growing up where it was once eliminated, then this form of eradication does not really work.

33. Answer: D

Hunting and habitat destruction are the only reasons mentioned for the depopulation of elk prior to the twentieth century.

34. Answer: D

According to the passage, in 1913, 50 elk were moved from Yellowstone to Pennsylvania. Two years later, 95 more were moved. The total shipped in those years comes to 145.

35. Answer: D

"At present," says the passage, "new herds are established in Arkansas, Kentucky, Michigan, and Wisconsin in addition to Pennsylvania." There is talk of moving herds to Tennessee (choice A) and the Adirondacks (choice C) in the future. Georgia (choice B) is mentioned only as the original southernmost range of eastern elk; it is not a place where they might be seen today.

36. Answer: B

As the passage states clearly, "All of the eastern subspecies are now extinct." The reintroduced subspecies is the western subspecies, the one found in Yellowstone. It is a different subspecies from the original Pennsylvania elk.

37. Answer: C

The author implies positive things about the reclamation of land (choice A) and the reintroduction of elk (choice D), and there is no support for choice B in the passage. Because reintroduction now includes careful monitoring of species and more concern about the animals' welfare, you can infer that the author believes it has improved (choice C).

38. Answer: D

Your answer must directly support the contention that elk repopulation is carefully monitored. Choices A and C have nothing to do with repopulation; they deal with animals in confined conditions. Choice B deals with wild elk but not with monitoring of the population. Choice D shows an example of monitoring that is taking place today.

39. Answer: C

The claim is that elk reintroduction benefits other species. Your answer must contradict this contention. Choice A shows a clear benefit to other populations, so it does not contradict the claim. Choice B shows a change in a species that does not live where elk live. Choice D does not refer to other species at all. Only choice C indicates a possible problem; the fact that deer are migrating northward may mean that elk are encroaching on their habitats.

40. Answer: D

A statement of opinion tells what someone thinks or believes. It cannot be checked or proved. The only statement here that fits that definition is choice D—whether the reintroduction of species is indeed "vastly improved" is something that may be debatable.

41. Answer: B

Locating the word in the passage is step one to determining the answer. "They would evacuate air from the tube, pass high voltage through it, and show audiences the patterns of light that appeared." The lecturers are removing the air from the tube, so choice B is correct.

42. Answer: A

George Thomson was J.J.'s son, and his work followed that of his father. Hertz and Lenard are described as working with waves but not as particles. Of the choices, only Johnstone Stoney is mentioned as having described the particle he called the *electron*.

43. Answer: C

Return to the passage and look for information on Thomson's first experiment. "The first experiment determined that the negative charge of cathode rays could not be separated from the rays themselves using magnetism." The negative charge (choice A) was discovered earlier by Jean Perrin. Thomson diverted the rays (choice B) in his second experiment, not the first, and he determined the tiny size and huge charge of the particles (choice D) in his third experiment. The fact that the charge could not be removed from the rays indicated that it was a property of particles. The answer is choice C.

44. Answer: B

Corpuscles are mentioned as a term of Isaac Newton's, which he used to describe particles of light long before his theories were proved. The same term was used by Thomson to describe the particles he found in cathode rays. The best answer is choice B.

45. Answer: B

Following this opening, the author goes on to name the variety of scientists whose work led to this important discovery. Even if you did not understand the opening sentence, you could tell that this was not a straightforward discovery but rather one that depended on many people's discoveries. The author never, however, goes so far as to imply that the discovery could never have been made by a single scientist (choice C)—only that it was not.

46. Answer: A

The author calls J.J. Thomson's experiments "elegant" and credits him with determining "the existence of a subatomic particle with a negative charge." There is no support in the passage for choices B, C, or D.

47. Answer: D

The answer is more straightforward than you might think. Newton's and Huygens's conflicting theories of light (choice A)—one particle theory, the other wave theory—are related to wave-particle duality, but obviously came far earlier than George Thomson's work. The results of gravity on waves (choice B) might have something to do with wave theory, but they are connected directly neither to Thomson nor to quantum mechanics. Similarly, de Broglie's equation (choice C) is connected to quantum mechanics, but it does not prove the author's contention. A definition connecting wave-particle duality to quantum mechanics (choice D) would support the author's statement.

48. Answer: C

An electron microscope uses streams of electrons to allow us to view things smaller than a beam of light. It relies on the connection between particles and waves in electrons. Although the other inventions mentioned rely on waves, they do not depend on the connection between those waves and the particles that make up those waves.

SECTION 7. QUANTITATIVE ABILITY

1. Answer: C

The mixed number $4\frac{5}{7}$ can be converted into a fraction as follows:

$$4\frac{5}{7} = \frac{4 \cdot 7 + 5}{7} = \frac{28 + 5}{7} = \frac{33}{7}.$$

2. Answer: B

To perform the subtraction $4\dfrac{5}{6} - 2\dfrac{3}{4}$, you should first convert each of the fractions

from a mixed number to its standard form and then find a common denominator to complete the subtraction process:

$$4\frac{5}{6} = \frac{4\cdot 6 + 5}{6} = \frac{24 + 5}{6} = \frac{29}{6} \qquad 2\frac{3}{4} = \frac{2\cdot 4 + 3}{4} = \frac{8 + 3}{4} = \frac{11}{4}$$

$$4\frac{5}{6} - 2\frac{3}{4} = \frac{29}{6} - \frac{11}{4} = \frac{58 - 33}{12} = \frac{25}{12}.$$

3. Answer: C

From the information in the problem,

$$\text{Average} = \frac{\text{Sum of Terms}}{\text{Number of Terms}}$$

$$86 = \frac{85 + 78 + 83 + 91 + 89 + 86 + x}{7} = \frac{512 + x}{7}$$

$$x = 86 \times 7 - 512 = 602 - 512 = 90.$$

4. Answer: B

To solve this problem, you must first determine the number of hours in a five-day week. With 24 hours in a day and 5 days in a work week, there are a total of 120 hours per week. The percentage that an employee is at work is:

$$\frac{40 \text{ hours / wk}}{120 \text{ hours / wk}} \times 100\% = 33.3\%.$$

5. Answer: A

To divide 2.4×10^6 by -1.2×10^3, first arrange in the proper form of division and then separately divide the coefficients and the exponents:

$$\frac{2.4 \times 10^6}{-1.2 \times 10^3} = -\frac{2.4}{1.2} \times \frac{10^6}{10^3} = -2 \times 10^3.$$

6. Answer: B

To determine the product of 35.2 and 4.16, the numbers should be arranged as:

$$
\begin{array}{r}
35.2 \\
\times 4.16 \\
\hline
2112 \\
3520 \\
+140800 \\
\hline
146.432
\end{array}
$$

7. Answer: B
In scientific notation, the number 13.9 is 1.39×10^1.

8. Answer: C
To find the total number of girls in the science class, we must first find the fraction of students in the class who are girls. For every set of 5 students, 2 students are girls, yielding a fraction of $\frac{2}{5}$. Thus, the total number of girls in the class is $\frac{2}{5} \times 430 = 172$.

9. Answer: C
The quotient of $6x^2y^5z^3$ divided by $3x^2y^3z^6$ or $\frac{6x^2y^5z^3}{3x^2y^3z^6}$ can be found by:

$$\frac{6x^2y^5z^3}{3x^2y^3z^6} = \frac{6}{3} \cdot \frac{x^2}{x^2} \cdot \frac{y^5}{y^3} \cdot \frac{z^3}{z^6} = 2 \cdot 1 \cdot y^2 \cdot \frac{1}{z^3} = \frac{2y^2}{z^3}$$

10. Answer: D
Simplifying the expression in terms of its factors,

$$\frac{x^2 + x - 42}{x+7} = \frac{(x+7)(x-6)}{x+7} = x - 6 = 1.$$

Solving for x yields $x = 6 + 1 = 7$.

11. Answer: A
This equation $x^2 - 7x - 18 = 0$ must be solved using the quadratic formula

$$x = \frac{-b \pm \sqrt{b^2 - 4ac}}{2a},$$

where $a = 1$, $b = -7$, and $c = -18$. Substituting into the formula yields:

$$x = \frac{-(-7) \pm \sqrt{(-7)^2 - 4(1)(-18)}}{2(1)} = \frac{7 \pm \sqrt{49 + 72}}{4} = \frac{7 \pm \sqrt{121}}{4} = \frac{7 \pm 11}{4}.$$

The roots of the quadratic equation are:

$$x = \frac{7+11}{4} = \frac{18}{4} = 4.5 \text{ and } x = \frac{7-11}{4} = \frac{-4}{4} = -1.$$

12. Answer: B
The product of $4a^2 b^4c$ and $-7a^5 b^3$ can be found by:

$$4a^2b^4c \times -7a^5b^3 = (4 \times -7) \cdot (a^2 \times a^5) \cdot (b^4 \times b^3) \cdot (c \times 1) = -28 \cdot a^7 \cdot b^7 \cdot c = -28a^7b^7c.$$

13. Answer: C
The sum of the polynomials, $5x + 3xy - 6y^2$, $9xy + 7y^2 - 4x$, and $-8y^2 + 7x + 12xy$ can be found by combining like terms:

$$5x + 3xy - 6y^2$$
$$9xy + 7y^2 - 4x$$
$$+ \quad \underline{-8y^2 + 7x + 12xy}$$
$$5x + 3xy - 6y^2 + 9xy + 7y^2 - 4x - 8y^2 + 7x + 12xy$$

Simplifying the above expression yields:

$$5x - 4x + 7x + 3xy + 9xy + 12xy - 6y^2 + 7y^2 - 8y^2 = 8x + 24xy - 7y^2.$$

14. Answer: C

Because the base is common, the product is obtained by simply adding the exponents and calculating the result or: $3^3 \cdot 3^2 \cdot 3^1 = 3^{3+2+1} = 3^6 = 729$.

15. Answer: D

The roots of a quadratic equation $3x^2 - x - 10 = 0$ can be found by using the quadratic formula:

$$x = \frac{-b \pm \sqrt{b^2 - 4ac}}{2a},$$

where $a = 3$, $b = -1$, and $c = -10$. Substituting into the formula yields:

$$x = \frac{-(-1) \pm \sqrt{(-1)^2 - 4(3)(-10)}}{2(3)} = \frac{1 \pm \sqrt{1 + 120}}{6} = \frac{1 \pm \sqrt{121}}{6} = \frac{1 \pm 11}{6}$$

yielding the roots

$$x = \frac{1 + 11}{6} = \frac{12}{6} = 2 \text{ and } x = \frac{1 - 11}{6} = \frac{-10}{6} = -\frac{5}{3}.$$

16. Answer: C

To solve this system of equations, begin by:

(1) $x + y = 4$

(2) $2x - 6y = 3$

Starting with Equation (1), solve for x which results in

(3) $x = 4 - y$

Substituting Equation (3) into Equation (2) yields:

(4) $2(4 - y) - 6y = 3$

$$8 - 2y - 6y = 3$$

$$8y = 8 - 3 = 5$$

(5) $$y = \frac{5}{8}.$$

Substituting Equation (5) into Equation (1) yields:

$$x + \left(\frac{5}{8}\right) = 4$$

$$x = 4 - \left(\frac{5}{8}\right) = \frac{32}{8} - \frac{5}{8} = \frac{27}{8}$$

The solutions for the system of equations are $x = \frac{27}{8}, y = \frac{5}{8}.$

17. Answer: A

You should note that $\sqrt[3]{x} = x^{\frac{1}{3}}$ and $x^{\frac{1}{3}} = y^4$. Taking the cube of both sides yields:

$$\left(x^{\frac{1}{3}}\right)^3 = \left(y^4\right)^3$$

$$x = y^{12}.$$

18. Answer: A

The probability of selecting a single orange-colored candy from a bag of Skittles® requires 8 successful outcomes out of 37 possible outcomes. So the probability of selecting a single orange-colored candy is: $p = \frac{8}{37}.$

19. Answer: B

To determine the probability that a randomly selected card is an ace of a red suit, you should first note that a card can be selected from a deck in $n = 52$ different ways. Since there are two such aces (ace of hearts and ace of diamonds), then an ace can be drawn from the deck in $s = 2$ different ways. Thus, the probability that the selected card is an ace is: $p = \frac{s}{n} = \frac{2}{52}.$

20. Answer: C

You are asked to determine the probability of randomly selecting one face card (king, queen, or jack) of a spade suit from two standard decks of cards. Because there are two decks of cards, a single card can be selected from two decks in $n = 104$ different ways. Since there are 3 face cards of a spade suit in one deck of cards, such a card can be drawn from the two decks in $s = 6$ different ways. Thus, the probability that the selected card is a face card of a spade suit is: $p = \frac{s}{n} = \frac{6}{104}.$

21. **Answer: D**

The number of total possible outcomes from the roll of two dice is 36. In other words, there are 36 different pairs of numbers that can be obtained. You first need to determine the number of possible outcomes yielding a sum of 7 and 12 from the two dice. The number of possible outcomes yielding a sum of 7 is 6 or

$$\{(1, 6), (2, 5), (3, 4), (4, 3), (5, 2), (6, 1)\}.$$

The probability of yielding a sum of 7 between the two dice is

$$P(A) = P(7) = \frac{6}{36} = \frac{1}{6}.$$

The number of possible outcomes yielding a sum of 12 is 1 or

$$\{(6, 6)\}.$$

The probability of yielding a sum of 12 between the two dice is

$$P(B) = P(12) = \frac{1}{36}.$$

Upon the roll of two dice, you cannot obtain a sum of 7 and a sum of 12 at the same time; thus the two outcomes are mutually exclusive. The probability that the sum of the two dice is either 7 or 12 is: $P(A \text{ or } B) = P(A) + P(B) = P(7) + P(12) = \frac{6}{36} + \frac{1}{36} = \frac{7}{36}$.

22. **Answer: B**

Because the two drawings are made from a complete deck of cards, the two events are independent of one another. You first need to determine the probability of drawing a card of two suits from a deck of cards. Out of a total of 52 cards, there are 13 cards of any suit and 26 cards of a black suit. The probability of drawing a card of a black suit, P(A), is $\frac{26}{52}$. Because the first card is replaced before the second drawing, the probability of drawing a card of the same suit, P(B), is also $\frac{26}{52}$. Thus, the probability of drawing two cards of the same suit is

$$P(A \text{ and } B) = P(A) \cdot P(B) = \frac{26}{52} \cdot \frac{26}{52} = \frac{676}{2704}.$$

23. **Answer: C**

The mean of a data set is the arithmetic average of the values of the data set or

$$\frac{2.4mL + 3.2mL + 3.7mL + 3.7mL + 4.5mL + 6.8mL + 7.3mL + 8.1mL + 12.2mL}{9}$$

$$= \frac{51.9mL}{9} = 5.8mL.$$

24. **Answer: B**
The median is the middle or center value of the data set arranged in ascending numerical order, or $4.5 \, \text{mL}$.

25. **Answer: A**
The mode is the measurement that is the most frequent or common value in the data set. In this example, the mode is $3.7 \, \text{mL}$, because it occurs twice, more than any of the other measurements that occur only once.

26. **Answer: D**
The range or the difference between the largest and smallest values in this data set is $12.2 \, \text{mL} - 2.4 \, \text{mL} = 9.8 \, \text{mL}$.

27. **Answer: D**
The first thing to do in solving the equation $x^2 - 12x = -36$ for x is to rewrite the equation by adding 36 to both sides and then to express the equation in terms of factors:

$$x^2 - 12x + 36 = 0$$

$$(x - 6) \cdot (x - 6) = 0$$

Solving the equation for x yields $x = 6$.

28. **Answer: A**
In order to solve the equation $x^3 - 64x = 0$ for x, you can apply factor analysis and solve for x in each term:

$$\frac{x^3}{x} - \frac{64x}{x} = \frac{0}{x}$$

$$x^2 - 64 = 0$$

$$x = \pm 8.$$

29. **Answer: C**
This equation can be solved by first taking the square root of both sides of the equation $(4x - 1)^2 = 121$ or

$$\sqrt{\left(4x - 1\right)^2} = \sqrt{121}$$

$$4x - 1 = 11$$

Solving for x yields $x = 3$.

30. **Answer: A**
The slope is defined as: $m = \dfrac{y_2 - y_1}{x_2 - x_1}$. If the first point $(5, 2) = (x_1, y_1)$ and the second point $(8, 3) = (x_2, y_2)$, then substituting these coordinate values into the definition for the slope yields

$$m = \frac{3 - 2}{8 - 5} = \frac{1}{3}.$$

31. **Answer: B**

The slope can be identified by adapting the equation to the formal equation of a line or $y = mx + b$ or

$$2y + 3x - 12 = 0$$
$$2y = -3x + 12$$
$$\frac{2y}{2} = \frac{-3x}{2} + \frac{12}{2}$$
$$y = -\frac{3}{2}x + 6$$

where the slope $m = -\frac{3}{2}$.

32. **Answer: C**

You can use the information provided by the specific point and the value of the slope to derive the equation for the line:

$$m = \frac{y_2 - y_1}{x_2 - x_1}$$
$$-\frac{2}{3} = \frac{y_2 - (-1)}{x_2 - (-3)} = \frac{y_2 + 1}{x_2 + 3}$$

$$y_2 + 1 = -\frac{2}{3} \cdot (x_2 + 3)$$
$$y_2 + 1 = -\frac{2}{3}x_2 - \frac{2}{3}(3)$$
$$y_2 + 1 = -\frac{2}{3}x_2 - 2$$
$$y = -\frac{2}{3}x - 3$$

33. **Answer: A**

When the equation $T_F = \frac{9}{5}T_C + 32$ is adapted to the equation of a line, it can readily be seen that the slope is $\frac{9}{5}$. However, because the equation has physical significance, it is important that the units associated with the slope are clearly indicated. Because the slope is the ratio of the change in the y-axis versus the change in the x-axis, the appropriate units for the slope are $\frac{°F}{°C}$.

34. **Answer: C**

For this problem, you need to, in essence, rearrange the equation to solve for T_c, or

$$T_C = \frac{5}{9}(T_F - 32) = \frac{5}{9}T_F - 17.8.$$

35. **Answer: D**

You know that $T_F = \dfrac{9}{5}T_C + 32$. Kelvin temperature can be incorporated through the conversion formula with Celsius temperature or:

$$T_C = T_K - 273$$
$$T_F = \frac{9}{5}\left(T_K - 273\right) + 32 = \frac{9}{5}T_K - \frac{9}{5} \cdot 273 + 32 = \frac{9}{5}T_K - 459.4$$
$$T_F = \frac{9}{5}T_K - 459.4.$$

36. **Answer: B**

Two lines are perpendicular if the product of their slopes is -1. The line that is perpendicular to the one given in the problem is $y - \dfrac{1}{3}x = -5$ because its slope of $+\dfrac{1}{3}$, when multiplied by the slope of the original line (-3), is equal to -1.

37. **Answer: C**

A line is parallel to another if they have the same slope. The slope of the line $y + 3x = 8$ is $m = -3$. The only choice that describes a line with the same slope of -3 is $y + 3x = -5$.

38. **Answer: A**

In evaluating the derivative, you should note that the function is a number or a constant because it has no dependence on the variable, x. Thus, the derivative of a constant is 0 or

$$\frac{d}{dx}\left(100\right) = 0.$$

39. **Answer: A**

Although you might be tempted to invoke the derivative formula of a power function $\dfrac{d}{dx}\left(x^n\right) = nx^{n-1}$ to solve the stated problem, you should note that the derivative can only be performed with respect to a differentiating variable, which in this case is x. Because there is no x in the function $5a^4$, it is a constant and the derivative of a constant is zero.

40. **Answer: C**

The derivative of a power function can be found according to the general equation:

$$\frac{d}{dx}\left(x^n\right) = nx^{n-1}$$

In the problem, $n = 5$ and therefore the derivative can now be calculated as:

$$\frac{d}{dx}\left(5x^4\right) = 4 \cdot 5x^{4-1} = 20x^3.$$

41. Answer: A

The function can first be simplified by dividing 15 by 3 and rewriting the differentiated function as a negative exponent, which simplifies the function as:

$$\frac{d}{dx}\left(\frac{5}{x^8}\right) = \frac{d}{dx}\left(5x^{-8}\right).$$

The derivative of a power function is defined as:

$$\frac{d}{dx}\left(x^n\right) = nx^{n-1}$$

$$\frac{d}{dx}\left(5x^{-8}\right) = \left(-8\right)\left(5\right)x^{-8-1} = -40x^{-9} = -\frac{40}{x^9}.$$

42. Answer: C

The derivative of a polynomial is the sum of the derivatives of the terms of the polynomial or:

$$\frac{d}{dx}\left(6x^4 - 4x^3\right) = \frac{d}{dx}\left(6x^4\right) + \frac{d}{dx}\left(-4x^3\right)$$

$$= \frac{d}{dx}\left(6x^4\right) - \frac{d}{dx}\left(4x^3\right)$$

$$= 24x^3 - 12x^2.$$

43. Answer: B

You first must calculate the derivative before you can evaluate the derivative at a given point.

$$\frac{d}{dx}\left(9x^5 - 3x^4 + 3x^2 - 10\right) = \frac{d}{dx}\left(9x^5\right) + \frac{d}{dx}\left(-3x^4\right) + \frac{d}{dx}\left(3x^2\right) + \frac{d}{dx}\left(-10\right)$$

$$= 45x^4 - 12x^3 + 6x$$

The derivative can now be evaluated at $x = 1$ by plugging in the value of 1 for x in the derivative or

$$(45x^4 - 12x^3 + 6x)\big|_{x=1} = 45(1)^4 - 12(1)^3 + 6(1) = 45 - 12 + 6 = 39.$$

44. Answer: A

You first must calculate the derivative before you can evaluate the derivative at a given point.

$$\frac{d}{dx}\left(24x^3 - 9x^2 + 3x - 11\right) = \frac{d}{dx}\left(24x^3\right) + \frac{d}{dx}\left(-9x^2\right) + \frac{d}{dx}\left(3x\right) + \frac{d}{dx}\left(-11\right)$$

$$= 72x^2 - 18x + 3$$

The derivative can now be evaluated at $x = 3$ by plugging in the value of 3 for x in the derivative or

$$(72x^2 - 18x + 3)\big|_{x=3} = 72(3)^2 - 18(3) + 3 = 648 - 54 + 3 = 597.$$

45. **Answer: B**

You begin by simplifying the function to be integrated or

$$\int t^2\left(\frac{5}{t} - \frac{t}{5}\right)dt = \int\left(\frac{5t^2}{t} - \frac{t^3}{5}\right)dt = \int\left(5t - \frac{t^3}{5}\right)dt = \int 5t\,dt - \int\frac{t^3}{5}\,dt = \frac{5t^2}{2} - \frac{t^4}{20} + C.$$

46. **Answer: C**

Evaluation of this integral proceeds by:

$$\int\left(8 - t^3\right)dt = \int 8\,dt - \int t^3\,dt = 8t - \frac{t^4}{4} + C.$$

47. **Answer: A**

You begin by solving the integral and then evaluating the result between the limits of 1 and 9.

$$\int_1^9 3t^3dt = \frac{3t^4}{4}\bigg|_1^9 = \frac{3(9)^4}{4} - \frac{3(1)^4}{4} = \frac{19683}{4} - \frac{3}{4} = \frac{19680}{4} = 4920.$$

48. **Answer: B**

You begin by solving the integral and then evaluating the result between the limits of 2 and 4.

$$\int_2^4\left(x^5 - 6x^3 + 8x + 2\right)dx = \left(\frac{x^6}{6} - \frac{6x^4}{4} + \frac{8x^2}{2} + 2x\right)_2^4$$

$$= \left(\frac{(4)^6}{6} - \frac{6(4)^4}{4} + \frac{8(4)^2}{2} + 2(4)\right) - \left(\frac{(2)^6}{6} - \frac{6(2)^4}{4} + \frac{8(2)^2}{2} + 2(2)\right)$$

$$= \left(\frac{4096}{6} - \frac{1536}{4} + \frac{128}{2} + 8\right) - \left(\frac{64}{6} - \frac{96}{4} + \frac{32}{2} + 4\right)$$

$$= \frac{4448}{12} - \frac{80}{12} = \frac{4368}{12} = 364.$$